Eating Disorders and Obesity

A Comprehensive Handbook

THIRD EDITION

EDITED BY

Kelly D. Brownell
B. Timothy Walsh

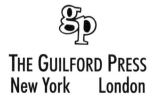

THE GUILFORD PRESS
New York   London

Copyright © 2017 The Guilford Press
A Division of Guilford Publications, Inc.
370 Seventh Avenue, Suite 1200, New York, NY 10001
www.guilford.com

Printed in the United States of America

This book is printed on acid-free paper.

Last digit is print number: 9 8 7 6 5 4 3 2 1

The authors have checked with sources believed to be reliable in their efforts to provide information
that is complete and generally in accord with the standards of practice that are accepted at the time
of publication. However, in view of the possibility of human error or changes in behavioral, mental
health, or medical sciences, neither the authors, nor the editors and publisher, nor any other party
who has been involved in the preparation or publication of this work warrants that the information
contained herein is in every respect accurate or complete, and they are not responsible for any errors
or omissions or the results obtained from the use of such information. Readers are encouraged to
confirm the information contained in this book with other sources.

Library of Congress Cataloging-in-Publication Data

Names: Brownell, Kelly D., editor. | Walsh, B. Timothy, 1946– editor.
Title: Eating disorders and obesity : a comprehensive handbook / edited
    by Kelly D. Brownell, B. Timothy Walsh.
Description: Third edition. | New York : The Guilford Press, [2017] |
Includes bibliographical references and index.
Identifiers: LCCN 2016028018 | ISBN 9781462529063 (hardcover)
Subjects: LCSH: Eating disorders—Handbooks, manuals, etc. | Obesity—
Handbooks, manuals, etc.
Classification: LCC RC552.E18 E2825 2017 | DDC 616.85/26—dc23
LC record available at *https://lccn.loc.gov/2016028018*

About the Editors

Kelly D. Brownell, PhD, is Dean of the Sanford School of Public Policy at Duke University, where he is also Robert L. Flowers Professor of Public Policy and Professor of Psychology and Neuroscience. Prior to joining the faculty at Duke, Dr. Brownell was the James Rowland Angell Professor of Psychology, Professor of Epidemiology and Public Health, and Director of the Rudd Center for Food Policy and Obesity at Yale University. His work focuses on obesity and food policy. Dr. Brownell has been named to the National Academy of Medicine (Institute of Medicine); has received numerous awards, including the Lifetime Achievement Award from the American Psychological Association; and in 2006 was named by *Time* magazine as one of the World's 100 Most Influential People.

B. Timothy Walsh, MD, is Ruane Professor of Pediatric Psychopharmacology at the College of Physicians and Surgeons of Columbia University and Director of the Division of Clinical Therapeutics at the New York State Psychiatric Institute. The clinical research group he founded and has led at Columbia has conducted studies of the etiology and treatment of eating disorders, with a particular focus on underlying pathophysiological mechanisms. Dr. Walsh has served as president of the Academy for Eating Disorders and of the Eating Disorders Research Society, and chaired the Eating Disorders Work Group for DSM-IV and DSM-5. He has received awards from the American Psychiatric Association, the Academy for Eating Disorders, the National Eating Disorders Association, and the Association for Behavioral and Cognitive Therapies.

Contributors

Karina L. Allen, PhD, Eating Disorders Service, Maudsley Hospital, South London and Maudsley NHS Foundation Trust, London, United Kingdom; School of Psychology, University of Western Australia, Crawley, Western Australia, Australia

David B. Allison, PhD, Nutrition Obesity Research Center and Office of Energetics, School of Public Health, University of Alabama at Birmingham, Birmingham, Alabama

Kelly C. Allison, PhD, Center for Weight and Eating Disorders, Department of Psychiatry, Perelman School of Medicine, University of Pennsylvania, Philadelphia, Pennsylvania

Tatiana Andreyeva, PhD, UConn Rudd Center for Food Policy and Obesity, Hartford, Connecticut; Department of Agriculture and Resource Economics, University of Connecticut, Storrs, Connecticut

Louis J. Aronne, MD, Comprehensive Weight Control Center, Weill Cornell Medical College, Cornell University, New York, New York

Nerys Astbury, PhD, Nuffield Department of Primary Care Health Sciences, University of Oxford, Oxford, United Kingdom

Arne Astrup, MD, Department of Nutrition, Exercise and Sports, University of Copenhagen, Copenhagen, Denmark

Evelyn Attia, MD, Department of Psychiatry, Weill Cornell Medical College, Cornell University, and New York State Psychiatric Institute, New York, New York

S. Bryn Austin, ScD, Division of Adolescent and Young Adult Medicine, Boston Children's Hospital, Boston, Massachusetts; Department of Social and Behavioral Sciences, Harvard T. H. Chan School of Public Health, Harvard University, Cambridge, Massachusetts

Linda M. Bartoshuk, PhD, Department of Food Science and Human Nutrition, University of Florida, Gainesville, Florida

Bryan C. Batch, MD, Division of Endocrinology, Metabolism and Nutrition, Department of Medicine, Duke University School of Medicine, Durham, North Carolina

Anne E. Becker, MD, PhD, Department of Global Health and Social Medicine, Harvard Medical School, and Department of Psychiatry, Massachusetts General Hospital, Boston, Massachusetts

Gary G. Bennett, PhD, Department of Psychology and Neuroscience and Duke Global Health Institute and Division of Nephrology, Department of Medicine, Duke University School of Medicine, Durham, North Carolina

Laura A. Berner, PhD, Eating Disorder Center for Treatment and Research, Department of Psychiatry, UC San Diego School of Medicine, University of California, San Diego, La Jolla, California

Leann L. Birch, PhD, Department of Foods and Nutrition, University of Georgia, Athens, Georgia

Heidi M. Blanck, PhD, Division of Nutrition, Physical Activity, and Obesity, National Center for Chronic Disease Prevention and Health Promotion, Centers for Disease Control and Prevention, Atlanta, Georgia

Jennie Brand-Miller, PhD, Charles Perkins Centre, University of Sydney, Sydney, New South Wales, Australia

Gerome Breen, PhD, Institute of Psychiatry, Psychology and Neuroscience and South London and Maudsley NHS Foundation Trust, King's College London, London, United Kingdom

Kelly D. Brownell, PhD, Sanford School of Public Policy, Duke University, Durham, North Carolina

Rachel Bryant-Waugh, MSc, DPhil, Department of Child and Adolescent Mental Health, Great Ormond Street Hospital for Children NHS Foundation Trust, London, United Kingdom

Cynthia M. Bulik, PhD, Departments of Psychiatry and Nutrition, University of North Carolina at Chapel Hill, Chapel Hill, North Carolina; Department of Medical Epidemiology and Biostatistics, Karolinska Institutet, Stockholm, Sweden

Meghan L. Butryn, PhD, Department of Psychology, Drexel University, Philadelphia, Pennsylvania

John Cawley, PhD, Department of Policy Analysis and Management and Department of Economics, Cornell University, Ithaca, New York

Frank J. Chaloupka, PhD, Health Policy Center, Institute for Health Research and Policy, University of Illinois at Chicago, Chicago, Illinois

Jamie F. Chriqui, PhD, MHS, Division of Health Policy and Administration, Institute for Health Research and Policy, University of Illinois at Chicago, Chicago, Illinois

Ilseung Cho, MD, Division of Gastroenterology, Department of Medicine, New York University School of Medicine, New York, New York

Philip Chuang, MD, Department of Medicine, New York University School of Medicine, New York, New York

Scott Crow, MD, Department of Psychiatry, University of Minnesota, Minneapolis, Minnesota

Christopher R. Daigle, MD, FRCSC, The Bariatric Center, Cleveland Clinic Akron General, Akron, Ohio

Michael J. Devlin, MD, Department of Psychiatry, New York State Psychiatric Institute and Columbia University Medical Center, New York, New York

William H. Dietz, MD, PhD, Redstone Global Center for Prevention and Wellness, Milken Institute School of Public Health, George Washington University, Washington, DC

Dawn M. Eichen, PhD, Center for Healthy Eating and Activity Research Center, UC San Diego School of Medicine, University of California, San Diego, La Jolla, California

Ivan Eisler, PhD, Institute of Psychiatry, King's College London, London, United Kingdom

Elissa S. Epel, PhD, Department of Psychiatry, School of Medicine, University of California, San Francisco, San Francisco, California

Leonard H. Epstein, PhD, Department of Pediatrics, University at Buffalo, State University of New York, Buffalo, New York

Christopher G. Fairburn, DM, FRCPsych, FMedSci, Department of Psychiatry, University of Oxford, and Warneford Hospital, Oxford, United Kingdom

Myles S. Faith, PhD, Department of Counseling, School and Educational Psychology, Graduate School of Education, University at Buffalo, State University of New York, Buffalo, New York

Thomas A. Farley, MD, MPH, Department of Public Health, City of Philadelphia, Philadelphia, Pennsylvania

Lucy F. Faulconbridge, PhD, Center for Weight and Eating Disorders, Department of Psychiatry, Perelman School of Medicine, University of Pennsylvania, Philadelphia, Pennsylvania

Jennifer Orlet Fisher, PhD, Center for Obesity Research and Education, Department of Social and Behavioral Sciences, Temple University, Philadelphia, Pennsylvania

Paul C. Fletcher, MD, Department of Psychiatry, School of Clinical Medicine, University of Cambridge, Cambridge, United Kingdom

Jennifer I. Flynn, PhD, Department of Exercise Science, Arnold School of Public Health, University of South Carolina, Columbia, South Carolina

Gary D. Foster, PhD, Weight Watchers International, New York, New York; Center for Weight and Eating Disorders, Perelman School of Medicine, University of Pennsylvania, Philadelphia, Pennsylvania; Center for Obesity Research and Education, College of Public Health, Temple University, Philadelphia, Pennsylvania

Alexis C. Frazier-Wood, PhD, Children's Nutrition Research Center, Baylor College of Medicine, Houston, Texas

Roberta R. Friedman, ScM, RFriedman Consulting, Hamden, Connecticut

Dympna Gallagher, EdD, New York Obesity Research Center, Columbia University, New York, New York

Ashley N. Gearhardt, PhD, Department of Psychology, University of Michigan, Ann Arbor, Michigan

Timothy Gill, PhD, Boden Institute and the Prevention Research Collaboration, Sydney Medical School, University of Sydney, Sydney, New South Wales, Australia

Neville H. Golden, MD, Division of Adolescent Medicine, Department of Pediatrics, Lucile Packard Children's Hospital, Stanford University School of Medicine, Stanford, California

Richard A. Gordon, PhD, Psychology Program, Bard College, Annandale-on-Hudson, New York

Steven L. Gortmaker, PhD, Department of Social and Behavioral Sciences, Harvard T. F. Chan School of Public Health, Harvard University, Cambridge, Massachusetts

Carlos M. Grilo, PhD, Program for Obesity, Weight, and Eating Research, Department of Psychiatry, Yale University School of Medicine, New Haven, Connecticut

Angela S. Guarda MD, Department of Psychiatry and Behavioral Sciences, Johns Hopkins University School of Medicine, Baltimore, Maryland

John Gunstad, PhD, Department of Psychological Sciences, Kent State University, Kent, Ohio

Kevin D. Hall, PhD, Laboratory of Biological Modeling, National Institute of Diabetes and Digestive and Kidney Diseases, National Institutes of Health, Bethesda, Maryland

Jennifer L. Harris, PhD, UConn Rudd Center for Food Policy and Obesity, Hartford, Connecticut; Department of Applied Health Sciences, University of Connecticut, Storrs, Connecticut

Corinna Hawkes, PhD, Centre for Food Policy, City University of London, London, United Kingdom

Misty A. W. Hawkins, PhD, Department of Psychology, Oklahoma State University, Stillwater, Oklahoma

Phillipa J. Hay, DPhil, MD, Centre for Health Research, School of Medicine, Western Sydney University, Sydney, New South Wales, Australia

Stephen T. Higgins, PhD, Vermont Center on Behavior and Health, Departments of Psychiatry and Psychological Science, University of Vermont, Burlington, Vermont

Andrew J. Hill, PhD, Institute of Health Sciences, Leeds University School of Medicine, Leeds, United Kingdom

Hans W. Hoek, MD, PhD, Parnassia Psychiatric Institute, The Hague, Netherlands; Faculty of Medical Sciences, University of Groningen, Groningen, Netherlands; Department of

Epidemiology, Mailman School of Public Health, Columbia University, New York, New York

Adela Hruby, PhD, MPH, Nutritional Epidemiology Program, Jean Mayer USDA Human Nutrition Research Center on Aging, Tufts University, Boston, Massachusetts

Frank B. Hu, MD, PhD, MPH, Departments of Nutrition and Epidemiology, Harvard T. H. Chan School of Public Health, Harvard University, Cambridge, Massachusetts

James I. Hudson, MD, ScD, Department of Psychiatry, Harvard Medical School, and Biological Psychiatry Laboratory, McLean Hospital, Boston, Massachusetts

John M. Jakicic, PhD, Physical Activity and Weight Management Center, Department of Health and Physical Activity, School of Education, University of Pittsburgh, Pittsburgh, Pennsylvania

Michelle A. Joyner, MS, Department of Psychology, University of Michigan, Ann Arbor, Michigan

Walter H. Kaye, MD, Eating Disorder Center for Treatment and Research, Department of Psychiatry, UC San Diego School of Medicine, University of California, San Diego, La Jolla, California

Pamela K. Keel, PhD, Department of Psychology, Florida State University, Tallahassee, Florida

Neha Khandpur, ScD, Department of Nutrition, Harvard T. H. Chan School of Public Health, Harvard University, Cambridge, Massachusetts

Samantha M. R. Kling, PhD, Department of Nutritional Sciences, Pennsylvania State University, Philadelphia, Pennsylvania

Judith Korner, MD, PhD, Division of Endocrinology and Metabolism, Department of Medicine, Columbia University Medical Center, New York, New York

Shiriki K. Kumanyika, PhD, MPH, African American Collaborative Obesity Research Network, Dornsife School of Public Health, Drexel University, Philadelphia, Pennsylvania

Rekha B. Kumar, MD, Comprehensive Weight Control Center, Weill Cornell Medical College, Cornell University, New York, New York

Robert F. Kushner, MD, Feinberg School of Medicine, Northwestern University, Evanston, Illinois

Jason M. Lavender, PhD, Neuropsychiatric Research Institute, Fargo, North Dakota

Hannah G. Lawman, PhD, Division of Chronic Disease Prevention, Philadelphia Department of Public Health, Philadelphia, Pennsylvania

Daniel Le Grange, PhD, Departments of Psychiatry and Pediatrics, School of Medicine, University of California, San Francisco, San Francisco, California

Rudolph L. Leibel, MD, Naomi Berrie Diabetes Center and Department of Pediatrics, Division of Molecular Genetics, Columbia University Medical Center, New York, New York

Tim Lobstein, PhD, World Obesity Federation, London, United Kingdom; Public Health Advocacy Institute, Curtin University, Bentley, Western Australia, Australia

Ruth J. F. Loos, PhD, Charles Bronfman Institute for Personalized Medicine and Mindich Child Health and Development Institute, Icahn School of Medicine at Mount Sinai, New York, New York

Katie A. Loth, PhD, MPH, RD, Department of Family Medicine and Community Health, University of Minnesota Medical School, Minneapolis, Minnesota

Michael R. Lowe, PhD, Department of Psychology, Drexel University, Philadelphia, Pennsylvania

Angela Makris, PhD, RD, private practice, Huntingdon Valley, Pennsylvania

Marsha D. Marcus, PhD, Department of Psychiatry, University of Pittsburgh School of Medicine, Pittsburgh, Pennsylvania

Ashley E. Mason, PhD, Osher Center for Integrative Medicine, University of California, San Francisco School of Medicine, San Francisco, California

Laurel E. S. Mayer, MD, New York State Psychiatric Institute and Department of Psychiatry, Columbia University Medical Center, New York, New York

Philip S. Mehler, MD, FACP, FAED, Eating Recovery Center, ACUTE at Denver Health, University of Colorado School of Medicine, Denver, Colorado

Marion Nestle, PhD, MPH, Department of Nutrition, Food Studies, and Public Health, New York University, New York, New York

Dianne Neumark-Sztainer, PhD, MPH, RD, Division of Epidemiology and Community Health, School of Public Health, University of Minnesota, Minneapolis, Minnesota

Meghan L. O'Connell, MPH, UConn Rudd Center for Food Policy and Obesity, Hartford, Connecticut

Cynthia L. Ogden, PhD, MRP, Division of Health and Nutrition Examination Surveys, National Center for Health Statistics, Centers for Disease Control and Prevention, Hyattsville, Maryland

Emily Oken, MD, MPH, Department of Population Medicine, Harvard Medical School, Boston, Massachusetts; Department of Nutrition, Harvard T. H. Chan School of Public Health, Harvard University, Cambridge, Massachusetts

Russell R. Pate, PhD, Department of Exercise Science, Arnold School of Public Health, University of South Carolina, Columbia, South Carolina

Lilia S. Pedraza, MSc, Department of Nutrition, Gillings School of Public Health, University of North Carolina at Chapel Hill, Chapel Hill, North Carolina; National Institute of Public Health of Mexico, Morelos, Mexico

Katharine A. Phillips, MD, Department of Psychiatry and Human Behavior, Alpert Medical School of Brown University, and Body Dysmorphic Disorder Program, Rhode Island Hospital, Providence, Rhode Island

Kathleen M. Pike, PhD, Department of Psychiatry, Columbia University Medical Center, and New York State Psychiatric Institute, New York, New York

Jennifer L. Pomeranz, JD, MPH, College of Global Public Health, New York University, New York, New York

Harrison G. Pope, Jr., MD, MPH, Department of Psychiatry, Harvard Medical School, and Biological Psychiatry Laboratory, McLean Hospital, Boston, Massachusetts

Lizzy Pope, PhD, RD, Department of Nutrition and Food Sciences, University of Vermont, Burlington, Vermont

Rebecca M. Puhl, PhD, UConn Rudd Center for Food Policy and Obesity, Hartford, Connecticut; Department of Human Development and Family Studies, University of Connecticut, Storrs, Connecticut

Claudia Ivonne Ramirez-Silva, PhD, National Institute of Public Health of Mexico, Morelos, Mexico

Eric Ravussin, PhD, Pennington Biomedical Research Institute, Louisiana State University, Baton Rouge, Louisiana

Graham W. Redgrave, MD, Department of Psychiatry and Behavioral Sciences, Johns Hopkins University School of Medicine, Baltimore, Maryland

Tirissa J. Reid, MD, Division of Endocrinology and Metabolism, Department of Medicine, Columbia University Medical Center, New York, New York

Juan A. Rivera, PhD, National Institute of Public Health of Mexico, Morelos, Mexico

Christina A. Roberto, PhD, Department of Medical Ethics and Health Policy, Perelman School of Medicine, University of Pennsylvania, Philadelphia, Pennsylvania

Thomas N. Robinson, MD, MPH, Departments of Pediatrics and Medicine, Stanford Solutions Science Lab, Division of General Pediatrics, and Stanford Prevention Research Center, Stanford University School of Medicine, Stanford, California

Renee J. Rogers, PhD, Department of Health and Physical Activity, School of Education, University of Pittsburgh, Pittsburgh, Pennsylvania

Barbara J. Rolls, PhD, Department of Nutritional Sciences, Pennsylvania State University, State College, Pennsylvania

Michael Rosenbaum, MD, Department of Pediatrics, Division of Molecular Genetics, Columbia University Medical Center, New York, New York

James F. Sallis, PhD, Department of Family Medicine and Public Health, University of California, San Diego, La Jolla, California

David B. Sarwer, PhD, Center for Obesity Research and Education, College of Public Health, Temple University, Philadelphia, Pennsylvania

Lauren Schaefer, MA, Department of Psychology, University of South Florida, Tampa, Florida

Philip R. Schauer, MD, Bariatric and Metabolic Institute, Cleveland Clinic, and Lerner College of Medicine, Case Western Reserve University, Cleveland, Ohio

Ulrike Schmidt, MD, PhD, FRCPsych, Department of Psychological Medicine, Institute of Psychiatry, Psychology and Neuroscience, King's College London, London, United Kingdom

Erica M. Schulte, MS, Department of Psychology, University of Michigan, Ann Arbor, Michigan

Gary J. Schwartz, PhD, Departments of Medicine and Neuroscience, Albert Einstein College of Medicine, New York, New York

Marlene B. Schwartz, PhD, UConn Rudd Center for Food Policy and Obesity, Hartford, Connecticut; Department of Human Development and Family Studies, University of Connecticut, Storrs, Connecticut

Gerard P. Smith, MD, Department of Psychiatry, Weill Cornell Medical College, New York, New York

Kendrin R. Sonneville, ScD, RD, Department of Nutritional Sciences, School of Public Health, University of Michigan, Ann Arbor, Michigan

Joanna E. Steinglass, MD, New York State Psychiatric Institute and Department of Psychiatry, Columbia University Medical Center, New York, New York

June Stevens, PhD, Departments of Nutrition and Epidemiology, Gillings School of Global Public Health, School of Medicine, University of North Carolina at Chapel Hill, Chapel Hill, North Carolina

Eric Stice, PhD, Oregon Research Institute, Eugene, Oregon

Robyn Sysko, PhD, Eating and Weight Disorders Program, Department of Psychiatry, Icahn School of Medicine at Mount Sinai, New York, New York

Marian Tanofsky-Kraff, PhD, Department of Medical and Clinical Psychology, Uniformed Services University of the Health Sciences, Bethesda, Maryland

Deborah F. Tate, PhD, Departments of Health Behavior and Nutrition, Gillings School of Global Public Health, University of North Carolina at Chapel Hill, Chapel Hill, North Carolina

Elsie M. Taveras, MD, MPH, Department of Pediatrics, Massachusetts General Hospital for Children, Boston, Massachusetts

Jennifer J. Thomas, PhD, Eating Disorders Clinical and Research Program, Massachusetts General Hospital, Harvard Medical School, Boston, Massachusetts

J. Kevin Thompson, PhD, Department of Psychology, University of South Florida, Tampa, Florida

Stephen W. Touyz, PhD, School of Psychology, University of Sydney, Sydney, New South Wales, Australia

Janet Treasure, OBE, PhD, FRCP, FRCPsych, Department of Psychological Medicine, King's College London, London, United Kingdom

Adam G. Tsai, MD, MSCE, Kaiser Permanente of Colorado and Division of General Internal Medicine, University of Colorado School of Medicine, Denver, Colorado

Dorothy J. Van Buren, PhD, Department of Psychiatry, Washington University School of Medicine in St. Louis, St. Louis, Missouri

Eric M. VanEpps, PhD, VA Center for Health Equity Research and Promotion and Department of Medical Ethics and Health Policy, Perelman School of Medicine, University of Pennsylvania, Philadelphia, Pennsylvania

Thomas A. Wadden, PhD, Center for Weight and Eating Disorders, Department of Psychiatry, Perelman School of Medicine, University of Pennsylvania, Philadelphia, Pennsylvania

Tracey D. Wade, PhD, School of Psychology, Flinders University, Adelaide, South Australia, Australia

Elizaveta Walker, MPH, Division of Bariatric Surgery, Oregon Health and Science University, Portland, Oregon

B. Timothy Walsh, MD, New York State Psychiatric Institute and Department of Psychiatry, Columbia University Medical Center, New York, New York

Y. Claire Wang, MD, ScD, Department of Health Policy and Management, Mailman School of Public Health, Columbia University, New York, New York

Brian Wansink, PhD, Charles H. Dyson School of Applied Economics and Management, Cornell University, Ithaca, New York

Theodore E. Weltzin, MD, FAED, CEDS, FAPA, Department of Psychiatry and Behavioral Medicine, Medical College of Wisconsin, Milwaukee, Wisconsin

Delia Smith West, PhD, Department of Exercise Science, Arnold School of Public Health, University of South Carolina, Columbia, South Carolina

Kitty Westin, MA, LP, The Emily Program Foundation, St. Paul, Minnesota

Denise E. Wilfley, PhD, Department of Psychiatry, Washington University in St Louis School of Medicine, St. Louis, Missouri

G. Terence Wilson, PhD, Department of Psychology, Rutgers, The State University of New Jersey, New Brunswick, New Jersey

Rena R. Wing, PhD, Weight Control and Diabetes Research Center, The Miriam Hospital, and Department of Psychiatry and Human Behavior, Alpert Medical School of Brown University, Providence, Rhode Island

Alexis C. Wojtanowski, BS, Weight Watchers International, New York, New York

Bruce M. Wolfe, MD, FACS, Division of Bariatric Surgery, Oregon Health and Science University, Portland, Oregon

Stephen A. Wonderlich, PhD, Neuropsychiatric Research Institute, Department of Psychiatry and Behavioral Science, University of North Dakota School of Medicine and Health Sciences, Fargo, North Dakota

Margo G. Wootan, DSc, Center for Science in the Public Interest, Washington, DC

Sonja Yokum, PhD, Oregon Research Institute, Eugene, Oregon

Yiying Zhang, PhD, Department of Pediatrics, Division of Molecular Genetics, Columbia University Medical Center, New York, New York

Hisham Ziauddeen, PhD, Department of Psychiatry, School of Clinical Medicine, University of Cambridge, Cambridge, United Kingdom

Preface

The previous two editions of this book were published in 1995 and 2002, both with Christopher G. Fairburn and one of us (Kelly D. Brownell) as coeditors. We are grateful for the pioneering role Chris has played in the creation of this book, and in the field overall. He continues to be a pioneer, an inspiring figure, and a wonderful colleague. B. Timothy Walsh has taken on Chris's role in this edition.

The preface of each of the prior editions noted the exciting possibilities and the glaring gaps that existed when considering the eating disorders and obesity fields as possible companions. We argued that an improved exchange of information between the two fields could expand the knowlege of both, and might yield new theories to be explored, a better understanding of mechanisms governing eating behavior and weight control, more effective treatments, and the ability to intervene in one area without causing harm in the other. It is informative to look now, some two decades after the first edition was published, at how things have changed, and to what degree these hopes have been realized.

The scientific underpinnings of our understanding of eating disorders and of obesity have advanced in impressive ways, leading to much better knowledge of causes, risk factors, pathophysiology, treatment, prevention, and, especially for obesity, policy. There have been stunning discoveries in genetics (and epigenetics), diagnostic advances have occurred, social causes and consequences are better understood, medical complications are better defined, and treatment options have expanded. These are exciting intellectual advances, but, most importantly, they offer more hope for those who suffer from eating disorders and obesity.

In both of the earlier editions of the book, strong calls were made to better connect the eating disorders and obesity fields. How much progress has there been?

Our sense is that although connections have improved in some ways, the fields remain largely distinct from one another. At most meetings on obesity, eating disorders are rarely mentioned, and obesity is rarely a major topic at meetings on eating disorders. However, there are signs of modest progress. The prior intense concern that recommendations to diet were a major causal factor in the development of eating disorders has largely subsided. It is increasingly recognized that a minority of obese individuals meet criteria for binge-eating disorder, which was officially recognized in DSM-5 in 2013, and that such individuals may benefit from specifically tailored treatments. Perhaps most promising is the growing focus on brain mechanisms in both the obesity and the eating disorders fields. There is increasing recognition that changes in behavior are an essential component of effective treatment interventions for both problems, and an improved understanding of how the brain regulates eating behavior is a critical common foundation in both areas.

This New Edition

This third edition follows the same model as the prior two. We asked leading authorities to write about the area they know best. To provide concise, easily "digestable" and accessible content, we limited the length of the chapters and eliminated the typical in-text references. Rather, we asked that each chapter have a Suggested Reading section, with very brief annotations. These principles have allowed us to assemble a volume of manageable size but containing more than 100 chapters, thereby providing what we hope is comprehensive coverage. The chapters have been organized into three broad sections, Foundations, Eating Disorders, and Obesity, each of which has several subsections.

Behind the theories, statistics, randomized trials, and policy proposals that comprise most of the content of the chapters is the desire and goal to provide assistance for people in need. Eating disorders and obesity bring a cascade of medical, social, and psychological consequences that can have a profound effect on affected individuals, their families, and friends. Our hope is that this book aids the important work of clinicians and researchers to help alleviate and prevent this suffering.

Acknowledgments

We are deeply grateful to the chapter authors for their willingness to contribute to this volume and for helping to describe, clarify, and synthesize complex ideas and vast areas of knowledge into brief chapters. We would also like to thank Jim Nageotte, Senior Editor, and Seymour Weingarten, Editor-in-Chief, and many of their colleagues at The Guilford Press for making this and previous editions possible.

We are especially grateful for the outstanding assistance of Ryan Smith, who was responsible for keeping us and the contributors on task and on time, and keeping track of the myriad details entailed in a volume with over 100 chapters and authors. His help has been invaluable.

We hope this book will help generate innovation and creativity in our fields, and provoke new thinking.

Contents

Epidemiology and Etiology of Eating Disorders

Clinical Characteristics of Obesity

Treatment of Obesity

Obesity Prevention and Policy

Part I

FOUNDATIONS

REGULATION OF BODY WEIGHT

Central Neural Pathways and Integration in the Control of Food Intake and Energy Balance

GARY J. SCHWARTZ

The transmission of gut neural signals related to the controls of food intake, such as gastric volume and gastrointestinal nutrient exposure, is primarily mediated by the afferent vagus nerves supplying the gut. Complete surgical transection of these gut afferent vagal nerves chronically increases meal size in rodent models, yet does not promote increases in body weight, because decreased meal number compensates for the additional caloric intake in each larger meal. Gut vagal afferents project first to central nervous system caudal brainstem sites important in the control of meal size, including the nucleus of the solitary tract (NTS) and area postrema (AP), then via distinct pathways to the brainstem lateral parabrachial nucleus (lPBN) and forebrain limbic and hypothalamic regions, including the amygdala, bed nucleus of the stria terminalis, and the lateral and paraventricular nuclei of the hypothalamus (PVN).

The Melanocortin Pathway

The PVN is a neuroanatomical crossroads between ascending control feeding signals arising from the brainstem, and feeding excitatory and inhibitory neuropeptide signals from hypothalamic arcuate nucleus (ARC) projection neurons, located within the base of the brain abutting the third intracerebral ventricle. ARC neurons include neurochemically distinct populations of feeding-stimulatory (orexigenic) agouti-related peptide (AgRP)/ neuropeptide Y (NPY), and feeding-inhibitory (anorexigenic) pro-opiomelanocortinergic (POMC) neurons. AgRP acts as a melanocortin receptor 3/4 (MC3/4R) antagonist in PVN neurons to promote food intake and body weight gain, while the POMC product alpha-melanocyte-stimulating hormone (alpha-MSH) acts as an agonist at PVN MC3/4R to reduce feeding and adiposity.

Results from molecular genetic studies support the relevance of brain melanocortin receptor signaling in obesity and food intake. Mutations in the *MC4R* gene, occurring in the obese population at approximately 6%, are the most common known cause of monogenic human obesity, characterized by early onset hyperphagia and increased meal size. Mice lacking *MC4R* demonstrate a similar profile of hyperphagia early in development that promotes obesity in adulthood, and mice unable to synthesize the endogenous *MC4R* agonist alpha-MSH are hyperphagic and obese. Furthermore, hypothalamic PVN and brainstem administration of *MC4R* agonists reduce food intake by limiting meal size, resulting in decreased body weight. In contrast, parenchymal administration of *MC4R* antagonists in these sites increases food intake, body weight, and adiposity.

Distinct brainstem projecting populations of MC3/4R neurons in the PVN produce glutamate and oxytocin, two neurochemicals with important feeding modulatory actions at caudal brainstem neurons that receive feeding control signals. Stimulation of glutamatergic projections from the PVN to neurons in the lPBN inhibits feeding, while oxytocinergic nerve projections from the PVN innervate NTS neurons that are activated by feeding inhibitory doses of the gut satiety peptide cholecystokinin (CCK), a negative feedback control of food intake. Brainstem application of oxytocin receptor (OR) antagonists blocks the ability of CCK to inhibit food intake, and brainstem administration of OR antagonists alone markedly increases meal size. In addition to the feeding modulatory PVN hypothalamic glutamatergic and oxytocinergic projections to the brainstem, alpha-MSH fibers arising from the ARC project directly to the NTS, where pharmacological activation of MCR3/4R reduces feeding and body weight. Together, these findings identify reciprocal functional connections between brainstem (NTS and lPBN) and hypothalamus (PVN, ARC) that can drive a recurrent loop to limit feeding by forebrain modulation of gut-derived control signals acting in the brainstem.

The relevance of AgRP for the control of body weight and feeding is highlighted by the consequences of selective stimulation or inhibition of AgRP neurons; neurochemically specific photo- or chemostimulation of AgRP neurons inhibits PVN oxytocin neurons and rapidly increases meal size, while photostimulation of ARC POMC neurons reduces feeding and body weight. Ablation of AgRP/NPY neurons in adult mice results in profound anorexia and starvation, accompanied by hyperactivation of lPBN neurons. Stimulation of inhibitory lPBN gamma-aminobutyric acid (GABA) A receptors prevents the anorexia produced by AgRP neuronal ablation, suggesting a descending hypothalamic modulatory pathway to limit the activation of the lPBN, a brainstem relay that processes negative feedback controls of ingestion.

Brainstem integration of peripheral meal-related controls and central feeding modulatory neurochemical signals is supported by the neuroanatomical convergence of gut feeding controls and central melanocortin action: alpha-MSH projections to the brainstem terminate on gut-sensitive, CCK-responsive NTS neurons, and brainstem application of *MC4R* antagonists block the satiety actions of peripheral feeding inhibitory doses of CCK. Taken together with the previously discussed consequences of hypothalamic melanocortin pathway activation, these data demonstrate that central melanocortins have neuroanatomically distributed, redundant effects that are important for the control of feeding behavior and energy balance.

Leptin

The adiposity signal leptin has been importantly implicated in both forebrain and brainstem control of food intake and body weight through both melanocortin-dependent and independent mechanisms. In very rare cases of human genetic leptin deficiency accompanied by severe obesity, pharmacological administration of leptin eliminates hyperphagia and normalizes body weight and adiposity. A central action of leptin in these effects is suggested by the dense distribution of leptin receptors in hypothalamic ARC POMC and AgRP neurons, as well as in brainstem NTS/AP neurons. Each of these populations is localized near circumventricular organs, characterized by a relatively porous blood–brain barrier that permits enhanced brain access to peripherally circulating factors. Leptin reaches hypothalamic ARC neurons via a highly selective transport system mediated by tanycytes, specialized glial cells lining the third ventricle. Hypothalamic leptin uptake is disrupted in both diet-induced obesity and genetic obesity in *db/db* mice lacking the leptin receptor. Given the morphological similarities shared among circumventricular organs, it is likely that leptin access to the brainstem relies on transport processes similar to those in the hypothalamic ARC.

Leptin injections into the ARC produce long-lasting suppression of meal size and total chow intake, and rats prone to develop diet-induced obesity have defective projections arising from ARC neurons, accompanied by reduced leptin signaling that persists into adulthood. The ability of ARC leptin signaling to reduce feeding is significantly blunted by brainstem injection of *MC4R* antagonists, suggesting a leptin-activated ARC–PVN–NTS melanocortin circuit. Genetically obese (*fa(k)/fa(k)*) rats lack functional leptin receptors and are consequently obese and hyperphagic; their hyperphagia is characterized by increased meal size and reduced feeding inhibitory actions of CCK. Selective restoration of leptin receptors confined to the ARC restores the ability of peripherally administered CCK to both activate brainstem NTS/AP neurons and to limit food intake by a reduction in meal size. Thus, neuroanatomical connectivity between leptin sensitive hypothalamic sites and the caudal brainstem is an important determinant of the brainstem processing of satiety signals.

The metabolic context provided by central signals of adiposity such as leptin also determines the magnitude of the neural response to gut negative feedback signals and their ability to reduce meal size. Gut-sensitive neurons in the NTS are dose-dependently activated by increasing gastric volume stimuli, and central leptin administration increases the neurophysiological potency of such stimuli. Thus, NTS neurons integrate central adiposity signals with peripheral controls of feeding. Such integration occurs not only at the level of the individual neuron but also at a population level, as central leptin also increases the number of NTS cells activated by gastric loads. From a behavioral standpoint, ventricular, lPBN, and NTS leptin administration reduces food intake and body weight in rats, and increases the degree of feeding suppression produced by gastric loads and duodenal nutrient infusions. Conversely, molecular genetic knockdown of brainstem leptin receptors increases food intake by increasing the size of spontaneous meals, increases body weight and adiposity, and blunts the feeding inhibitory effects of CCK. Taken together, these demonstrate the ability of leptin acting at both the brainstem and hypothalamus to modulate the brainstem control of food intake, meal size, body weight, and adiposity.

However, the metabolic milieu determined by either dietary or genetic obesity does not strictly limit the inhibitory potency of all feeding and body weight regulatory stimuli. For example, the ability of oxytocin to (1) reduce food intake and body weight and (2) activate brainstem NTS and AP is preserved in hyperleptinemic, leptin-resistant rats with diet-induced obesity and in Koletsky *fa/fa* rats lacking leptin receptors. In this way, leptin- and obesity-independent determinants of feeding and body weight may also engage brainstem sites that process direct control signals.

Nutrient Sensing

Finally, nutrient sensing by neuronal populations in hypothalamic–brainstem circuits provides another avenue for the integrated and distributed central controls of food intake and body weight. Feeding or gastrointestinal infusion of the essential branched-chain amino acid leucine rapidly elevates its appearance in cerebrospinal fluid, hypothalamus, and brainstem, and hypothalamic activation of leucine signaling pathways, either by leucine itself or downstream mediators, reduces food intake, meal size, and body weight gain. Several genes involved in branched-chain amino acid metabolism have been suggested as candidate genes in human obesity. Furthermore, in humans, single-nucleotide polymorphisms in leucine transporters have been associated with body mass index, and mice with deficient leucine transporter expression have reduced leucine-inhibited food intake and weight gain during high-fat diet maintenance. Leucine directly activates hypothalamic POMC neurons that express oxytocin, and the ability of hypothalamic leucine to reduce feeding is blocked by brainstem administration of oxytocin receptor antagonists, demonstrating that hypothalamic nutrient sensing engages oxytocin brainstem pathways important in the control of meal size. Leucine sensing also appears to be redundantly expressed, as direct brainstem application of leucine and its downstream signaling mediators also reduce food intake, meal size, and body weight gain.

Summary

In summary, brainstem and hypothalamic neuronal interconnections form the basis for a distributed and redundant set of pathways to modulate the control of feeding and body weight (see Figure 1.1). Meal-related sensorineural signals generated by the presence of nutrients along the gastrointestinal tract project to a circuit of brainstem and hypothalamic neurons localized in brain regions with preferred access to circulating factors, including individual nutrients, as well as hormones whose circulating levels reflect the availability of stored nutrients (the adiposity hormones leptin and insulin) and the availability of gastrointestinal nutrients (e.g., ghrelin). Each of these signals of nutrient availability, the gastrointestinal presence of nutrients, circulating nutrients, adiposity hormones, and gut peptides determines the activity of neurons in gut-recipient brainstem and hypothalamic sites, and such activation is strongly associated with the control of food intake and body weight. The unknown functions of the redundant sensitivity to these stimuli in hypothalamic and brainstem sites represent an important gap in our understanding of the neurobiology of energy balance. In physiologically relevant settings, none of these factors acts on feeding or body weight control in isolation; the neurobiological environment of these neuronal populations is characterized by distinct levels of each class of stimuli at any given time. The biological responses of brainstem and hypothalamic neurons to nutritionally relevant stimuli are determined by the metabolic context or milieu in which a stimulus occurs. Accordingly, both neuronal populations also have the capacity to respond to combinations of sensorineural, hormonal, and nutrient stimuli in an integrative fashion. This integrative capacity within and across gut-sensitive neurons appears to be an important index of the feeding and body weight consequences of these interactions. Neuroanatomical connectivity and communication among brainstem and hypothalamic sites suggest that they work in a coordinated fashion to determine energy balance. Progress will depend on the identification of the ways in which physiologically relevant constellations of nutrient-related signals jointly determine the activity

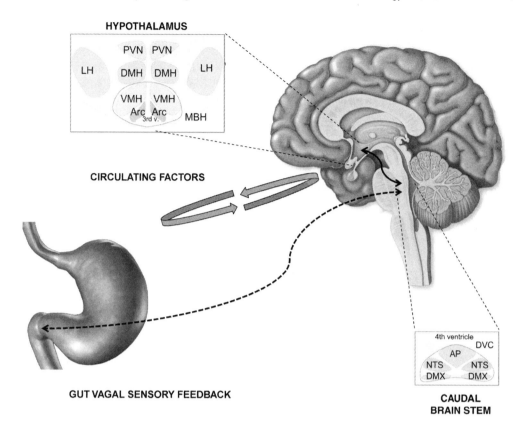

FIGURE 1.1. Schematic of discussed hypothalamic–brain stem circuits involved in controlling energy balance. The diagram depicts a subset of the neuronal connections reported to influence feeding and body weight. Sensory meal-related signals are transmitted via gut sensory vagal afferent projections to the brain stem–hypothalamic axis. Humoral factors, including circulating nutrients, adiposity hormones, and gut peptides also impinge on this axis. Note that the black dashed arrows reflect connectivity between hypothalamic and brain stem regions, and not any specific anatomical pathway. MBH, mediobasal hypothalamus; PVN, paraventricular nucleus of the hypothalamus; ARC, arcuate nucleus of the hypothalamus; AP, area postrema; NTS, nucleus of the solitary tract.

of hypothalamic and brainstem neuronal circuits in the service of food intake and body weight control.

Acknowledgment

This work was supported by Grant Nos. NIH P30 DK26687 and NIH R01 DK105441 to Gary J. Schwartz.

Suggested Reading

Blouet, C., & Schwartz, G. J. (2010). Hypothalamic nutrient sensing in the control of energy homeostasis. *Behavioral Brain Research, 209*(1), 1–12.—A discussion of the hypothalamic and brainstem circuits capable of detecting nutrients and the physiological and metabolic consequences of this detection important for the control of energy balance.

Grill, H. J., & Hayes, M. R. (2012). Hindbrain neurons as an essential hub in the neuroanatomically distributed control of energy balance. *Cell Metabolism, 16*(3), 296–309.—A comprehensive view of the wide ranging structural and functional influences of hindbrain neurons on hypothalamic function and multiple effectors of energy homeostasis.

Moran, T. H., & Ladenheim, E. E. (2011). Adiposity signaling and meal size control. *Physiology and Behavior, 103*(1), 21–24.—A critical discussion of mechanisms and modes of action of adiposity signals and the control of meal size.

Morton, G. J., Blevins, J. E., Williams, D. L., Niswender, K. D., Gelling, R. W., Rhodes, C. J., et al. (2005). Leptin action in the forebrain regulates the hindbrain response to satiety signals. *Journal of Clinical Investigation, 115*(3), 703–710.—Demonstration of the importance of hypothalamic signaling to brainstem processing of meal-related negative feedback signals important in the control of ingestion.

Sadaf Farooqi, I., & O'Rahilly, S. (2014). 20 years of leptin: Human disorders of leptin action. *Journal of Endocrinology, 223*, T63–T70.—An important characterization of the progress in evaluating the metabolic consequences of leptin deficiency and leptin therapy.

Schwartz, G. J., & Zeltser, L. M. (2013). Functional organization of neuronal and humoral signals regulating feeding behavior. *Annual Review of Nutrition, 33*, 1–21.—A recent review of the integrative neuroanatomy and neurobiology underlying the control of food intake.

2

Decreased Peripheral Hormonal Negative-Feedback Control of Food Intake and Body Weight in Obesity

GERARD P. SMITH

In 1922, Curt Richter published the first meal patterns of rats living alone in cages with free access to food and water. The meal patterns demonstrated that eating occurred in bouts (meals) separated by intervals of noneating (intermeal intervals). These data established two axioms for investigating eating and food intake: First, the meal is the functional unit of analysis of eating and, second, food intake in any interval is the result of the size and number of meals. The second axiom predicts that an increase of food intake is the result of increased meal size, increased meal number, or both. Genetic and diet-induced obesity (DIO) are characterized by increased meal size. Meal number is usually decreased. Thus, increased meal size must be due to changes in the peripheral positive and negative feedback(s), central processing of peripheral feedback information, or central integrative controls of meal size (see Chapter 2).

Resistance to Peripheral Negative-Feedback Control of Meal Size in DIO

Larger meals in DIO have been suggested to be the result of increased peripheral positive feedback produced by ingestion of energy-dense, palatable, hedonic diets. Extensive investigation has shown, however, that larger meals in DIO rats are associated with normal or decreased central rewarding effects of ingested diet rather than increased rewarding effects. Thus, larger meals in DIO rats must be due to decreased potency of peripheral negative feedback. This is due to the decreased inhibitory potency of leptin, insulin, cholecystokinin (CCK-8), glucagon-like peptide 1 (GLP-1), and peptide tyrosine tyrosine (peptide YY) released from the small intestine by the stimulation of ingested foods and their digestive products. Amylin is the only exception; its release from the pancreatic islets and its circulating concentration are normal.

This widespread loss of inhibitory potency is referred to as *resistance*. The cellular mechanisms of leptin and insulin resistance are partially known, but the mechanisms of the resistance to other hormones are not.

The possibility that the loss of peripheral negative-feedback control of meal size accounts for the hyperphagia and obesity of the DIO rat has been tested by administering these hormones to DIO rats. Continuous subcutaneous infusions of amylin for 12–14 days produced a significant reduction of food intake and body weight in male rats with DIO. When identical infusions of leptin, PYY, or CCK-8 were administered alone, however, there was little or no decrease of food intake or body weight.

Peripheral circulating peptides for decreasing meal size circulate simultaneously during and after the ingestion of food, and they interact synergistically in *lean* rats. To exploit this synergism for therapeutic purposes in DIO, simultaneous infusions of amylin and leptin or amylin and PYY were tested. These peptide combinations decreased food intake and body weight significantly more than the additive effect of the individual peptides infused alone. Furthermore, when amylin, leptin, and CCK-8 were infused simultaneously, the decreases of food intake and body weight were larger than those produced by the combination of amylin and leptin.

A similar synergism has been obtained by infusing a stabilized form of CCK-8 and the GLP1 agonist exanetide. This synergism is dependent on the action of stabilized CCK-8 because the synergism is blocked by a selective antagonist of the CCK1 receptor (CCK-1R). Furthermore, the synergism is not dependent on endogenous leptin because it occurs in the leptin-deficient *ob/ob* (obese) mouse.

The infusions of the combinations of peptides decreased body weight about 15% in 12–14 days. This is equivalent to the decreases of body weight produced by gastrointestinal surgery in DIO rats, the largest current therapeutic effect (see below).

The synergistic inhibitory effect of these peptide combinations on food intake and body weight in DIO rats is important for two reasons. First, it supports the possibility that the loss of peripheral negative-feedback potency due to the development of resistance to these peptides is *sufficient* to produce DIO in rats. Second, peripheral combination-peptide therapy is feasible in humans. These effects of combination-peptide therapy are the most promising nonsurgical therapy of DIO available for translation to obese humans.

Synergism between Diet Therapy and CCK-8

CCK-8 also increased the effect of diet therapy in DIO rats. Male and female DIO rats were restricted to three meals per day. This produced a significant weight loss. When the weight loss stabilized, CCK-8 was administered intraperitoneally prior to each of the three daily meals. The addition of CCK-8 to diet treatment for 3 weeks decreased food intake and body weight significantly more than dietary restriction alone.

Genetic Obesity: The Osaka Long–Evans Tokashima Fatty Rat

The Osaka Long–Evans Tokashima Fatty (OLETF) rat has a spontaneous loss-of-function mutation of the CCK-1R. The mutant rat has increased meal size, increased food intake, and obesity. The absence of CCK-1R in the stomach, small intestine, and vagal afferent nerves prevents the negative-feedback effect of CCK released from the small intestine by postingestive, preabsorptive stimuli of ingested food and its digestive products.

In addition to the decreased negative feedback, there is increased positive feedback. This was detected by increased intake of sucrose solutions in sham feeding. Because sham feeding allows ingested sucrose to drain out of the stomach through a gastric cannula, it eliminates the negative-feedback effects of ingested sucrose as an explanation of the increased sham-fed intake. Further investigation demonstrated that the absence of CCK-1R in the dorsomedial hypothalamic nucleus was necessary for the increased positive feedback. Note that decreased negative feedback produces hyperphagia and obesity in the DIO rat, but hyperphagia and obesity in the OLETF rat is due to the combined effects of decreased negative feedback and increased positive feedback. This distinction is important for further investigation of the pathophysiology of DIO and the genetic obesity of the OLETF rat.

Bariatric Surgery and Peripheral Hormonal Negative Feedback

The rationale for bariatric surgery is to decrease food intake and body weight by increasing the negative feedback control of meal size and food intake. Adjustable gastric banding (AGB), vertical sleeve gastrectomy (VSG), and Roux-en-Y gastric bypass (RYGB) are the most commonly used procedures (see Chapters 87, 88, and 89). AGB increases gastromechanical negative feedback by decreasing the functional volume of the stomach. RYGB and VSG produce numerous changes in appetite and metabolism. The change most relevant to the negative-feedback control of food intake is the changed profile of gut hormones released from the stomach and small intestine by ingested food and its digestive products. RYGB and VSG decrease body weight more than AGB and produce a larger and more rapid resolution of type 2 diabetes (T2D). Circulating levels of GLP-1 and PYY increase after RYGB and VSG, but not after AGB. The increase of GLP-1 has been suggested as the major mediator of the larger effects of RYGB on body weight and T2D than AGB because GLP-1 agonists have been efficacious in the clinical treatment of T2D and obesity.

Discussion

Recent research in rats and humans has demonstrated the importance of peripheral hormonal negative-feedback control of food intake in the development and treatment of obesity. The development and maintenance of DIO in rats is associated with a loss of inhibitory potency of a number of peripheral hormones released from the small intestine, adipose tissue, and pancreatic islets by ingested food and its digestive products. Amylin released from the pancreatic islets is an important exception. Although subcutaneous infusion of amylin decreases food intake and body weight in rats with DIO, the effect is small compared to the loss of weight produced by RYGB or VSG. When amylin is combined with leptin or PYY, however, the loss of body weight is equivalent to that produced by RYGB or VSG. The inverse relationship between increased food intake and body weight and the negative-feedback potency of circulating peripheral hormones suggests that the widespread decrease of potency of the hormones is *sufficient* to cause the development and maintenance of DIO in the rat. That inference requires testing in the rat. Furthermore, the similar efficacy of RYGB and VSG for decreasing body weight and food intake in rat and human DIO suggests that the increased circulating GLP-1 and PYY after these human surgeries may be an important experimental bridge for translation of hormonal-combination therapy from rat to human.

Suggested Reading

Heppner, K. M., & Perez-Tilve, D. (2015). GLP-1 based therapeutics: Simultaneously combating T2DM and obesity. *Frontiers in Neuroscience, 9,* 1–11.—Good review of the therapeutic effects of GLP-1.

Johnson, P. M., & Kenny, P. J. (2010). Addiction-like reward dysfunction and compulsive eating in obese rats: Role for dopamine D_2 receptors. *Nature Neuroscience, 13,* 645–651.—Compelling demonstration of decreased rewarding effect of food in DIO rats.

Lutz, T. A. (2013). The interaction of amylin with other hormones in the control of eating. *Diabetes, Obesity, and Metabolism, 15,* 99–111.—Authoritative review of amylin and its interaction with other satiating peptides in the negative-feedback control of eating.

Moran, T. H. (2008). Unraveling the obesity of OLETF rats. *Physiology and Behavior, 94,* 71–78.—A classic analysis of a genetic obesity produced by a mutation of the receptor for the negative feedback control of food intake by CCK.

Smith, G. P. (2000). The controls of eating: A shift from nutritional homeostasis to behavioral neuroscience. *Nutrition, 16,* 814–820.—The author discusses the evidence for the paradigm shift and the importance of peripheral positive- and negative-feedback control of eating.

Stefater, M. A., Wilson-Perez, H. E., Chambers, D. A., Sandoval, D. A., & Seeley, R. J. (2012). All bariatric surgeries are not created equal: Insights from mechanistic comparisons. *Endocrine Reviews, 33,* 595–622.—A thorough and critical discussion of the effects of bariatric surgeries in rats and humans.

Trevaskis, J. L., Sun, C., Altanacio, J., D'Souza, L., Samant, M., Tatarwiecz, K., et al. (2015). Synergistic metabolic benefits of an exenatide analogue and cholecystokinin in diet-induced obese and leptin deficient rodents. *Diabetes, Obesity, and Metabolism, 17,* 61–73.— First report of a significant synergism between a GLP-1 agonist and CCK for decreasing food intake and body weight in DIO in rats and in ob/ob mice. CCK-1 receptors are necessary for the synergism, and endogenous leptin is not.

Troke, R. C., Tan, T. M., & Bloom, S. R. (2014). The future role of gut hormones in the treatment of obesity. *Therapeutic Advances in Chronic Disease, 5,* 4–14.—An informed look at the potential for gut hormonal therapy of human DIO.

Leptin and Body Weight

YIYING ZHANG
RUDOLPH L. LEIBEL

Body weight, specifically fat, in mammals is regulated by homeostatic mechanisms operating primarily in service of "tuning" the gonadal axis to sufficiency of caloric stores for successful parturition, and provision of stored energy against environmental vicissitudes.

The *lipostatic* model—formulated by Kennedy, Hervey, and others—speculated that fat mass, via a humoral factor, provides an afferent signal that is sensed and responded to (via alterations in energy intake–expenditure) by the hypothalamus. Efforts to identify this fat-based humoral signal continued through much of the second half of the previous century, culminating in the discovery of the *leptin* gene by positional cloning in 1994. Two autosomal recessive mouse obesity mutations, *ob* and *db,* which exhibit virtually identical phenotypes, including hyperphagia, reduced energy expenditure, and preferential deposition of stored calories as fat, provided the keys. The *leptin* gene, which is inactivated by a mutation in the *ob* mouse, encodes a secreted protein produced in adipocytes in proportion to fat cell size. The *leptin receptor* gene, which is mutated in the *db* mouse, encodes the cognate receptor that functions primarily in the brain, particularly the hypothalamus. The discovery and characterization of the leptin signaling pathway in humans and rodents provided a compelling molecular genetic mechanism for control of body fat, vindicating the lipostatic model.

Leptin Production in Relation to Fat Mass, Adipocyte Size, and Acute Energy Status

Adipocytes are the primary source of circulating leptin. Several types of stomach cells also contribute a small amount of circulating leptin. Plasma leptin concentrations are highly correlated with fat mass and adiposity. In adipose tissue, leptin messenger RNA (mRNA) levels and protein secretion rates are positively correlated with adipocyte size.

Plasma leptin concentrations are generally higher in adult females than in males. The gender-related differences likely result from the differences in body fat distribution between men and women and depot-specific differences in leptin expression (higher per cell in subcutaneous fat). Plasma leptin concentrations per unit of fat mass are not significantly different between prepubertal boys and girls, but increase in girls and decrease in boys as the pubertal process progresses, and are significantly higher in girls than boys by Tanner Stages IV and V. Individual differences in plasma leptin concentration per unit of fat mass—controlled for factors alluded to earlier—have also been observed, but the physiological causes and consequences of these differences are unclear. Plasma leptin concentration is extremely sensitive to acute energy deficits—short-term caloric restriction markedly suppresses leptin expression even when there has been little and no fat loss. On the other hand, energy surpluses or infusions of insulin have little acute effect on plasma leptin concentrations in humans, although similar treatments result in small increases in plasma leptin levels in rodents. The molecular mechanisms underpinning these features of *leptin* gene expression are key unresolved questions in the biology of leptin; their elucidation could provide novel therapeutic approaches to obesity. The asymmetric responses of leptin concentrations to acute energy surpluses (minimal) and deficits (strong) reflect the major physiological role of this hormone in defense of body fat.

Molecular Mechanisms of Leptin Signaling

The leptin receptor (LEPR) is a member of the type I cytokine receptor family, closely related to the interleukin-6 receptor (Figure 3.1). Multiple LEPR isoforms are produced through alternative splicing of a single primary transcript. These isoforms differ only in their C-terminal cytoplasmic sequences. The "long" isoform of LEPR (LEPRb), which is absent in the *db* mouse, contains the binding sites for the signaling molecules, Janus kinase 2 (JAK2) and signal transducer and activator of transcription 3 (STAT3). The functions of the shorter LEPR isoforms, which are devoid of most of the cytoplasmic sequences of the long isoform, are unclear. LEPRb is expressed at much higher levels in the hypothalamus and several other regions of the brain than in peripheral tissues. Central leptin actions mediated by LEPRb are essential to normal body weight homeostasis.

Leptin activates the protein tyrosine kinase JAK2, which phosphorylates LEPR and many downstream effectors, including STAT3. All three cytoplasmic tyrosine (Y) residues of LEPR (Y985, Y1077, and Y1138 in mouse, which are conserved across all known mammalian LEPR) can be phosphorylated, and serve as the interaction sites for downstream effectors. The LEP–JAK2–STAT3 signaling pathway, mediated by Y1138, plays an especially prominent role in the regulation of energy metabolism. Disruption of this pathway leads to an obesity phenotype similar to that of the *db* mouse. SH2B1 is a positive regulator of leptin signaling that enhances JAK2 activity and promotes LEPR–JAK2 interactions with various downstream effectors, including insulin receptor substrate 2 (IRS2). Deletion or mutation of SH2B1 leads to hyperphagia and morbid obesity in both humans and rodents. The Y985 tyrosine residue of LEPR is involved in the feedback inhibition of leptin signaling by suppressor of cytokine signaling 3 (SOCS3). Mutation of Y985 to leucine results in resistance to diet (high-fat)-induced obesity in female but not male mice, underscoring the importance of both this feedback inhibitory mechanism and sexual dimorphism in leptin physiology. The effects of leptin on glucose homeostasis and reproduction are not entirely dependent on these cytoplasmic tyrosine residues. Mice

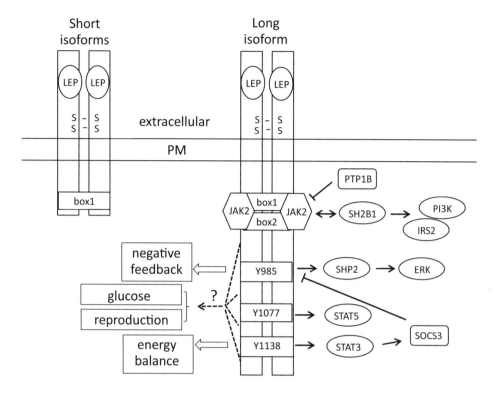

FIGURE 3.1. The long and short isoforms of mouse leptin receptor (LEPR) and the major leptin-activated signaling pathways that affect energy balance. Two LEPR molecules form preexisting (i.e., before LEP binding) dimers through disulfide bonds, and each dimer binds two leptin molecules. The binding of leptin to the receptor dimer activates multiple signaling pathways; the major signaling pathways activated by leptin are shown here. Leptin is a permissive factor for normal pubertal development and reproduction, which provide a critical link between adipose tissue energy stores and reproductive integrity. Leptin also plays an important role in glucose metabolism. Although Y1077 and PI3 kinase have been implicated, respectively, in leptin's regulation of reproduction and glucose metabolism, the molecular mechanisms for these effects of leptin are not fully understood. LEP, leptin; JAK2, Janus kinase 2; box1 and box2; conserved sequences of JAK binding site; Y985, tyrosine at 985 position of mouse LEPR; Y1077, tyrosine at 1077 position of mouse LEPR; Y1138, tyrosine at 1138 position of mouse LEPR; PTP1B, protein tyrosine phosphatase 1B; SH2B1, SH2B adaptor protein 1; IRS2, insulin receptor substrate 2; PI3K, phosphoinositide 3-kinase; SHP2, SHP2 tyrosine phosphatase; ERK, extracellular signal-regulated kinase; STAT3 and STAT5, signal transducer and transcription activators 3 and 5; SOCS3, suppressor of cytokine signaling 3; PM, plasma membrane. From Allison & Myers (2014). Copyright © 2014 by the Society for Endocrinology. Adapted by permission.

lacking all three tyrosine residues are as obese as *db* mice but exhibit relatively normal glucose homeostasis and reproductive function.

LEPR signaling is negatively regulated by two mechanisms: (1) Activation of the JAK2–STAT3 pathway increases the expression of SOCS3, which binds to Y985 of LEPR and provides feedback inhibition of leptin signaling, and (2) protein tyrosine phosphatase 1B (PTP1B) dephosphorylates JAK2 and negatively regulates leptin signaling. Expression levels of SOCS3 and PTP1B are both increased in the hypothalami of obese mice. Deletion or knockout of SOCS3 or PTP1B leads to increased leptin sensitivity, resistance to diet-induced obesity, and lean phenotypes in mice. Other potential mechanisms affecting leptin signaling include the regulation of expression and posttranslational modification of LEPR, and the access of circulating leptin to LEPR in the central nervous system (CNS). Impairments in the function of second-order neurons in leptin-regulated neural circuits constitute a separate category of impaired leptin action. Mc4R neurons in the paraventricular hypothalamus (PVH), which regulate food intake and energy homeostasis, are affected by leptin indirectly through POMC and AgRP neurons in the arcuate nucleus of the hypothalamus (ARH). Obese individuals with mutations affecting the Mc4R signaling pathway are resistant to leptin therapy.

Leptin-Regulated Neural Circuits and Their Effects on Energy Intake and Body Weight

The long form of LEPR (LEPRb) is expressed in brain regions involved in the regulation of energy homeostasis (Figure 3.2). High densities of LEPR are found in neurons in the ARH, ventromedial and dorsomedial nuclei of the hypothalamus (VMH and DMH), ventral premammillary nucleus (PMV), and medial preoptic nucleus (MEPO) of the hypothalamus, underscoring the prominent role of the hypothalamus in mediating leptin action. The ARH POMC and AgRP neurons, which are the prototypes of LEPR-expressing neurons, are regulated by leptin in opposite directions. Leptin activates glutamatergic POMC neurons and stimulates the production of the anorexigenic peptide alpha-melanocyte-stimulating hormone (alpha-MSH; derived from POMC) while inhibiting gamma-aminobutyric acid (GABA)ergic AgRP neurons, thus suppressing the production of orexigenic peptides AgRP and neuropeptide Y (NPY). The increase of alpha-MSH and decrease of AgRP activates Mc4R neurons in the PVH. The ARH POMC and AgRP neurons also directly innervate and regulate—through synaptic signaling—PVH Mc4R neurons and many other neuronal groups in other regions of the hypothalamus and the brainstem. ARH POMC neurons themselves are also regulated by leptin indirectly via excitatory (glutamatergic) inputs from LEPR-expressing VMH neurons and inhibitory (GABAergic) inputs from the neighboring AgRP neurons. Direct leptin action in ARH neurons acutely suppresses food intake but has relatively minor effects on the long-term energy balance in mice. Outside of the hypothalamus, neurons in the nucleus of solitary tract (NTS) of the brainstem also express LEPRb and respond to leptin directly, in addition to receiving excitatory inputs from hypothalamic POMC neurons. The NTS receives input signals from the gut as well, including circulating anorexigenic gut peptides such as glucagon-like peptide 1 (GLP-1) and cholecystokinin (CCK), and direct neural inputs from vagal afferents. Leptin action sensitizes NTS neurons to gut signals, increasing their satiating effects. To regulate food intake, leptin and other signals are further relayed from NTS neurons via excitatory inputs to the anorexigenic neurons in the lateral parabrachial nucleus (PBN) of the hindbrain, which also receive strong inhibitory inputs from ARH AgRP neurons.

Leptin also plays an important role in the mesolimbic dopamine system that mediates pleasure and reward ("hedonic") responses. Leptin-deficient children have impaired ability to discriminate reward properties of foods; leptin replacement corrects this defect. In the mouse, leptin acts directly on the dopaminergic and nondopaminergic neurons in

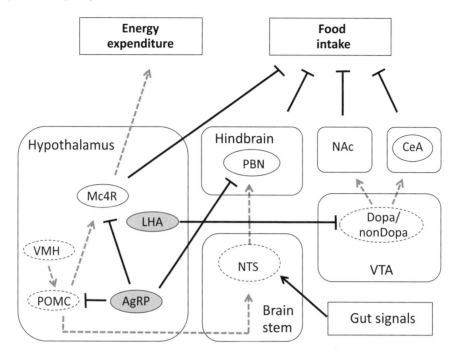

FIGURE 3.2. Leptin-regulated neural circuits in the control of food intake and energy expenditure. The dotted-line ovals represent neurons activated by leptin, which are primarily glutamatergic; the gray ovals represent those suppressed by leptin, which are primarily GABAergic; the white ovals are those indirectly regulated by leptin. The dotted-line arrows indicate stimulation and the solid-lines suppression. The solid-line arrow indicates that leptin sensitizes NTS neurons to afferent gut signals. Mc4R, Mc4R neurons of the paraventricular nucleus; POMC, pro-opiomelanocortin neurons of the arcuate nucleus; AgRP, agouti-related peptide neurons of the arcuate nucleus; VMH, ventromedial nucleus; LHA, lateral hypothalamic area; PBN, lateral parabrachial nucleus; NTS, nucleus of solitary tract; NAc, nucleus of accumbens of the ventral striatum; CeA, central nucleus of the amygdala. Gut signals include peptide hormones, such as GLP-1, CCK, as well as vagal inputs. Dopamine is shown here as having suppressive effects on food intake by the pathways shown, but may have orexigenic effects in other circuits. Based on Gautron and Elmquist (2011).

the ventral tegmental area (VTA), which innervate the nucleus of accumbens (NAc) of the ventral striatum and central nucleus of the amygdala (CeA), the major reward centers. Leptin also regulates dopamine production in VTA neurons via LEPR-expressing neurons in the lateral hypothalamic area (LHA) that innervate these VTA neurons (see Figure 3.2).

Pathophysiology of Leptin Deficiency and Leptin Replacement Therapy

While extremely rare, complete deficiency of leptin or LEPR leads to profound hyperphagia and early-onset obesity in humans. The hyperphagia is associated with increased hunger and decreased satiety. Energy partitioning is also markedly altered: Excess energy is preferentially deposited as fat in both humans and rodents. Energy expenditure (adjusted for metabolic mass) is decreased in LEPR-deficient rodents, primarily due to impaired thermoregulatory thermogenesis, but is not significantly affected in leptin- or LEPR-deficient humans. As a measure of the long-term energy status (the size of expendable energy reserves of the organism), leptin is a permissive factor for normal pubertal development, reproduction, and immunity in both humans and rodents. Patients homozygous for loss-of-function mutations of leptin or LEPR genes have normal birth weight but rapidly gain weight (fat) a few months after birth due to hyperphagia. Early cognitive development and linear growth are usually normal. Normal pubertal development is absent or severely impaired due to hypogonadotropic hypogonadism. Hypothalamic hypothyroidism is also characteristic of these patients. Lipodystrophy represents a major form of secondary partial leptin deficiency. Patients with lipodystrophy develop metabolic and neuroendocrine abnormalities that resemble those in patients with complete leptin deficiency, including hyperphagia, dyslipidemia, and, in females, hypoamenorrhea.

Leptin replacement was first administered to 3- and 9-year-old congenitally leptin-deficient children in 1997. In these two children, daily injections of recombinant leptin markedly decreased hunger, increased meal-related satiety, and increased their ability to discriminate rewarding properties of foods. Functional magnetic resonance imaging studies showed that in the leptin-deficient state, food cues strongly activated neurons in brain areas associated with pleasure and reward, such as the ventral striatal region, and that this activation was attenuated by leptin treatment even before weight loss occurred. Leptin replacement normalized thyroid function, caused preferential loss of fat, and allowed the normal development of puberty in these children. In 2014, leptin was approved by the U.S. Food and Drug Administration specifically for the treatment of metabolic disorders associated with lipodystrophy. As in patients with congenital leptin deficiency, leptin suppresses food intake and markedly improves dyslipidemia, hepatic steatosis, and glucose–insulin homeostasis in lipodystrophic patients.

Physiology and Pathophysiology of Leptin in the Obese State

Obesity in general is associated with elevated plasma leptin concentrations. In contrast to the profound metabolic benefits of leptin administration in patients with complete or partial leptin deficiency, leptin, as high-dose monotherapy or combined therapy, has very little efficacy in suppressing energy intake or inducing long-term weight loss in obese patients. Leptin administration acutely suppresses food intake in lean mice but not in overfed obese mice, suggesting an impairment in the acute response to leptin in the obese mice. However, leptin administration also has limited long-term effects on body weight in normal-weight humans and rodents. On the other hand, functional blockade of endogenous leptin by a leptin antagonist markedly increases food intake and body weight to similar extents in lean and obese mice. And decreases in plasma leptin concentrations resulting from weight loss or acute energy deficits evoke strong physiological responses, including increased hunger and decreased energy expenditure, in both obese and lean individuals. These physiological changes associated with negative energy balance can be reversed by low-dose leptin replacement that restores plasma leptin to the pre-weight-loss level. These observations suggest that the leptin signaling system is more physiologically sensitive to energy deficits than to energy surpluses, and responds to negative energy balance similarly in lean and in obese individuals. Thus, the physiology of leptin signaling system is well suited to detect and signal energy deficits and to defend against loss of fat mass, the primary energy reserve of all mammals.

Suggested Reading

Allison, M. B., & Myers, M. G., Jr. (2014). 20 years of leptin: Connecting leptin signaling to biological function. *Journal of Endocrinology, 223,* T25–T35.—This review summarizes the signaling pathways engaged by LEPRb and their effects on energy balance, glucose homeostasis, and reproduction.

Farooqi, I. S., & O'Rahilly, S. (2014). 20 years of leptin: Human disorders of leptin action. *Journal of Endocrinology, 223,* T63–T70.—This review summarizes characteristic clinical features of leptin deficiency, human obesities caused by defects in the pathways downstream of leptin signaling within the brain, and the effects of leptin replacement on energy intake, energy expenditure, immunity, and neuroendocrine functions in leptin-deficient patients.

Gautron, L., & Elmquist, J. K. (2011). Sixteen years and counting: An update on leptin in energy balance. *Journal of Clinical Investigation, 121,* 2087–2093.—This review provides an update on current understanding of leptin-sensitive neural pathways in terms of both anatomical organization and physiological roles.

Grill, H. J. (2010). Leptin and the systems neuroscience of meal size control. *Frontiers in Neuroendocrinology, 31,* 61–78.—This review summarizes the neural control of meal size, focusing on the role of the neurons of the NTS in the integration of two principal sources of that control: satiation signals arising from the gastrointestinal tract and adipose signal leptin.

Kennedy, G. C. (1953). The role of depot fat in the hypothalamic control of food intake in the rats. *Proceedings of the Royal Society of London [Biology], 140,* 578–592.—This work, together with work by Hervey, Coleman, and others, led to the formulation of lipostatic theory and the speculation that the *ob* and *db* mutations affect the ligand and its receptor, respectively, of a signal pathway that regulates satiety and energy balance.

Oral, E. A., Simha, V., Ruiz, E., Andewelt, A., Premkumar, A., Snell, P., et al. (2002). Leptin-replacement therapy for lipodystrophy. *New England Journal of Medicine, 346,* 570–578.—The authors describe the first leptin replacement study in patients with lipodystrophy, demonstrating the powerful therapeutic benefits of leptin replacement in this group of patients.

Park, H. K., & Ahima, R. S. (2015). Physiology of leptin: Energy homeostasis, neuroendocrine function and metabolism. *Metabolism, 64,* 24–34.—This review summarizes current understanding of the physiology of leptin in regulating energy homeostasis, neuroendocrine function, metabolism, immune function, and other systems through its effects on the central nervous system and peripheral tissues.

Rosenbaum, M., & Leibel, R. L. (2014). 20 years of leptin: Role of leptin in energy homeostasis in humans. *Journal of Endocrinology, 223,* T83–T96.—This review summarizes the major role of leptin in the physiology of the weight-reduced state and argues that the major physiological function of leptin is to signal states of negative energy balance and decreased energy stores; an inference is that leptin, and pharmacotherapies affecting leptin signaling pathways, are likely to be most useful in sustaining rather than inducing weight loss.

Rosenbaum, M., Nicolson, M., Hirsch, J., Heymsfield, S. B., Gallagher, D., Chu, F., et al. (1996). Effects of gender, body composition, and menopause on plasma concentrations of leptin. *Journal of Clinical Endocrinology and Metabolism, 81,* 3424–3427.—This work, together with similar work by others, elucidated the effects of adiposity, gender, and acute nutritional status on plasma leptin concentration.

Zhang, Y., Proenca, R., Maffei, M., Barone, M., Leopold, L., & Friedman, J. M. (1994). Positional cloning of the mouse *obese* gene and its human homologue. *Nature, 372,* 425–432.—This work described the positional cloning of the leptin (*ob*) gene and discussed the possible role of leptin as a fat-based humoral signal in the feedback regulation of energy balance.

4

Genetics of Obesity and Related Traits

RUTH J. F. LOOS
RUDOLPH L. LEIBEL

Over the past four decades, the prevalence of obesity has almost doubled world-wide. While the sharpest increases are seen in high-income countries, the prevalence is also rising at alarming rates in middle- and low-income countries, particularly in populous nations, such as India and China. While a major driver of the obesity epidemic is undoubtedly a westernized lifestyle—characterized by an abundance of energy-dense foods coupled with a reduced need for daily physical activity—not everyone exposed to the present-day obesogenic environment becomes overweight or obese. In fact, a substantial number of individuals seems protected from weight gain altogether, an indication that the extent to which people respond to the obesogenic environment is determined, at least in part, by innate genetic factors. Indeed, obesity is a common condition that is the result of an intricate interplay between genes and environment. In only a very few, extreme cases is obesity due solely to genetic defects. Here, we review current insights into the genetics of common forms of obesity.

Familial Risk and Heritability of Obesity

The notion that the susceptibility to gaining weight and becoming obese is partially determined by genetic factors has been supported by family and twin studies since the 1920s.

Individuals *with* a family history of obesity have a 1.5–8 times higher risk of becoming obese themselves compared to individuals *without* a family history. The risk increases with genetic proximity of family members and with increasing severity of their obesity; for example, an individual whose identical twin is severely obese is more than five times more likely to be severely obese compared to someone whose identical twin is of normal weight. Individuals whose parents were obese as children have a five to 15 times higher risk of becoming obese adults themselves, compared to those whose parents were of normal weight. While these studies provide support for a familial component in obesity risk, they do not allow for a breakdown of the contribution of genetic relatedness versus shared environment.

Heritability studies aim to quantify the contribution of genes and environment to variation in obesity susceptibility, and heritability estimates are dependent on the environment (e.g., time period, geographical region) in which they are assessed. Large-scale twin and family studies have estimated that 40–70% of the interindividual variation in obesity susceptibility is due to genetic differences between individuals, whereas the remainder of the variation is explained by differences in environment and lifestyle. Heritability estimates tend to increase throughout childhood and adolescence until the onset of adulthood, after which they decrease with age.

Insights from Animal Models

Heritability estimates the contribution of genes to specific phenotypes but does not implicate specific genes or their modes of inheritance. An important strategy adopted early on in the search for genes and pathways controlling body weight has been the molecular cloning of mutations causing monogenic obesity in mice. The genes for leptin (mouse *ob*) and its receptor (mouse *db*; rat *fa*), as well as the melanocortin 4 receptor (mouse yellow mutation interferes with action at MC4R), carboxypeptidase E/proconvertase 1 (mouse *fat*), *Bdnf*, *Sim1*, and a ciliary protein (mouse *tub*) are prominent examples. The importance of these efforts has been the demonstration of an incontestable contribution of single genes and their constituent pathways to the regulation of body weight, and insights into the molecular physiology of their effects, virtually all of which, importantly, are conveyed through the central nervous system (CNS). In all instances, human orthologs of these genes have been identified in which inactivating mutations lead to obesity. These individuals confirm the inferences reached from the gene cloning/manipulation studies in mice.

Insights from Monogenic Forms of Obesity

Though they represent only a small fraction of clinical instances, research into monogenic forms of human obesity has shed light on the biology that underlies common obesity. The first patients with single-gene defects leading to extreme and early-onset obesity were identified in the mid-1990s. Consistent with the observations in animal models, most mutations are in genes expressed in the brain, participating in both so-called *homeostatic* and *hedonic/cognitive* aspects of ingestive behaviors. To date, the most prevalent causes of monogenic severe obesity have been mutations in the melanocortin 4 receptor (*MC4R*), accounting for 3–5% of extreme early-onset obesity in many populations.

Identifying Genes for Common Obesity

Despite strong evidence for a genetic contribution to obesity susceptibility and convincing insight from cases of extreme obesity in humans and animal models, identifying genes and genetic variants that cause *common* obesity has—until now—been a slow, arduous task.

However, advances in high-throughput genotyping technology and availability of detailed information on the sequence and organization of the human genome have greatly accelerated gene discovery over the past decade. Two major approaches have been employed to identify genes that affect obesity susceptibility: the candidate-gene approach and the genomewide approach.

Candidate-Gene Studies

The candidate gene approach, applied since the early 1990s, is hypothesis-driven and assumes a priori insights into the biology that underlies obesity susceptibility. Genes that are thought to be involved in energy balance and weight gain, based on animal models, cellular systems, or extreme/monogenic instances in humans, are considered "candidate genes."

Over the years, hundreds of genes have been proposed as *candidates,* but only a half-dozen have been firmly established as *true* obesity genes. The reasons for the limited success of this approach have to do with the small sample size of candidate-gene studies, limited a priori insights regarding the biology of the gene, and the scarcity of information on genetic variation in the 1990s, when this approach was predominantly applied.

To date, few large-scale studies ($N > 5,000$) have identified robust associations of genetic variants in candidate genes with obesity traits. They include nonsynonymous (i.e., that change amino acid sequence) variants in *MC4R* (V103I, I251L), beta-3-adrenergic receptor (*ADRB3*; W64R), proprotein convertase subtilisin/kexin type 1 (*PCSK1*; N221D, Q665E-S690T), brain-derived neurotrophic factor (*BDNF*; V66M), melanotonin receptor type 1B (*MTNR1B*; G24E), and a functional variant near lactase (*LCT*; C/T_{-13910} (rs4988235)). The fact that hundreds of other proposed candidate genes have not been confirmed does not mean that they do not affect obesity risk. Larger studies that interrogate all functional variants in and near these candidate genes are needed to convincingly confirm or refute their role in body weight regulation.

Genomewide Studies

Genomewide approaches are hypothesis-generating. By screening the whole genome, they aim to identify new, unanticipated genetic variants associated with obesity traits. Experimental follow-up on the newly identified genetic variants is needed to reveal the novel pathways that, in turn, increase our understanding of body weight regulation.

Genomewide Linkage Approach

The genomewide linkage approach, used since the mid-1990s, requires populations of related individuals and tests whether chromosomal regions across the genome co-segregate with obesity from one generation to the next. To date, more than 80 genomewide linkage studies have reported at least 300 loci that show suggestive linkage with obesity-related traits. These loci are typically large chromosomal regions that harbor hundreds of genes. So far, none of these loci has been narrowed down enough to pinpoint the causal gene(s). A well-powered meta-analysis of 37 genomewide linkage studies, including data for more than 31,000 individuals from 10,000 families, did not identify any obesity or body mass index (BMI) loci. The genomewide linkage approach has not been successful in identifying genes that affect obesity susceptibility, due to the small sample sizes that are typical of family studies and the relatively low statistical power this approach has for common multifactorial diseases such as obesity.

Genomewide Association Studies

Genomewide association studies (GWAS) have been available since 2005 and have increased the pace of gene discovery immensely. These studies screen the genome at a much higher resolution than genomewide linkage studies, testing associations of millions of single-nucleotide polymorphisms (SNPs) with obesity traits. GWAS can be performed with both related and unrelated individuals, allowing for larger sample sizes than linkage studies. They generally employ a two-stage design, requiring that loci reach highly statistically significant associations in the first stage, before they are confirmed in second stage analyses of a separate collection of subjects. Loci for which the association reaches the genomewide significance threshold ($P < 5 \times 10^{-8}$) are considered *established*. The stringent significance threshold accounts for the millions of SNP-association tests that are performed across the whole genome.

In 2007, two GWAS independently identified variants in *FTO* (fat mass and obesity-associated gene) to be strongly associated with BMI. Since the identification of the *FTO* locus, many more GWAS have been performed for a number of obesity traits, including BMI, extreme and early-onset obesity, waist circumference, BMI-adjusted waist-to-hip ratio (WHR_{adjBMI}), body fat percentage, visceral adipose tissue (VAT) and subcutaneous adipose tissue (SAT), weight loss after surgery, and circulating leptin levels. Most GWAS have been performed in populations of European ancestry, with many fewer in populations of exclusively African or East Asian ancestry. The majority of gene associations have been made in adults, but at least three GWAS have been performed in children and/or adolescents. Since height, weight, and waist and hip circumference are inexpensive and noninvasive measurements, the most studied obesity traits are BMI, as a proxy for overall adiposity, and WHR_{adjBMI} as a proxy for body fat distribution. As the cost of genomewide genotyping has plummeted and more GWAS have become available, GWAS meta-analyses have grown larger over the years. The most recent GWAS meta-analyses by the Genetic Investigation of Anthropometric Traits (GIANT) consortium comprised ~340,000 individuals for BMI and ~225,000 individuals for WHR_{adjBMI}, predominantly of European ancestry.

Other Genomewide Approaches

Driven by advances in high-throughput sequencing technology, genomewide studies are no longer confined to common genetic variants. Whole-genome (WGS) and whole-exome sequencing (WES) studies allow investigation of the role of every single base-pair of the genome and exome, respectively. While GWAS identify common variants with small effects, it has been speculated that WGS and WES studies will identify rare variants that are more likely to have larger effects and to affect the function of genes and their proteins. Yet results from the first sequencing studies suggest that effects of rare variants may not be as large as expected, and that large samples sizes will still be needed to identify robust associations.

Besides interrogation of genetic variation, genomewide studies have also started to examine the role of other -omics exposures on obesity risk, such as gene and protein expression, metabolite levels, epigenetic markers, among others. The integration of these multilayered data will be needed to elucidate the molecular processes underlying body weight regulation.

Insights from GWAS-Associated Loci

To date, large-scale GWAS have identified more than 180 loci associated with obesity traits across different ancestries and ages (Figure 4.1). The majority of loci were first identified for BMI or WHR$_{adjBMI}$, for which large-scale, well-powered GWAS are available. Fewer loci have been identified for more refined obesity traits, which tend to be available in smaller numbers of individuals and in select populations. Loci identified in European ancestry populations typically show association with obesity traits in populations of African and Asian ancestry, and vice versa. Furthermore, loci identified in adulthood often show association with BMI and obesity in childhood and adolescence, whereas no obesity loci have shown association with birth weight so far. Longitudinal and birth cohort studies have shown that, in aggregate, the effect of genetic variants on obesity risk increases during childhood and adolescence, peaks in early adulthood, and decreases with age from there.

Despite their large number, robustly associated loci explain less than 3% of the inter-individual variation in obesity traits and, even when combined, cannot predict whether someone will become obese. Furthermore, the causal gene(s) or genetic variant(s) within most loci have yet to be pinpointed. Most obesity-associated variants have no immediate implications to the function of nearby genes, but they tag the—still unknown—causal variant(s) that change the sequence of the causal gene and alter its expression and/or

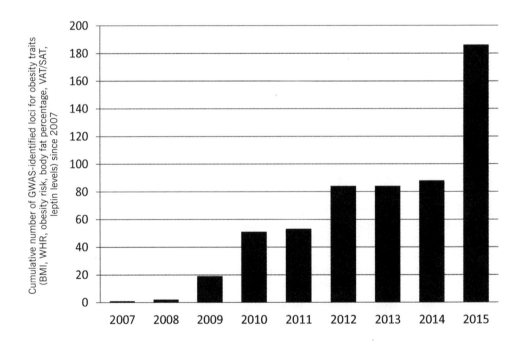

FIGURE 4.1. Cumulative number of GWAS-identified loci for obesity traits (BMI, WHR, obesity risk, body fat percentage, VAT/SAT, leptin levels) since 2007.

protein levels. Identifying the causal variant(s)/gene(s) is a critical step in the translation of a GWAS-locus to gain insight into the underlying biology.

Insights from BMI-Associated Loci

At least 100 BMI-associated loci have been identified, of which variants in the *FTO* locus have the largest effect; that is, each *FTO* risk-allele increases body weight by ~1 kg for a 1.70-m-tall person. Even though the *FTO* locus was identified in 2007, it remains unclear how these intronic variants affect body weight regulation. Some assume that *FTO* is the causal gene, whereas others believe *FTO*'s intronic variants influence genes downstream (*RPGRIP1L*) and/or upstream (*IRX3*) that, in turn, affect energy intake and/or expenditure.

Tissue and gene set enrichment analyses have shown that genes harbored in the ~100 BMI-associated loci are more often expressed in brain tissues (Figure 4.2, Panel A) and implicated in central regulatory pathways, as compared to genes elsewhere in the genome. This discovery provides strong support for the predominant role of the CNS in body weight regulation, in particular through control of appetite, reward, and satiety.

Insights from WHR$_{adjBMI}$-Associated Loci

Of the 50 loci that have been associated with WHR$_{adjBMI}$, 20 show more pronounced effects in women than in men. The reasons for the marked sexual dimorphism remain unclear, but may be attributed, in part, to the influence of sex hormones on body fat distribution. Because WHR is adjusted for BMI, none of the WHR loci overlap with those identified for BMI. Also, the expression profiles and pathways of the genes within the ~50 WHR$_{adjBMI}$ loci are from those observed for the BMI-associated loci. They are predominantly expressed in white adipose tissue, and the pathways in which they are implicated include adipogenesis, angiogenesis, transcriptional regulation, and insulin resistance (Figure 4.2, Panel B).

Insights from More Refined Obesity Traits

So far, fewer loci have been identified for refined traits such as body fat percentage, VAT/SAT, and circulating leptin levels. Since their measurement is substantially more invasive and expensive than BMI and WHR, they are available in fewer studies, which limits the statistical power for discovery. Nevertheless, GWAS meta-analyses for these refined traits have revealed several new loci that had not been identified before in much larger GWAS of BMI or WHR$_{adjBMI}$, providing unique new insights. For example, in a GWAS for body fat percentage, a variant near *IRS1* was identified, in which the body-fat-*increasing* allele is associated with a *protective* effect on type 2 diabetes and cardiovascular disease. Detailed follow-up analyses showed that the body-fat-increasing allele influenced only the subcutaneous fat depots and not the metabolically harmful visceral fat tissue.

Gene–Environment Interaction

Genes and lifestyle factors do not simply act additively or independently; rather, they interact synergistically and in time- and gender-dependent ways. The most convincing

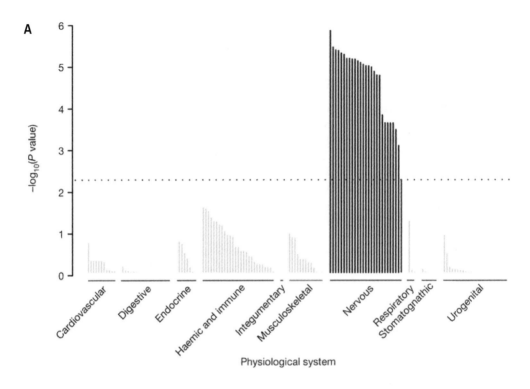

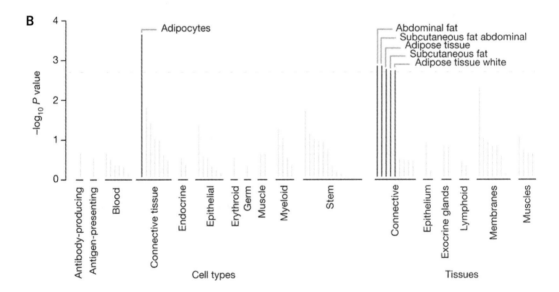

FIGURE 4.2. Tissue-specific expression of genes located in BMI-associated loci (Panel A) and WHR-adjBMI-associated loci (Panel B). The Y-axis shows significance of enrichment. Significantly enriched tissues are in black; the dotted line represents statistically significant enrichment.

evidence for this type of interaction has been provided for the *FTO* locus. Several studies, including a large-scale meta-analysis of more than 218,000 individuals, found that the BMI-increasing effect of *FTO* variants is ~30% lower among physically active individuals than among inactive individuals. A similar interaction has been reported with dietary factors; that is, *FTO*'s effect on obesity is reduced in individuals with a healthy diet.

Furthermore, the genetic susceptibility to obesity, broadly assessed as the aggregate of numerous established BMI-associated loci, is also sensitive to environmental influences. Large-scale studies have shown that a physically active lifestyle attenuates the genetic susceptibility to obesity by 30–40%, compared to an inactive lifestyle. Thus, even the most genetically predisposed individuals benefit from adopting a healthy lifestyle.

Conclusions and Future Directions

Advances in high-throughput genotyping technology and insights into the architecture of the human genome have accelerated gene discovery over the past 10 years. As current sequencing efforts increase the resolution with which the genome is being interrogated, gene discovery advances focus on the identification of rare (coding) variants, with the expectation that they have functional implications on a gene (and its protein) and larger effects on obesity risk.

Despite the large number of loci identified thus far, they explain only a fraction of the heritability factor, and for most loci, the causal genes and/or variants remain elusive. Future research needs to focus on prioritizing and annotating the putative candidate genes/variants within each locus, which are needed for an in-depth functional characterization of the pathways involved in body weight regulation.

Suggested Reading

Berthoud, H. R., & Morrison, C. (2008). The brain, appetite, and obesity. *Annual Review of Psychology, 59,* 55–92.—Review of the role of the CNS in the control of body weight regulation through its influence on appetite and reward.

Elks, C. E., den Hoed, M., Zhao, J. H., Sharp, S. J., Wareham, N. J., Loos, R. J., et al. (2012). Variability in the heritability of body mass index: A systematic review and meta-regression. *Frontiers in Endocrinology, 3,* 29.—Large-scale meta-analyses estimate the heritability of BMI to be ~75%, when using twin studies and 46%, when using family studies.

Kilpeläinen, T. O., Qi, L., Brage, S., Sharp, S. J., Sonestedt, E., Demerath, E., et al. (2011). Physical activity attenuates the influence of FTO variants on obesity risk: A meta-analysis of 218,166 adults and 19,268 children. *PLoS Medicine, 8*(11), e1001116. Large-scale meta-analyses that shows that physical activity attenuates the BMI-increasing effect of *FTO* by 40%.

Kilpeläinen, T. O., Zillikens, M. C., Stančákova, A., Finucane, F. M., Ried, J. S., & Langenberg, C., et al. (2011). Genetic variation near IRS1 associates with reduced adiposity and an impaired metabolic profile. *Nature Genetics, 43*(8), 753–760.—First large-scale GWAS meta-analysis for body fat percentage identifies a variant near *IRS1* of which the body fat increasing allele is protective for type 2 diabetes and cardiovascular disease.

Locke, A., Kahali, B., Berndt, S. I., Justice, A. E., Pers, T. H., Day, F. R., et al. (2015). Large-scale genetic studies of body mass index provide insight into the biological basis of obesity. *Nature, 518,* 197–206.—Latest genomewide association study for BMI in ~340,000 individuals from 125 studies, reporting 97 associated loci, of which more than half are novel, that point toward a role of the central nervous system in body weight regulation.

Loos, R. J. (2012). Genetics determinants of adiposity. In M. E. Symonds (Ed.), *Adipose tissue biology* (pp. 317–378). New York: Springer.—Comprehensive review of the genetic contribution to obesity susceptibility.

Lu, Y., & Loos, R. J. (2013). Obesity genomics: Assessing the transferability of susceptibility loci across diverse populations. *Genome Medicine, 5*(6), 55.—Review of the GWAS-identified loci for obesity traits supporting the notion that they affect obesity risk across populations of different ancestry.

Myers, M. G., & Leibel, R. L. (2015). Lessons from rodent models of obesity. (2015). In L. J. De Groot, P. Beck-Peccoz, G. Chrousos, K. Dungan, A. Grossman, J. M. Hershman, et al. (Eds.), *Endotext*. South Dartmouth, MA: MDText.com, Inc. Retrieved from *http://www.endotext. org/?s=lessons+of+rodent+models+of+obesity*.—Review of the insights gained regarding the genetics of obesity through the study of rodent models.

Shungin, D., Winkler, T. W., Croteau-Chonka, D. C., Ferreira, T., Locke, A. E., Mägi, R., et al. (2015). New genetic loci link adipose and insulin biology to body fat distribution. *Nature, 518,* 187–196.—Latest genomewide association study for WHR_{adjBMI} in ~225,000 individuals from 125 studies, reporting 49 associated loci, of which 44 are novel, that point toward pathways involved in adipogenesis and insulin resistance.

Tung, Y. C., Yeo, G. S., O'Rahilly, S., & Coll, A. P. (2014) Obesity and FTO: Changing focus at a complex locus. *Cell Metabolism, 20*(5), 710–718.—Review of a broad spectrum of research that has been performed for the *FTO* locus, illustrating the complexity of functionally characterizing GWAS loci.

5

The Epigenetics of Obesity

ALEXIS C. FRAZIER-WOOD
DAVID B. ALLISON

The term *epigenetic factors* refers to changes in structure of DNA that do not change the sequence of the DNA but may have phenotypic consequences. Epigenetic changes are lead candidate mechanisms for explaining why genetically identical mice, raised concurrently within the same litter, can show extreme differences in coat color and body size. Similarly, cloned mice show increases in body size that are not attributed to the DNA sequence and are not passed to offspring. However, some epigenetic effects are transgenerationally inherited, and this may be one explanation why highly heritable conditions such as obesity have shown increases in prevalence beyond that which can be presumably explained by the rate of de novo DNA mutations.

Epigenetic processes are a vital part of normal human development. For example, *imprinting,* the silencing of genes dependent on the parent from which they were inherited, prevents asexual reproduction by silencing maternal genes necessary for life, such that viable offspring only arise when these genes are inherited paternally. Males and females are distinguished by their sex chromosomes; males carry an X and a Y chromosome, while females carry two X chromosomes. X-inactivation (lyonization) is the inactivation of one of the two X chromosomes in females, such that the constituent genes no longer have biological effects (*silencing*). *Methylation,* the most common epigenetic change studied in the context of human obesity, refers to the addition of a carbon atom bonded to three hydrogen atoms (a methyl group) to a location in DNA—most commonly to a cytosine–guanine nucleotide pair bonded by a phosphate bond (a CpG site). Methylation, in concert with other mechanisms, underlies imprinting and, in concert with histone acetylation, is responsible for X-inactivation. Methylation also has important direct effects on human development; in the immediate postconception period, DNA methylation allows the temporary activation of differentiation-specific genes in pluripotent cells, forming cells with different functionality despite having the same DNA sequence.

The role of "aberrant" epigenetic factors in disease was first elucidated in the field of cancer. While the importance of epigenetic processes to other diseases states is slowly being appreciated, challenges in studying epigenetic processes in human chronic diseases, as opposed to in tumors, have led to a slower development of epigenetics in obesity.

Epigenetic Effects on Adipose Tissue Function

There is a known involvement of epigenetic changes in adipose tissue differentiation and function. Adipose tissue depots have a specific gene expression profile compared to other cell types, and noncoding RNAs are critical in the regulation of adipogenesis. Methylation in early embryogenesis is partly responsible for the differentiation of pluripotent stem cells into three different types of adipocytes that are thought to have differing effects on overall adiposity levels: brown, beige and white. However, whether individual differences in epigenetic marks across the lifespan are responsible for, or even correlated with, individual differences in the relative proportion of these adipocyte cells and/or the interindividual differences in the functioning of these cell types (e.g., differences in the thermogenic potential of brown vs. white adipose tissue) is unknown. Epidemiological studies have offered alternative insights into the association of epigenetic changes with obesity risk, but these need to be understood within the confines of methodological difficulties inherent in studying epigenetic processes in humans in observational research.

Syndromic Obesity and Epigenetic Changes

A distinction is often made between three types of obesity: monogenic, syndromic, and polygenic. Polygenic obesity, sometimes called common obesity, has a complex etiology involving many genes of small effect that act in addition to, and interact with, environmental contributors to obesity. Common obesity is considered to account for most of the current obesity prevalence, is the subject of most epidemiological epigenetic research, and is the focus of this chapter. However, syndromic obesity, obesity that arises as part of a more complex disorder that often includes severe intellectual disability, dysmorphic features, and/or morphological changes in organ development, provides one of the best-described human models of epigenetic changes in obesity.

Prader–Willi syndrome, a condition characterized by severe intellectual disability, accompanied by obesity arising from hyperphagia, arises from a deletion at 15q11.2–q12; however, the Prader–Willi phenotype is seen only when the deletion is inherited from the paternal allele. When the maternal allele contains the same deletion (or a mutation in the same region), the Angelman syndrome phenotype is seen. Despite originating from the same genetic mutation, hyperphagia does not arise in Angelman syndrome, nor is Angelman syndrome associated with obesity.

Such "parent-of-origin" effects are known as imprinting. The expression of imprinted genes differs based on the mode of inheritance: Co-segregation of certain alleles with maternal or paternal origin alters the DNA methylation in the promoter regions of the gene, altering gene transcription. While it was hoped that syndromic obesity would provide a model for understanding common obesity, few such parent-of-origin effects have been reported and validated in humans with common obesity.

Methodological Difficulties with Human Epigenetic Studies of Common Obesity

Studying the effects of epigenetic variation on health outcomes in humans has many challenges. First, most epigenetic marks are tissue-specific. Once gastrulation has occurred *in utero*, epigenetic effects will be conserved at least across the three germ layers. Later on in development (pre- or postnatally) epigenetic marks will be conserved via mitosis, and so are usually organ-specific. To conserve methylation across cell replications, DNA methyltransferase 1 (DNMT1) binds to the parent, methylated strand of DNA and methylates the new strand. Other DNMTs do not bind to methylated DNA but rather are involved in de novo methylation, a process that DNMT1 less commonly completes. While some tissues that are highly relevant to understanding the pathogenesis of obesity are more or less readily available in human studies (e.g., adipose tissue), others are prohibitive to collect, such as pancreatic, liver, and brain tissue.

A second concern is the poorly understood dynamic nature of many epigenetic marks. Methylation changes in response to several known environmental factors, such as stress, nutrition, and exercise, and it is not yet understood how quickly these changes occur and how long they persist, in both a tissue-specific and a global sense.

Third, epigenetic changes can be both a cause and a consequence of health conditions such as obesity. Untangling these may require expensive longitudinal studies or intervention studies that need to be conducted in animals but make inferences to human populations difficult. Finally, while the ability to survey the whole genome for epigenetic differences (epigenomewide association studies; EWAS) associated with a trait allows the development of new hypotheses and the detection of methylation loci–trait associations, there remain statistical problems with this approach. A costly correction for multiple testing makes it difficult to detect small effect sizes without extremely large samples; it is not known whether epigenetic effects on adiposity are large enough to survive this.

Fetal Programming Studies of Obesity in Humans

Two times in human development are characterized by widespread demethylation and are therefore particularly sensitive to epigenetic changes: gametogenesis and early embryogenesis. The "fetal programming hypothesis" suggests that due to changes during these early stages of development, the risk of subsequent chronic disease is partially set *in utero*, the effects of which are manifest later in life. One of the earliest demonstrations of the fetal programming hypothesis was studies of the offspring of Dutch famine victims. Epidemiological follow-up studies of the Dutch famine survivors of 1944–1945 reported that exposure to maternal caloric restriction occurring as a result of the famine and subsequent rationing, during the third trimester of pregnancy, and reduced food supply in the first year of life was associated with decreased obesity rates of the offspring up to 30 years after birth.

However, neither caloric restriction in the third trimester nor caloric restriction in the postnatal period were, on their own, associated with obesity differences. In addition, the epigenetic changes were inferred (at that time, attributed to effects on the differentiation of hypothalamus cells *in utero,* which are involved in the regulation of food intake) and not directly observed. Finally, although the natural experiment provided a unique opportunity to study the effects of famine on unselected, free-living individuals, the lack of scientific control makes it hard to disentangle other factors, such as uterine growth rate or the effects of early life stress on subsequent obesity. Nonetheless, the idea that nutritionally mediated epigenetic changes occurring *in utero* are associated with a host of chronic diseases remains one of the most popular hypotheses when examining the association between intrauterine exposures and subsequent obesity risk in the offspring.

Other Nutritional Influences on Epigenetic Changes *In Utero*

While other aspects of maternal dietary intake have been associated with offspring epigenetic changes, these have mostly been observed in animal studies and are less well characterized than metastable epialleles, which makes it hard to know whether the changes are linked to offspring adiposity. Studies with mechanistic links to obesity are accumulating; for example, fatty acid supplementation in pregnant rat dams influences microRNA (miRNA) expression in offspring liver and adipose tissue, providing a potential mechanistic pathway to obesity. A maternal diet high in methyl donors is associated with hypermethylation of the leptin (*Ob*) promoter, which reduces leptin in the offspring, presumably via reduced expression of the leptin gene. However, while this should lead to obesity via metabolic or behavioral changes associated with leptin deficiency obesity, food intake was only increased in young pups, and only males show the obese phenotype into adulthood.

Metastable Epialleles

Metastable epialleles (MEs) are one form of epigenetic change that occur *in utero* at the very early postconception stage. MEs are methylation switches that occur early on in embryonic development before gastrulation; therefore, as the separation of the three germ layers has not yet occurred, they are conserved throughout all body tissues. There is no evidence that methylation status at MEs can be altered; thus, they appear static rather than dynamic. However, while a tempting target for examining the effects of epigenetic changes on obesity, MEs on their own have limited utility because they are thought to be rare compared to other epigenetic marks, and any role in human obesity, if it exists, is likely to be small compared alternative epigenetic changes, often termed *cell-type-specific differentially methylated loci*.

One of the first and subsequently the most well characterized example of an ME is the murine agouti viable yellow (A^{vy}) ME. In mice, the *Agouti* gene encodes a paracrine signaling molecule that encodes for two different types of melanin: either black eumelanin or yellow phaeomelanin. Expression of agouti in mice is dynamic throughout life, and temporary phaeomelanin production in hair follicles leads to a yellow band on each black hair shaft, which looks brown. Transposition of the intracisternal A particle upstream of the transcription start site of *Agouti* alters the expression of *Agouti* and is responsible for the yellow mouse fur seen in these mice. When this intracisternal A particle transposition occurs in early embryonic development, the altered gene expression is not cell-type specific (i.e., not seen only in hair follicle cells) and so has other outcomes. In mice, the agouti protein is not only part of melanin formation but it also binds to the melanocortin

4 receptor (*MC4R*), known to influence appetite. Mice with the intracisternal A particle transposition that express agouti protein, in addition to having yellow fur, are hyperphagic and have obesity, while their genetically identical counterparts, which do not express the protein, are brown (called *pseudoagouti*), do not display increased appetite, and consequently are without obesity. This demonstration of epigenetic effects, in which altered adiposity is a "side effect" of the protein expression related to coat color, was one of the first, and remains one of the most compelling, demonstrations that epigenetic processes may play a role in obesity.

Influences on the Development of MEs In Utero

The murine A^{vy} ME has been replicated and confirmed in numerous studies and serves as one of the most popular models to examine factors that influence the development of MEs *in utero*. Methylation requires a methyl donor, and several dietary factors, notably those that contain methionine (choline, methyltetrahydrofolate, soy isoflavones, and vitamins B_6 and B_{12}) supply methyl for methylation. Maternal supplementation of these factors, and of the neuroendocrine disrupter bisphenol A (BPA) preconception, leads to increased methylation of CpG sites across A^{vy} in offspring and changes offspring coat color in a stochastic fashion; the distribution of coat colors in the offspring is shifted away from predominantly agouti offspring toward greater numbers of pseudoagouti offspring. Following the expectations of ME definitions, the methylation of CpG sites across A^{vy} in offspring are found across the three germ layers, including brain, kidney, and liver tissue, reinforcing the notion that these changes appear early on in embryonic development and are maintained into adulthood. Thus, if they play a functional role in the development of human obesity, they may have effects across many organs that are pervasive across the lifespan. However, in maternal supplementation studies, offspring do not show the expected changes in offspring body weight; thus, the phenotypic effects of MEs in human obesity remain under study.

Nutritional Effects *In Utero* on the Development of MEs in Humans

The seasonal variation in rural Gambia, which coincides with agricultural load, demonstrated the association of perinatal nutritional status with MEs. The change in climate across the year divides the nutritional intake of women into two seasons: (1) the "rainy" season, in which women work hard, eat more, and have higher plasma concentrations of folate, vitamin B_2, methionine, and betaine, and lower plasma-active B_{12}, dimethyl glycine, homocysteine, and S-adenosylhomocysteine compared to (2) the "dry" season, in which work is scarce and the stored food is eaten. Children conceived during the rainy season have higher levels of methylation at CpG sites at six genes. The methylation was maintained with a high correlation across hair follicles and peripheral blood cells, suggesting that it was systemic, not tissue-specific. Validation studies in tissues after autopsy showed that methylation at these sites is maintained across all three germs layers, again suggesting that it develops early on in embryonic development and is different between pairs of identical twin pairs, suggesting the methylation is not genetically mediated and established probabilistically. Due to the association of methylation status at MEs with obesity in mice, and the association of maternal prenatal nutrition status with obesity risk in humans, MEs are a leading candidate for being the mechanism between maternal nutrition at the time of conception and obesity, via a known epigenetic mechanism, but follow-up studies on the adiposity status of offspring are needed to confirm this.

The decreasing cost of whole-genome methylation arrays has made screening the genome agnostically possible both for new studies and for existing epidemiological cohorts with stored samples. This approach is appealing, but, as we mentioned earlier, is not without statistical limitations, and the literature is fraught with a lack of replication across studies and study-specific associations that are hard to interpret as a whole.

Summary and Synthesis

Maternal nutrition at the time of conception and during pregnancy is considered a factor for individual differences in having obesity. The mechanisms underlying this association are likely partially epigenetic in nature, but pinning down the exact nature, location, and timing of these changes remains a challenge. This knowledge, when gained, will have to be integrated into studies that consider the effects of these epigenetic changes *in utero* in conjunction with epigenetic changes that occur across the lifespan in response to age or environmental factors such as stress, exercise, and food intake. Currently, there is optimism for identifying epigenetic changes that underlie not only the formation and differentiation of adipose tissue cells but are also responsible for individual differences in adiposity and obesity risk. This is far from a known conclusion, however, and this remains an exciting area of research.

Glossary of Terms

CpG site. A site in the genome where a cytosine nucleotide is joined to a guanine nucleotide by a phosphate bond; a common site for methylation.

DNA. Deoxyribonucleic acid.

Embryogenesis. The formation and development of the embryo.

Epigenetic change. The specific alteration responsible for an epigenetic process.

Epigenetic mark. A change in the DNA that does not alter DNA sequence, such as the addition of a methyl group, but affects gene expression.

Epigenetic process. A process that alters DNA structure and consequently gene expression independent of the DNA sequence.

Epigenomewide association study (EWAS). Interrogation of the genome for sites where methylation associates with a trait of interest, without prior hypothesis as to the location of such associations.

Fetal programming hypothesis. That the risk of chronic disease across the lifespan is partially in response to the uterine environment.

Gastrulation. When the blastocyst changes from a single-layered organism to a trilayered organism.

Imprinted genes. Expression changes that are dependent on the parent from whom a given allele is inherited.

Metastable epiallele. A locus in the genome where methylation potential is set *in utero* across all tissues in response to perinatal factors.

Methyl donor. A molecule containing a methyl group that can be transferred.

Methylation. The addition of a methyl group to a cytosine in the genome sequence.

Micro-RNA (MiRNA). An RNA molecule with effects on gene expression.

Silencing. The process by which genes are rendered inert, such that they have no biological effects.

Transgenerational effects. The effect of some exposure or stimulus in one generation on the phenotype in a subsequent generation.

X-inactivation. The silencing, or nonexpression, of genes on the X chromosome. Also known as **lyonization.**

Acknowledgments

Alexis C. Frazier-Wood is funded by the American Heart Association (Grant No. 14BGIA18740011) and the U.S. Department of Agriculture/Agricultural Research Service (USDA/ARS; Grant No. CRIS 309-5-001-058). This work is a publication of the USDA/ARS Children's Nutrition Research Center, Department of Pediatrics, Baylor College of Medicine, Houston, Texas, and is funded in part with federal funds from the USDA/ARS under Cooperative Agreement No. 58-6250-0-008. David B. Allison is supported by Award No. P30DK056336 from the National Institute of Diabetes and Digestive and Kidney Diseases. The content is solely the responsibility of the authors does not necessarily reflect the views or policies of the USDA, the National Institutes of Health, or any other organization.

Suggested Reading

D'Addario, C., Dell'Osso, B., Palazzo, M. C., Benatti, B., Lietti, L., Cattaneo, E., et al. (2012). Selective DNA methylation of BDNF promoter in bipolar disorder: Differences among patients with BDI and BDII. *Neuropsychopharmacology, 37*(7), 1647–1655.—This was one of the first studies where the results suggested that methylation associated with a behavioral phenotype, and so presumably originating from the brain could be detected in blood; this is seen by some as a demonstration of whole body coordination across epigenetic changes.

Davies, M. N., Volta, M., Pidsley, R., Lunnon, K., Dixit, A., Lovestone, S., et al. (2012). Functional annotation of the human brain methylome identifies tissue-specific epigenetic variation across brain and blood. *Genome Biology, 13*(6), R43.—Highlighting the role of methylation in different tissue function, this study shows that tissues from different brain regions can be distinguished, in part, by their patterns of DNA methylation.

Dick, K. J., Nelson, C. P., Tsaprouni, L., Sandling, J. K., Aïssi, D., Wahl, S., et al. (2014). DNA methylation and body-mass index: A genome-wide analysis. *Lancet, 383*, 1990–1998.—An example of a study which interrogates the genome for evidence that methylation at distinct loci associate with body mass index.

Dominguez-Salas, P., Moore, S. E., Baker, M. S., Bergen, A. W., Cox, S. E., Dyer, R. A., et al. (2014). Maternal nutrition at conception modulates DNA methylation of human metastable epialleles. *Nature Communications, 5*, 3746.—The first human study to explicitly link methyl donors at the time of conception with the development of MEs *in utero.*

Ravelli, G. P., Stein, Z. A., & Susser, M. W. (1976). Obesity in young men after famine exposure in utero and early infancy. *New England Journal of Medicine, 295*(7), 349–353.—Epidemiological follow-up of the Dutch famine victims, reporting that *in utero* exposure to severe malnutrition, in the first trimester only, resulted in increased adiposity in adulthood when food was abundant; exposure in the third trimester/early postnatal period had the opposite association.

Reik, W. (2007). Stability and flexibility of epigenetic gene regulation in mammalian development. *Nature, 447,* 425–432.—Review of the role of epigenetic processes, especially methylation, during gametogenesis and embryogenesis in early development.

Waddington, C. H. (1940). *Organisers and genes.* Cambridge, UK: Cambridge University Press.— A more in-depth look at the role of genes, and epigenetic processes across the lifespan; this remains one of the seminal articles laying out the "epigenetic landscape" and its potential to influence development.

Waterland, R. A., & Jirtle, R. L. (2003). Transposable elements: Targets for early nutritional effects on epigenetic gene regulation. *Molecular and Cellular Biology, 23*(15), 5293–5300.— This study shows that periconceptional supplementation of methyl donors in rat dams skews the ratio of methylated versus unmethylated CpG bonds at the A^{vy} ME locus in offspring; methylation at this locus is associated with increased adiposity in adult offspring, providing a promising target for examining associations between methylation and adiposity.

6

Prenatal Effects on Body Weight

EMILY OKEN

The idea that factors present before birth might influence later health has its foundations in the concept of programming, in which an exposure at a critical or sensitive period of development can set lifelong health trajectories. This chapter summarizes current knowledge on prenatal programming of growth and adiposity.

Intrauterine Growth and Later Size

A number of epidemiological studies, especially since the 1980s and 1990s, have examined associations of weight at birth with later body size and risk for cardiometabolic disease. Most of the earlier publications were from retrospective studies that took advantage of previously existing public health or clinical records from birth or early life, and related them to measurements in adolescence or adulthood. The advantage of this approach has been the opportunity to follow individuals well into adulthood. However, several limitations exist, including concern about generalizing results to modern populations from those born in the early to mid-20th century, when social and nutritional conditions were likely quite different. Also, limited information about pregnancy experiences and gestational age at birth was available, such that it is difficult to know whether the smaller babies were born prematurely, or experienced intrauterine growth restriction. Furthermore, not all babies survived to adulthood, which might bias results.

More recently, prospective studies have been established to follow children longitudinally from (or even before) birth. These studies, while more expensive and time consuming to conduct, can provide more detail about prenatal experiences, including maternal diet, smoking, and other behaviors, as well as gestational age at birth. Since most researchers have commenced recruitment more recently, the data represent populations growing up within the obesity epidemic. As several of these cohorts now are entering their second and even third decades, they can now begin to reveal outcomes in early adulthood that include not only biological intermediates but also disease outcomes.

Despite the different types of limitations of the retrospective and prospective studies, almost all have shown a direct linear relationship between size at birth and attained size in childhood, adolescence, and adulthood. That is, individuals who had been born small tend to be shorter and lighter, on average, and children born larger tend to be heavier. These findings are supported by animal studies, in which experimental manipulations such as early life over- or underfeeding lead to persistent changes in body size throughout life, even when the animals are exposed to a similar environment after weaning. The other important contribution from animal studies has been confirmation that there are likely to be critical periods for these exposures. For example, in one study, rodents that had been underfed in the period just after birth (which is developmentally similar to the third trimester of gestation in humans) remained much smaller throughout their lives, whereas those that experienced a similar period of underfeeding in later life regained their body weight once food was again freely available. The importance of timing of exposure is also highlighted in the findings of what has been called the "Dutch Famine study." Males in the Netherlands whose mothers had been exposed to severe caloric restriction during the first trimester of gestation had higher weights at age 18 compared with those who were born before the famine, whereas those exposed in later gestation did not.

Most of the epidemiological studies measured attained size via weight, height, and calculated body mass index (BMI), which incorporate both fat and lean mass. Increasingly, studies are directly assessing adiposity, often via measurement of skinfold thicknesses, bioelectrical impedance, or dual X-ray absorptiometry (DXA) scans, all of which provide similar estimates of body fat. These more detailed assessments have shown that large babies tend to be larger because of both greater fat mass and greater lean mass. Because of their greater adiposity, individuals who had been larger at birth tend to have higher risk for obesity-related disorders. Interestingly, although small babies tend to remain smaller and thinner, they are at higher risk for cardiometabolic diseases, including type 2 diabetes, high blood pressure, and cardiovascular disease, especially after adjustment for their attained BMI. There is also some evidence that those who had been smaller at birth have a higher proportion of fat versus lean mass and greater central adiposity at any given BMI.

Ongoing research has sought to investigate upstream factors, especially those that are potentially modifiable, that might underlie differences in size at birth and "program" later size and health outcomes. Certainly, genetic factors might explain tracking of weight throughout a lifetime, but genes are unlikely to explain the worldwide secular trends in birth weight and body weight that have occurred quite rapidly, even within a generation. The following sections briefly summarize the research into modifiable prenatal factors that might influence growth and adiposity.

Maternal Weight Entering Pregnancy and Weight Gain during Pregnancy

Higher maternal weight entering pregnancy and greater gestational weight gain are each linearly related to both higher weight at birth and higher offspring weight. For example, compared with normal weight mothers, mothers who are obese entering pregnancy are almost 2.5 times more likely to have a baby born at high birth weight, and three to five times more likely to have a child who is obese. The relationship between higher gestational weight gain and greater infant weight at birth is equally strong. These interrelationships likely derive from a number of factors, including shared genetics between mother and child, shared maternal and child eating and physical activity behaviors, and shared environment.

While prepregnancy weight and gestational weight gain are both theoretically modifiable, the fact that half of all pregnancies are unplanned, and that many women do not routinely seek care before pregnancy, has led most intervention efforts to focus on limiting gestational weight gain. Current guidelines recommend weight gain ranges specific to maternal BMI entering pregnancy: 25–35 pounds for women of normal BMI, greater gain for those who are underweight, and less gain for those who are overweight or obese. However, almost half of mothers gain more than recommended, and rates of excessive weight gain are especially high among overweight and obese mothers.

Lifestyle interventions that target nutrition and exercise can succeed at lowering rates of excessive gestational weight gain. Some interventions were also effective at decreasing risk for poor obstetric outcomes that include being large for gestational age, or *macrosomia*, especially in women who were high risk by virtue of being overweight or obese, or having gestational diabetes mellitus. None of these studies has followed children long enough to demonstrate any long-term effect on offspring obesity.

While similar trials are not yet available for prepregnancy lifestyle interventions, indirect evidence for a direct, causal relationship between a mother's weight and that of her child comes from several streams of evidence. Children born to mothers who were morbidly obese but had bariatric surgery prior to conception are less likely to be obese and have improved cardiometabolic risk markers compared with children born to similar mothers who had their bariatric surgery after pregnancy. Also, numerous animal studies have revealed that maternal overfeeding before pregnancy can result in offspring adiposity—even, in one creative experiment, if the embryo is removed after conception and implanted via *in vitro* fertilization into an unexposed, normal weight mother.

Maternal Diet Quality

It is less clear whether the quality—as opposed to the overall quantity—of a mother's diet is important for offspring growth and health. Some evidence points to specific macro- and micronutrients that might have relevance, but there has been little consistency about which particular dietary factors have been studied. Furthermore, nutrient intake does not often vary in isolation, but as part of a larger dietary pattern; thus, it can be difficult to tease out whether it is the overall pattern, or specific foods or nutrients, that are most important.

Gestational Diabetes Mellitus

While there is not strong evidence for a relationship between maternal glucose or carbohydrate intake during pregnancy and offspring size, it has long been recognized that higher maternal circulating glucose concentrations during pregnancy predict higher birth weight, as well as greater weight and adiposity in later childhood and adulthood. This relationship was first recognized in the 1950s as "Pedersen's hypothesis," which posits that glucose transfer between the mother and fetus across the placenta stimulates fetal secretion of insulin, leading to greater fetal growth and neonatal fat mass. Both animal and human studies have been consistent in showing this relationship. Newer human data suggest a key role for the placenta, which may up-regulate macronutrient transport to the fetus in response to high circulating levels of glucose or other nutrients in the maternal circulation. What is less clear is whether the relationship between diabetes during pregnancy and offspring attained size is solely attributable to the fact that mothers with diabetes tend to have higher weight and gestational weight gain before the time of glycemic screening, or whether there is an additional independent contribution from the changes associated with dysglycemia.

Maternal Smoking

Maternal smoking during pregnancy is associated with slower fetal growth. This relationship is so well established that in decades past, when operative deliveries were less safe and routine, anecdotal evidence suggests that obstetricians recommended that their patients smoke to prevent traumatic delivery of a large baby. It has therefore been somewhat surprising that several dozen published observational studies have now found that children who were exposed to maternal smoking *in utero* are more likely to be obese in later life. However, there is likely to be substantial confounding given that (at least in modern developed settings) women who smoke tend to be of lower socioeconomic status, which also predicts obesity. Unfortunately, there have been no randomized trials of smoking cessation in pregnancy that followed children after birth, the most rigorous approach to eliminating confounding. Many studies, now summarized in meta-analyses, have statistically adjusted for social factors, and have continued to show the association between maternal smoking and childhood obesity. These findings are also supported by rodent studies, in which offspring of dams injected prenatally with nicotine are larger, with higher body fat. Mechanisms remain unclear but likely include effects on hypothalamic appetite centers.

Emerging Research

Emerging areas of inquiry have identified additional potential culprits. Synthetic chemicals are being released into the environment at an astounding rate. Some identified chemicals inappropriately stimulate adipogenesis and fat storage, the so-called "environmental obesogens." Evidence already exists for a number of chemicals, including bisphenol A, tribytultin, per- and polyfluorinated compounds, and air pollution; many more likely exist that remain unstudied. These chemicals may even have intergenerational influences.

The microbiome is another potentially important factor. For example, some evidence suggests that delivery by cesarean section is associated with higher risk for later obesity, and babies who are born via cesarean section have, at least in the short term, marked differences in the intestinal microbiome compared with those delivered vaginally. Infant diet is likely another source of influence on the microbiome, as intestinal microbiota differ between babies that are breast milk or formula fed. Several investigators, including those at infant formula companies, are putting intensive effort into identifying beneficial *prebiotics,* nondigestible carbohydrates, and other nutrients that promote colonization of beneficial microbes.

Summary

In summary, abundant animal and human observational research links prenatal exposures with later size and growth. Some exposures, such as maternal prepregnancy BMI, are likely mediated by greater intrauterine growth that tracks into later life; others, such as maternal smoking, can have opposing effects on intrauterine and extrauterine growth. Future evidence from well-designed human randomized trials will be helpful in not only confirming causality but also identifying behavioral or other targets for intervention and thus prevention. Additional animal and basic human studies will also be essential for teasing out potential mechanisms by which these exposures can result in lasting changes.

Acknowledgments

Emily Oken received grant support from the National Institutes of Health (Grant Nos. K24 HD069408 and P30 DK092924).

Suggested Reading

Boeke, C. E., Oken, E., Kleinman, K. P., Rifas-Shiman, S. L., Taveras, E. M., & Gillman, M. W. (2013). Correlations among adiposity measures in school-aged children. *BMC Pediatrics*, *13*(1), 99.—In school-age children, BMI, sum of skinfolds, and other adiposity measures were strongly correlated with DXA fat mass, suggesting that BMI and skinfolds are adequate surrogate measures of relative adiposity in children when DXA is not practical.

Gaudet, L., Ferraro, Z. M., Wen, S. W., & Walker, M. (2014). Maternal obesity and occurrence of fetal macrosomia: A systematic review and meta-analysis. *BioMed Research International*, *2014*, 640291.—Results from the meta-analysis showed that maternal obesity is associated with fetal overgrowth, defined as birth weight ≥ 4,000 g (odds ratio = 2.17, 95% confidence interval = 1.92, 2.45), birth weight ≥ 4,500 g (odds ratio = 2.77, 95% confidence interval = 2.22, 3.45), and birth weight ≥ 90%ile for gestational age (odds ratio = 2.42, 95% confidence interval = 2.16, 2.72).

Gillman, M. W., & Ludwig, D. S. (2013). How early should obesity prevention start? *New England Journal of Medicine*, *369*(23), 2173–2175.—This perspective summarizes modifiable early life predictors of obesity, including prenatal and postnatal factors, and includes recommendations for early life obesity prevention.

Institute of Medicine. (2009). *Weight gain during pregnancy: Reexamining the guidelines*. Washington, DC: National Academies Press.—This report summarizes existing evidence on pregnancy and longer-term maternal and child health outcomes associated with gestational weight gain, and includes recommendations for adequate gain.

Janesick, A. S., Shioda, T., & Blumberg, B. (2014). Transgenerational inheritance of prenatal obesogen exposure. *Molecular and Cellular Endocrinology*, *398*(1–2), 31–35.—This review summarizes evidence that xenobiotic chemicals may not only promote excess adiposity in the exposed offspring, but also may have transgenerational health effects.

Muktabhant, B., Lawrie, T. A., Lumbiganon, P., & Laopaiboon, M. (2015). Diet or exercise, or both, for preventing excessive weight gain in pregnancy. *Cochrane Database of Systematic Reviews*, Issue 6 (Article No. CD007415).—This meta-analysis summarized 49 randomized trials involving 11,444 women that included interventions on diet, exercise, or both, to limit gestational weight gain.

Oken, E., Levitan, E. B., & Gillman, M. W. (2008). Maternal smoking during pregnancy and child overweight: Systematic review and meta-analysis. *International Journal of Obesity*,

32(2), 201–210.—Based on results of 84,563 children reported in 14 observational studies, children whose mothers smoked during pregnancy were at elevated risk for overweight (pooled adjusted odds ratio = 1.50, 95% confidence interval = 1.36, 1.65) at ages 3–33 years, compared with children whose mothers did not smoke during pregnancy.

Perng, W., Gillman, M. W., Mantzoros, C. S., & Oken, E. (2014). A prospective study of maternal prenatal weight and offspring cardiometabolic health in midchildhood. *Annals of Epidemiology, 24*(11), 793–800.—In this study of 1,090 mother–child pairs followed from pregnancy to child ages 6–10 years, children born to heavier mothers had more overall and central fat and greater cardiometabolic risk, and those born to women with higher gestational weight gain had greater adiposity and higher leptin levels.

Ravelli, G. P., Stein, Z. A., & Susser, M. W. (1976). Obesity in young men after famine exposure *in utero* and early infancy. *New England Journal of Medicine, 295*(7), 349–353.—In a historical cohort study of 300,000 19-year-old men exposed to the Dutch famine of 1944-1945 and examined at military induction, the authors found less obesity with exposure to famine in later pregnancy, but greater obesity in those with early gestational exposure.

Tarry-Adkins, J. L., & Ozanne, S. E. (2011). Mechanisms of early life programming: Current knowledge and future directions. *American Journal of Clinical Nutrition, 94*(Suppl. 6), 1765S–1771S.—In this review, the authors summarize current knowledge regarding mechanisms by which early life programming might occur.

Taste, Eating, and Body Weight

LINDA M. BARTOSHUK

Do foods taste the same to people who are obese? Do they like food better than do nonobese people? These questions have fascinated investigators for years. But a psychophysical error has compromised decades of research devoted to answering them. The psychophysical error, a solution, and the resulting changes in our views are described in this chapter.

Affect (Pleasure–Displeasure) of Taste, Olfaction, and Flavor

Taste affect is hardwired in the brain. Babies are born liking sweet and disliking bitter and sour; salt receptors require some weeks to mature, but when they do, babies like dilute salt but dislike strong salt (which stings the tongue). Evaluative conditioning studies show that olfactory affect can be transferred. Pairing neutral odors with positive affect (e.g., sweet, liked foods, liked faces) can render them positive; pairing with negative affect (e.g., nausea) can render them negative. It is unclear whether any olfactory affect is hardwired in humans, but some negative olfactory affect is believed to be hardwired in lower animals (e.g., cadaverine is negative in zebrafish).

Olfactory stimuli enter the nose by two routes. In *orthonasal olfaction*, sniffing brings volatiles from the environment through the nostrils and into the nasal cavity. In *retronasal olfaction*, chewing and swallowing force volatiles from the mouth up behind the palate and into the nasal cavity from the rear. Retronasal olfaction and taste project to common brain regions, where they are integrated into flavor.

Taste sensations fall into a small number of categories. The classics are sweet, salty, sour, and bitter. Over the years, other sensations have been proposed (e.g., metallic, fatty, umami, alkaline) but are not universally accepted. There are many qualitatively different olfactory sensations; these tend to be the names of the objects that emit the odorants (e.g., smoky, minty, chocolate, vanilla, roast beef). The identity of foods comes primarily from olfaction; food pleasure is a combination of hardwired taste pleasure and acquired olfactory pleasure.

Measurement Error: Invalid Psychophysical Comparisons

S. S. Stevens

In 1940, a committee of the British Association for the Advancement of Science (BAAS) published "The Problem of Measurement." Some of the physical scientists on the committee apparently could not conceive of any legitimate measures of sensation and S. S. Stevens's sone scale for loudness came in for special criticism. In 1946, Stevens responded with the now classic "On the Theory of Measurement," an article defining the properties of nominal, ordinal, interval, and ratio measurement. Magnitude estimation became his most popular ratio scale; subjects assigned numbers to reflect the perceived intensity of stimuli, such that one sensation twice as intense as another was assigned a number twice as large. Cross-modality matching instructed subjects to assign the same number to sensations of different quality that matched in intensity. The work resulting from these advances established modern sensory and hedonic psychophysics.

Practical Category and Visual Analogue Scales: Within-Subject Comparisons

The practical measurement of sensations has been going on for many years, in spite of the BAAS. The Greek astronomer Hipparchus (190–120 B.C.E.) devised a 6-point scale for the brightness of stars. The Quartermaster Corps of the U.S. Army devised the Natick 9-point scale for food (sensory and hedonic versions). Clinicians devised the 10-point scale for pain. These category scales (ordinal measurement) did not have ratio properties (e.g., 4 on a category scale is not twice as intense as 2), but over the years, category scales morphed into visual analogue scales that do have ratio properties.

Stevens's magnitude estimation, category scales, and visual analogue scales can all provide within-subject comparisons. For example, one might use a hedonic version of the Natick scale to determine whether one type of coffee is liked more than another.

How Can We Make Valid Across-Group Comparisons?

As time went on, investigators began to propose hypotheses that required comparisons across groups—for example, do women like coffee better than do men? These investigators simply used the available scales to make these across-group comparisons. However, such comparisons are not valid.

Some reflection reveals the problem. We each live in our own subjective world; in the absence of the ability to read minds, we cannot compare experiences directly with others. Yet we may seem to do this. For example, if I describe my headache as strong and you describe yours as moderate, this might seem to suggest that my pain is more intense than yours. However, intensity descriptors (e.g., moderate, strong) may denote different absolute intensities to different people.

The following experiment illustrates the challenge and offers a solution. Consider a visual analogue scale for sweet: a line labeled "no sensation" at one end and "sweetest you have ever tasted" at the other. Suppose we sort subjects by the number of taste buds: One group has the most and another group has the fewest. Now we ask all subjects to rate the sweetness of a soft drink on our sweet scale. Most subjects will rate the sweetness about the same, roughly two-thirds of the way above "no sensation." This suggests that perceived sweetness intensity does not relate to the number of taste buds.

However, do the experiment a different way. Each subject puts on headphones and adjusts a sound generator, so that the loudness of the sound matches the sweetness of the soft drink (cross-modality matching). Now our two groups will behave differently. Those with the most taste buds will set the sound around 90 db (about the loudness of a train whistle). Those with the fewest taste buds will set the sound intensity around 80 db (about the loudness of a telephone's dial tone). Based on Stevens's sone scale, we know that an increase of 10 db reflects a doubling of loudness. Thus, those with the most taste buds matched their sweetness to a sound twice as loud as did those with the fewest taste buds. If both groups perceive loudness the same, we have just shown that those with the most taste buds experience twice the sweetness as those with the fewest. This method is called *magnitude matching*. Experiments such as the soft drink study led to the discovery of supertasters: those who experience the most intense taste sensations.

Global Sensory Intensity Scales (GSIS)

Magnitude matching is now easier because of the development of labeled scales devised to meet its requirements. In our laboratory, for sensory comparisons, one end of a line is labeled "no sensation," and the other end, "strongest sensation of any kind ever experienced." We ask subjects to note the experience that is the strongest to them. This permits us to be certain that the sensation we wish to compare across groups is not the sensation the subject finds the "strongest" (i.e., this ensures that the top label, which serves as the standard, is independent of the sensations to be compared).

Global Hedonic Intensity Scales (GHIS)

For hedonic comparisons, one end of our scale is labeled "strongest dislike of any kind," and the other end, "strongest like of any kind"; the center is labeled "neutral." Similar to the sensory scale, we ask subjects to note the experiences that determine the outer boundaries. Valid comparisons require that the affective experience to be compared across groups be independent of that comprising the most intense affect (positive or negative). For example, we are able to compare liking–disliking of foods across groups because the strongest liking–disliking is rarely a food experience.

Sweet–Fat Preferences and the Body Mass Index

Studies dating back to the 1950s appeared to show no sensory difference associated with sweet or fat in individuals of varying BMI. Hedonically, obesity was thought to be associated with enhanced liking for fat but not for sweet. We revisited these conclusions in 2006. Magnitude matching confirms the early conclusions for fat: Fat evokes more pleasure in people who are obese. The story is different for sweet. Sweet sensations are reduced slightly in people who are obese; correcting for this and using magnitude matching shows that sweet is liked more by obese people than by nonobese people.

Pleasure from Food and the Body Mass Index

Several older reviews concluded that obese and nonobese people get similar pleasure from food. We revisited this conclusion in 2008 with magnitude matching. We found that when food liking is assessed with a food questionnaire, the liking ratings correlate with the body mass index (BMI): Obese persons like food more than do nonobese persons.

A variety of functional magnetic resonance imaging (fMRI) studies have examined the neural mechanisms underlying food pleasure. One interesting hypothesis (anhedonia) argues that reduced liking for food leads to overconsumption. This hypothesis rests on the empirical observation of reduced dopamine activity in the brain reward circuits of obese individuals, as well as the assumption that dopamine activity in these areas mediates liking. This assumption was apparently based on the faulty psychophysics of an earlier era.

In general, some fMRI studies use within-subject comparisons to relate brain activity to sensory or hedonic experiences (e.g., correlating variation in brain activity with increasing concentration of a taste solution). However, other fMRI studies require across-subject comparisons (e.g., associating variation in brain activity with magnitude of liking–disliking a stimulus in both obese and nonobese individuals). Such comparisons require psychophysical methods capable of rendering valid comparisons. How many associations between functional imaging and behavior have been compromised because of invalid psychophysical comparisons?

Taste Genetics and the BMI

The first genetic variation in taste was discovered in 1931; PTC (phenythiocarbamide) and its chemical relative PROP (6-*n*-propylthiouracil) are bitter to most individuals (tasters), but tasteless or nearly so to some (nontasters). We now know that the gene that expresses the receptors that bind PTC and PROP is only one of 25 bitter genes.

Supertasting is more complex in that it is likely to result from several genes. Supertasters perceive the most intense tastes, have the most taste buds, and perceive the most intense sensations from fats and irritants, chiefly because of anatomical associations between taste buds and receptors conveying touch and pain. Supertasters are more likely to be female and not European American.

The meaning of associations between PROP status and BMI is not always clear. Is PROP bitterness itself associated with BMI, or is the association actually with aspects of supertasting (e.g., oral anatomy)?

Taste Pathology and the BMI

One of the possible reasons that we see sensory differences between obese and nonobese people is that some taste pathologies result in sensory alterations that can enhance the palatability of energy dense foods.

Taste pathology is common, because some of the nerves mediating taste are especially susceptible to damage. The chorda tympani nerve (taste on the anterior tongue) exits the tongue with a branch of the trigeminal nerve (pain and touch on the anterior tongue), so dental anesthesia for pain control can damage the chorda tympani. Next, the chorda tympani passes through the middle ear, where it is vulnerable to middle ear infections (otitis media). Head injuries can damage the chorda tympani as it travels through bone to the brainstem. The glossopharyngeal nerve (taste and somatosensation on the posterior tongue) is adjacent to the tonsils. The nerve is normally protected by a muscle layer, but that muscle is missing in some individuals; in these cases, the glossopharyngeal nerve may be damaged during tonsillectomy.

Nerve signals from the chorda tympani and glossopharyngeal nerves mildly inhibit one another centrally. Damage to one nerve releases its inhibition on the central projection of the other nerve; increased neural response from that central projection area compensates for the damage, resulting in stable whole-mouth sensation (taste constancy). In certain individuals, this release of inhibition overcompensates: Some patients with mild taste damage show intensified whole-mouth taste sensation, which in turn elevates retronasal olfaction. Taste damage can also release inhibition on oral touch and pain, thereby intensifying sensations evoked by fats (creaminess, oiliness, viscosity, thickness) and irritants (spiciness, burn). These alterations in the sensory properties of foods may enhance palatability of energy-dense foods, leading to BMI gain. Also, the taste stimulation provided by eating can reduce pain, leading to yet another motive to overeat.

Conclusions

Earlier studies appeared to show that food tastes the same and is equally liked by obese and nonobese individuals. A new look at how we make psychophysical comparisons has shown that both of these conclusions are false. Psychophysical scales were devised for within-subject comparisons: Is caffeinated coffee liked better than decaf? As the importance of differences in perception began to emerge, investigators used those same scales to make across-group comparisons: Do obese people experience less pleasure from food than do nonobese people? These comparisons are invalid, because we cannot experience the sensations of others. Apparent comparisons (e.g., "That lemonade tastes strong to me; is it strong to you?") are illusory, because intensity descriptors (e.g., strong) can denote different intensities to different people. The solution we favor, magnitude matching, involves relationships between sensations of interest and a standard that is independent of the sensation of interest. We now know that food does not taste the same to obese and nonobese individuals. One compelling reason is that taste damage can alter the sensations evoked by food, such that energy-dense foods become more palatable, leading to weight gain.

Acknowledgments

Preparation of this chapter was supported, in part, by Grant Nos. DC283, DC8620, and DC13751 and the University of Florida Plant Innovation Center.

Suggested Reading

Bartoshuk, L. (2014). The measurement of pleasure and pain. *Perspectives on Psychological Science, 9*(1), 91–93.—Psychophysical advances now permit the quantification of pleasure and pain.

Bartoshuk, L. M., Duffy, V. B., Fast, K., Green, B. G., Prutkin, J. M., & Snyder, D. J. (2002). Labeled scales (e.g., category, Likert, VAS) and invalid across-group comparisons: What we have learned from genetic variation in taste. *Food Quality and Preference, 14,* 125–138.— Scales (category, VAS, Likert) developed for within-subject comparisons cannot make valid across-group comparisons.

Bartoshuk, L. M., Duffy, V. B., Hayes, J. E., Moskowitz, H. R., & Snyder, D. J. (2006). Psychophysics of sweet and fat perception in obesity: Problems, solutions and new perspectives.

Philosophical Transactions of the Royal Society B: Biological Sciences, 361, 1137–1148.—Reevaluation of the earlier idea that fat but not sweet is more palatable to the obese shows that fat and sweet are both more palatable to obese individuals.

Bartoshuk, L., & Snyder, D. J. (2016). The affect of taste and olfaction: The key to survival. In L. F. Barrett, M. A. Lewis, & J. M. Haviland-Jones (Eds.), *Handbook of emotions* (4th ed., pp. 235–252). New York: Guilford Press.—Evaluative conditioning insights reveal how affect is transferred to and from olfactory to other stimuli.

Berridge, K. C., Ho, C.-Y., Richard, J. M., & DeFeliceantonio, A. G. (2010). The tempted brain eats: Pleasure and desire circuits in obesity and eating disorders. *Brain Research, 1350,* 43–64.—The anhedonia hypothesis of obesity (that the obese eat more because they experience less pleasure from food) present logical difficulties.

Marks, L. E., Stevens, J. C., Bartoshuk, L. M., Gent, J. G., Rifkin, B., & Stone, V. K. (1988). Magnitude matching: The measurement of taste and smell. *Chemical Senses, 13,* 63–87.—The term *magnitude matching,* coined by Marks and Stevens, was applied to show that tasters (by threshold) experienced greater bitterness from PROP, as well as greater sweetness from sucrose.

Michell, J. (1999). *Measurement in psychology.* Cambridge, UK: Cambridge University Press.—An account of the British Association for the Advancement of Science's committee on "The Problem of Measurement."

Snyder, D. J., & Bartoshuk, L. M. (2008). The logic of sensory and hedonic comparisons: Are the obese different? In E. M. Blass (Ed.), *Obesity: Causes, mechanisms, prevention and treatment* (pp. 139–161). Sunderland, MA: Sinauer.—Empiracle evidence that the obese experience more pleasure from food.

Stevens, S. S. (1946). On the theory of scales of measurement. *Science, 103,* 677–680.—This classic article S. S. Stevens's paper introduces the classication of scales of measurement into nominal, ordinal, interval and ratio scales.

Tepper, B. J., Banni, S., Melis, M., Crnjar, R., & Barbarossa, I. T. (2014). Genetic sensitivity to the bitter taste of 6-n-propylthiouracil (PROP) and its association with physiological mechanisms controlling body mass index (BMI). *Nutrients, 6,* 3363–3381.—BMI and taste associations are complex and depend on a variety of variables.

Physiological Adaptations Following Weight Reduction

MICHAEL ROSENBAUM
RUDOLPH L. LEIBEL

Despite the development of numerous pharmacological, mechanical, and lifestyle interventions, the ~85% recidivism rate following otherwise successful nonsurgical weight loss has remained relatively constant for over three decades. For example, in the Look AHEAD Study, only 38% of subjects were able to lose at least 10% of their weight within the first year of the intervention, and only 16% were able to sustain a 10% or greater weight loss for 4 year(s), even with intense lifestyle intervention.

The physiological responses to alterations in body weight in the context of the relative long-term constancy of body weight in adults suggest that body weight (stored fat) is "regulated" (see Figure 8.1). This regulation reflects evolutionary forces promoting defense of body fat in service of reproductive integrity and survival in circumstances of restricted access to food. The tenacity and strength with which the body defends its fat content, compensating for fat loss by lowering energy expenditure and increasing hunger, accounts for a substantial portion of weight regain. These compensatory processes are suitable candidates for pharmacological and other interventions.

Evidence That Body Weight Is Regulated

Heritability quantifies the proportion of the variance in a given trait that is attributable to genes in individuals living in a specified environment. In children and adults, body fatness, weight change in response to overfeeding and underfeeding, and multiple other key factors in energy homeostasis (energy expenditure, food choice, growth patterns, etc.) are all strongly heritable (heritability estimates range from approximately 0.30 to 0.75). In adults, the remarkable constancy of body weight and composition over long periods of time (the average American gains 0.5–1.5 kg/year or about 4,000 kcal of stored energy), representing an approximately 0.4% positive "error" relative to a total caloric intake of approximately 900,000–1,000,000 kcal/year. The "coupling" of energy intake and output necessary to achieve this constancy is evident when one considers that simply

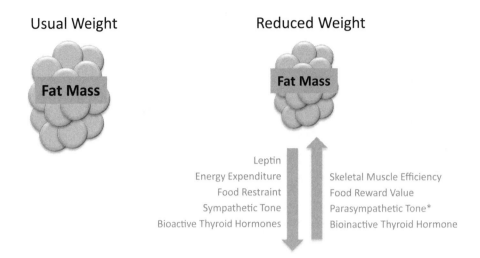

Usual Weight   **Reduced Weight**

Fat Mass   Fat Mass

Leptin
Energy Expenditure   Skeletal Muscle Efficiency
Food Restraint   Food Reward Value
Sympathetic Tone   Parasympathetic Tone*
Bioactive Thyroid Hormones   Bioinactive Thyroid Hormone

FIGURE 8.1. Physiological and behavioral adaptations to reduced weight maintenance. *Not at least partially reversed by leptin repletion in subjects maintaining a 10% or greater reduced body weight.

increasing or decreasing energy expenditure by 50 kcal/day (roughly equivalent to the energy expended in walking half a mile) without changing energy intake would result in a net energy imbalance of 25,000 kcal (about 4.5 kg of body weight) over 1 year.

Stored energy (fat) is a key component of survival and of reproductive integrity in circumstances of restricted access to food. Therefore, the pressures of natural selection and predation have likely favored genetic enrichment for alleles favoring energy ingestion, storage, and conservation. As a consequence of such evolutionary forces, genetic–physiological mechanisms for defense of body fat are more potent than those for resisting its accretion.

Physiological Response to Sustained Weight Loss

Conventional wisdom holds that "behavioral" issues related to persistence of "bad habits" that provoke weight gain in the first place account for much or all of the virtually inexorable weight regain following dietary weight loss. However, the control of energy stores is achieved through coordinated regulation of energy intake and expenditure mediated by signals emanating from adipose, gastrointestinal, and other endocrine tissues, and integrated by the liver and by regulatory (hypothalamus, brainstem), hedonic–emotional (amygdala, ventral striatum, orbitofrontal cortex], and executive–restraint (cingulate, middle frontal, supramarginal, precentral, and fusiform gyri) elements of the central nervous system (CNS). Changes in these signals are not voluntary and are largely due to the reduction in circulating leptin that accompanies a reduction in fat mass. These physiological responses to maintenance of a reduced body weight are relieved by administration of "replacement" doses of exogenous leptin, and constitute the physiological basis for the high recidivism to obesity of otherwise successfully treated patients. For individuals successfully sustaining weight loss, the "price" is a lifetime of conscious effort to decrease energy intake and increase expenditure beyond the respective levels required of individuals who are "naturally" at the same weight. Considerations of therapy should be tempered by the fact that these responses are highly heterogeneous and that a "one-size-fits-all" approach to behavioral, surgical, or pharmacotherapeutic interventions is not likely to be successful. Though this is a discussion of the physiology of responses to attempts to sustain weight loss, it should also be noted that there is a strong underlying genetic basis for many of these responses, as evidenced by studies of the responses of identical twin pairs to over- and underfeeding.

Energy Intake

Weight-reduced humans display increased region-specific functional magnetic resonance imaging (fMRI) signaling in response to visual food cues in brain areas related to reward (mainly the orbitofrontal cortex) and decreased signaling in the hypothalamus and brain areas related to restraint (mainly the prefrontal cortex). Interestingly, studies of subjects in the National Weight Control Registry indicate that successful maintenance of reduced body weight is associated with extremely high levels of dietary restraint. Similarly, in studies such as Look AHEAD Study and the Diabetes Prevention Trials (DPT), dietary restraint has been positively associated with the degree of weight loss, and negatively associated with the rate of weight regain during a supervised lifestyle intervention in adults with type 2 diabetes or prediabetes. Autonomic nervous system (ANS) tone may possibly modulate feeding behavior by effects on gut peptides such as cholecystokinin (CCK), glucagon-like peptide 1 (GLP-1), nesfatin-1, peptide YY (PYY), and pancreatic polypeptide.

Energy Expenditure

Components of Energy Expenditure

Maintenance of a 10% or greater reduction in body weight by lean or obese individuals is accompanied by a decline in energy expenditure that is approximately 300–400 kcal/day below that predicted by the new body weight and composition. In controlled inpatient studies, we have found that this hypometabolism persists in individuals successfully maintaining reduced weight for periods from 3 months to 6 years. Similarly, outpatient studies, such as the National Weight Control Registry, report that individuals who are successful at keeping weight off for periods of over 10 years still need to increase exercise and decrease caloric intake to compensate for a similar decrease in energy expenditure compared to those who are naturally the same weight. The degree of *adaptive thermogenesis* (changes in energy expenditure beyond those predicted by changes in body weight and composition) following weight loss is quite variable (approximately +5% to −35% below predicted following a 10% or greater dietary weight loss, with most adaptive thermogenesis occurring in response to early (10%) weight loss. Even in sedentary individuals who do not alter their level of physical activity, *nonresting energy expenditure* (NREE; the energy expended in physical activity), accounts for the majority (~150–250 kcal/day) of the disproportionate decline in energy expenditure; the remainder is accounted for by declines in resting energy expenditure (REE). Notably, additional weight loss (>10%) results in further declines (adjusted for metabolic mass) in NREE but not REE. The decline in NREE is due mainly to an approximate 20% increase in skeletal muscle che-momechanical contractile efficiency during low levels of muscle work. This increased efficiency is correlated with increased relative expression in muscle of the more efficient myosin heavy chain (MHC) and sarcoplasmic endoplasmic reticulum Ca^{2+}-dependent ATPase (SERCA) isoforms (MHC I and SERCA2). These responses are apparent conse-quences of the neuroendocrine and autonomic changes described below. The simultane-ous declines in both energy expenditure and satiety following weight loss conspire to create the optimal biological circumstances for weight regain. Of note, some, but not all, studies of subjects following bariatric surgery show a "blunting" of this disproportionate decline in energy expenditure resulting—in humans—from relative increases in REE or the thermic effect of feeding (TEF). In mice and rats, compensatory decreases in energy expenditure following weight loss caused by bariatric surgery are minimal, perhaps due to a lack of effect of surgical weight loss on sympathetic nervous system (SNS) tone and the importance of SNS tone in regulating brown adipose tissue (BAT) thermogenesis in rodents (see below).

Autonomic Nervous System

Parasympathetic and sympathetic branches of the ANS provide major outflow tracts linking afferent biochemical signals regarding energy stores (e.g., leptin) to efferent tracts regulating energy expenditure via the CNS. Increased parasympathetic nervous system (PNS) output from the nucleus ambiguus in the dorsal motor nucleus of the vagus slows heart rate and decreases resting energy expenditure. Activation of the SNS augments hypothalamic–pituitary–thyroid (HPT) axis activity centrally and production of epi-nephrine in the adrenal medulla peripherally. In white adipose tissue (WAT), increased SNS tone increases lipolysis by direct innervations of WAT. Increased SNS tone is asso-ciated with increased heart rate, decreased skeletal muscle work efficiency and, espe-cially in rodents, increased thermogenesis by BAT due to uncoupling of mitochondrial substrate oxidation from adenosine triphosphate (ATP) generation. Recent advances in positron emission tomography (PET) scanning technology have allowed detailed imag-ing of human BAT, but the magnitude of its thermogenic role in adult humans remains unclear. SNS stimulation of both BAT and WAT has been shown to result in retrograde sympathetic signaling to multiple hypothalamic areas involved in the regulation of energy intake and output in rodents. The maintenance of a reduced body weight is associated with reduced SNS tone and increased PNS tone, accounting for some of the dispropor-tionate declines in both REE and NREE.

Neuroendocrine Function

The primary neuroendocrine effect of weight loss and maintenance of a reduced body weight is lower activity of the hypothalamic–pituitary–thyroid axis as a consequence of reduced circulating leptin. After more extreme reductions in fat mass, hypothalamic–pituitary–gonadal (HPG) axis activity declines, as is seen in individuals with very low body fat content due to exercise or eating disorders. The leptin-responsive hypothalamic pro-opiomelanocortin (POMC)–melanocortin 4 receptor (MC4R) and neuropeptide Y (NPY)/agouti-related peptide (AgRP) pathways in the paraventricular nucleus (PVN) of the hypothalamus provide a nexus for the effects of relative hypoleptinemia, negative energy balance, and decreased energy stores on energy intake and expenditure. Decreased circulating (and CNS concentrations) of leptin during and following weight loss result in decreased activity of the HPT axis (decreased thyroid-stimulating hormone [TSH], triiodothyronine [T3], and thyroxine [T4], and increased reverse T3 [rT3]) and, in cases of extreme weight loss or leptin deficiency, decline in activity of the HPG axis. The decline in thyroid hormone decreases REE and also decreases the relative expression in muscle of the less chemomechanically efficient molecular isoforms: MHC II and SERCA1. Despite the fact that leptin-deficient or resistant animals are hypercortisolemic and the obese phenotype can be prevented by adrenalectomy, studies of the hypothalamic–pituitary–adrenal (HPA) axis after weight loss in humans have not consistently found changes in cortisol production.

Leptin

Circulating concentrations of the adipocyte-derived hormone leptin are dependent on energy balance and fat mass. During active weight loss (negative energy balance), circulating concentrations of leptin are disproportionately (~50%, dependent on the degree and duration of caloric restriction) reduced relative to levels anticipated for that fat mass in a weight-stable individual. In animals, these decreases in circulating leptin result in decreased POMC/cocaine- and amphetamine-related transcript (CART) and increased NPY/AgRP in respective cells of the arcuate nucleus (ARC) of the hypothalamus. The subsequent declines in the POMC-cleavage products alpha-melanocyte-stimulating hormone (alpha-MSH) and beta-endorphin (beta-EP) result, respectively, in decreased hypothalamic (PVN) expression of pro-thyrotropin-releasing hormone (TRH) and increased cortisol production. The efficacy of leptin in altering energy intake and expenditure in humans is dependent on the levels of energy stores (fat) relative to their "customary" levels for that individual, and the status of energy balance (weight loss vs. maintenance). Administration of leptin to congenitally leptin-deficient rodents and humans in doses that restore circulating leptin concentrations to "normal" increases energy expenditure, decreases energy intake, increases SNS activity, and normalizes HPA, HPT, and HPG axis function. These effects are severely attenuated in humans during dynamic weight loss (small decline in appetite), and almost nonexistent in obese or never-obese humans at their customary body weights. Based on these observations, we and others have suggested that each person has an individualized brain "threshold" for leptin signaling. This "threshold" is the consequence of genetic, developmental, and metabolic influences on the cells and molecules that constitute the leptin-sensing and response mechanisms in the brain (primarily hypothalamus and brainstem). This threshold determines that the concentration of leptin is biologically "sufficient" for that individual. The threshold is higher in obese than in lean individuals, resulting in obese individuals' need for higher amounts of body fat (leptin) to generate a sufficient signal to the brain. When concentrations of leptin are below this threshold, anabolic metabolic and behavioral responses are triggered. This model of leptin as a hormone whose effects are "asymmetrical" is consistent with its lack of efficacy in subjects at usual weight.

Implications for the Future

Recent advances in the study of human physiology before, during, and after weight loss raise important questions regarding possible directions for new therapeutic approaches to obesity. It is clear from data such as the relative leptin-unresponsiveness of individuals losing weight versus individuals attempting to maintain a reduced weight, and the association of different genotypes and phenotypes with the degree of weight loss and weight regain in large studies such as Look AHEAD and DPT that dynamic weight loss (negative energy balance) and reduced weight maintenance (energy balance) are physiologically distinct states. Expansion of inquiry into therapies specifically designed to delay or prevent weight regain after otherwise successful weight loss may identify new approaches to reduced weight maintenance treatment, the goals of which would be to "reverse" the physiological responses to weight loss.

Acknowledgments

Preparation of this chapter was supported, in part, by Grant Nos. UL1TR000040 and DK64773 from the National Institutes of Health.

Suggested Reading

Bouchard, C., & Tremblay, A. (1997). Genetic influences on the response of body fat and fat distribution to positive and negative energy balances in human identical twins. *Journal of Nutrition, 127*(5), 943S–947S.—Individual differences in susceptibility to chronic overfeeding or in sensitivity to negative energy balance seem to be largely explained by genetic factors.

Rosenbaum, M., & Leibel, R. L. (2014). Adaptive response to weight loss. In R. F. Kushner & D. H. Bessesen (Eds.), *Treatment of the obese patient* (2nd ed., pp. 97–112). New York: Springer.—A review of the metabolic and behavioral responses to both dynamic weight loss and static reduced weight maintenance.

Rosenbaum, M., & Leibel, R. L. (2014). 20 years of leptin: Role of leptin in energy homeostasis in humans. *Journal of Endocrinology, 223*(1), T83–T96.—A review of the role of leptin in human energy homeostasis.

Ryu, V., & Bartness, T. J. (2014). Short and long sympathetic–sensory feedback loops in white fat. *American Journal of Physiology: Regulatory, Integrative and Comparative Physiology, 306*(12), R886–R900.—Demonstration of short feedback loops via the spinal cord and longer feedback loops via the brainsteam linking white adipose tissue with the sympathetic nervous system.

Wadden, T. A., Neiberg, R. H., Wing, R. R., Clark, J. M., Delahanty, L. M., Hill, J. O., et al. (2011). Four-year weight losses in the look AHEAD Study: Factors associated with long-term success. *Obesity, 19*(10), 1987–1998.—Intensive lifestyle intervention in overweight or obese adults with type 2 diabetes results in sustained weight loss of 5% or greater in 46% of subjects with significant weight regain between years 1 and 4.

Wing, R. R., & Phelan, S. (2005). Long-term weight loss maintenance. *American Journal of Clinical Nutrition, 82*(1), 222S–225S.—Individuals who are successful at sustaining weight loss engage in significantly more moderately vigorous physical activity and consume fewer calories per day than individuals who are "naturally" at the same level of fatness.

9

Body Composition

NERYS ASTBURY
DYMPNA GALLAGHER

The relative importance of knowing the composition of the body greatly depends on the question of interest. The need to assess body composition commonly arises in investigations of obesity and malnutrition, weight loss composition following bariatric surgery, muscle wasting, sarcopenia, lipodystrophy, altered states of hydration, and osteopenia/osteoporosis. Established gender differences in body composition influence treatment; compared with men, women have more adiposity and less muscle mass, adjusted for height and weight, and have proportionally less visceral adipose tissue (VAT). These differences are attenuated in postmenopausal women. There are also metabolic consequences (e.g., insulin resistance) associated with high and low levels of body fat and with fat distribution. From a nutritional perspective, interest in body composition has increased multifold with the global increase in the prevalence of obesity and its complications.

Body Composition Measurement Methods

No single body composition measurement method provides information on all body tissues. Body composition measurement methods vary in complexity, cost, and precision, and range from simple field-based methods (e.g., anthropometry, bioimpedance analysis) to more technically challenging laboratory-based methods (e.g., dual-energy X-ray absorptiometry, air plethysmography, and magnetic resonance imaging). Unlike in animals, on which dissections or carcass analysis can be conducted to determine and confirm the mass of a specific tissue or depot, in living humans, in order to prioritize participant safety, only noninvasive estimates can be performed.

Body Mass Index

The body mass index [BMI = weight (kg)/height (m)^2] continues to be the most commonly used index of weight status, in which normal weight is a BMI of 18.5–25.9 kg/m^2; overweight is a BMI of 25.0–29.9 kg/m^2; and obese is a BMI > 30.0 kg/m^2. The BMI is a commonly used index of fatness due to the high correlation between BMI and percent body fat in children and adults. The accuracy of the prediction of percent body fat is dependent on age (higher in older persons), sex (higher in females), and race (higher in Asians compared to African Americans and European Americans).

Anthropometry

For routine clinical use, anthropometric measurements (circumference measures and skinfold thickness) have been preferred due to ease of measurement and low cost. Waist circumference and waist–hip ratio measurements are commonly used surrogates of fat distribution, especially in epidemiological studies. Waist circumference is highly correlated with visceral fat, a clinical risk factor for the development of the metabolic syndrome. Specifically, waist circumferences greater than 102 cm (40 inches) in men and greater than 88 cm (35 inches) in women are suggestive of elevated risk. Skinfold thicknesses, which estimate the thickness of the subcutaneous fat layer, are highly correlated with percent body fat. Since the subcutaneous fat layer varies in thickness throughout the body, a combination of site measures is recommended, reflecting upper and lower body distributions. Predictive percent body fat equations based on skinfold measures are age and sex specific in adults and children.

Bioelectrical Impedance Analysis

Bioelectrical impedance analysis (BIA) is a simple, inexpensive, and noninvasive body composition measurement method. BIA is based on the electrical conductive properties of the human body. Measures of bioelectrical conductivity are proportional to total body water and the body compartments with high water concentrations, such as fat-free and skeletal muscle mass. BIA assumes that the body comprises two compartments, fat and fat-free mass (FFM; body weight = fat + FFM). Although BIA is best known as a technique for the measurement of percent body fat, more recently it has been used for estimating skeletal muscle mass as well. The equations developed to estimate body composition by any BIA system are population-specific, such that they are most valid in populations similar to the population in which a specific equation was developed. The validity of BIA in very obese persons is questioned, since total body water (TBW) and extracellular water relative to TBW are both greater in obese subjects compared with normal-weight individuals.

Air Displacement Plethysmography and Hydrodensitometry

One of the oldest methods of measuring body composition, the determination of body volume by water displacement (Archimedes' principle), allows for the estimation of FFM density (in which an assumption is made that densities of fat and FFM are constant across individuals) from which percent body fat is calculated using a two-compartment body composition model. A more commonly used method today for measuring body volume is air displacement plethysmography. Limitations with the body volume approach include the assumptions of stable densities of fat and FFM across the age range, which may not be true in older individuals, and across racial/ethnic groups given that it is now known that the density of FFM in black individuals is higher.

Dual-Energy X-Ray Absorptiometry

Dual-energy X-ray absorptiometry (DXA) systems contain an X-ray source that, after appropriate filtration, emits two photon energy peaks. The attenuation of the two energy peaks relative to each other depends on the elemental content of tissues through which the photons pass. Bone, fat, and lean soft tissues are relatively rich in calcium/phosphorus, carbon, and oxygen, respectively. DXA systems are designed to separate pixels, based on appropriate models and relative attenuation, into these three components. There are known factors, including hydration effects, that significantly influence the validity of DXA fat and bone mineral estimates. Excessive or reduced fluid volume would be interpreted as changes in lean soft tissue. The radiation exposure is minimal, and DXA can be used in children and adults of all ages. DXA measures in persons who fit within the DXA field-of-view have good reproducibility for total body and regional components. For persons whose body size extends beyond the DXA field-of-view, half-body scans have been proposed; however, due to the inability to validate the half-body scan in large-size individuals, the accuracy of the results remains unknown, and this approach is not recommended.

Dilution Techniques

Because fat is relatively anhydrous, the body's water is found primarily in the body's FFM compartment; approximately 73% of the FFM compartment is water in healthy, non-obese adults. The body's water pool can be measured using tracers, which, after administration, dilute throughout the body. Plasma or saliva samples are obtained at baseline and 3 hours after administering the tracers in adults. Basic assumptions involved with tracer dilution for body composition determination include equal distribution throughout the pool of interest and complete dilution within a specific period of time without any loss. Examples of commonly used tracers include deuterium oxide for total body water and sodium bromide for extracellular water. These isotope dilution techniques allow for the evaluation of fat and FFM without making the assumption that the hydration of FFM is constant and therefore stable.

Quantitative Magnetic Resonance

The quantitative magnetic resonance (QMR) approach is a nonimaging technique that uses a static magnetic field to detect the hydrogen atoms of fat, lean tissue, and water by their particular spin characteristics, determined by their environment or by the tissue to which they are attached. The radiofrequency relaxation signal from the hydrogen atoms in the whole body is obtained to estimate fat mass, FFM, free water (water not bound to tissues) and TBW. Using various pulse sequences, the QMR system (EchoMRI-AH; Echo Medical Systems, Houston, TX) provides estimates of fat mass, lean tissue mass, free water, and total body water. The QMR approach has important advantages over currently available methods because it provides body composition estimates with high precision and without the use of ionizing radiation. The adult system can accommodate subjects up to 250 kg, almost double than that of the widely used DXA approach.

Models in Body Composition

The use of models in the assessment of body composition allows for the indirect assessment of compartments in the body. Typically, a compartment is assumed to be homogenous in composition (e.g., fat); however, the simpler the model, the greater the assumptions made and the greater the likelihood of error. The sum of components in each model is equivalent to body weight. These models make assessments at the whole-body level and do not provide for regional or specific organ/tissue assessments. The basic two-compartment (2C) model is derived by measuring FFM by hydrodensitometry and subtracting FFM from total body weight, thereby deriving fat mass (body weight – FFM = fat mass). FFM is a heterogeneous compartment that comprises numerous tissues and organs. A 2C approach becomes inadequate when the tissue of interest is included within the FFM compartment. Nevertheless, the 2C model is routinely and regularly used to calculate fat mass from air displacement plethysmography/hydrodensitometry, TBW, and total body potassium.

A three-compartment (3C) model consists of fat, fat-free solids, and water. The water content of FFM is assumed to be between 70 and 76% for most species, and results from cross-sectional studies in adult humans show no evidence of change in the hydration of FFM with age. The fat-free solids component of FFM refers to minerals (including bone) and proteins. The 3C approach involves the measurement of body density (usually by air displacement plethysmography/hydrodensitometry) and TBW by an isotope dilution technique. Assumptions are made that both the hydration of FFM and the solids portion of FFM are constant. Because bone mineral content is known to decrease with age, the 3C approach is limited in its accuracy in persons or populations where these assumptions are incorrect.

A four-compartment (4C) model involves the measurement of body density (for fat), TBW, bone mineral content by DXA, and residual [residual = body weight – (fat + water + bone)]. This model allows for the assessment of several assumptions that are central to the 2C model. The 4C approach is frequently used as the criterion method against which new body composition methods are compared in both children and adults. The more complex 4C model involves neutron activation methods for the measurement of total body nitrogen and total body calcium, where total body fat = body weight – [total body protein (from total body nitrogen) + total body water (dilution volume) + total body ash (from total body calcium)].

A six-compartment (6C) model is calculated as follows: fat mass (measured from total body carbon) = body weight – (total body protein + total body water + bone mineral + soft tissue mineral [from a combination of total body potassium, total body nitrogen, total body chloride, total body calcium] + glycogen [total body nitrogen] + unmeasured residuals). However, the availability of neutron activation facilities is limited; therefore, the more complex 4C and the 6C models are not readily obtainable by most researchers.

At the organizational level, a five-level model was developed in which the body can be characterized at five levels. The following are the levels and their constituents: atomic = oxygen, carbon, hydrogen, and other (Level 1); molecular = water, lipid, protein, and other (Level 2); cellular = cell mass, extracellular fluid, and extracellular solids (Level 3); tissue-system level = skeletal muscle, adipose tissue, bone, blood, and other (Level 4); and whole body (Level 5).

Insights into the Composition of Weight Loss and Weight Gain

Weight loss induced by bariatric surgery causes substantial losses in total and regional adipose tissue within the first year of surgery, with continued losses between 12 and 24 months in women, despite no significant changes in body weight. Therefore, bariatric surgery has an important effect on reducing adipose tissue depots even after body weight has begun to stabilize. In both men and women, there was 77% reduction in VAT at 12 months postsurgery. In women at 24 months postbariatric surgery, VAT mass was lower than that in age-matched women controls.

In adult females with anorexia nervosa, there is a greater loss in extremity fat compared to central truncal fat during the weight loss or illness phase. Studies assessing short-term weight restoration in adult females with anorexia nervosa show a greater gain in trunk or abdominal fat. In fully weight-restored women, with long-term weight maintenance, body fat distribution is normal.

Conclusions and Future Directions

In summary, a range of techniques is now available to assess body composition safely and accurately in living humans from birth through senescence. The more sophisticated the model of body composition employed, the greater the complexity of the techniques required. While there is a great demand for a simple, safe, accurate, and inexpensive measurement method, such a technique does not yet exist.

Research efforts should concentrate on identifying the importance of monitoring fetal and infant body composition for the tailoring of nutrition during pregnancy and postpartum (energy, nutrient, and fluid requirements of the premature infant) and of treatment interventions for the infant or child (drug dosing). There is a growing consensus that phenotyping obese patients in the intensive care unit (ICU) could aid in their treatment. However, many of the conventional body composition measurement methods are based on assumptions that are violated in the very obese state that is further confounded when the patient is nonambulatory, ill (trauma, sepsis), and receiving medications and parenteral nutrition.

Monitoring the effects of interventions (behavioral, pharmacological, surgical) to promote a healthy weight and a healthy body composition includes longitudinal measurement of changes in body weight. In recent years, there has been a notable increase in the number of apps that allow individuals to track weight, physical activity, and food intake/eating habits on their smartphones. However, more important is the need to monitor the composition of that weight change (e.g., in terms of fat and FFM).

Suggested Reading

Al-Gindan, Y. Y., Hankey, C., Govan, L., Gallagher, D., Heymsfield, S. B., & Lean, M. E. (2014). Derivation and validation of simple equations to predict total muscle mass from simple anthropometric and demographic data. *American Journal of Clinical Nutrition, 100*(4), 1041–1051.—Anthropometric prediction equations for whole-body muscle mass are presented here (including for men, body weight, waist, hip, and age, and for women, body weight, hip, age, and height) that lack predictive power for use in individuals or for clinical purposes but have sufficient accuracy for use to estimate skeletal muscle in groups and for research and survey purposes within mixed populations, without the need to adjust for race.

Davidson, L. E., Kelley, D. E., Heshka, S., Thornton, J., Pi-Sunyer, F. X., Boxt, L., et al. (2014). Skeletal muscle and organ masses differ in overweight adults with type 2 diabetes. *Journal of Applied Physiology, 117*(4), 377–382.—Compared with healthy controls adults with type 2 diabetes mellitus had less lean body mass and less skeletal muscle mass and larger kidneys, liver, and spleen masses, suggesting a specific relationship between the relative size of these organs and the diabetic state.

El Ghoch, M., Calugi, S., Lamburghini, S., & Dalle Grave, R. (2014). Anorexia nervosa and body fat distribution: A systematic review. *Nutrients, 6*(9), 3895–3912.—This article provides a review of body fat distribution before and after partial and complete weight restoration in individuals with anorexia nervosa.

Gallagher, D., Heshka, S., Kelley, D. E., Thornton, J., Boxt, L., Pi-Sunyer, F. X., et al. (2014). Changes in adipose tissue depots and metabolic markers following a 1-year diet and exercise intervention in overweight and obese patients with type 2 diabetes. *Diabetes Care, 37*(12), 3325–3332.—Weight loss of 7–10% from an intensive lifestyle intervention over 1 year reduced subcutaneous adipose tissue and visceral adipose tissue and prevented an increase in intermuscular adipose tissue; reductions in adipose tissue depots were associated with improvements in biomarkers.

Mayer, L. E., Klein, D. A., Black, E., Attia, E., Shen, W., Mao, X., et al. (2009). Adipose tissue distribution after weight restoration and weight maintenance in women with anorexia nervosa. *American Journal of Clinical Nutrition, 90*(5), 1132–1137.—This study shows that adipose tissue is not distributed normally during weight recovery; it is disproportionately deposited around the waist and in the abdominal cavity in women with anorexia nervosa, but among patients who maintain normal body weight over a 1-year period, adipose tissue distribution normalizes.

Toro-Ramos, T., Goodpaster, B. H., Janumala, I., Lin, S., Strain, G. W., Thornton, J. C., et al. (2015). Continued loss in visceral and intermuscular adipose tissue in weight-stable women following bariatric surgery. *Obesity, 23*(1), 62–69.—Bariatric surgery resulted in significant losses in total and regional adipose tissue at 12 and 24 months postbariatric surgery, with continued losses between 12 and 24 months in women, when body weight change was not significant.

Wang, Z., Pi-Sunyer, F. X., Kotler, D. P., Wielopolski, L., Withers, R. T., Pierson, R. N., et al. (2002). Multicomponent methods: Evaluation of new and traditional soft tissue mineral models by *in vivo* neutron activation analysis. *American Journal of Clinical Nutrition, 76*(5), 968–974.—Provides insights into multicomponent body composition models.

Widen, E. M., Strain, G., King, W. C., Yu, W., Lin, S., Goodpaster, B., et al. (2014). Validity of bioelectrical impedance analysis for measuring changes in body water and percent fat after bariatric surgery. *Obesity Surgery, 24*(6), 847–854.—Study results suggest that clinically meaningful differences exist between BIA estimates of total body water and percent body fat and reference values; BIA estimates may be more appropriate for use in measuring change over time at the group level rather than at the individual level.

Energy Expenditure and the Regulation of Energy Balance

ERIC RAVUSSIN

Body weight is the result of an intricate balance between energy intake (calories consumed) and energy expenditure (calories burned) but, more importantly, between protein, carbohydrate, and lipid ingested and oxidized (Figure 10.1). When energy intake exceeds energy expenditure over an extended period of time, body weight is gained and may lead to overweight and obesity. Whether the culprit of this weight gain is increased energy intake or reduced energy expenditure is unknown, but it is likely to be a combination of both, with proportions of each varying from case to case.

Since Lavoisier's famous statement *"la réspiration est donc une combustion"* (respiration is therefore combustion) in 1790, generations of scientists have actively studied how the human body metabolizes energy and how to precisely measure this metabolism. Progressing toward the development of metabolic chambers in the 1970s and doubly labeled water (DLW) in the 1980s, many research laboratories in the world can now precisely and accurately measure energy expenditure of organisms in laboratory and free-living conditions. After a brief description of the methods to measure energy metabolism, this chapter reviews the physiological and molecular mechanisms linking energy expenditure and excess weight gain and discusses whether pharmacological approaches targeting energy expenditure are feasible for the control of body weight.

Methods of Measuring Energy Expenditure

Several methods have been developed to measure daily energy expenditure in humans. The most accurate methods involve continuous measurement of heat output (direct calorimetry) or gas exchange (indirect calorimetry) in individuals who, confined to small metabolic chambers, are unable to continue true activities of daily living. The DLW method has been developed and validated and is now the method of choice to measure energy expenditure in free-living conditions.

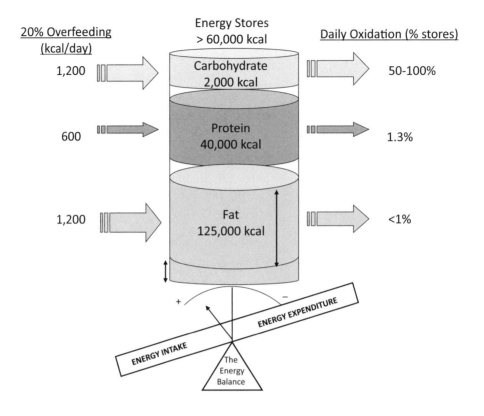

FIGURE 10.1. Energy balance equation. Body weight is an intricate balance between energy intake (calories consumed) and energy expenditure (calories burned). However, calories are consumed on a daily basis as proteins, carbohydrates, and fats (plus alcohol), and it is important to consider the energy balance as the sum of the different ingested macronutrients. For someone requiring 2,500 kcal/day, approximately 20% of the intake comes from proteins, whereas carbohydrates and fats each account for 40%. Interestingly, the ingested carbohydrates represent a 50–100% turnover of the stored carbohydrates, whereas protein and fat intake represent approximately 1% each. I have previously described how the different macronutrient balances are impacted by a surplus or a deficit in energy. In conditions of energy surplus such as 20% overfeeding (3,000 kcal/day), carbohydrate and protein stores appear to be well maintained and the surplus is stored mostly as fat (~500 kcal/day). In conditions of energy deficit, once again, stores of protein and carbohydrate are defended, and the energy deficit is accounted for by loss of fat mass.

Indirect Calorimetry

Under normal physiological conditions, neither oxygen nor carbon dioxide is stored in the body. Therefore, an indirect way of measuring energy expenditure is to measure oxygen consumption, carbon dioxide production, and nitrogen excretion. Presently, indirect calorimetry is widely used in normal and diseased conditions, and is mainly performed using open-circuit systems that can measure energy expenditure over several hours or days. Metabolic chambers are large enough (12,000–30,000 L) for an individual to live comfortably for up to a few days and can measure the various components of daily energy expenditure, including sleeping metabolic rate, the energy cost of arousal and of spontaneous physical activity, and the thermic effect of food.

Doubly Labeled Water

The DLW method is a form of "indirect" indirect calorimetry based on the differential elimination of two nonradioactive isotopes, deuterium (^{2}H) and ^{18}oxygen (^{18}O) from body water, following a single dose of these isotopes. Since ^{2}H is lost from the body only in H_2O, while ^{18}O is lost in both H_2O and CO_2, the difference between the two elimination rates (^{18}O $- ^2$H) is a measure of CO_2 production, from which total daily energy expenditure in the free-living state can be calculated. The major advantage of the DLW method is that it provides an integrated measure of energy expenditure over 1–3 weeks with excellent accuracy (1–3%) and precision (3–8%), yet requires only periodic sampling of urine.

Portable Smart Devices

Accelerometers provide a count value that describes the intensity, frequency, and duration of physical activity. However, the reliability of accelerometers in estimating daily energy expenditure is quite variable and often disappointing. The rapid development of commercially available motion sensors coupled with GPS technology on smartphones or watches will soon revolutionize the way individuals can assess their activity-related or even total daily energy expenditure. Coupled with wireless scales, such technology will even allow the calculation of daily energy intake in free-living individuals, using the principle of the energy balance equation, without relying on the erroneous assumption that a change in body weight of 1 pound signifies a net change in energy expenditure versus intake of 3,500 kcal.

Components of Energy Expenditure and Their Relevance for Human Obesity

Total daily energy expenditure (TDEE) varies substantially in humans, such that two adults with the same body size and body composition can have TDEEs that vary by as much as 1,500 kcal/day. Understanding the inherent variability in energy expenditure will potentially assist in elucidating dynamics of excess weight gain and obesity. Such variability in daily energy requirements may be attributed to differences in the three components of energy expenditure: basal metabolic rate (BMR), the thermic effect of food (also termed *diet-induced thermogenesis*), and the energy cost of physical activity that comprises both exercise and nonexercise activity thermogenesis (Figure 10.2).

Resting metabolic rate (RMR) accounts for 60–70% of TDEE and represents the energy required to maintain essential functions of the body's vital organs. It has long been recognized that there is a close relationship between RMR and body size; this association has led to the development of widely used equations to predict RMR using sex, weight, and height. Up to three quarters of the variance in RMR is determined by fat-free mass and to a lesser extent, by fat mass, sex and age. Together, these four components explain up to 85% of the inter-individual variance in RMR.

The *thermic effect of food* (TEF) is the increase in energy expenditure associated with the digestion, absorption, and storage of food. It is the smallest component, accounting

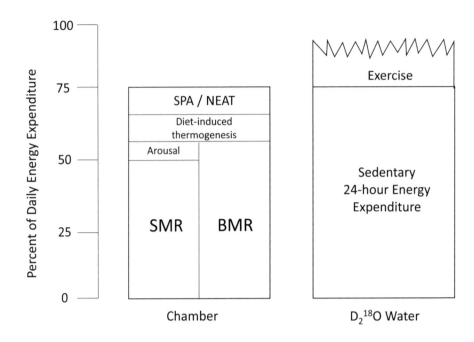

FIGURE 10.2. The components of daily energy expenditure. Basal metabolic rate (BMR; 60–70%) includes the energy cost required to maintain the integrated systems of the body and homeostatic temperature at rest, and can be divided into sleeping metabolic rate (SMR), the energy cost of arousal, diet-induced thermogenesis, and activity thermogenesis during volitional and nonvolitional activities. The latter is termed spontaneous physical activity (SPA) or nonexercise activity thermogenesis (NEAT), and includes the energy cost of sitting, maintaining posture, fidgeting, and so forth. Total daily energy expenditure and its components can be measured in the laboratory in standard conditions and in free-living conditions. The left panel indicates the measurement of daily energy expenditure for 24 hours in an indirect room calorimeter, and the right depicts the total daily energy expenditure measured over 7–14 days using doubly labeled water.

for 5–10% of TDEE. Given the difficulty and variability in measuring TEF, its role in the etiology of obesity is not clear. However, prospective studies have not identified a relationship between TEF and weight change.

In distinction to the thermic effect of food of a single meal, *diet-induced thermogenesis* (DIT) is more related to the cumulative response to prolonged overfeeding. In classical studies reported in *Nature* in 1979, Rothwell and Stock described that overfeeding resulted in less weight gain than anticipated, probably related to the activation of the sympathetic system, with concomitant increases in brown adipose tissue (BAT) mass and activity. After the "rediscovery" of BAT in humans during the past few years, it has been debated whether BAT can be stimulated in humans to induce a larger DIT and therefore be involved in the resistance to weight gain. Unfortunately, our recent data in humans seem to indicate that unlike cold-induced thermogenesis (CIT), DIT is probably not mediated by BAT in humans.

Activity thermogenesis comprises two distinct types of energy thermogenesis—the energy expended during exercise or structured physical activity (normally planned activities) and the energy expended in all other nonexercise activities (normally unplanned activities). The latter, originally described as spontaneous physical activity and subsequently called nonexercise activity thermogenesis (NEAT), includes activities such as the energy cost of sitting, standing, talking, fidgeting, and pacing a room, and has been suggested as a determinant of body weight control. The hypothesis that reduced physical activity is the cause of the worldwide obesity epidemic is an attractive one. Since the amount of structured physical activity has remained relatively stable over the years, some have hypothesized that the decrease in occupational physical activity may have been one of the factors that has tilted the energy balance toward weight gain across populations.

The Role of Energy Metabolism in the Etiology of Obesity

Cross-sectional studies that compare lean and obese individuals have added little to our understanding of the role of energy expenditure in the progression of obesity. Understanding the pathogenesis of human obesity demands longitudinal studies to reveal predictors or risk factors. The Pima Indians living in southwestern Arizona comprise one of the most obese populations in the world, with the highest reported prevalence of type 2 diabetes and, as such, provide opportunities to examine predictors of weight gain. Risk factors related to energy expenditure include a low metabolic rate, low activity thermogenesis, low sympathetic nervous system activity, and low fat oxidation.

Low Metabolic Rate

In prospective studies among nondiabetic Pima Indians, we found that a low metabolic rate (adjusted for body size, age, and sex) correlated with subsequent weight gain years later. Even if such a relationship was not found in other populations, our results demonstrate that low rates of energy expenditure are significant predictors of weight gain, at least in a population prone to obesity. Importantly, a low metabolic rate explains a relatively low percentage of the variance in weight gain; therefore, other factors, such as excessive energy intake and reduced activity levels, are likely culprits. After weight gain, the *metabolic adaptation* (defined as a greater increase in energy expenditure than predicted on the basis of the changes in fat mass and fat-free mass) was highly variable between individuals. Similarly, my colleagues and I recently reported that a reduction in energy expenditure in response to weight loss can counteract further weight loss or even predispose to weight regain. Importantly, a recent report indicated that greater decreases in energy expenditure during caloric restriction and/or less increase during overfeeding predict less weight loss in weight loss attempts, thus confirming the presence in obese people of "thrifty" and "spendthrift" phenotypes and their roles in weight control.

Low Fat Oxidation

The choice of nutrient substrate (carbohydrate vs. fat oxidation, as assessed by the ratio between carbon dioxide production and oxygen consumption; respiratory quotient [RQ]) may be an important factor in the etiology of obesity. After controlling for diet composition, recent energy balance, sex, adiposity, and family membership, the 24-hour RQ measured in a metabolic chamber was correlated with changes in body weight 3 years later among Pima Indians. Similar results have also been reported in European Americans.

Low Activity Thermogenesis

The most variable component of activity thermogenesis may be NEAT, also known as spontaneous physical activity (SPA). Using whole-room calorimetry, longitudinal studies in Pima Indians demonstrated that SPA correlated inversely with the rate of weight change 3 years later in males only. Even if several longitudinal studies have clearly demonstrated the association between reduced NEAT–SPA and weight gain, the jury is still deciding whether a similar association exists for habitual or structured physical activity.

Low Sympathetic Nervous System Activity

Reduced sympathetic nervous system (SNS) activity plays a causative role in several rodent models of obesity and is related to energy expenditure. In Pima Indians, 24-hour urinary epinephrine excretion rates were negatively associated with weight gain after a 3-year follow-up.

In summary, cross-sectional studies have not been informative about the determinants of weight gain, since low metabolic rate, low activity energy expenditure, low SNS activity, and low fat oxidation are all predictive of weight gain, whereas people with obesity have high metabolic rate, high energy expenditure for activity, high SNS activity, and high fat oxidation.

Molecular Mechanisms of Energy Expenditure Variability and Avenues for Treatment

Leptin

Leptin, a hormone predominantly secreted by adipocytes, primarily binds to receptors in the entire central nervous system and plays a key role in regulating long-term energy homeostasis. Humans with the *ob* mutation lack circulating levels of leptin and therefore develop severe, early-onset obesity with associated metabolic and behavioral consequences, including hyperphagia, defective thermogenesis, and type 2 diabetes. Leptin replacement therapy using daily subcutaneous injections has been shown to completely reverse these symptoms in patients with congenital leptin deficiency. These early findings in leptin-deficient patients suggested that administering leptin in obese patients would be a stand-alone "magic bullet" for the treatment of obesity. However, disappointingly, the results from a randomized controlled trial of daily subcutaneous recombinant leptin injection showed similar marginal amounts of weight loss over the initial 4-week of the study in both lean and obese subjects. In a small number of obese subjects studied for a further 20 weeks, weight change varied widely among patients, from a loss of about 15 kg to a gain of 5 kg in the group treated with the highest dose. Moreover, these doses induced skin irritation and swelling at the injection site in 62% of patients and headache in half the patients. The potential of leptin therapy as a panacea for obesity was a failure.

Leptin replacement therapy may be more pertinent for patients during weight loss maintenance. In calorie-restricted animals and humans, exogenous leptin replacement has been shown to reverse the metabolic adaptation induced by caloric restriction and to restore energy expenditure, catecholamine and thyroid hormone levels, and skeletal muscle efficiency to baseline values. Some of the recent studies of my colleagues and myself showed drastic metabolic adaptation (drop in RMR beyond what is expected on the basis of the losses in fat-free and fat masses) in response to massive weight loss by bariatric surgery (201 ± 182 kcal/day) or by intense behavioral changes among participants in *The Biggest Loser* TV program (504 ± 171 kcal/day). Interestingly, the metabolic adaptation was strongly related to the decrease in plasma leptin concentration ($r = .47$; $p = .02$; see Figure 10.3). Such adaptation is what makes the simple 3,500 kcal per pound of weight loss rule wrong.

Beta-3 Adrenergic Receptors

Beta-3-adrenergic receptor (ADRB3) agonists are very effective thermogenic and antiobesity and insulin-sensitizing agents in rodents. Testing in humans with the first generation of ADRB3 agonists revealed promising results on energy metabolism but poor selectivity versus the beta-1 and beta-2 adrenergic receptor subtypes, leading to many undesired effects. The second generation of ADRB3s had improved selectivity but poor oral availability or pharmacokinetics. Given these problems, we are not aware of any ADRB3s that have progressed beyond Phase II clinical trials. However, given the recent findings that BAT is present in adult humans, the potential of ADRB3 agonists for increasing the amount and activity of BAT remains an active area of exploration.

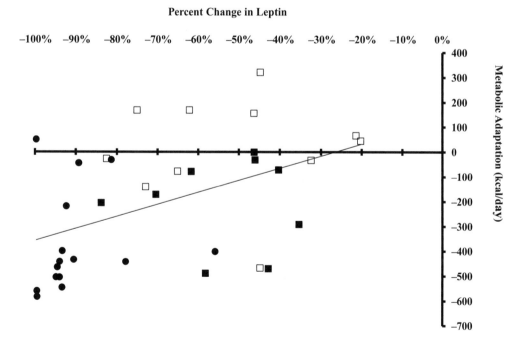

FIGURE 10.3. Correlation between metabolic adaptation and the percent decrease in circulating leptin ($r = .47$, $p = .02$) among participants in *The Biggest Loser* TV program after 7 months of weight loss (●) and among individuals after 6 (□) and 12 months (■) of weight loss following bariatric surgery.

Uncoupling Proteins and Activation of BAT

The uncoupling proteins (UCPs) gene and especially UCP1 encode for mitochondrial protein carriers, which uncouple respiration from adenosine triphosphate (ATP) production, thus stimulating heat production. Activation of such proteins may therefore be important to decrease metabolic efficiency and therefore help in weight control. Studies using ^{18}F-fluorodeoxyglucose in positron emission tomography/computed tomography (PET/CT) revealed the presence of BAT in adult humans. Currently, there is intense investigation into mechanisms for stimulating existing BAT or to induce BAT in white adipose tissue as means to promote thermogenesis and energy expenditure.

Conclusions

The global obesity epidemic has stimulated intense interest in the genetic and molecular basis of body weight regulation. Changes in the components of energy expenditure, which comprises BMR, TEF, and physical activity thermogenesis have important roles in energy balance. However, what ultimately determines "metabolic efficiency" is extremely complex. All components of energy expenditure are likely influenced by interactions between our individual genes and the environment, affecting many physiological and biochemical processes. Recent progress in gene targeting and other technologies has pushed mouse models to the forefront of this effort. Whether these preclinical findings will translate into therapeutic utility for human obesity is not yet known. There is no doubt that the field of energy expenditure has developed tremendously over the years, and understanding the homeostatic balance between energy intake and energy expenditure will continue to be an active research endeavor.

Suggested Reading

Church, T. S., Thomas, D. M., Tudor-Locke, C., Katzmarzyk, P. T., Earnest, C. P., Rodarte, R. Q., et al. (2011). Trends over 5 decades in US occupation-related physical activity and their associations with obesity. *PLoS ONE, 6*(5), e19657.—Over the past 50 years, daily occupation-related energy expenditure has decreased in parallel to the increased prevalence of obesity.

Hall, K. D., & Chow, C. C. (2013). Why is the 3500 kcal per pound weight loss rule wrong? *International Journal of Obesity, 37*(12), 1614.—The 3,500-kcal per pound rule fails to account for the dynamic changes in energy expenditure during weight loss.

Jéquier, E. (1981). Long-term measurement of energy expenditure in man: Direct or indirect calorimetry. In P. Björntorp, M. Cairella, & A. N. Howard (Eds.), *Recent advances in obesity research III* (pp. 130–135). London: John Libbey.—Description of methods to measure energy expenditure.

Knuth, N. D., Johannsen, D. L., Tamboli, R. A., Marks-Shulman, P. A., Huizenga, R., Chen, K. Y., et al. (2014). Metabolic adaptation following massive weight loss is related to the degree of energy imbalance and changes in circulating leptin. *Obesity (Silver Spring), 22*(12), 2563–2569.—Metabolic adaptation among participants in *The Biggest Loser* TV program and in individuals with obesity following bariatric surgery.

Peterson, C. M., Lecoultre, V., Frost, E. A., Simmons, J., Redman, L. M., & Ravussin, E. (2016). The thermogenic responses to overfeeding and cold are differentially regulated. *Obesity* (Silver Spring), 24(1), 96–101.—This study shows a dissociation between the changes in cold-induced thermogenesis and dietary-induced thermogenesis in response to cold acclimation.

Ravussin, E., Lillioja, S., Knowler, W. C., Christin, L., Freymond, D., Abbott, W. G., et al. (1988). Reduced rate of energy expenditure as a risk factor for body-weight gain. *New England Journal of Medicine, 318*(8), 467–472.—A low resting metabolic rate is associated with significant weight gain over years. However, only part of the weight gain can be attributed to a low RMR.

Ravussin, E., & Swinburn, B. A. (1996). Energy expenditure and obesity. *Diabetes Reviews, 4*(4), 403–422.—This publication summarizes all the "energy metabolic predictors" of weight gain in humans.

Reinhardt, M., Thearle, M. S., Ibrahim, M., Hohenadel, M. G., Bogardus, C., Krakoff, J., et al. (2015). A human thrifty phenotype associated with less weight loss during caloric restriction. *Diabetes, 64*(8), 2859–2867.—Description of thrifty and spendthrift phenotypes in obese humans.

Tam, C. S., Lecoultre, V., & Ravussin, E. (2012). Brown adipose tissue: Mechanisms and potential therapeutic targets. *Circulation, 125*(22), 2782–2791.—This chapter reports on the feasibility of therapeutically targeting the amount and activity of brown adipose tissue for weight control management.

Zurlo, F., Lillioja, S., Esposito-Del Puente, A., Nyomba, B. L., Raz, I., Saad, M. F., et al. (1990). Low ratio of fat to carbohydrate oxidation as predictor of weight gain: Study of 24-h RQ. *American Journal of Physiology: Endocrinology and Metabolism, 259*(5), E650–E657.—In prospective studies, a low relative rate of fat oxidation is associated with significant weight gain.

Macronutrients, Energy Balance, and Body Weight Regulation

KEVIN D. HALL

When the rate of energy intake from eating food differs from the energy expended to maintain life and perform physical work, the resulting energy imbalance is accounted for by changes in the body's energy stores. This energy balance concept is merely a reiteration of the law of energy conservation and provides a quantitative framework for understanding body weight regulation. This chapter provides an overview of human energy balance, macronutrient metabolism, and examines the question of whether body weight and energy balance are actively regulated.

Energy Balance Confusion

Unfortunately, the energy balance concept has often been identified with the "calories in, calories out" theory of obesity and misinterpreted to imply that obesity is caused by some combination of gluttony or sloth—a conclusion that is overly simplistic and leads to weight bias, stereotyping, and stigma. Perhaps as a reaction to such false conclusions, along with the fact that the omnipresent advice to eat less and exercise more has been ineffective at reversing obesity, there has been a recent trend to deny that humans are subject to the energy balance equation.

Energy balance deniers argue that humans do not metabolize foods in the same way that bomb calorimeters measure energy. They propose that the energy content of the diet is much less important than the quality of the diet when it comes to body weight regulation. The obesity epidemic is argued to be primarily caused by a change in diet quality and not increased energy intake or decreased expenditure. In particular, increased consumption of refined carbohydrates is purported to be particularly fattening because of their effect on insulin secretion and its well-known role in regulating adipose tissue fat storage. While these assertions have become quite common in recent years, is there really any solid evidence that the energy balance concept does not apply to humans?

Macronutrient Metabolism and Energy Balance

The complex metabolic physiology that derives energy from oxidation of macronutrients obeys the law of energy conservation. Furthermore, Hess's law of path independence dictates that the same net enthalpy change occurs in both the bomb calorimeter and the human body. In other words, "a calorie is a calorie" when it comes to macronutrients being oxidized in the calorimeter through combustion or via the intricate biochemical pathways of oxidative phosphorylation inside cells. However, rather than equating the abstract concept of body energy stores with body weight, as sometimes implied by the energy balance equation, it is important to recognize that metabolizable energy is stored in the body as protein, fat, and glycogen, which is a form of carbohydrate. Any imbalance between the intake and net metabolic utilization of these macronutrients will lead to an alteration of body composition, since the stored protein, fat, or glycogen must change to account for the imbalance.

The energy stored per unit mass of carbohydrate, fat, and protein varies considerably, especially when accounting for the intracellular water associated with stored glycogen and protein. Furthermore, dietary carbohydrates have an impact on renal sodium excretion via insulin, which results in concomitant changes of extracellular fluid. So cutting carbohydrates is expected to result in greater losses of sodium and associated body water than cutting other macronutrients. Therefore, changes of body weight are expected when the macronutrient composition of a diet is altered, even when its energy content is constant.

One could theoretically imagine the possibility of disassociating body fat balance from carbohydrate and protein balance, such that body weight and composition could be altered by manipulating the composition of the diet, without changing energy intake. However, most human studies with adequately controlled diets have shown little impact of diet composition on body weight and fat mass changes when calories are held constant, and thereby demonstrate the exquisite regulation of metabolic fuel selection to adjust to the macronutrient content of the diet.

Another way that diet composition could impact body weight and composition is if the body's energy expenditure rate depends on the macronutrient mix of the diet. For example, it is well known that consumption of dietary protein elicits a significantly larger increment of energy expenditure for several hours after a meal in comparison to dietary fat or carbohydrate. Furthermore, the fluxes through various energy-requiring metabolic pathways depend on the macronutrient composition of the diet. For instance, the breakdown and resynthesis of body fat requires eight molecules of adenosine triphosphate (ATP) per molecule of triglyceride, and the flux through this pathway is strongly influenced by dietary carbohydrate via insulin's inhibition of lipolysis. Similarly, other energy-requiring metabolic processes, such as gluconeogenesis, de novo lipogenesis, and protein turnover, can be significantly influenced by isocaloric changes in diet composition.

Calculating the expected net impact of diet changes on overall energy expenditure can be done using mathematical models that simulate how the various metabolic fluxes are altered by changing diet composition. Despite the attractive theoretical possibility of a significant "metabolic advantage" of one diet over another, the overall calculated impact of diet composition on total energy expenditure appears to be relatively modest, especially when dietary protein is unchanged. Specifically, large isocaloric exchanges of dietary carbohydrate and fat result energy expenditure changes of less than ~500 kJ/day, which corresponds to only about a 10 g/day difference in the rate of body fat change. Using current body composition methods, it would require a sustained period of many months to detect such a difference in body fat directly.

Therefore, the energy balance concept that "a calorie is a calorie" is a reasonable first approximation, since any differences in body fat due to varying diet composition are likely to be so small in the real world that they will be lost in the sea of noise attributable to the usual fluctuations in food intake.

Body Weight Stability Does Not Necessarily Imply Active Regulation of Energy Balance

In his classic 1927 metabolism textbook, Eugene Dubois observed that "there is no stranger phenomenon than the maintenance of a constant body weight under marked variation in bodily activity and food consumption" (p. 228).This remarkable stability of human body weight is often used as an argument for the active regulation of energy balance over time scales longer than a day. Indeed, daily energy intake is almost never equal to energy expenditure, and the energy balance concept is only apparent when averaged over some prolonged time period. What is the appropriate time scale for human energy balance?

Mathematically, the equation representing human body weight dynamics has the same form as that of an electric circuit with a resistor and a capacitor. The characteristic time scale for such a circuit is given by the product of the resistance and capacitance, and the circuit acts as a low-pass filter such that high-frequency fluctuations of the input voltage are damped to result in smaller and smoother fluctuations in the output. The longer the characteristic time scale, the greater the damping of the rapid input fluctuations. The analogous equation for human body weight dynamics has recently been shown to have a characteristic time scale of years. Therefore, the relatively large fluctuations in day-to-day energy intake are damped by several hundredfold, such that long-term body weight is strangely stable. Therefore, mechanisms other than the active regulation of energy balance are sufficient to explain Eugene Dubois's observation.

A similar argument for active regulation of human energy balance was made by Jeffery M. Friedman in his commentary in *Nature Medicine*: "The average human consumes one million or more calories per year, yet weight changes very little in most people. These facts lead to the conclusion that energy balance is regulated with a precision of greater than 99.5%" (2004, p. 567). This observation may be explained by the self-limiting nature of body weight change as a result of weight-related changes in energy expenditure. In other words, if energy intake increases in a stepwise fashion, body weight and energy expenditure will increase in parallel, until a new steady state of energy balance is achieved after several years. Typically, each kilogram of eventual weight change requires a sustained increase of ~100 kJ/day (~24 kcal/day) above a previously energy-balanced baseline diet. About 50% of the eventual weight change occurs within 1 year, and 95% within 3 years. Therefore, if a weight-maintaining person who was consuming 11 MJ/day (~2,600 kcal/day) in energy balance adds an average of 100 kJ/day (~24 kcal/day) to his or her daily diet, then he or she will gain about 0.5 kg after 1 year. This is equivalent to storing less than 4,000 kJ (<1,000 kcal) despite consuming more than 4 million kJ (>4 million kcal) over the year. Therefore, active regulation of energy balance is not required to explain Jeffery Freidman's observation.

While active regulation of energy balance is not required to explain the relative stability of human body weight, this does not mean that energy balance is unregulated. Rather, our ability to explain much of the observed body weight stability by passive mechanisms means that active regulatory mechanisms need not be as precise as previously believed.

Evidence for Energy Balance Regulation

Active regulation of energy balance is likely to be observed in response to perturbations that act to change body weight. For example, altering energy intake results in changes in energy expenditure that are often beyond what would be expected based on the body weight or composition changes alone. This phenomenon, called *metabolic adaptation* or *adaptive thermogenesis,* has been repeatedly demonstrated in humans, and both resting energy expenditure and activity energy expenditure are altered in parallel. Furthermore, the magnitude of metabolic adaptation appears to be proportional to the change in energy intake, the degree of energy imbalance, and may be mediated by changes in leptin and thyroid hormones.

The evidence is less clear that human energy intake is actively regulated, but the limited evidence base may be partially due to the difficulty in obtaining accurate measurements of energy intake in free-living humans. In laboratory conditions, a small number of experimental underfeeding studies in lean adults have consistently demonstrated weight loss, decreased energy expenditure, and a subsequent increase in *ad libitum* energy intake over short durations. A few experimental overfeeding studies in lean adults have found that subsequent *ad libitum* energy intake was quite variable between subjects but tends to return to near-baseline levels. These studies appear to suggest an asymmetry in the control of energy intake, with increased intake following underfeeding and weight loss but inconsistent decreases following overfeeding and weight gain. Nevertheless, human laboratory studies utilize a contrived food environment over short durations, thereby limiting their ability to assess the control of energy intake more realistic settings over the long term.

When people undertake an exercise program in free-living conditions, body weight losses are typically less than would be expected based on the added energy expenditure of exercise. This suggests that energy intake may have increased to compensate for the increased expenditure. However, it is also possible that other components of energy expenditure, including nonexercise activity thermogenesis (NEAT) or spontaneous physical activity, may have decreased, or sedentary time may have increased to compensate for the added exercise. Furthermore, even if energy intake does increase with the addition of an exercise program, this may be a result of people rewarding themselves with food rather than via a homeostatic increase in energy intake per se.

Better evidence for the active control of energy intake in free-living people requires a means of covertly changing energy output in a manner unlikely to evoke central mechanisms directly. For example, the recently approved class of diabetes drugs that inhibit the sodium/glucose cotransporter 2 (SGLT2 inhibitors) result in consistent increases in urinary glucose excretion, which thereby augments energy output by >1 MJ/day (>200 kcal/day). These drugs result in significant weight loss that plateaus after ~6 months and is sustained thereafter. However, the observed weight loss is much less than would be predicted based solely on the increased energy output in urinary glucose. Therefore, energy intake likely increased in these patients in response to either the increased energy output or the weight loss itself.

Active regulation of human energy intake may also be responsible for the typical pattern of weight change following lifestyle interventions: initial weight loss, a plateau after ~6–8 months, followed by slow regain (Figure 11.1). The model-simulated time course of energy intake underlying these weight changes exhibits an exponential decay of diet adherence, such that initial reduction in energy intake rapidly wanes and returns to baseline levels. By the time of maximum weight loss success, intake is already very close to baseline levels, and weight regain lags behind energy intake.

Summary

Despite the popularity of recent claims to the contrary, the human body obeys the principle of energy balance. Diets with the same energy content that differ in their macronutrient composition typically have a similar impact on energy expenditure and body fat. Nevertheless, diet composition may play an important role in modulating hunger, satiety, and adherence to an intervention, thereby altering net energy intake and energy balance, resulting in differences in body weight and composition.

The remarkable stability of human body weight does not necessarily imply that energy balance itself is actively regulated. However, experiments that have perturbed body weight from baseline suggest that both human energy expenditure and intake are subject to active regulation. Much work remains to better understand the quantitative strength of the feedback control mechanisms that regulate human body weight and their potential variability between people.

Acknowledgments

This research was supported, in part, by the Intramural Research Program of the National Institutes of Health, National Institute of Diabetes and Digestive and Kidney Diseases.

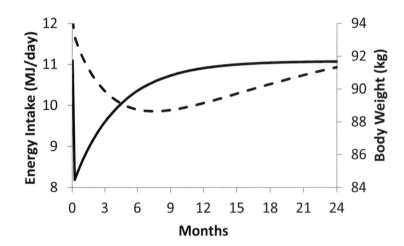

FIGURE 11.1. Model-simulated time course of energy intake (solid curve) and body weight (dashed curve) following a typical outpatient lifestyle intervention for weight loss.

Suggested Reading

Buchholz, A. C., & Schoeller, D. A. (2004). Is a calorie a calorie? *American Journal of Clinical Nutrition, 79*(5), 899S–906S.—This review provides a comprehensive overview of the evidence for energy balance in humans and provides an interpretation of the results of various weight loss studies with diets varying in macronutrient composition.

Chow, C. C., & Hall, K. D. (2014). Short and long-term energy intake patterns and their implications for human body weight regulation. *Physiology and Behavior, 134,* 60–65.—This study demonstrated mathematically that active control of human food intake on short time scales is not required for body weight stability.

Friedman, J. M. (2004). Modern science versus the stigma of obesity. *Nature Medicine, 10*(6), 563–569.—This article provides a review of biological responses to weight loss efforts and presents an argument for active regulation of human energy balance.

Hall, K. D. (2012). Modeling metabolic adaptations and energy regulation in humans. *Annual Review of Nutrition, 32,* 35–54.—This review provides an overview of the various approaches that have been used to mathematically model body weight dynamics and energy regulation in humans, highlights several insights that these models have provided, and suggests how mathematical models can serve as a guide for future experimental research.

Hall, K. D., Heymsfield, S. B., Kemnitz, J. W., Klein, S., Schoeller, D. A., & Speakman, J. R. (2012). Energy balance and its components: Implications for body weight regulation. *American Journal of Clinical Nutrition, 95*(4), 989–994.—This review provides an enumeration of the interacting components of energy expenditure and intake that comprise the energy balance equation.

Hall, K. D., Sacks, G., Chandramohan, D., Chow, C. C., Wang, Y. C., Gortmaker, S. L., et al. (2011). Quantification of the effect of energy imbalance on bodyweight. *Lancet, 378,* 826–837.—This study provides a quantification of the relationship between changes in energy intake, body weight, and energy expenditure in adults, and includes an interactive, Web-based tool that allows the user to simulate how diet and physical activity changes impact body weight and composition over time (*http://bwsimulator.niddk.nih.gov*).

Taubes, G. (2007). *Good calories, bad calories: Challenging the conventional wisdom on diet, weight control, and disease.* New York: Knopf.—This popular book presents a fascinating investigation into the history of body weight regulation and obesity research, and includes many of the arguments suggesting that dietary carbohydrates are primarily responsible for obesity and that the energy content of the diet is less important.

Sanghvi, A., Redman, L. M., Martin, C. K., Ravussin, E., & Hall, K. D. (2015). Validation of an inexpensive and accurate mathematical method to measure long-term changes in free-living energy intake. *American Journal of Clinical Nutrition, 102*(2), 353–358.—This study validates a new mathematical method for measuring changes in energy intake over long time periods in free-living people using repeated body weight measurements, and offers an alternative to self-report methods, which tend to greatly underestimate energy intake, and to laboratory measurements that can cost thousands of dollars to obtain a single data point.

12

Cognitive Neuroscience and the Risk for Weight Gain

ERIC STICE
SONJA YOKUM

Researchers have focused on the role of reward circuitry in obesity because eating high-fat/high-sugar food increases activation in reward regions (e.g., striatum, orbito-frontal cortex [OFC]) and causes dopamine (DA) release in the striatum, with the amount released correlating with meal pleasantness ratings and caloric density of the food.

Our purpose in this chapter is to review the primary neural vulnerability theories for excessive weight gain and evidence (in)consistent with these theories. We focus mainly on prospective studies and randomized experiments, as cross-sectional studies do not permit unambiguous conclusions regarding temporal precedence and the directions of effects.

The Reward Surfeit Theory of Obesity

The reward surfeit theory of obesity posits that reward region hyperresponsivity to food intake, which is presumably an inborn characteristic, increases risk for overeating and consequent weight gain. In support, prospective functional magnetic resonance imaging (fMRI) studies have found that reward region hyperresponsivity to high-calorie food receipt predicts future weight gain. Two studies did not find a main effect, but they did find that elevated caudate response to milkshake receipt predicted weight gain for individuals with a genetic propensity for greater DA signaling capacity by virtue of possessing the *TaqIA* A2/A2 allele, and lower caudate response predicted weight gain for those with a genetic propensity for lower DA signaling capacity by virtue of possessing a *TaqIA* A1 allele. These latter results converge with evidence that a genetic propensity for elevated DA signaling capacity in reward circuitry predicts future weight gain, as well as significantly less weight loss in response to obesity treatment. Healthy-weight adolescents at high versus low risk for future weight gain based on parental obesity status showed greater reward activation in response to receipt of high-calorie food and monetary reward, suggesting that this reward region hyperresponsivity is general rather than specific to food reward.

The Incentive Sensitization Theory of Obesity

The incentive sensitization model posits that repeated intake of high-calorie, palatable foods results in reward region hyperresponsivity to cues that are repeatedly associated with palatable food intake via conditioning, which prompts overeating when these cues are encountered. Animal experiments indicate that firing of striatal and ventral pallidum DA neurons initially occurs in response to receipt of a novel palatable food but that after conditioning, DA neurons begin to fire in response to food-predictive cues and no longer in response to food receipt. Theorists posit that this shift during cue–reward learning acts either to update knowledge regarding the predictive cues or attribute reward value to the cues themselves, thereby guiding behavior. This theory implies that a period of overeating palatable foods is necessary for the conditioning process that gives rise to reward region hyperresponsivity to food cues, suggesting that this might be better viewed as a maintenance model of overeating rather than a process that contributes to the initial emergence of overeating.

In support, adults who were randomly assigned to consume high-calorie foods daily over 2- to 3-week periods showed an increased willingness to work for their assigned food relative to controls, echoing findings with rodents, as well as increased *ad lib* consumption of the foods after habitual intake. Healthy-weight adolescents eating beyond objectively measured basal metabolic needs showed greater response during cues predicting impending palatable food receipt in regions encoding visual and gustatory processing, attention, salience, and reward. These latter findings suggest that overeating, even if it has not yet resulted in excess weight gain, may be accompanied by hyperresponsivity of reward, attentional, and gustatory regions to food-predictive cues.

Reward region hyperresponsivity to food cues has reliably predicted future weight gain. One study indicated that these effects are significantly stronger for individuals with a genetic propensity for greater DA signaling capacity due to possessing an A2/A2 *TaqIA* allele. However, the samples in these studies contained overweight individuals, raising the possibility that a period of overeating may be necessary to give rise to these predictive effects.

As noted, animal experiments indicate that after repeated pairings of palatable food receipt and cues that predict palatable food receipt, DA signaling increases in response to predictive cues but decreases in response to food receipt. In humans, we found an increase in caudate response during exposure to milkshake-predictive cues over repeated exposures, demonstrating a direct measure of *in vivo* cue–reward learning. A simultaneous decrease in putamen and ventral pallidum response during milkshake receipt occurred over repeated exposures, putatively reflecting reward receipt habituation. Critically, individuals who exhibited the greatest escalation in ventral pallidum responsivity to cues and those with the greatest decrease in caudate response to milkshake receipt showed significantly larger weight gain. Individuals who showed the strongest initial caudate response to the first few tastes of milkshake showed the greatest habituation, suggesting that the predictive relation between food habituation propensities may be at least partially rooted in reward region hyperresponsivity to novel palatable foods. We observed no relation between individuals showing the greatest cue–reward learning and those showing the greatest receipt habituation, which indicates that there may be two qualitatively distinct vulnerability pathways to weight gain. These results suggest that there may be important individual differences in food cue–reward learning and food reward habituation that may give rise to reward region hyperresponsivity that underlies the incentive sensitization process.

The Reward Deficit Theory of Obesity

The reward deficit model of obesity posits that individuals with lower sensitivity of DA-based reward regions overeat to compensate for this deficiency. Although cross-sectional data indicate the obese versus lean individuals show reduced reward region response to palatable food taste, prospective and experimental findings suggest that reward region hyporesponsivity is simply a consequence of overeating. Individuals who gained weight over a 6-month period showed a reduction in striatal responsivity to palatable food receipt relative to those whose weight remained stable. Rats randomized to overeating conditions that result in weight gain versus control conditions showed down-regulation of postsynaptic D_2 receptors, reduced D_2 sensitivity, and lower sensitivity of DA reward circuitry to food intake, electrical stimulation, amphetamine administration, and potassium administration.

The evidence that weight gain is associated with down-regulation of DA-based reward circuitry dovetails with evidence that weight loss increases D_2 receptor availability and responsivity of reward circuitry to food cues, though one study indicated that weight loss was associated with a reduction in D_2 receptor availability. Furthermore, mice in which reduced striatal DA signaling from food intake was experimentally induced through chronic intragastric infusion of fat worked *less* for acute intragastric infusion of fat and consumed *less* rat chow *ad lib* than control mice.

The data suggest that it is intake of energy-dense foods versus a positive energy balance per se that causes plasticity of reward circuitry. High-calorie food intake resulted in down-regulation of striatal D_1 and D_2 receptors in rats relative to isocaloric intake of low-calorie rat chow. In humans, habitual intake of ice cream was associated with reward region hyporesponsivity to the taste of an ice-cream-based milkshake. Yet total kilocalorie intake over the past 2 weeks did not correlate with reward response to milkshake receipt.

None of the prospective fMRI studies described earlier indicated a main effect of reward region hyporesponsivity on future weight gain, but the data suggest that weaker striatal response to palatable food receipt and weaker putamen and OFC response to palatable food images predict future weight gain for individuals possessing the *TaqIA* A1 allele. These interactive effects suggest the possibility of qualitatively distinct reward surfeit and reward deficit pathways to obesity: Both too much or too little DA signaling capacity and reward region responsivity may increase risk for overeating.

The Inhibitory Control Deficit Model of Overeating

It has been proposed that individuals with inhibitory control deficits and, by extension, lower activation of brain regions implicated in inhibitory control are more sensitive to food cues, which increases overeating. In support, rats that showed behavioral disinhibition in response to food reward on a serial reaction time task exhibited greater future sucrose-seeking behaviors and enhanced sensitivity to sucrose-associated stimuli after extinction relative to rats that exhibited behavioral inhibition. Individuals with inhibitory control deficits show poorer response to weight loss treatment. Furthermore, inhibitory control deficits in response to high-calorie foods in delay discounting tasks, which reflect an immediate reward bias, reliably predicted future weight gain. Similar results have emerged from studies that examined the relation of self-report measures of inhibitory control to future weight gain.

In terms of neuroimaging findings, individuals who showed less recruitment of inhibitory control regions (e.g., inferior frontal gyrus) during difficult versus easy choices on a delay discounting task showed greater weight gain, though in one study there was no significant relation between less recruitment of inhibitory regions when trying to inhibit responses to high-calorie food images and future weight gain. Another study revealed a marginal trend for reduced gray-matter volume in the prefrontal cortex to predict weight gain.

The Working Etiological Model of Neural Vulnerability Factors That Predict Weight Gain

Collectively, the prospective and experimental results we have reviewed appear to support the reward surfeit model of obesity, the incentive sensitization theory of obesity, and the inhibitory control deficit model of overeating. However, the data have provided little support for the reward deficit theory of obesity.

Findings suggest that a biphasic etiological process may give rise to initial overeating and subsequent maintenance of overeating, which represents a refinement on our dynamic vulnerability model of overeating. In Figure 12.1, the solid black arrows represent well-established relations, and the thickness of these arrows represents the number of studies that found such a relation. Dotted lines represent provisional hypotheses. The data suggest that reward region hyperresponsivity to palatable food tastes predicts future weight gain. Preliminary data suggest that this reward region hyperresponsivity is general, rather than specific to food reward. Findings also imply that repeated high-calorie food intake leads to hyperresponsivity of reward and attention regions to food-predictive cues, which predicts further overeating and weight gain. Emerging data suggest that the effects of reward region hyperresponsivity on future weight gain are stronger for individuals with a genetic propensity for elevated DA signaling. Furthermore, overeating

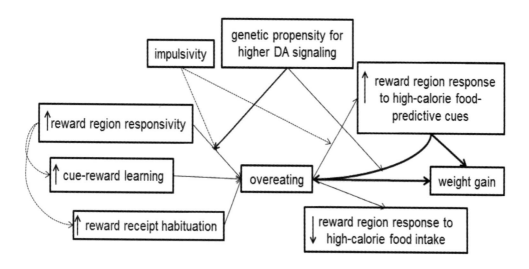

FIGURE 12.1. The biphasic etiological model.

contributes to reward region hyperresponsivity to food predictive cues and hyporesponsivity to high-calorie food receipt. Finally, emerging findings suggest that individual differences in food cue–reward learning and food reward habituation increase the risk of overeating, resulting in future weight gain. We hypothesize that reward region hyperresponsivity and inhibitory control deficits may interact in the prediction of future weight gain, and that reward region hyperresponsivity predicts increases in cue–reward learning and reward receipt habituation.

Future Research Directions

This literature review suggests several directions for research on neural vulnerability factors that predict the onset and maintenance of overeating. First, it will be useful for future prospective studies to test whether reward region hyperresponsivity, reward–cue learning, and reward receipt habituation predict future weight gain. Second, prospective studies should test whether the relation between reward region hyperresponsivity to palatable food receipt and future weight gain is significantly amplified among individuals with versus without inhibitory control deficits. Third, future fMRI studies should test whether individuals who show more pronounced food reward–cue learning are at elevated risk for initial excess weight gain. Fourth, it will be important for additional prospective repeated-measures fMRI studies to test whether, after obesity onset, individuals show a reduction in reward response to high-calorie food intake relative to baseline and comparison participants who do not gain weight. Fifth, future prospective research should test whether genotypes associated with DA signaling moderate the relation between reward region response to high-calorie food intake/cues and future weight gain because there is evidence that there may be two qualitatively distinct pathways to obesity that conform to the reward surfeit and reward deficit models. Finally, it will be crucial for human experiments to test whether assignment to habitual intake of high-calorie foods results in reduced reward region responsivity to high-calorie foods, and whether this leads to reduced caloric intake and willingness to work for high-calorie foods, as suggested by the animal studies.

Suggested Reading

Berridge, K. C., Ho, C. Y., Richard, J. M., & DiFeliceantonio, A. G. (2010). The tempted brain eats: Pleasure and desire circuits in obesity and eating disorders. *Brain Research, 1350,* 43–64.—Describes the incentive sensitization model of obesity and reviews animal research consistent with this etiological model.

Burger, K. S., & Stice, E. (2014). Greater striatopallidal adaptive coding during cue-reward learning and food reward habituation predict future weight gain. *NeuroImage, 99,* 122–128.— First study to capture individual differences in reward-cue learning and reward receipt habituation *in vivo,* and to show that a greater propesity of both predicted future weight gain.

Demos, K. E., Heatherton, T. F., & Kelley, W. M. (2012). Individual differences in nucleus accumbens activity to food and sexual images predict weight gain and sexual behavior. *Journal of Neuroscience, 32,* 5549–5552.—The first study to show that elevated reward region response to palatable food images predicts future weight gain.

Nederkoorn, C., Smulders, F., Havermans, R., Roefs, A., & Jansen, A. (2006). Impulsivity in obese women. *Appetite, 47,* 253–256.—One early study that documented that obese versus lean individuals show response inhibition deficits on a behavioral task, extending evidence that the former exhibit an immediate reward bias.

Stice, E., Spoor, S., Bohon, C., & Small, D. M. (2008). Relation between obesity and blunted striatal response to food is moderated by TaqIA A1 allele. *Science, 322,* 449–452.—First brain imaging study to link reward region responsivity to palatable food receipt to future weight gain and show that relations are moderated by genetic risk for greater dopamine signaling capacity in reward regions.

Stice, E., Spoor, S., Bohon, C., Veldhuizen, M. G., & Small, D. M. (2008). Relation of reward from food intake and anticipated food intake to obesity: A functional magnetic resonance imaging study. *Journal of Abnormal Psychology, 117,* 924–935.—First study to show that obese versus lean individuals show greater reward region responsivity to palatable food cues, but blunted reward region response to palatable food tastes.

Stice, E., Yokum, S., Burger, K. S., Epstein, L. H., & Small, D. M. (2011). Youth at risk for obesity show greater activation of striatal and somatosensory regions to food. *Journal of Neuroscience, 31,* 4360–4366.—First study to show that lean youth at risk for future obesity, by virtue of parental obesity, show greater rather than weaker reward region response to receipt of palatable food and monetary reward relative to youth at low risk for obesity.

Wang, G. J., Volkow, N. D., & Fowler, J. S. (2002). The role of dopamine in motivation for food in humans: Implications for obesity. *Expert Opinion on Therapeutic Targets, 6,* 601–609.—Describes the reward deficit theory of obesity.

Yokum, S., Gearhardt, A., Harris, J., Brownell, K., & Stice, E. (2014). Individual differences in striatum activity to food commercials predicts weight gain in adolescence. *Obesity (Silver Spring), 22,* 2544–2551.—First study to show that greater reward region response to commercials for unhealthy foods predicts future weight gain, making it one of the more ecologically valid brain imaging studies on neural vulnerability factors for obesity.

Yokum, S., Marti, C. N., Smolen, A., & Stice, E. (2015). Relation of the multilocus genetic composite reflecting high dopamine signaling capacity to future increases in BMI. *Appetite, 87,* 38–45.—First study to document that youth with a genetic propensity for greater dopamine signaling show elevated future weight gain, a finding that replicated in three independent studies.

Body Weight and Neurocognitive Function

MISTY A. W. HAWKINS
JOHN GUNSTAD

Body weight can be represented on a spectrum, with the range for optimal human health located between excess body weight (i.e., adiposity) on one end and insufficient body weight on the other. As a burgeoning literature supports the link between unhealthy weight levels and poorer functioning of multiple organ systems, there is little surprise that the brain and its corresponding neurocognitive functions are also impacted. This chapter addresses the associations between neurocognitive function and unhealthy body weight, with a focus on the extremes of the weight spectrum. Given that conditions of excess body weight (i.e., overweight and obesity) are far more common than insufficient weight, they receive greater attention.

The Impact of Excess Weight on Cognitive Function

Excess body weight, particularly obesity, has been linked with indices of poorer neurocognitive function in both healthy and patient populations. We briefly summarize the findings from these studies then discuss possible mechanisms. Together, the findings support an independent relationship of excess body weight with relative impairments in cognitive function.

Neurodegenerative Disease Risk

Excess weight during midlife is an independent risk factor for a range of neurodegenerative diseases, including Alzheimer's disease and vascular dementia. Indeed, meta-analytic findings of prospective studies support a "dose–response-type" relationship, with higher levels of excess weight conferring higher risk for dementia. For example, individuals who are overweight in midlife have a 35% greater relative risk for Alzheimer's disease and a

26% greater risk for all-cause dementia relative to their normal weight peers, whereas those who are obese have even higher relative risk at 104% and 64%, respectively. These effects appear to be independent of the medical comorbidities commonly found in obese persons, such as hypertension, cardiovascular disease, and diabetes.

Neuropsychological Test Performance

The cognitive deficits associated with excess adiposity can be detected at subclinical levels long before the manifestation of severe neurodegenerative diseases such as dementia. Indeed, relative deficits in cognitive function can be found in pediatric populations, as overweight and obese children between ages 6 and 10 years show greater deficits in inhibitory cognitive control compared to normal-weight age- and gender-matched peers. These deficits continue into adulthood, with obese adults exhibiting impairments in executive functions, learning and memory, processing speed, and other neurocognitive functions relative to normative data or to nonobese comparison groups. Severe obesity is linked to even greater impairments: Studies indicate that nearly one-fourth of bariatric surgery candidates exhibit clinically meaningful impairments on neuropsychological testing. Excess adiposity is also longitudinally associated with more rapid cognitive decline, with data indicating that multiple anthropometric indices (e.g., body mass index, waist-to-hip ratio) predict accelerated declines in global cognitive function, executive function, and memory across several assessment time points. Interestingly, recent studies indicate that a small amount of weight loss in otherwise healthy individuals leads to improved cognitive function, and that the dramatic weight loss after bariatric surgery is associated with rapid and sustained improvements in multiple cognitive domains.

Neuroanatomical and Functional Brain Changes

Researchers are beginning to identify the anatomical and functional neural mechanisms linking obesity to adverse neurocognitive outcomes. With regard to brain structure, higher body mass index (BMI), waist circumference, and/or visceral adiposity have been associated with smaller whole-brain volume, as well as diffuse reduction in gray-matter volume, including areas of the prefrontal, temporal, and parietal cortices; the hypothalamus; and the cerebellum. In addition to smaller brain volumes, visceral fat and higher BMI have also been associated with cortical thinning and damage to white-matter microstructural integrity, as indicated by decreased white matter in the corpus callosum and fornix, reduced white-matter fiber bundle length, and neuronal and myelin abnormalities of the frontal lobe. These observational data are strengthened by prospective evidence demonstrating that obesity in midlife predicts greater reductions in gray-matter volume, precuneus, and cingulate and orbitofrontal gyri. Weight gain is also associated with hippocampal atrophy in the Framingham Offspring Cohort and other prospective studies. In addition to these abnormalities on neuroimaging, obesity has also been directly linked to other pathophysiological hallmarks of Alzheimer's disease, including higher levels of amyloid-beta precursor protein, plasma amyloid proteins, and tau expression. Last, indices of excess body weight have been linked to a variety of other structural factors implicated in neurodegenerative disease development, including disruption of the blood–brain barrier and disrupted astrocyte and microglia expression.

In regard to changes in brain function, a growing number of studies indicate abnormalities on functional magnetic resonance imaging (fMRI) and positron emission tomography (PET). For example, working-memory-related activity assessed using the blood-oxygen-level-dependent response (BOLD) was reduced in the right superior frontal gyrus and the left middle frontal gyrus as waist circumference increased. This effect remained after adjusting for demographics, blood pressure, and total cholesterol. Similarly, a PET study indicated that greater body mass was associated with reduced baseline metabolic activity in the prefrontal cortex and cingulate gyrus. fMRI data also demonstrate that severely obese persons have greater deficits in connectivity of the networks controlling appetite when compared to normal weight peers. The accumulating imaging data combined with evidence of impaired neuropsychological test performance and greater risk of neurodegenerative disease support a clear and consistent relationship between excess body weight and deficits in neurocognitive function. Accordingly, the mechanisms of these effects on the brain urgently need to be clarified, and likely contributors are briefly discussed below.

Mechanisms

Existing literature on obesity-related cognitive impairment suggests a cyclical model of obesity (Figure 13.1) in which excess body weight or adiposity causes physiological changes (Path A) that impair cognitive function (Path B). Cognitive deficits contribute to reduced self-regulation abilities (Path C), resulting in unhealthy behaviors (Path D) that further promote obesity progression (Path E). More specifically, obesity is linked to dysregulation of many physiological systems, including metabolic, vascular, respiratory, inflammatory, and neurohormonal processes. Such dysregulation leads to a host of clinical conditions (e.g., type 2 diabetes, coronary artery disease). In combination, these physiological changes impair the cognitive functions needed for successful regulation of behaviors such as eating and exercise, which can lead to the deposition of additional adipose tissue.

The Impact of Insufficient Weight on Cognitive Function

The literature examining insufficient body weight and cognition is limited given that underweight is less common and most typically occurs in conjunction with another medical condition. The populations generally affected include low-birth-weight infants or failure-to-thrive children and individuals with anorexia nervosa, as well as unintentional weight loss in older adults.

Existing data indicate that low-birth-weight children or failure-to-thrive children exhibit moderate-to-severe cognitive deficits and developmental lags that follow this group into adulthood. Individuals with anorexia nervosa exhibit altered brain structure and metabolism, as well as deficits in various neurocognitive domains that may or may not be reversible with weight gain. Persons with low body weight in midlife also have increased risk of dementia (96% greater) when compared to their normal-weight peers, and accelerated weight loss has been identified as a potential marker of impending Alzheimer's disease.

However, given that the populations in which insufficient weight occurs are so diverse, research is needed to clarify whether these poor cognitive outcomes are attributable to (1) factors independent of low body weight, (2) medical conditions that produce

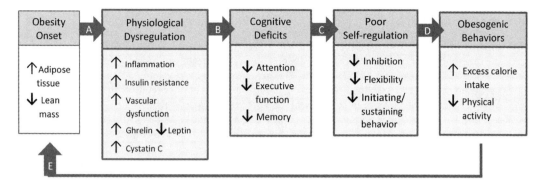

FIGURE 13.1. The cyclical model of obesity and cognitive function.

weight loss and/or malnourishment, or (3) other factors not yet identified. Even if a common risk factor is discovered, it is likely to have different effects at various stages of the lifespan. For example, malnourishment leading to low body weight during childhood may alter patterns of brain maturation, whereas malnourishment in an older adult may accelerate pathological, degenerative processes. Additional work in this area is urgently needed.

Cognitive Function and the Obesity Paradox

The "obesity paradox" has received much attention in recent years (so much that a book on the topic was published in 2014), and the topic warrants brief mention as part of this chapter. The *obesity paradox* refers to a phenomenon in which higher body mass confers neutral or even positive effects on health outcomes rather than the more commonly expected adverse outcomes. Recent findings on the possibility of an obesity paradox for neurological outcomes have been mixed. Although most studies have shown that elevated BMI is associated with greater risk for cognitive decline and dementia, others have not. Methodological issues complicate understanding of this topic. For example, many studies fail to include severely obese persons in analyses due to their premature death (survival bias) or inability to participate because of illness burden (selection bias). Similarly, given that Alzheimer's-related neuropathology develops years prior to dementia diagnosis and is known to produce weight loss, it is possible that many older persons with a normal BMI are exhibiting a more advanced stage of the disorder at the time of study entry (lead-time bias).

Conclusions

Despite methodological challenges, a better understanding of the possible effects of body weight on neurological outcomes is much needed. At the time of this writing, more than two-thirds of American adults are overweight or obese, and more than 1 in 10 adults are expected to be severely obese by 2030. When combined with the expected increased proportion of older adults, determining the influence of insufficient and excess body weight on conditions such as Alzheimer's disease and vascular dementia is of significant financial and societal importance.

Suggested Reading

Aarnoudse-Moens, C. S. H., Weisglas-Kuperus, N., van Goudoever, J. B., & Oosterlaan, J. (2009). Meta-analysis of neurobehavioral outcomes in very preterm and/or very low birth weight children. *Pediatrics, 124*(2), 717–728.—These meta-analytic results indicate that 4,125 very preterm or children with insufficient weight show decrements in executive function (–0.36 to –0.57 standard deviation) in comparison to 3,197 term-born controls.

Alosco, M. L., Galioto, R., Spitznagel, M. B., Strain, G., Devlin, M., Cohen, R., et al. (2014). Cognitive function following bariatric surgery: Evidence for improvement 3 years' post-surgery. *American Journal of Surgery, 207,* 870–876.—Results of this study show that patients who received bariatric surgery saw sustained improvements in their memory function at 36-months postsurgery.

Anstey, K. J., Cherbuin, N., Budge, M., & Young, J. (2011). Body mass index in midlife and late-life as a risk factor for dementia: A meta-analysis of prospective studies. *Obesity Reviews, 12,* e426–e437.—A meta-analytic summary of 15 longitudinal studies examining the effect of excess adiposity in mid-life on dementia risk with pooled relative risks ratios ranging from 1.26 to 2.04.

Cournot, M., Marquie, J., Ansiau, D., Martinaud, C., Fonds, H., Ferrières, J., et al. (2006). Relation between body mass index and cognitive function in healthy middle-aged men and women. *Neurology, 67*(7), 1208–1214.—This study reports that higher BMI was related to poorer cognitive function and greater cognitive decline after adjusting for demographic, medical, and psychosocial variables among healthy, middle-aged adults without dementia.

Driscoll, I., Beydoun, M. A., An, Y., Davatzikos, C., Ferrucci, L., Zonderman, A. B., et al. (2012). Midlife obesity and trajectories of brain volume changes in older adults. *Human Brain Mapping, 33,* 2204–2210.—This study reports on the associations between global and central excess adiposity in midlife and subsequent trajectories of regional brain atrophy in 152 individuals.

Gunstad, J., Lhotsky, A., Rice Wendell, C., Ferrucci, L., & Zonderman, A. B. (2010). Longitudinal examination of obesity and cognitive function: Results from the Baltimore Longitudinal Study of Aging. *Neuroepidemiology, 34,* 222–229.—Multiple obesity indices were associated with several cognitive domains including global screening measures, memory, and verbal fluency tasks in this prospective study.

Kerem, N. C., & Katzman, D. K. (2003). Brain structure and function in adolescents with anorexia nervosa. *Adolescent Medicine, 14*(1), 109–118.—This article provides a literature review of key studies of neuroimaging and cognitive function in adolescents with anorexia nervosa.

Nguyen, J. C. D., Killcross, A. S., & Jenkins, T. A. (2014). Obesity and cognitive decline: Role of inflammation and vascular changes. *Frontiers in Neuroscience, 8,* 375.—This review presents the clinical and preclinical effects of obesity on cognitive performance as well as a discussion of the potential mechanisms, especially inflammation and vascular and metabolic factors.

Prickett, C., Brennan, L., & Stolwyk, R. (2015). Examining the relationship between obesity and cognitive function: A systematic literature review. *Obesity Research and Clinical Practice, 9*(2), 93–113.—This review presents the current state of evidence for domain-specific cognitive deficits in obesity as well as methodological limitations of the current literature.

Whitmer, R. A., Gunderson, E. P., Barrett-Connor, E., Quesenberry, C. P., Jr., & Yaffe, K. (2005). Obesity in middle age and future risk of dementia: A 27 year longitudinal population based study. *British Medical Journal, 330,* 1360.—This large prospective study of 10,276 adults indicates that persons with excess adiposity had a 35–74% increased risk of dementia compared to those with normal weight.

PSYCHOLOGICAL AND SOCIAL FACTORS

14

Acquisition of Food Preferences and Eating Patterns in Children

JENNIFER ORLET FISHER
LEANN L. BIRCH

There is great need to understand the behaviors and processes that lead to excessive energy intake. Food preferences are major determinants of food intake, and both food and flavor preferences have significant learned components. This learning begins *in utero* and continues into adulthood, involving a complex interplay between biology and the social and physical contexts in which eating occurs.

The first years of life bring dramatic changes in development of eating behaviors. Humans begin life subsisting on a single food—milk—typically consumed on demand. By the end of the first year, a modified adult meal and snack pattern emerges, and the typical child has been exposed to more than 100 foods. Infants also begin milk and complementary feeding completely dependent on their caregivers but rapidly gain the motor skills to self-feed and, subsequently, the cognitive and communication skills to have greater independence in eating, including food choices, preparation, self-serving, and social rituals (e.g., setting the table). Children's experiences with food are deeply rooted in the values, norms, and behaviors of the sociocultural contexts in which they eat.

By the time children reach preschool, their dietary intake patterns resemble those of adults, and involve the same problems. U.S. preschoolers snack more frequently than in previous decades, and consume much higher levels of solid fats and added sugars than recommended. Vegetable intake is uniformly low and french fries are among the most frequently consumed vegetables. These patterns are thought to be produced by a combination of biological predispositions that favor the consumption of energy-rich foods and current dietary environmental conditions that exploit such predispositions, providing intense marketing of and ubiquitous access to foods high in sugar and fat, often in large portion sizes.

Development of Food Preferences

The development of food preferences is important because children tend to eat what they like. Food preferences, as well as food intake, also show modest tracking (consistency) during childhood, underscoring the need to understand factors that influence food acceptance in early development.

Biology of Taste Preference

The biology of basic taste preferences is thought to have evolved to promote the consumption of energy and nutrients, as well as to protect against the ingestion of toxins and spoiled food. Liking of sweet, umami, and salty tastes, and rejection of bitter and sour tastes is evident in early postnatal development. These predispositions explain, in part, why children tend to prefer foods high in sugar, salt, and fat, while foods with bitter or sour notes, such as vegetables, are not readily accepted. Interestingly, though treated somewhat interchangeably in health promotion efforts, fruits and vegetables are very different from an acceptance perspective; due to its sweetness, fruit tends to be among the most preferred food groups among young children. There is growing appreciation of genetic variation in bitter and sweet taste perception that may partially explain individual differences in food acceptance patterns. Complicating the acceptance of healthful foods such as vegetables is the fact that food *neophobia,* the fear of new foods, is normative during the toddlerhood and preschool years. Despite this neophobia, many children go on to learn to like, consume, and enjoy a variety of foods, including vegetables. This observation underscores the fact that children can learn to like healthful foods that may not be immediately accepted.

The Role of Experience

While children's food likes and dislikes may be readily perceived by caregivers, many may fail to recognize food acceptance as a learned process that occurs through experiences surrounding eating. Familiarization is a fundamental form of learning that plays a key role in children's early learning and is central in the development of food preferences and intake patterns. Children become familiar with foods through repeated exposure, and they may require several exposures to a new food before they begin to accept and consume the food. In general, acceptance of new foods has been observed to occur with 5–10 exposures. Caregivers who are unaware of the importance of familiarization in the development of food preferences, however, may not offer a new food again if it is initially rejected by the child.

Effects of repeated exposure on acceptance are seen very early in development, well before children experience the first taste of complementary foods. Exposure to flavors of the maternal diet during pregnancy and during breast-feeding promote acceptance of those flavors during the transition to complementary feeding. Fundamental issues regarding the role of early experience in promoting acceptance of healthful foods, however, remain unclear, such as sensitive developmental windows for exposing children to vegetables (e.g., before food neophobia emerges), the frequency and timing of introducing different types of vegetables (e.g., daily or weekly), the optimal preparation (e.g., raw or mixed with other foods), and context (e.g., meals or snacks).

It is not only the quantity of exposure, however, but also the quality of children's experiences with food during, following, and surrounding ingestion that influence acceptance. Dimensions of positive experience with foods that appear to promote acceptance include social modeling and use of feeding practices that are responsive rather than coercive and generate positive affect at mealtimes. Other associative conditioning processes also have an important role in liking; acceptance of foods is facilitated if they are associated with preferred flavors, postingestive consequences, and positive social contexts.

Children learn myriad bits of information from watching others eat, including which foods to consume, when to consume particular foods, and how much of those foods to consume. Evidence of this type of learning has been well established in other mammalian species. In primates, for example, this type of social influence is thought to increase foraging efficiency and prevent ingestion of toxins for diets that may consist of hundreds of species of plants and animals. There are numerous associational studies of parent–child similarities in preferences and dietary intake. However, those studies do not directly assess modeling. There are probably not many more than a dozen experimental studies on social modeling of eating among children. However, the evidence is fairly consistent about effects of acceptance of new foods. Social modeling both increases children's willingness to try new foods and promotes liking and intake, even when foods are originally disliked. And this type of learning is most successful in promoting acceptance when the model is eating the same food as the child and the model is enthusiastic about eating that food. While there have been studies of both adults and children as models, few studies have involved parents per se.

Food Preferences and Obesity and/or Appetite

The evidence base regarding the role of food liking and preference in obesity is still limited, but there are individual differences among children that emerge early to affect intake patterns. "Infant temperament," defined as differences in regulation and reactivity, is trait-like and related to differences in children's responses to food, eating patterns, and risk of obesity. Children who are seen as "picky eaters" tend to weigh less, whereas those with greater enjoyment of food tend to be heavier. Recent research has focused on associations of sweet taste perception and preferences with obesity. Exposure of the gastrointestinal tract to sweet tastes in foods activates food reward signaling pathways that are thought to reinforce pleasure in eating, as well as food preferences. There are large individual differences in sweet sensitivity that are thought to have both genetic and environmental bases. Limited evidence suggests that obese individuals may have decreased sensitivity to but higher preferences for sweet than other individuals. These findings point to the potential intersection of developmental influences on taste and food preference with appetite regulation among children.

Appetite, Food Liking, and Obesogenic Eating Behaviors

Definition

As a problem of energy imbalance, understanding influences on the development of appetite regulation is central to understanding obesity risk among children. *Appetite* is typically defined in terms of hunger, satiation, and satiety. *Hunger* refers to processes and feelings that lead to the initiation of eating, whereas *satiation* refers to processes and feelings that lead to the termination of eating. *Satiety* refers to postabsorptive effects of food to suppress hunger and increase the interval between eating occasions. Historically, short-term appetite regulation among children has been measured situationally, using subjective assessments (e.g., pictoral scales), food intake methods (e.g., measured intake at test meals), and more globally by parental questionnaire. Dimensions of appetite, such as eating rate, food responsiveness, and eating in the absence of hunger, appear to have a strong genetic component, demonstrating significant heritability and tracking across childhood.

Modification of Eating Self-Regulation by Environmental Influences

Experimental research has demonstrated the capacity of infants and young children to self-regulate short-term energy intake by adjusting food intake in response to covert changes in energy content of foods consumed. However, appetite during infancy and childhood is also responsive to and modified by the environmental conditions in which ingestion occurs. In particular, offering children large portions of energy-dense foods can interfere with satiation at meals and elicit eating in the absence of hunger. There is some suggestion that offering large portions of energy-dense foods at meals can also decrease children's intake of less preferred foods at the meal, such as vegetables. Children's susceptibility to the influence of external cues on eating increases with age, although there have been few studies using longitudinal designs. One hypothesis is that these age differences reflect a developmental shift in the complexity of social cues and in norms that affect intake and cumulative exposure to environmental factors that promote intake.

Individual Differences in Appetite Regulation

Environmental influences on appetite do not have uniform effects, however, as evidenced by the observation that a majority of youth are not obese in the current environment. There is evidence that these individual differences are linked to trait-like dimensions of general self-regulation and appetitive drive. "General self-regulation" refers to internal or transactional processes that guide goal-directed activities over time and across contexts. Impulsivity and reward responsiveness have been associated with child body mass index and obesity. The evidence regarding extent to which children's regulation of eating reflects general self-regulatory development is mixed. Emerging evidence indicates that children with poorer satiety responsiveness and greater food responsiveness may be more vulnerable to obesogenic dietary environments, consuming larger food portions at meals and greater intakes from snacks than other children. Recent brain imaging studies also reveal increased neural processing activity in food reward centers among obese children. Other findings indicate that lower levels of inhibitory control are associated with higher weight status and greater weight gain in childhood.

Implications for Supporting Healthy Food Preferences and Appetite

Despite strong biological underpinnings, food preferences and eating behaviors show great plasticity in early development and have the potential to be positively shaped by early experiences with foods and eating. The study of children's eating behaviors is still relatively new, but research in this rapidly growing field clearly points to the powerful role of family and child care environments in shaping children's eating behaviors and establishing early habits. There are several features of dietary environments that support appetite regulation and children's preference of healthful foods:

- *Provide repeated exposure.* Offering repeated exposure to foods is the most effective, and perhaps easiest route to food acceptance. Cross-cultural variation in cuisine rules and what is considered comfort food highlights the powerful role of familiarity in establishing eating norms. This process begins *in utero* and during breast-feeding, and continues into early childhood through caregiver decisions that shape the family food environment and the foods to which children are exposed. Acceptance may be reinforced when repeated exposure is accompanied by positive social, flavor, and postingestive consequences that become associated with foods

- *Structure the food environment.* Human biology has evolved to protect against energy deficits to a greater extent than surfeits. The current dietary environment is thought to provide numerous types of cues that stimulate reward pathways and overwhelm internal hunger and satiety signals. These observations highlight the need to structure children's eating environment in a way that minimizes exposure to a variety of energy-dense foods and large portion sizes, and that establishes routines that impose structure on the timing and frequency of eating occasions and set limits on what foods are available. In the same vein, because children eat what they like and like what is familiar, eating environments should maximize the availability and accessibility of healthful foods. Structuring the food environment to drive healthy choices may be particularly important for children with greater motivation to eat and greater susceptibility to obesogenic dietary influences.

Suggested Reading

Anzman-Frasca, S., Stifter, C. A., & Birch, L. L. (2012). Temperament and childhood obesity risk: A review of the literature. *Journal of Developmental and Behavioral Pediatrics, 33*(9), 732–745.—This article reviews the dimensions and contribution of child temperament that modulate risk of obesity.

Birch, L. L., & Doub, A. E. (2014). Learning to eat: Birth to age 2 y. *American Journal of Clinical Nutrition, 99*(3), 723S–728S.—This review details how infants' and toddlers' experiences and learning shape the development of eating behavior through the child–caregiver feeding relationship. This article was written as a contribution to the National Institute of Child Health and Human Development "B-24" project aimed at establishing an evidence base to inform the development of dietary guidelines for children under 2 years of age.

Blissett, J., & Fogel, A. (2013). Intrinsic and extrinsic influences on children's acceptance of new foods. *Physiology and Behavior, 121,* 89–95.—This article reviews social and biological influences on young children's food acceptance.

Carnell, S., Benson, L., Pryor, K., & Driggin, E. (2013). Appetitive traits from infancy to adolescence: Using behavioral and neural measures to investigate obesity risk. *Physiology and Behavior, 121,* 79–88.—This review describes behavioral and neural measures assessing dimensions of child appetite relevant to obesity risk.

Faith, M. S., Carnell, S., & Kral, T. V. (2013). Genetics of food intake self-regulation in childhood: Literature review and research opportunities. *Human Heredity, 75*(2–4), 80–89.—This article details emerging scientific understanding of the genetic basis for appetite and behavioral aspects of food intake regulation.

Frankel, L. A., Hughes, S. O., O'Connor, T. M., Power, T. G., Fisher, J. O., & Hazen, N. L. (2012). Parental influences on children's self-regulation of energy intake: Insights from developmental literature on emotion regulation. *Journal of Obesity, 2012,* Article No. 327259.—This article draws from literature on general parenting and child development to lend perspective to research on parental influences on children's appetite and self-regulation of energy intake.

Mennella, J. A. (2014). Ontogeny of taste preferences: Basic biology and implications for health. *American Journal of Clinical Nutrition, 99*(3), 704S–711S.—This article describes taste biology and its role in food acceptance and health.

Nicklaus, S. (2011). Children's acceptance of new foods at weaning: Role of practices of weaning and of food sensory properties. *Appetite, 57*(3), 812–815.—This review details factors that influence food acceptance during the transition from a milk-based diet to complementary feeding and foods of the family diet.

Parental Food Rules and Children's Eating

Intended and Unintended Consequences

MYLES S. FAITH

This chapter reviews "food rules" that parents use to leverage child eating behavior and the extent to which these rules promote or protect against childhood obesity. What are the most commonly used food rules and how do these impact child food intake and weight status? Which rules are most effective? Which, if any, appear to backfire? This is a fascinating yet understudied topic with very practical implications for caregivers.

There has been a dearth of conceptual models to organize this literature. Thus, a food rules model (FRM) is introduced for this chapter. The FRM strives to organize and facilitate interpretation of existing data. It also offers a heuristic for parents, to encourage self-reflection and self-evaluation when implementing food rules at home. The FRM is summarized below, along with a discussion of the impact of food rules explicitly directed to children and research needs and practical parenting implications.

The Food Rules Model

Figure 15.1 presents the food rules model (FRM), which differentiates two broad categories of caregiver food rules: (1) "deeper" cognitions, beliefs, and values regarding feeding relations that are internal to the caregiver and (2) verbal prompts and instructions explicitly directed to the child. In principle, these should be related.

The first category is likely be shaped by multiple factors, including culture, peer groups, media, health professionals, and personal life experiences. Research on this topic, however, is greatly lacking. In fact, very little is known about the origins of deeply held parenting attitudes about feeding. Validated questionnaires and interviews are needed, among other priorities, to assess feeding-related cognitions. One of the few tools in this realm is the Feeding Demands Questionnaire, which assesses parental demand cognitions

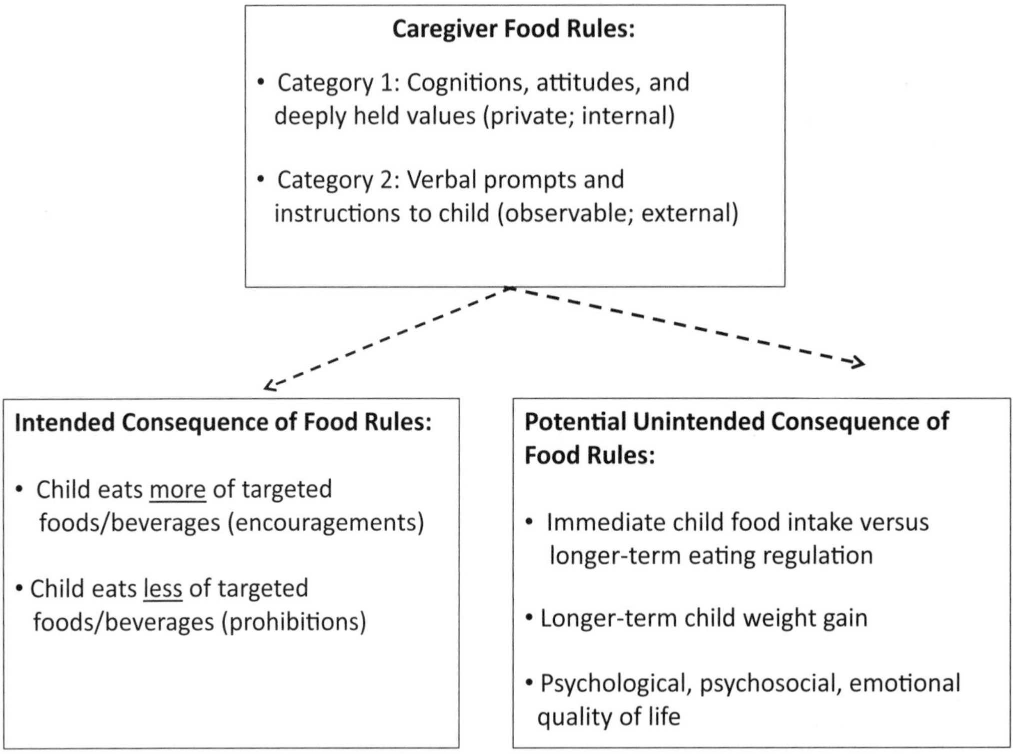

Caregiver Food Rules:

- Category 1: Cognitions, attitudes, and deeply held values (private; internal)

- Category 2: Verbal prompts and instructions to child (observable; external)

Intended Consequence of Food Rules:

- Child eats <u>more</u> of targeted foods/beverages (encouragements)

- Child eats <u>less</u> of targeted foods/beverages (prohibitions)

Potential Unintended Consequence of Food Rules:

- Immediate child food intake versus longer-term eating regulation

- Longer-term child weight gain

- Psychological, psychosocial, emotional quality of life

FIGURE 15.1. The food rules model.

about feeding relationships with children. Specifically, it assesses (1) anger/frustration during feeding, (2) caregiver demands about the types of foods their child should eat, and (3) caregiver demands about the amount of food their child should eat. We found that individual differences in feeding demand cognitions correlated in expected directions with parental feeding practices, such as restriction and encouragements to eat.

The second general category in the FRM refers to overt verbal prompts or mandates directed to children. Such feeding rules have received greater study.

The FRM differentiates intended consequences and potential unintended consequences of food rules. *Intended consequences* are what parents strive to achieve and generally fall into two categories: increase child intake of targeted foods (e.g., eat more vegetables) and reduce intake of targeted foods (e.g., drink less sugar-sweetened beverages). Equally important are potential *unintended consequences*, which can include detrimental effects on longer-term child eating regulation, weight gain, and psychological well-being. Only by considering *both* intended and unintended consequences, immediately and over the longer term, can the impact of food rules be fully evaluated.

Effects of Food Rules Directly Conveyed to Children

The second category of the FRM refers to explicit prompts or instructions directed to children. Use of these statements is an attempt to get children to eat more food or less food.

Verbal Prompts and Instructions to Eat More Food

Caregivers often instruct their children to eat more food, especially "healthier" choices such as fruits and vegetables. Indeed, only a minority of children in the nation consume sufficient servings of fruits and vegetables. Thus, many parents find themselves encouraging, prompting, coaxing, pressuring, or cajoling their children to eat healthier foods. These prompts fall into two categories: prompts to eat *without* contingencies, and prompts to eat *with* reward contingencies.

Prompts to eat *without contingencies* do not involve rewards. These are mandates or "orders" that children are expected to follow. Examples include "Clean your plate" or "Finish all your vegetables." Although parental mandates often succeed in getting children to eat, this strategy can have unintended consequences for self-regulation of eating. Wansink, Payne, and Werle (2008) studied parents of 63 preschoolers, who rated the extent to which "I tell my child to clean [his or her] plate." Children of parents who more strongly endorsed this statement requested more cereal *ad libitum* during a preschool breakfast. Specifically, researchers dispensed cereal into their breakfast bowls, instructing children to ask if they want more. In fact, parents who more strongly endorsed the "clean your plate" philosophy had boys and girls who portioned out greater amounts of cereal. This association did not depend on whether the cereal bowls were small or large (16 vs. 32 oz.). The authors concluded that "for a physician who is counseling a family with potential obesity issues, a clean-your-plate strategy may lead to unwanted consequences" (p. 994).

Ordering children to eat might also disrupt healthy weight gain, at least among girls. In a secondary data analysis of the National Longitudinal Survey of Youth, we examined whether coercive feeding by parents predicted excess body mass index (BMI) z-score gain and obesity risk over time. Specifically, parents responded to the following two questions in 1986: "When it is mealtime, how often does your child eat what you want him or her to eat?" and "When your child doesn't eat what you want him or her to eat and you tell him or her to do so, how often does he or she obey and eat?" Response options ranged from 1 = almost never to 5 = almost always. Among girls, higher parental scores on these questions predicted greater BMI z-score gain over 10 years. Hence, coercion may be "effective" in the short run of a meal to of induce eating, but potentially ineffective over the long haul for healthy weight gain.

Interestingly, parental prompts for children to clean their plate appear to be common. In a population-based survey of parents of adolescents residing in Minneapolis–St. Paul, Minnesota, 61% of fathers and 51% of mothers endorsed the statement, "My child should always eat all of the food on his or her plate." The percentage of parents endorsing this statement was higher among parents with less education (e.g., 70% for those without a high school degree vs. 38% for those who completed college) and from racial/ethnic minority groups (e.g., 70% for Hispanic/Latino vs. 35% for European American respondents). Hence, many parents prompt their children to eat more food, without accompanying rewards.

Certain food rules, however, *do* involve rewards. This is called "instrumental feeding," and it is based on operant learning (i.e., positive reinforcement). Examples include offering small trinkets, prizes, and even verbal praise for eating target foods. In fact, a number of experiments show that incentivizing children to eat target foods successfully gets children to eat more of those foods. This has been used in social media campaigns to increase fruit and vegetable consumption. Specifically, "Food Dudes" was launched as a pilot program across 150 schools across Ireland; then, starting in 2007, it was introduced to all primary schools across Ireland and rolled out over 7 years (*http://publichealth.gwu.edu/departments/pch/phcm/casesjournal/volume3/showcase/cases_3_10.pdf*). Hence, data show that incentives can increase child food consumption of fruits and vegetables. Perhaps the best evidence for rewarding food choices comes from family treatment research using "behavioral contracts." In the hands of highly motivated parents, these contracts stipulate contingencies (typically rewards) for meeting behavioral change goals—including dietary changes. Behavioral contracts set clear expectations for all family members, ideally are "negotiated" with full family buy-in, and set a positive tone for goal attainment and fostering success.

Instrumental feeding, however, can have an unintended detrimental effect on child preferences for targeted foods. In studies with preschool children that used a diverse array of incentives (e.g., movies, verbal praise, toys), incentivizing children to eat fruits and vegetables reduced liking of those. This is an important finding because food preference is one of the strongest predictors of child food intake. This is based on the psychological theory of *overjustification*, which purports that external rewards can diminish internal valuing or liking of something—including food.

Verbal Prompts and Instructions to Eat Less Food

Caregivers often prompt their children to eat less food, especially energy-dense foods. Such prohibitions can occur in the home and, perhaps more pernicious, may include foods in home cupboards. This latter form of restriction can have a "look but do not touch" feel. Explicit rules may include "Only on the weekends" or "Only on special occasions." These rules may be effective if communicated in the context of a fuller family discussion about health, and if appropriately negotiated (e.g., using behavioral contracts). However, if treats are perpetually accessible but "off limits" at home, or if prohibitions are unilaterally dictated by parents, this may be very frustrating for children.

Restricting access to high-fat, high-sugar foods, almost by definition, curbs child intake of those foods. This should protect against child overconsumption and positive energy balance in principle. However, there is evidence that restriction can have unintended consequences—both for physical health and psychological well-being. Regarding physical health, restrictive feeding by parents is associated with poorer eating self-regulation and increased BMI gain over time in children. Children whose access to palatable foods at home is restricted show greater *eating in the absence of hunger (EAH)*, which is the tendency to snack on accessible foods following a meal and despite being full. EAH is a risk factor for excess weight gain and obesity among children. Hence, restriction may compromise longer-term eating and weight regulation, potentially because the "forbidden fruit" becomes so tempting, and self-control is compromised when children eventually do have access.

There may also be unintended psychological consequences to restrictive feeding. Across a number of studies, restrictive feeding by parents is associated with greater child emotional eating and more negative child feelings about eating (sadness, shame, guilt). Moreover, restriction moderates the relationship between girls' weight status and their perceived cognitive ability. Among girls whose parents are high (but not low) in restriction, heavier weight status is associated with poorer academic self-concept. Hence, restrictive feeding may have unintentional consequences compromising happiness and emotional well-being.

The prevalence of restrictive feeding also appears to be relatively common in the population. From the aforementioned study of parents of adolescents residing in Minneapolis–St. Paul, Minnesota, 33% of fathers and 34% of mothers endorsed the statement "I intentionally keep some foods out of my child's reach."

Research Needs

There are many scientific questions yet to be answered. Research needs to include the development of new measures (e.g., for parent cognitions and attitudes about child feeding, technology to evaluate food rules articulated in real time); experimental studies that manipulate the specific food rules to which children are exposed; prospective studies examining child exposure to parental food rules and their impact on weight gain trajectories; and the interaction of food rules × child eating styles. There is mounting evidence that children differ in fundamental eating styles or attributes (e.g., "food cue responsiveness"—or the tendency to eat in response to foods in the environment). Future research should explore whether exposure to particular food rules interacts with these eating phenotypes to promote overeating and obesity.

Considerations for Caregivers

The data reviewed in this chapter, in the context of the FRM, have implications for caregivers. These include the following:

1. Being mindful of deeply held attitudes and beliefs about feeding relationships, as well as the specific mandates directed to children. Audio-recording interactions during meals and listening back could raise awareness.
2. Carefully monitoring potential unintended consequences of invoked food rules. Are there any detrimental influences on child food preferences, emotions, or family relations? Are caregivers winning the battle but losing the war of healthy eating regulation and weight gain?
3. Keeping it positive. Whether children respond positively or negatively to implemented food rules may depend on nuanced parental behavior (e.g., affect, facial expression, and emotional climate).

Indeed, these factors are important aspects of empirically supported parenting interventions for child behavioral disorders.

Suggested Reading

Birch, L., Marlin, D. W., & Rotter, J. (1984). Eating as the "means" activity in a contingency: Effects on young children's food preference. *Child Development, 55*(2), 431–443.—This is one of the earliest experiments to demonstrate that rewarding children to eat healthy foods decreases preference for those foods.

Cooke, L. J., Chambers, L. C., Añez, E. V., Croker, H. A., Boniface, D., Yeomans, M. R., et al. (2011). Eating for pleasure or profit: The effect of incentives on children's enjoyment of vegetables. *Psychological Science, 22*(2), 190–196.—This randomized controlled trial demonstrated that reinforcing children to eat a disliked vegetable, with either a monetary or social reward, increased both intake and liking of that vegetable.

Davison, K. K., & Birch, L. L. (2001). Weight status, parent reaction, and self-concept in five-year-old girls. *Pediatrics, 107*(1), 46–53.—This study found that restrictive feeding moderates the association between child weight status and self-concept.

Faith, M. S., Heo, M., Kral, T. V., & Sherry, B. (2013). Compliant eating of maternally prompted food predicts increased body mass index *z*-score gain in girls: Results from a population-based sample. *Child Obesity, 9*(5), 427–436.—This prospective analysis of the National Longitudinal Survey of Youth finds that greater use of maternal coercive feeding practices was associated with greater BMI *z*-score gain over 10 years in girls.

Faith, M. S., Storey, M., Kral, T. V., & Pietrobelli, A. (2008). The Feeding Demands Questionnaire: Assessment of parental demand cognitions concerning parent–child feeding relations. *Journal of the American Dietetic Association, 108*(4), 624–630.—This is a validation study of a questionnaire assessing parents' demand cognitions about how children should be fed.

Farrow, C. V., Haycraft, E., & Blissett, J. M. (2015). Teaching our children when to eat: How parental feeding practices inform the development of emotional eating—a longitudinal experimental design. *American Journal of Clinical Nutrition, 101*(5), 908–913.—This study found an association between restrictive feeding practices and the development of emotional eating in early childhood.

Fisher, J. O., & Birch, L. L. (2000). Parents' restrictive feeding practices are associated with young girls' negative self-evaluation of eating. *Journal of the American Dietetic Association, 100*(11), 1341–1346.—This was the first study to find that young girls whose mothers use restrictive feeding practices tend to have more sadness, guilt, and shame about eating those foods.

Loth, K. A., MacLehose, R. F., Fulkerson, J. A., Crow, S., & Neumark-Sztainer, D. (2013). Eat this, not that!: Parental demographic correlates of food-related parenting practices. *Appetite, 60*(1), 140–147.—This study examined the prevalence of parents' common food practices in Minnesota.

Maimaran, M., & Fishbach, A. (2014). If it's useful and you know it, do you eat?: Preschoolers refrain from instrumental food. *Journal of Consumer Research, 41*(3), 642–655.—This series of experiments shows that young children consume less of a food when the food is presented as being "instrumental" to achieving specified goals—including health or educational goals (e.g., reading, counting).

Wansink, B., Payne, C., & Werle, C. (2008). Consequences of belonging to the "clean plate club." *Archives of Pediatrics and Adolescent Medicine, 162*(10), 994–995.—This study found that mothers who were more likely to have children "clean their plate" had children who self-served greater portions of breakfast cereal.

Prevalence and Demographics of Dieting

ANDREW J. HILL

In the developed world the malnutrition of poverty appears to have given way to the malnutrition of affluence. Externally imposed food shortage has been superseded by self-imposed food restriction. For some sections of society, dieting and attendant body dissatisfactions have become normal, even normative. This chapter examines what is meant by dieting and the drivers of dieting, summarizes research on prevalence, identifies who is most likely to engage in dieting, considers the commerce of dieting, and looks to the future.

Assessment of Dieting

Research interest in the levels and reasons for dieting started in the mid-1960s. This has continued, enabled by health-directed population surveys and energized by global increases in obesity prevalence. Generalizable conclusions can be problematic, since prevalence estimates vary widely according to what is asked and how. General questions (e.g., about trying to lose weight) produce higher levels of endorsement than those with more specific meaning (whether one is currently dieting to lose weight). Epidemiological surveys tend to use single, more general questions, since assessment of weight control is a subsidiary part of the administered package. In contrast, surveys with smaller samples are more often designed for the purpose of detailing dieting but are directed at higher-risk subgroups.

A useful working definition of *dieting* is the intentional restriction of caloric intake for the purpose of weight loss or weight maintenance. This highlights that dieting is both deliberate and goal-directed, and that weight reduction is not the objective for all dieters. It follows that while engagement in dieting can be captured in a single question, the act of inhibition over eating is behaviorally complex. Dietary restraint offers a theoretical perspective on dieting, behavioral validation for the concept, and a widely used assessment: the Restraint Scale developed by Herman and Polivy. It has been extremely influential in demonstrating the difficulties that many dieters encounter in their efforts to control weight. Adding to this perspective on dieting, Lowe has offered an elaborated model. He argues that a complete account of a person's dieting should address three parts of the behavior: dieting history (past frequency and success of dieting), current dieting, and weight suppression (weight difference between current and previous highest weight). Unfortunately, this more comprehensive view of dieting is absent in much of the research literature on dieting.

Motivation for Dieting

Dieting is not uniform in its implementation. For some dieters, it signifies a simple desire to lose weight. For others, it is a collective term for different behaviors aimed at weight control. As noted earlier, some take dieting to represent attempts to maintain current weight and prevent weight gain, rather than to lose weight. These differences in purpose are mirrored by differences in the composition of weight loss diets, their duration, and intensity.

What might be expected, however, is greater agreement regarding the reasons why people engage in dieting. Analysis of the 1994–1996 Continuing Survey of Food Intakes by Individuals in the United States revealed that over 70% of all dieters were dieting to improve health, many on the advice of a doctor or dietitian. Interestingly, only half reported dieting to lose weight. The health focus of the survey is likely to have guided responses, and it certainly contrasts with more recent research that places appearance improvement as the main driver for dieting. Health improvement is a bonus, a secondary gain. The following clusters of dieting approaches illustrate how appearance and health can coexist as drivers of dieting. In one cluster, "thin, quick, and easy," dieters used calorie counting, special foods, meal plans, and supplements. The alternative, "thin, natural lifestyle," also had thinness as the primary goal, but the strategies included dietary integration into lifestyle and lifelong changes, and generally more healthy approaches. We currently know little about how these motivations and choices are related to past weight management behavior or likelihood of future success.

Prevalence of Dieting

Despite the cautions regarding how dieting is asked about or assessed, it is still possible to make reasonable prevalence estimates. Summarizing the many studies of Western adults shows 40–60% of women and 20–40% of men report currently trying to lose weight. Not all should be assumed to be dieting, since asking who is *currently dieting* to lose weight approximates to 25% of adult women and 10% of men. Extending the time period and asking whether respondents have dieted in the past 12 months increases this to over 50% of adult women and 25% of men. The highest rates are from questions on lifetime prevalence. Estimated at 75% of women and nearly 50% of men in the early 1990s, engagement in dieting at any point in one's lifetime is likely to be even higher in people surveyed today. What is consistent is that compared to men, women are nearly twice as likely to have a history of dieting or to report current dieting for weight loss. In contrast, men are more likely to endorse physical activity or exercise for weight control. This gender difference is not apparent in dieting for weight maintenance or to avoid weight gain. "Watching what I eat" is reported by some 10–30% of women and 10–25% of men.

There have been a number of studies comparing dieting prevalence between coun-tries, most often directed at young people in education. They are an accessible section of the population for surveys of health and well-being. Older teenagers and university students from countries across the developed and developing world show similar levels of dieting to those noted earlier: some 40–50% of all females and 20–25% of males. These figures are lower when surveys are restricted to non-overweight respondents, even when the focus is on losing weight rather than dieting: 35% of females and 15% of males. There is wide variation between countries. Young women from the Caribbean, parts of South America, sub-Saharan Africa, and the Mediterranean report lower levels of attempted weight loss. Those from Asian countries such as Bangladesh, Pakistan, the Philippines, Singapore, and Thailand report the highest. Indeed, one survey revealed that 70% of its sample of Japanese female students (and 63% of males) were currently trying to lose weight. One caution regarding university students is that they are not representa-tive of all young people in low-income countries. University education is not available to the majority. Consequently, these levels of weight loss engagement describe those who are more affluent, with easy access to food, and most directly exposed to Western values.

Regarding within-country variation by ethnicity or culture, the few studies available involve cohorts within the United States. Weight loss generally, and dieting specifically, is lowest in black American and highest in white American women, with Hispanic women closer to the latter. Whether dieting prevalence has changed over recent years is uncer-tain. Few studies are able to take more than a 10-year view, they tend to start during adolescence, and most are cross-sectional and therefore open to cohort effects. Dieting by young males has remained constant. Small but statistically significant increases and decreases have been reported in different cohorts of young females. More importantly perhaps is evidence of "tracking" (i.e., those dieting in adolescence are likely to continue this behavior into young adulthood).

Demographics of Dieting

Body weight, age, and social class all influence prevalence estimates. Alongside gender differences, the relationship with body weight is the most consistent factor in studies of dieting. Trying to lose weight and dieting are strongly related to body mass index (BMI). Overweight women are four times more likely to be currently trying to lose weight, and women with obesity, six times. Repeated attempts at dieting are also more common in people who are obese. However, the relationship between BMI and dieting is not linear. Contrary to expectation, some studies report proportionately more normal-weight cur-rent dieters than dieters who are obese. Most of these studies neglect individuals' dieting history, which for people who are obese is often both extensive and broadly unsuccessful.

With regard to age, older adolescent girls report slightly higher levels of dieting and younger adolescents report slightly lower levels, compared to adult women. Dieting increases in girls between ages 11 and 16, although up to one-fourth of 11-year-olds have already made one dieting attempt. The average age to start dieting in today's adolescent girls is 12–13. But awareness of dieting occurs at a much earlier age. For example, it has been observed that between one- and two-thirds of 5-year-olds in the United States com-prehend dieting as a mechanism for weight loss. This is especially the case in those whose mothers are currently or recently dieting. Dieting is also familiar to older women, with more than 50% of over 60s having a history of dieting to lose weight. This proportion may well increase as members of generations that are well versed in the dieting culture get older. A general principle that is applicable to all age groups is that dieting is more strongly related to perceived overweight than to actual weight in normal-weight females.

Many studies have observed a positive association between dieting and indicators of socioeconomic status (SES). This is true for adolescents and adults, and is observed in all countries. This is interesting given the inverse relationship between SES and prevalence of obesity in women. Looking at change over time, a decrease in dieting in teenage girls from lower-SES backgrounds has been reported. Again, they are likely to be most susceptible to future overweight.

Social context is relevant to dieting. Someone who overtly restricts his or her eating exerts a powerful inhibitory influence on other diners. A clustering of interest in physical activity, particular food choices, or dieting behavior can define friendship groups and is seen in more diverse social networks. The social context of dieting is relevant to both eating disorders and obesity. The possibly unhelpful role of friends in making teenage dieting normative contrasts with the motivating social support gained through regular attendance at slimming groups.

Dimensions of Dieting

Uncertainty over the validity of reported dieting has led some to operationalize the variety of dietary behaviors associated with intentional weight control. These include limiting the amount eaten at meals, avoiding fats and fatty foods, not eating between meals, and avoiding confectionery and sweet drinks. They are frequently endorsed and distinguish dieters from nondieters. Many of the commercially available dieting approaches use combinations of these behaviors. However, it is notable that some 10–30% (possibly more) of dieters are self-guided, using approaches they have heard about but dieting independently. While they may periodically use commercial products or services, self-guided dieters are generally successful in losing weight on their own. Unfortunately, we know little about them because they are invisible in the dieting literature. Dieting has also been linked with vegetarianism. For some, this is a pragmatic way of restricting the range of acceptable foods in the face of overwhelming choice. Semivegetarianism is more strongly linked to dieting than is full vegetarianism.

In contrast to these healthy dieting behaviors are unhealthy weight control practices such as skipping meals, fasting, vomiting, and using diet pills and laxatives. Individually, they are much less common (e.g., 12% of teenage girls fasting, 4% vomiting or using laxatives), although around 20% of young women report using at least one during the past year. They cluster, in that dieters are more likely to use extreme weight control methods, and those who use one are more likely to use several. Furthermore, those who engage in extreme weight control are more likely to smoke, binge-drink, or have suicidal thoughts.

Commerce of Dieting

A growing number of market research companies publish extremely expensive reports for industry on the performance of the weight loss market by region, by country, and globally. This information is sourced very differently than that in academia and adds a valuable perspective. The global weight loss market was valued at $148 billion in 2014, and at $60.5 billion in the United States alone. The latter is split evenly between weight loss products and services. These reports note that 80% or more of dieting consumers use these from home, accessing materials online or via books or diet plans. This is much larger than the proportion of self-guided dieters reported earlier.

The Future of Dieting

It is no surprise that dieting is recognized and attempted by girls at younger ages than ever before. Women now in their 60s started dieting in their early 20s. Today's adolescent girls start before they are teenagers. They are growing up in an appearance-focused and health-conscious environment in which weight loss offers benefit all round. The diet market is adaptable and increasingly profitable. Current predictions by analysts are that dieting consumers will increase their demand for natural and "free from" products, and use technology to personalize weight loss. The diet market global value is forecast to be $206 billion by 2019. The greatest growth is seen in emerging (rather than developed) markets, with Asia highlighted. The reasoning is unsurprising. This part of the world will see the greatest increases in obesity and diabetes. Disposable income will increase, and people will continue to be locked into sedentary lifestyles. On the global stage, dieting is in rude health and its future is assured.

Suggested Reading

Andreyeva, T., Long, M. W., Henderson, K. E., & Grode, G. M. (2010). Trying to lose weight: Diet strategies among Americans with overweight or obesity in 1996 and 2003. *Journal of the American Dietetic Association, 110,* 535–542.—The Behavioral Risk Factor Surveillance System (BRFSS) is typical of the large U.S. national surveys and the excellent data they generate.

Brown, C. S., Kola-Palmer, S., & Dhingra, K. (2015). Gender differences and correlates of extreme dieting behaviours in US adolescents. *Journal of Health Psychology, 20,* 569–579.—A very good entry into the literature on the relationship between extreme dieting behaviors and psychosocial and behavioral risk.

Calder, R. K., & Mussap, A. J. (2015). Factors influencing women's choice of weight-loss diet. *Journal of Health Psychology, 20,* 612–624.—A novel study attempting to relate women dieters' motivations to diet with their choice of diet methods.

de Ridder, D., Adriaanse, M., Evers, C., & Verhoeven, A. (2014). Who diets?: Most people and especially when they worry about food. *Appetite, 80,* 103–108.—Relating dietary restraint scores from a large community sample to measures of dietary concerns and food consumption, this invites the reader to think differently about present-day dieting.

Dwyer, J. T., Feldman, J. J., & Mayer, J. (1967). Adolescent dieters: Who are they?: Physical characteristics, attitudes and dieting practices of adolescent girls. *American Journal of Clinical Nutrition, 20,* 1045–1056.—One of the first studies documenting adolescent dieting and a reminder that this is not a new phenomenon.

Herman, C. P., & Polivy, J. (1980). Restrained eating. In A. J. Stunkard (Ed.), *Obesity* (pp. 208–225). Philadephia: Saunders.—An overview of the newly established research concept of dietary restraint, important in establishing a protocol for laboratory investigation, demonstrating both restrained and counter-regulatory (or disinhibited) eating and providing a cognitive perspective.

Neumark-Sztainer, D., Wall, M., Larson, N. I., Eisenberg, M. E., & Loth, K. (2011). Dieting and disordered eating behaviours from adolescence to young adulthood: Findings from a 10-year longitudinal study. *Journal of the American Dietetic Association, 111,* 1004–1011.—Illustrative of the quality information gathered on adolescents from cohorts such as Project EAT.

Peltzer, K., & Pengpid, S. (2015). Trying to lose weight among non-overweight university students from 22 low, middle and emerging economy countries. *Asia Pacific Journal of Clinical Nutrition, 24,* 177–183.—A good example of the new interest in global patterns of overweight and weight loss behavior with diverse countries included in the data collection.

Wardle, J., Haase, A. M., & Steptoe, A. (2006). Body image and weight control in young adults: International comparisons in university students from 22 countries. *International Journal of Obesity, 30,* 644–651.—A high-quality comparison of attempted weight loss by university students from across the world.

Witt, A. A., Katterman, S. N., & Lowe, M. R. (2013). Assessing the three types of dieting in the three-factor model of dieting: The Dieting and Weight History Questionnaire. *Appetite, 63,* 24–30.—Provides an entry to both the vast and influential literature on dietary restraint and Lowe's model of dieting.

17

The Impact of Dieting

DIANNE NEUMARK-SZTAINER
KATIE A. LOTH

Dieting for the purpose of weight loss is highly prevalent among adolescents and adults in societies in which a cultural ideal of thinness coexists alongside overweight and obesity. Indeed, dieting, or selling diet plans, is big business, and an ever-changing array of diet books regularly holds a place on best-seller lists. However, the long-held assumptions that dieting will yield long-term benefits of improved health and sustained weight loss have only recently been examined with empirical studies. Research findings have raised questions about the effectiveness of dieting for weight management and concerns about the potential for dieting to lead to unintentional weight gain, disordered eating behaviors, and eating disorders.

While many questions still remain, dieting has been identified as a shared risk factor for the development of both eating disorders and obesity. As such, there has begun a shift away from recommendations for individuals to engage in dieting for the purpose of weight management; instead, public health recommendations focus on the adoption of healthful eating and physical activity behaviors that are sustainable over long periods of time. That said, the overall prevalence of dieting remains high, particularly among individuals who are overweight, suggesting a need for continued public health efforts aimed at providing individuals with alternative options for achieving sustainable weight loss.

One key issue regards what the terms "dieting" or "going on a diet" really mean. Unfortunately, a clear definition cannot be provided because dieting means different things to different people. In a book for parents, *"I'm, Like, SO Fat": Helping Your Teen Make Healthy Choice about Eating and Exercise in a Weight-Obsessed World*, Neumark-Sztainer (2005, p. 103) defines dieting as "an eating plan that includes rigid rules about what to eat, how much, in what combinations, or at what times, that is usually followed for a specified period, for the purpose of weight loss." This definition emerged out of numerous research studies, conversations with young people and adults who have dieted, a review of many diet plans, and feedback from health care professionals. It stresses two separate and important tenets of dieting: the lack of flexibility (e.g., set rules that do not allow for eating more or different types of foods in different situations) and the short-term nature of the behaviors (e.g., a diet is something one does for a period of time before terminating the diet). Of note, this definition does not assume that fewer calories are eaten while dieting; the omission of this requirement is purposeful, as self-imposed dieting may or may not involve the consumption of fewer calories over an extended period of time.

Dieting, Disordered Eating, and Eating Disorders

Dieting often precedes the onset of disordered eating behaviors, including binge eating and extreme weight control practices, clinical eating disorders, and subthreshold eating disorders. These findings do not suggest that dieting on its own will lead to these problems; rather, dieting needs to happen in conjunction with other genetic, physiological, psychological, or social risk factors. Nor do these findings suggest that every dieter will develop a clinical eating disorder; the majority of dieters will not progress to such a severe state. It is commonly stated that dieting is a necessary, but not sufficient, condition for eating disorders; it is rare for a clinician to report on clients with eating disorders who have not dieted in the past.

On the one hand, retrospective data from individuals with eating disorders provides evidence of the association between dieting and eating disorders. A number of studies involving clinical samples have found that the majority of individuals with eating disorders report that they started to diet before they initiated more severe disordered eating behaviors. Further evidence of the association is provided by prospective studies within community samples of adolescents. Within prospective, observational studies, self-reported dieting has been shown to predict increased risk of disordered eating behaviors and subthreshold eating disorders. These results suggest that dieting may lead to more severe eating pathology.

On the other hand, it is important to note that results from a small number of experimental studies have produced seemingly conflicting results; these studies have shown that female participants randomly assigned to a low-calorie diet demonstrated a decrease in bulimic symptoms compared to participants assigned to a control condition. A plausible explanation for these inconsistent findings is that these experimental studies promoted healthy, structured, and sustainable dietary behaviors (e.g., increasing fruit and vegetable consumption, decreasing consumption of sugar-sweetened beverages, eating a balanced diet) that have a protective effect for bulimic behaviors, whereas dieting implemented within community-based samples looks quite different.

Questions remain about *how* dieting increases risk for disordered eating and eating disorders. Some investigators believe that dieting might simply be an antecedent, with no true causal significance in the development of eating disorders. In other words, we know that anorexia nervosa is a very complex illness, and it might be that dieting is an early symptom of the illness rather than a cause. We believe that for certain individuals, within certain social contexts, dieting reinforces problematic attitudes and behaviors in the person and his or her environment. For example, for a young girl struggling with low self-esteem and high levels of body dissatisfaction and perfectionism, who lives within a social context that encourages thinness, dieting may lead to a sense of control, weight loss, and appearance-related compliments that in turn may reinforce more extreme weight loss behaviors.

Our ability to understand more fully the role of dieting in the development of eating disorders will likely require a better understanding of the many different types of dieting and dieters. It has been suggested that some forms of dietary restraint are more likely to disrupt eating habits than others, and that the more chaotic the everyday eating pattern, the higher the risk of developing an eating disorder. An important question to consider is why, in some individuals, dieting sets up a pathway for continuous, extremely restricted eating and resultant weight loss, whereas in others, as discussed below, dieting can lead to overeating and subsequent weight gain over time.

Dieting, Weight Gain, and Obesity

Although dieting is often touted as the solution to excessive weight gain and obesity, a number of prospective studies suggest that dieting is not effective in preventing weight gain; rather, engaging in dieting has been found to predict weight gain over time. For example, in Project EAT, a 10-year longitudinal study of young people transitioning from adolescence to young adulthood, at both baseline and 5-year follow-up, those who dieted increased their body mass index (BMI) by twice as much as those who did not diet during this time period. These results were not due to higher baseline BMI values because the analyses adjusted for baseline BMI. Participants self-reported their dieting behaviors by responding to the global question, "How often have you gone on a diet in the past year? By 'diet' we mean changing the way you eat so that you can lose weight." This wording allowed for participant interpretation of the term "diet" but clarified that we were interested in dieting for weight loss. Interestingly, in analyses that examined associations between the use of specific unhealthy weight control behaviors that were listed (e.g., fasting, self-induced vomiting) and weight gain over time, similar associations were found.

The finding that dieting predicts weight gain over time raises questions about potential mechanisms of action. We propose four possible explanations for these associations. These explanations are not mutually exclusive of each other, and it is highly likely that they occur in combination. One explanation is that dieting behaviors are adopted on a short-term basis at the expense of more sustainable behavioral lifestyle choices that are likely to impact weight management positively, such as regular breakfast consumption, fruit and vegetable intake, and physical activity. A second explanation is that dieting leads to hunger, which leads to overeating, then to feelings of failure at "breaking one's diet," then back to dieting again. Thus, the cycle of dieting continues but is not effective at weight management. A third, and related, explanation, proposed by Polivy and Herman (1985), is that dieting causes binge eating by promoting the adoption of a cognitively regulated eating style. Through the use of cognitive control, rather than physiological controls (e.g., internal signs of hunger or satiety), dieting increases risk for disinhibition, whereby if one overeats and is then exposed to forbidden foods, overeating is likely to occur. Finally, if dieting is associated with decreased energy intake, metabolic efficiency may increase. Dieting may alter metabolism such that fewer calories are needed to maintain weight. When a diet ends, a person may struggle to reduce daily caloric intake to the new level required for weight maintenance in the face of these metabolic changes. Given that many individuals go on repeated diets, then overeat in between, metabolic efficiencies, even if small, may be problematic. While evidence to support this last explanation is scant, this claim is often made by repeat dieters.

The question remains about what types of behaviors do lead to healthy, sustained weight loss, at least for some individuals, and if any of these behaviors might be viewed as dieting. Data from the National Weight Control Registry, an ongoing research study that gathers information from people who have successfully lost weight and kept it off, helps to answer this question. Individuals are invited to join the National Weight Control Registry if they are 18 years or older, have lost at least 30 pounds, and have maintained this loss for 1 year or more. Among these, 98% report that they modified their food intake in some way in order to lose weight. With regard to sustaining their weight loss, most members report that they continue to maintain a low-calorie, low-fat style of eating and also engage in high levels of physical activity, watch less than 10 hours of TV per week, eat breakfast regularly, and regularly monitor their weight. It is unclear whether these individuals would describe the changes they made as dieting or as a change in lifestyle behaviors.

It is important to know what "counts" as dieting. If individuals view their behaviors as dieting, they may see these behaviors as rigid, short-term, to be utilized until the desired weight loss is achieved. In contrast, lifestyle behaviors tend to be more long term and allow for greater flexibility; thus, one might be less likely to make comments such as "I will start my diet on Monday " or "I already broke my diet so I might as well have another piece of cake." We would venture to guess that many people who lose weight and maintain the loss view their behaviors as lifestyle behaviors and that their more long-term vision contributes, at least in part, to their success. Other questions of interest include the following: Are there people for whom dieting is likely to lead to long-term weight management, and if so, what behaviors and/or attitudes contribute to their success? Why do most dieters gain weight, and why for others does dieting represent the first rung on the ladder to excessive dietary restriction?

Clinical Recommendations

Given that research demonstrates that dieting has relevance for a broad spectrum of eating and weight-related problems, we believe that it is important for health care providers to screen for dieting behaviors and discuss healthful alternatives to dieting. Providers should inquire about past and current dieting efforts. Suggested questions include the following: "Are you doing anything to lose or maintain your weight? If so, what? Have you gone on a diet in the past year to lose or maintain your weight? If so, please describe. Are you currently dieting to control your weight? If so, tell me what you are doing and how it is going for you." Among those individuals who report recent or current dieting efforts, clinicians should explore carefully what these individuals are actually doing, given that dieting can encompass different attitudes and behaviors for different individuals.

If clients are overweight and there are health reasons that justify weight control practices, clinicians should discuss healthful alternatives to short-term dieting to ensure long-term weight management and the avoidance of disordered eating behaviors and/or inadvertent weight gain over time. It may be useful to share with clients relevant research findings that indicate dieting is paradoxically associated with weight gain over extended periods. It may also be worthwhile to explore the client's thoughts on why dieting does not seem to be successful in long-term weight management, given that the client probably has had unsuccessful dieting experiences that can serve as a basis for discussion. Recommended behaviors may include engaging in physical activities that the client enjoys, eating more fruits and vegetables, limiting energy-dense foods, watching portion sizes, limiting or eliminating sugar-sweetened beverages, and eating breakfast on a regular basis. In addition, clients should be encouraged to pay attention to internal signs of hunger and satiety, and engage in more intuitive eating. Flexibility should be encouraged to avoid an overly rigid plan that may result in feelings of failure when the plan does not go as intended. Given that most overweight individuals have experienced weight stigmatization or some type of related mistreatment, care should be taken in discussing weight status; thus, it may be best to focus less on weight and more on behaviors for overall health. That said, since the time spent within the clinician's office offers a safe space to discuss experiences of weight stigma and body image concerns, it can be helpful for the clinician to ask openly about these experiences and feelings.

Regardless of a client's weight status, clinicians should explore reasons for, and consequences of, dieting behaviors. It is important to know what prompts dieting behaviors; for example, was the decision to go on a diet the result of a comment by someone at school or one's significant other? The behavioral consequences should also be explored to determine whether the dieting is leading to binge eating or ongoing restrictions beyond what is appropriate. It may also be appropriate to explore psychological (e.g., feelings of loss of control) and social (e.g., reactions by others to dieting behaviors or weight loss) consequences. In cases in which there is concern about the client's risk for developing disordered eating behaviors or an eating disorder, further assessment and possible referral to an eating disorders treatment team may be necessary.

Recommendations for Prevention

An important step is to develop interventions to reduce dieting and evaluate the effectiveness of such interventions in the prevention of related problems, particularly in young people. Risk factors for dieting, such as body dissatisfaction, internalization of cultural ideals of thinness, and possibly inaccurate information about the effects of dieting, should be addressed. Given the ubiquitous nature of diet information and advertisements within our culture, such interventions should aim to provide young people with the information they need to be critical consumers when they encounter such information. Within obesity prevention programs, we must seek out ways to reach youth effectively with messages likely to improve their eating and physical activity behaviors, such as healthful alternatives to dieting. Furthermore, it is crucial to consider the social contexts within which young people live and to address relevant family and peer norms. For example, parents should be made aware of the potentially harmful effects of modeling dieting behaviors or making weight-related comments. Schools and workplaces should avoid efforts that are likely to increase dieting (e.g., weight loss competitions) and, instead, ensure the availability and accessibility of resources (e.g., BMI report cards, weight loss competitions). likely to enhance healthful eating and physical activity behaviors. Finally, at the policy level, regulations regarding the false promises of diets are needed.

Suggested Reading

Haines, J., & Neumark-Sztainer, D. (2006). Prevention of obesity and eating disorders: A consideration of shared risk factors. *Health Education Research, 21*(6), 770–782.—The authors propose that there may be shared risk factors for obesity and eating disorders. Specifically, they describe preliminary evidence that dieting, media use, body image dissatisfaction, and weight-related teasing may have relevance for the development of the spectrum of weight-related disorders.

MacLean, P. S., Bergouignan, A., Cornier, M. A., & Jackman, M. R. (2011). Biology's response to dieting: The impetus for weight regain. *American Journal of Physiology: Regulatory, Integrative and Comparative Physiology, 301*(3), R581–R600.—This review article summarizes the body of evidence on biology's response to dieting, therefore helping to explain the role of dieting in the problem of weight regain.

Neumark-Sztainer, D. (2005). *"I'm, like, SO fat!": Helping your teen make healthy choices about eating and exercise in a weight-obsessed world.* New York: Guilford Press.—This book provides evidence-based recommendations for parents who want to raise children to have a positive body image, healthy eating and physical activity behaviors, and be at the weight that is best for them. The authors discusses how parents can respond constructively to "fat talk"; counteract negative media messages; provide a healthy home environment; and talk with their children about nutrition and calories, the dangers of dieting, and other weight-related topics.

Neumark-Sztainer, D. (2005). Can we simultaneously work toward the prevention of obesity and eating disorders in children and adolescents? *International Journal of Eating Disorders, 38*(3), 220–227.—The author strives to answer the overarching question: Can we simultaneously work toward the prevention of obesity and eating disorders? She specifically asks whether (1) there is a need for integrated approaches, (2) we can bridge the fields of obesity and eating disorders, (3) we can foster the development of environments that promote healthy eating and physical activity choices and the acceptance of diverse body shapes and sizes, and (4) we can work toward the development of interventions that have relevance to a broad spectrum of weight-related conditions and behaviors.

Neumark-Sztainer, D., Wall, M., Story, M., & Standish, A. R. (2012). Dieting and unhealthy weight control behaviors during adolescence: Associations with 10-year changes in body mass index. *Journal of Adolescent Health, 50*(1), 80–86.—The authors discuss findings from a 10-year longitudinal study (Project EAT) that examined associations between dieting and unhealthy weight control behaviors, and changes in body mass index from adolescence to young adulthood. Study findings clearly indicate that dieting and unhealthy weight control behaviors, as reported by adolescents, predict significant weight gain over time.

Polivy, J., & Herman, C. P. (1985). Dieting and binging: A causal analysis. *American Psychologist, 40*(2), 193–201.—The authors discuss the association between binge eating and dieting and present sequence data indicating that dieting usually precedes binge eating chronologically. Implications for therapy and the societal consequences of regarding dieting as a solution to the problem of bingeing are discussed.

Presnell, K., & Stice, E. (2003). An experimental test of the effect of weight-loss dieting on bulimic pathology: Tipping the scales in a different direction. *Journal of Abnormal Psychology, 112*(1), 166–170.—The authors discuss the findings from their experimental test of the dietary restraint model, in which individuals were assigned to a low-calorie diet or a waiting-list control; changes in bulimic symptoms were assessed. Contrary to the restraint model, the experiment demonstrated that dieting resulted in significant decreases in bulimic symptoms relative to the control condition. Overall, results provide evidence that dieting does not promote bulimic pathology; rather, effective decreases in caloric intake appear to reduce bulimic symptoms.

Stice, E., Presnell, K., Groesz, L., & Shaw, H. (2005). Effects of a weight maintenance diet on bulimic symptoms in adolescent girls: An experimental test of the dietary restraint theory. *Health Psychology, 24*(4), 402–412.—The authors describe the findings from their randomized experiment, in which they examined the effects of a weight maintenance diet on bulimic symptoms in a sample of adolescent girls. The weight maintenance diet intervention resulted in significantly greater decreases in bulimic symptoms and negative affect than observed in controls. These experimental findings appear antithetical to dietary restraint theory and suggest instead that dietary restriction curbs bulimic symptoms.

Wing, R. R., & Phelan, S. (2005). Long-term weight loss maintenance. *American Journal of Clinical Nutrition, 82*(1), 222S–225S.—The authors discuss findings from an examination of the data provided by National Weight Control Registry members. Information from this database provides evidence that long-term weight loss maintenance is possible and helps to identify the specific approaches associated with long-term success.

Weight Suppression

MICHAEL R. LOWE

For most of human history, whenever an adequate food supply has existed, people have typically maintained highly stable body weights despite the intake and expenditure of millions of calories over a lifetime. This stability is accomplished in an unconscious, automatic manner, not appreciably different from the maintenance of a constant body temperature. People were concerned with avoiding energy deficits and weight loss but had little reason to lose weight intentionally. As modern cultures developed—with their profusion of energy-rich foods and labor-saving devices—many people gained excessive weight to the point that dieting to lose weight has become commonplace. As a result, many people weigh less, and some people weigh much less, than their highest past body weight. The term *weight suppression (WS)* defines the difference between an individual's highest past weight at adult height (not due to pregnancy or medical conditions) and his or her current weight. Although there have been a number of observational studies of semistarvation in humans, until recently there was no research examining how individual differences in WS affect people biologically or psychologically. There are now about three dozen studies of WS. The extensive literature on the effects of weight loss on metabolism and eating behavior in animals and humans appears to implicate WS as a *cause,* not simply a correlate, of the outcomes with which it has been associated. This research is relevant to eating disorders and to the feasibility of overweight individuals maintaining weight loss over the long term, which comprise the topics of this chapter.

WS and Eating Disorders

The classic semistarvation study by Keys and colleagues provided a scientific basis for the impact of a major weight loss in producing adverse psychological, appetitive, and metabolic consequences, and offers the best evidence that large weight losses can cause binge eating in nonobese (and psychiatrically normal) people. Most individuals with anorexia nervosa (AN) or bulimia nervosa (BN) lose substantial amounts of weight (sometimes 20 kg or more) during the development of their eating disorder, and most remain well below their highest premorbid weight for years. The average level of WS in BN is 7–11 kg, and it is somewhat higher in those with AN. Although this fact has long been known, the possibility that *individual differences* in the discrepancy between past highest and current body weight would be related—independently of current body mass index (BMI)—to eating disorder symptoms and prognosis had not been considered until recently. WS research initially focused on those with BN but it has now been extended to those with AN. Three studies have found that the degree of WS is related to symptoms and weight gain in AN, even after the current state of emaciation is taken into account. Findings on the relation of WS and disordered eating (while controlling for current BMI) include the following:

• One study on BN found that higher WS predicted worse treatment outcome, but three subsequent studies failed to replicate this finding. In a 5-year observational study, those with the highest WS required the longest time to recover. The pattern of results across these studies suggests that WS may undermine treatment outcome only among those with the greatest WS (e.g., the upper third of the distribution).

• In some but not all studies, WS predicts frequency of binge eating and/or purging in BN; it is also positively related to the reinforcing value of food in BN and the size of binge episodes.

• In nearly all of the studies in which it has been examined, WS has robustly predicted the amount and/or the rate of future weight gain in both AN and BN for periods ranging from 4 weeks to 18 years.

• WS is positively related to exercise frequency in BN.

• In a 10-year follow-up study of college students, WS at baseline predicted the development of BN among students asymptomatic at baseline and the maintenance of BN in those who were symptomatic.

• In healthy individuals, WS correlated inversely with resting metabolic rate and total energy expenditure over 2 weeks. In eating disordered individuals, WS was inversely related to leptin level and directly related to menstrual irregularities.

• The importance of simultaneously considering both WS and BMI in research on AN is reflected in a recent cross-sectional analysis, in which higher WS and higher BMI were both independently associated with increased eating pathology, general distress, and physiological abnormalities.

• In the same study, the interaction of WS and absolute BMI was the best predictor of residential treatment outcome: At lower admission BMIs, greater weight suppression predicted better scores at discharge, while, at higher admission BMIs, greater weight suppression predicted worse scores at discharge.

• In a treatment study for binge eating disorder, WS was positively related to the frequency of binge eating. In the same study, higher WS also predicted smaller percent weight losses in a cognitive-behavioral weight loss treatment condition.

Research has revealed that, premorbidly, the average BMIs of individuals who go on to develop AN or BN are higher than those of same-age peers. Therefore, many individuals with BN who are of normal weight or even overweight may simultaneously have a high level of WS. In addition, the meaning of WS in early-onset AN is often ambiguous because if AN begins before adult height is reached, WS may be low despite the fact that the affected individual would have reached a higher BMI had the development of AN not interrupted normal development. These findings suggest that the body may be capable of sensing, and be "invested in" two types of weight reduction—that relative to a highest previous weight (sometimes called *relative WS*) and that involving weight loss below a healthy weight for height (called *absolute WS*). We have used the midpoint (a BMI of 21.7) of the range of normal BMIs (18.5–24.9) as a point estimate of a healthy weight for height, based on the assumption that most females require a minimum percentage of body fat to evince normal physiological function. Using this definition, a woman with BN with a BMI between 18.5 and 21.7 would be considered underweight in absolute terms.

The independent and interactive effects of WS and BMI can be studied because the two measures show little if any correlation. One study found that both WS and current BMI predicted future weight gain, and another found that the highest frequency of binge eating occurred among individuals with BN who were simultaneously high in relative and absolute WS (e.g., an individual whose past highest BMI was 26 kg/m^2 and whose current BMI is 19 kg/m^2). Finally, in a recent study, the interaction of WS and BMI was the most consistent predictor of outcome during the treatment of AN.

To date, the role of weight loss and WS has not been accounted for in cognitive and behavioral models of disordered eating. These models focus on sociocultural pressures toward slimness and the internalization of these pressures, especially among young women with anxiety or self-esteem problems. As noted earlier, research on individuals with eating disorders indicates that their premorbid BMIs are generally higher than those of their peers. Vulnerability to developing an eating disorder may therefore stem not just from an exaggerated sense of the importance of a thin body, but from the real-world stress of having a body mass that is higher than one's peers. Weight loss from these elevated premorbid body weights may improve the self-esteem of individuals with eating disorders but simultaneously creates metabolic and behavioral pressures that makes eventual weight regain very likely. Thus, even if an individual is in the healthy weight range, a high degree of WS will exert pressure toward weight regain. When such regain occurs in those with eating disorders, it is highly distressing and may prompt renewed weight loss efforts or purging behaviors that perpetuate this unhealthy cycle. Because even successfully treated patients are often still well below their highest previous weight, vulnerability to relapse may remain high. The recent identification of WS as central to the etiology, maintenance, and course of eating disorders opens new avenues of psychopathology and psychotherapy research.

WS and Weight Regain Following Weight Loss

WS has primarily been studied in eating disorders, where it has been shown to predict future weight gain. WS has also predicted weight gain in at least two studies of individuals without psychiatric or weight disorders. This evidence, along with numerous studies showing that overweight individuals routinely regain the weight they lose in weight loss programs, has implications for the more general question of the feasibility of maintaining a significant weight loss over the long term. It appears that when an individual gains weight and remains at the elevated weight for an extended period, the body treats the higher weight as its "new normal." That is, the highest weight becomes a new benchmark; downward deflections from this benchmark provoke responses similar to those following weight reductions below a healthy body weight—that is, they are strenuously resisted. A recent study followed a group of dieters who had lost weight and had kept off at least 5% of the lost weight 3 years later. The correlation between these individuals' starting BMI and their BMI after 3 years was .96. This suggests that the initial BMIs of these individuals functioned much like an "acquired set point," and that the body was exquisitely sensitive to deviations from this starting weight, so that these individuals' future weights were closely tied to their starting weights. Although a tenacious defense of an achieved body weight was once beneficial for survival, in the modern environment it appears, unfortunately, to have a very different impact. This is distressing news for the millions of overweight individuals who are trying to lose weight and keep it off.

These findings indicate that it would be wise to redirect some of the resources that are currently devoted to the treatment of obesity to the prevention of unhealthy weight gain among the nonobese. There are two reasons for this. First, weight gain predicts vulnerability to additional weight gain; though initially gaining a few kilograms is likely harmless, the fact that such weight gain usually presages future additional weight gain indicates it should be taken seriously in the early stages. Second, the popular assumption that overweight can be reversed whenever one is sufficiently motivated to do so is now known to be simplistic and misguided. Preventing unhealthy weight gain is likely to be far easier, and to have far fewer negative consequences, than trying to permanently lose extra weight after it has been gained.

Future Research Directions

A number of questions remain about why WS has the effects it does and how treatments for eating disorders and obesity might be modified in light of research on WS. First, little is known about how long an individual needs to be at a higher weight for the body to treat that weight as a newly established benchmark. A study of rats found that the duration of dietary obesity affects its reversibility: Those fed a high-fat diet for 17 weeks and then switched to chow feeding reversed their obesity, whereas those kept on the high-fat diet for 30 weeks did not. Similarly, little is known about whether the effects of weight loss change as a new, lower weight is maintained over time. The best-controlled research on this topic suggests that behavioral and metabolic resistance to weight loss is maintained over long periods, perhaps permanently. This does not mean that some individuals cannot successfully maintain weight loss, but it does help explain why this outcome is so rare. Additionally, although WS is a continuous measure, it is not known whether the body's behavioral and metabolic responses to weight loss are proportional to the weight loss. For instance, one group has suggested that individuals have different weight loss thresholds that must be crossed before powerful defensive reactions to weight loss (e.g., a drop in metabolic rate and leptin levels) are induced, suggesting that metabolic reactions to weight loss may be sudden and discontinuous.

Another potentially fruitful topic for investigation is whether the reason for WS determines the body's response. Emerging research in young adults has suggested that roughly 30% of those who experience more than 2 kg of WS report that the weight loss was not intentional. Nothing is known about whether the age at which a highest weight is reached, or the age at which weight is lost, has implications for the impact of WS. Finally, it is important to remember that the highest past weight and current weight that define WS can occur anywhere along the dimension of BMI. The consequences of WS may depend on the BMI level reached at the highest past weight (e.g., the impact of a WS of 10 kg on an individual whose initial BMI is 30 kg/m² may differ from the impact of the same WS on an individual with an initial BMI of 25 kg/m²), and on the BMI level reached following weight loss (a weight loss that reduces body fat to a subnormal level may have a greater impact than a similar weight loss that still leaves an individual with surplus body fat). Similarly, it is important to determine whether it may be better to measure WS relative to an individual's past highest weight (by dividing WS values by the highest past weight) rather than using unadjusted WS scores.

Suggested Reading

Berner, L. A., Shaw, J. A., Witt, A. A., & Lowe, M. R. (2013). Weight suppression and body mass index in the prediction of symptomatology and treatment response in anorexia nervosa. *Journal of Abnormal Psychology, 122,* 694–708.—Greater WS was related to greater psychopathology and interacted with BMI to predict treatment outcome.

Butryn, M. L., Juarascio, A., & Lowe, M. R. (2011). The relation of weight suppression and BMI to bulimic symptoms. *International Journal of Eating Disorders, 44,* 612–617.—Those with higher WS and lower BMIs showed the highest rate of binge eating.

Butryn, M. L., Lowe, M. R., Safer, D. L., & Agras, W. S. (2006). Weight suppression is a robust predictor of outcome in the cognitive-behavioral treatment of bulimia nervosa. *Journal of Abnormal Psychology 115,* 62–67.—Higher WS at the beginning of cognitive-behavioral therapy for BN predicted higher rate of dropout and reduced abstinence from binge eating and purging at the end of treatment.

Herzog, D. B., Thomas, J. G., Kass, A. E., Eddy, K. T., Franko, D. L., & Lowe, M. R. (2010). Weight suppression predicts weight change over 5 years in bulimia nervosa. *Psychiatry Research, 177,* 330–334.—In those with BN, WS, independent of starting weight, significantly predicted the direction and extent of weight change over a 5-year follow-up.

Keel, P. K., & Heatherton, T. F. (2010). Weight suppression predicts maintenance and onset of bulimic syndromes at 10-year follow-up. *Journal of Abnormal Psychology, 119*(2), 268–275.—Among college students, those higher in WS were most likely to develop a BN-spectrum disorder 10 years later; among those initially showing a BN-spectrum disorder, those with higher WS were more likely to remain in this category 10 years later.

Lowe, M. R., Berner, L. A., Swanson, S. A., Clark, V. L., Eddy, K. T., Franko, D. L., et al. (2011). Weight suppression predicts time to remission from bulimia nervosa. *Journal of Consulting and Clinical Psychology, 79*(6), 772–776.—Individuals with BN with the highest levels of WS took the longest to remit from their disorder.

Lowe, M. R., Davis, W., Lucks, D., Annunziato, R., & Butryn, M. (2006). Weight suppression predicts weight gain during inpatient treatment of bulimia nervosa. *Physiology and Behavior, 87,* 487–492.—WS level in individuals with BN starting residential treatment predicted amount of weight gain at discharge.

Shaw, J. A., Herzog, D. B., Clark, V. L., Berner, L. A., Eddy, K. T., Franko, D. L., et al. (2012). Elevated pre-morbid weights in bulimic individuals are usually surpassed post-morbidly: Implications for perpetuation of the disorder. *International Journal of Eating Disorders, 45*(4), 512–523.—Individuals with BN have elevated premorbid BMIs, and most eventually reach even higher BMIs during their disorder.

Stice, E., Durant, S., Burger, K. S., & Schoeller, D. A. (2011). Weight suppression and risk of future increases in body mass: Effects of suppressed resting metabolic rate and energy expenditure. *American Journal of Clinical Nutrition, 94*(1), 7–11.—Among psychiatrically normal, female college freshmen, WS predicted future weight gain and reduced metabolic rates and total energy expenditures.

Witt, A. A., Berkowitz, S. A., Gillberg, C., Lowe, M. R., Råstam, M., & Wentz, E. (2014). Weight suppression and body mass index interact to predict long-term weight outcomes in adolescent-onset anorexia nervosa. *Journal of Consulting and Clinical Psychology, 82*(6), 1207–1211.—Among adolescents with AN, high WS and low BMIs predicted the largest weight gains up to 18 years later.

Origins of Binge Eating

Pediatric Loss-of-Control Eating

MARIAN TANOFSKY-KRAFF

Risk for binge eating may be programmed as early as conception, although binge-type eating typically manifests in middle childhood. Most empirical data are in preadolescents and adolescents, and it is during these developmental periods that binge eating is typically referred to as *loss-of-control (LOC)* eating, which is likely the most evident precursor to binge-type eating disorders. LOC eating is the subjective experience of being unable to control what or how much is eaten, regardless of the amount reportedly consumed. By definition, LOC eating encompasses objectively large binge episodes, as well as smaller, ambiguously large binges. LOC eating is often used to describe binge eating in childhood due to difficulty in determining what constitutes an "objectively large" amount of food in growing boys and girls with vastly differing energy needs. Indeed, the presence of LOC regardless of episode size appears to be the most salient feature of binge eating patterns among children and adolescents. Therefore, this chapter focuses on the literature from these developmental periods as opposed to retrospective studies in adult samples, and makes use of the term "LOC" eating throughout. Correlational, phenotypic, and prospective data are presented. Last, areas for future exploration are discussed.

Prevalence of LOC Eating

At least one recent (within the past 1–3 months) episode of LOC eating is reported by 15 to 50% of youth, with the highest estimates among overweight and obese adolescent girls seeking weight loss treatment. Prior to adolescence, boys and girls appear to be at equivalent risk for reporting LOC. Reports of LOC are common among youth of diverse racial/ethnic backgrounds; more specifically, non-Hispanic white, white Hispanic, and black youth have comparable prevalence rates of LOC.

121

Correlates of LOC Eating

Physiological Correlates

Across studies, findings are generally consistent that youth with reported LOC are heavier and have more adiposity than their peers without LOC. As a result, studies rendering the most compelling findings are those that account for the contribution of body composition. Only such studies are considered in this section.

Data suggest that pediatric LOC eating is heritable; children with LOC are likely to have a parent with binge eating, a finding that suggests genetic and environmental influences. Only one pediatric study examined a candidate gene, namely, the *FTO* (fat mass and obesity associated) gene (*16q12.2*). Findings showed that youth with at least one high-risk allele were more likely to report LOC than those with the wild-type allele. Since *FTO* is highly expressed in hypothalamic regions important for appetite regulation, the relationship between LOC and appetitive hormones warrants investigation. However, only one pediatric study has examined leptin, an adipose-tissue-derived hormone that influences energy homeostasis, eating behaviors, and appetite regulation. Findings indicate higher levels of fasting serum leptin in youth with LOC eating compared to those without LOC. Elevated leptin levels may suggest either a persistent compensation mechanism in response to LOC eating episodes, or may reflect leptin resistance, which in turn might promote sensations of hunger and LOC eating. There are limited data on LOC and components of the metabolic syndrome. Some, but not all, data show a link between insulin resistance and LOC. Recent data suggest that youth with LOC may have higher systolic blood pressure and higher low-density lipoprotein cholesterol than youth without LOC.

There is some preliminary evidence for neural correlates of LOC eating. A functional magnetic resonance imaging (fMRI) study of overweight female adolescents found that, following a social rejection task, girls with LOC experienced blunting in the ventromedial prefrontal cortex compared to girls without LOC, who experienced *increased* activity, a response that might be expected in healthy samples. Moreover, only among girls with LOC, activity of the fusiform face area was positively associated with intake during a test meal immediately following the social rejection task. Such data support the notion that LOC may be promoted by neural mechanisms similar to those of social anxiety models in youth.

Psychological Correlates

The vast majority of research on pediatric LOC has been in the area of psychological associations. The temperamental trait of impulsivity appears to confer vulnerability for LOC. Compared to youth without LOC eating, those who report LOC also report lower self-directedness, which is indicative of the tendency for behavior to be driven by reactive impulses rather than thoughtful, goal-directed decision making. The temperamental trait of *negative urgency*—the tendency to act rashly or impulsively in response to distress—has been associated with self-reported LOC eating. Heightened trait reward sensitivity, especially in relation to palatable food, has also been linked to pediatric LOC. Youth with LOC are prone to eat in response to external food cues, such as the sight or smell of food, and LOC severity is associated with tendencies to have a strong desire to eat and preoccupation with food. Data also show that youth with LOC frequently report a range of disinhibited eating traits, such as emotional eating and eating in the absence of hunger.

Negative affect is also a distinguishing feature of youth with LOC eating; youth with LOC tend to report more symptoms of depression and anxiety and lower self-esteem compared to those without LOC. Data also consistently demonstrate that youth with LOC eating report greater disordered eating cognitions than do youth without LOC. Clinical overvaluation of weight and shape is reported by a substantial subset (~50%) of those with LOC. Yet it should be noted that data across studies suggest that elevations in all of these psychological variables typically do not reach clinical significance.

Behavioral Phenotype

Pediatric LOC eating has been phenotyped in several laboratory studies. Data are mixed on whether youth with LOC consume more total calories in the laboratory, and findings may vary based on sex, age, and body weight status. By contrast, youth with LOC tend to consume meals that comprise more calories from carbohydrates and fewer calories from protein than their peers who do not report LOC. Additionally, youth with LOC consistently tend to consume more highly palatable, energy-dense foods in the laboratory and based on self-reports.

Supporting several negative affect theories of binge eating (e.g., escape theory), in laboratory settings, not only do youth with LOC generally report greater premeal state negative affect than youth without LOC, but such mood states typically predict greater subsequent consumption of palatable foods and carbohydrates. Consistent with models of affect regulation, some laboratory studies found that overall reductions in negative affect occur from pre- to postmeal.

Differences in familial attachments and interactions also provide support for a distinct LOC phenotype. For instance, children with LOC frequently exhibit insecure attachment styles relative to non-LOC controls. Observational studies found that relative to those without LOC, children with LOC were subject to more critical comments about their eating, weight, and shape from parents, and general familial discord in both labora-tory and natural environments. These parent–child interaction patterns were associated with observed dysregulated eating patterns in the laboratory. In a separate laboratory study, youth with LOC eating reported a greater degree of hunger, more hostility, and greater preoccupation with family issues when an internalized family image was activated in comparison to nonclinical controls without LOC. It is possible that the interpersonal model may account for these relationships, such that unsatisfying familial relationships give rise to feelings of negative affect that precipitate LOC eating.

Prospective Data
Predictors

Numerous longitudinal studies have examined predictors of LOC eating behaviors in pediatric samples. Several have shown that weight-based teasing and critical comments by family members are robust risk factors for the onset of LOC eating. Similarly, longi-tudinal studies found that lower levels of perceived parental care and role differentiation within the family were predictive of LOC onset during adolescence. Additionally, social isolation and childhood experiences of peer teasing and bullying, particularly about weight and shape, are predictive of the initiation of LOC eating. Longitudinal studies in adolescent girls suggest that low social support is related to LOC eating onset. Depressive symptoms and negative self-esteem during early adolescence predict the onset and persistence of LOC eating during later adolescence and young adulthood. Psychosocial factors have also been found to predict the exacerbation or persistence of LOC eating patterns, for instance, trait negative urgency and insecure attachment style.

Existing data consistently support the dual-pathway model (i.e., that dietary restraint aimed to achieve a cultural "thin ideal" and negative affect interact to promote binge eating) to explain risk for LOC eating in pediatric samples. A large cohort study of pre-adolescent girls and boys found that a composite measure of thin ideal internalization and perceived social pressures about weight was predictive of the onset of LOC eating at 2-year follow-up. Perceived sociocultural pressure to be thin or to lose weight, as well as body dissatisfaction, were related to the subsequent onset of LOC eating in adolescents. In a prospective epidemiological study of adolescents, females reporting that they were trying to look like persons in the media were more likely to develop recurrent LOC eating. Similarly, parents' or peers' modeling of body image dissatisfaction, dieting, or disordered eating behavior predicts the onset of LOC eating in adolescent girls. Prospective tests of the dual-pathway model in children and adolescents provide support for the proposed mechanisms. However, most of these data are limited to primarily non-Hispanic white samples. Given that pediatric studies show that nonwhite Hispanic and black youth are less likely to ascribe to the "thin ideal," mechanistic data are required to elucidate how underrepresented groups develop LOC eating.

Course and Outcome

Following initial LOC onset, the natural course of LOC eating appears to involve both remission and relapse throughout childhood and adolescence. While the presence of LOC eating *ever* (in one's lifetime) has been associated with adverse outcomes, only about 50% of youth with LOC go on to experience persistent and exacerbated LOC eating patterns during middle to late adolescence and beyond. Persistent LOC eating throughout childhood has been shown to transition to partial- or full-syndrome binge eating disorder. Despite a somewhat variable course, a distinct subset of youth with LOC appears to be vulnerable to a persistent and exacerbated course of symptoms.

Across longitudinal studies, reports of LOC eating in childhood and adolescence consistently predict excess body weight and adiposity gain, as well as obesity onset. Moreover, LOC has been shown to predict worsening of metabolic syndrome components, including increased triglycerides, after accounting for the contribution of body weight gain, as well as central adiposity. With regard to psychological outcomes, over time, youth with LOC are at greater risk than those without LOC to experience a worsening of mood symptoms and the development of partial- and full-syndrome binge eating disorder.

Future Directions

Despite a considerable literature supporting the pernicious nature of pediatric LOC eating, the current data render more questions than answers. Given that approximately half of youth who report LOC eating remit over time, more specific characterization of the behavior is required. An important area for future exploration will be determination of which variables interact to promote persistence or exacerbation of LOC eating over time. Another important area for future research will involve disentangling LOC eating from other appetitive traits and behaviors. Indeed, numerous overlapping disinhibited eating conceptualizations are being studied around the globe in isolation of one another. It remains unclear to what extent LOC differs from other behaviors, including, but not limited to, emotional eating, eating in the absence of hunger, and food addiction. Taken together, and consistent with calls for more precise models of psychiatric diagnoses and presentations, LOC eating requires more accurate endophenotyping. Indeed, a number of diagnostic conceptualizations of LOC and related eating patterns that have been proposed may better predict which youth require early identification and intervention. Moreover, given its focus on underlying neural circuits, genetics, and physiology in the context of development, the Research Domain Criteria project may play an important role in clarifying LOC eating behaviors. It is likely that LOC eating is a manifestation of disinhibited eating behaviors that are driven by physical, psychological, and environmental factors that occur along a developmental trajectory. As children grow older, a subset with LOC will experience a worsening of symptoms that result in adverse psychiatric outcomes such as binge-type eating disorders and excessive weight gain and obesity.

Conclusions

The clearest initial manifestation of binge eating appears to be LOC eating. While a proportion of youth with LOC eating experience spontaneous remission, for many others, LOC eating persists and worsens throughout development. In susceptible youth, the presence of LOC increases risk for adverse physical and psychological outcomes, including the onset of obesity, full-syndrome eating disorders, and mood disturbances. Future research is required to better characterize children at greatest risk for adverse outcomes.

Suggested Reading

Hilbert, A., Hartmann, A. S., Czaja, J., & Schoebi, D. (2013). Natural course of preadolescent loss of control eating. *Journal of Abnormal Psychology, 22,* 684–693.—A community sample of children (ages 8–13 years) with and without LOC eating was assessed every 6 months over a 2-year follow-up. LOC eating predicted a partial binge eating disorder but not depressive symptoms.

Shomaker, L. B., Tanofsky-Kraff, M., Elliott, C., Wolkoff, L. E., Columbo, K. M., Ranzenhofer, L. M., et al. (2010). Salience of loss of control for pediatric binge episodes: Does size really matter? *International Journal of Eating Disorders, 43,* 707–716.—Among a sample of healthy boys and girls (ages 8–12 years), this study supports the notion that size of a binge episode is less salient than the experience of loss of control for distinguishing youth along physical, psychological and eating-related parameters.

Sonneville, K. R., Horton, N. J., Micali, N., Crosby, R. D., Swanson, S. A., Solmi, F., et al. (2013). Longitudinal associations between binge eating and overeating and adverse outcomes among adolescents and young adults: Does loss of control matter? *JAMA Pediatrics, 167*(2), 149–155.—A very large sample of 9- to 15-year-old boys and girls were surveyed every year or every other year from 1996 to 2006. Results showed that those with binge eating, but not overeating, were at greater odds for overweight/obesity onset and high depressive symptoms over time.

Tanofsky-Kraff, M., Goossens, L., Eddy, K. T., Ringham, R., Goldschmidt, A. S., Yanovski, S. Z., et al. (2007). A multi-site investigation of binge eating behaviors in children and adolescents. *Journal of Consulting and Clinical Psychology, 75,* 901–913.—In data from four U.S. and one European research site, boys and girls with reported LOC were distinguished from those without LOC with regard to qualitative physical, behavioral, contextual, and emotional aspects of eating episodes.

Tanofsky-Kraff, M., McDuffie, J. R., Yanovski, S. Z., Kozlosky, M., Schvey, N. A., Shomaker, L. B., et al. (2009). Laboratory assessment of the food intake of children and adolescents with loss of control eating. *American Journal of Clinical Nutrition, 89*(3), 738–745.—Healthy community boys and girls (ages 8–17 years) who reported LOC eating consumed more calories from carbohydrate, less calories from protein, and more highly palatable foods than youth without LOC eating during laboratory test meals.

Tanofsky-Kraff, M., Shomaker, L. B., Roza, C. A., Wolkoff, L. E., Columbo, K. M., Racite, G., et al. (2011). A prospective study of pediatric loss of control eating and psychological outcomes. *Journal of Abnormal Psychology, 120,* 108–118.—Compared to preadolescent boys and girls without reported LOC eating, those with LOC eating were at greater risk of developing partial- or full-syndrome binge eating disorder and worsening mood symptoms 5 years later.

Tanofsky-Kraff, M., Yanovski, S. Z., Schvey, N. A., Olsen, C. H., Gustafson, J. & Yanovski, J. A. (2009). A prospective study of loss of control eating for body weight gain in children at high risk for adult obesity. *International Journal of Eating Disorders, 42,* 26–30.—Preadolescent boys and girls who reported LOC eating had significantly higher BMI gain per year over a 4.5-year interval than youth without LOC eating.

Vannucci, A., Nelson, E. E., Bongiorno, D. M., Pine, D. S., Yanovski, J. A., & Tanofsky-Kraff, M. (2015). Behavioral and neurodevelopmental precursors to binge-type eating disorders: Support for the role of negative valence systems. *Psychological Medicine, 45*(14), 2921–2936.—This review article provides evidence for LOC eating as a precursor to binge-type eating disorders with a Research Domain Criteria negative valence system conceptualization.

20

Sociocultural Influences on Body Image and Eating Disturbance

ANNE E. BECKER

Diversity in body ideals across time, geography, and other kinds of social contexts is exhaustively documented in the scientific literature. Likewise, the prevalence of eating disorders has shown remarkable historical and cross-cultural variation. This fluctuation in the setting of shifting social mores and values has at various times raised the question of whether either anorexia nervosa or bulimia nervosa was uniquely associated with modern, Western cultures. Additional evidence of elevated risk for body dissatisfaction and disordered eating within some populations undergoing social transition through urbanization, economic development, transnational migration, and other modernization has been salient to understanding the complexity of pathogenesis and maintenance of eating disorders, as well as informing preventive strategies.

Sociocultural influences on eating disorder risk figure importantly in models that link diffusion and adoption of values and norms for body weight and shape, body dissatisfaction, and eating disturbances. Such conceptual models do not exclude the contributions of other social, biological, and psychological vulnerabilities as risk factors, moderators, and mediators, nor do they overwrite the consensus that eating disorders have multifactorial etiology. The relevance of sociocultural influences to eating disorders extends well beyond pathogenesis and maintenance factors, however, since they are also germane to the distribution of associated health burdens, differential access to care, challenges to diagnostic assessment, and therapeutic strategies.

Sociocultural influences on body image and eating disturbances fall into three principal domains. First, cultural factors shape body experience, body practices, aesthetic ideals, and dietary patterns through their configuration of core values and premises about selfhood. Second, local social structural factors mediate exposures to ideas, values, images, and products associated with outside cultural groups. For instance, regional political and economic events may result in urban and transnational migration; food insecurity; and ethnic, religious, or racial discrimination and/or differential access to housing and health services. And finally, large-scale global processes have provided the infrastructure for increased connectivity through advances in communications technology, transportation, and the extended reach of multinational corporations in marketing products and services. The latter processes promote the accelerated and widespread diffusion of a particular set of ideas, images, and values associated formerly with modern "Western" cultures, but increasingly with uptake among youth. These mechanisms, in turn, multiply the diversity of cultural exposures and social environments that shape identity, experience, and behavior. Culture is no longer fixed to place, nor is social identity fixed over time. The complex and multifold interactions across each of these domains also obviate a simple correspondence between any particular ethnic or social identity and body image or eating disturbances. For these reasons, it is intellectually and pragmatically most informative to consider how sociocultural factors may influence body image and eating disturbance as processes operating at local, regional, and sometimes global levels, rather than as characteristics inhering in any particular community, population, or sociodemographic group.

Cultural Diversity in Body Ideals

A robust anthropological and sociological literature documents considerable cultural diversity in aesthetic ideals, body practices, and embodied experience. This variation extends well beyond body size and shape ideals, encompassing dimensions such as how the body is adorned, inscribed, remolded, dressed, and otherwise cultivated and presented, as well as preferences relating to facial features, complexion, and hair. Posture and movement are also culturally scripted and imbued with social meanings. Although there are some striking commonalities in beauty ideals across widely different cultures, substantial variation illustrates their local contextualization. In addition, ethnographic evidence also demonstrates how body shape ideals reflect and encode core cultural values and draw on local symbols of social prestige. Because of the role that the drive for thinness and body dissatisfaction play in the pathogenesis and maintenance of eating disturbance, cultural variation in body shape ideals has been a particular focus of inquiry on differential risk across ethnic and cultural contexts.

Converging lines of evidence indicate that as social norms and exposures change, so does risk for body dissatisfaction and eating pathology. Studies reporting elevated risk for disordered eating in the setting of transnational migration, urbanization, and modernization are consistent with this premise. Other observed temporal changes in eating pathology concomitant with economic development across distinct cultural contexts lend credence to the hypothesis that eating disorders are linked to cultures of "modernity" rather than to a specific region or tradition. For example, historians have traced the emergence of the female body ideal of slenderness in 20th-century U.S. popular culture from the previous social valuation of corpulence within a nexus of concurrent influences, including the beauty industry, the ready-to-wear fashion industry, and the increasingly broad distribution of a narrow range of body shapes through print and televised media that have been presented as ideal, routinized, and associated with social prestige. The migration of body weight and shape ideals for women toward a broad cultural preference for thinness coincided with increased prevalence of the eating disorders anorexia nervosa and bulimia nervosa, both with core psychopathology relating to body image.

Changes in the prevalence and presentation of eating disorders in China since the 1980s also illustrate an association of social change with risk. Beginning at that time, Sing Lee and colleagues described a prevalent local variant of an eating disturbance characterized by low weight and entrenched restrictive pattern eating, but without the intense fear of fatness associated with the conventional presentation of anorexia nervosa (AN). They demonstrated the clinical severity of this phenotype and argued that the alternative rationales for dietary restriction were more salient than fat phobia in the local cultural context. Over the ensuing decades, they documented a proportional decline in the presentation of the "non-fat-phobic AN" cases, whereas conventional presentations of AN and also bulimia nervosa (BN) became relatively more common. These shifts were attributed to the emerging salience of thinness and appearance among Hong Kong Chinese women.

Similarly, a series of coordinated studies within a small-scale indigenous population in Fiji supports increasing risk for eating pathology among adolescent women that corresponds with rapid modernization over the past 25 years. Traditional body ideals for robust size and weight in Fiji reflected the social prestige associated with a community's generosity and capacity to procure and distribute food. Weight gain was viewed as an indicator of social connection and a number of cultural practices reinforced feasting and weight gain and also constrained personal agency over appetite and weight control. Eating disorders were absent from the indigenous nosology and rare, if present at all. However, following a period of brisk social and economic development, which included electrification of rural villages and the introduction of broadcast television, eating pathology began to emerge. Social norms for weight and body shape ideals changed noticeably. That is, in contrast to the preference for robust body weight rooted in long-standing local traditions, Fijian women started to express admiration for the lifestyles and slender body size associated with characters portrayed in television dramas. As this social norm changed, there was a concomitant uptick of dieting and, increasingly, young women purged to manage their weight. Distinctive patterning of eating disturbances in both Fiji and Hong Kong further illustrates the social contextualization of symptoms.

Social Identities, Body Image, and Eating Disturbances

Whereas some studies report variation in body image and eating disturbances across major ethnic groups in the United States, others support clinically important commonalities. However, the frequent conflation of heterogeneous ethnic identities with socially constructed broad categories (e.g., those corresponding to major U.S. census groups) limits the relevance of these studies. Social identity, furthermore, comprises numerous additional dimensions, including gender, religion, class, occupation, and generation, any of which may underpin body image, perceived social norms, values, and help seeking in the health care sector. Social identities may be plural and concurrent, and assimilation to a perceived dominant culture, global culture, or postmigration culture may be orthogonal to retention of aspects of ethnic identity tied to a community of origin. Notwithstanding cultural patterning of body experience and body ideals, there is epidemiological evidence of comparable risk for eating disorders across major ethnic groups. However, evidence of clinician bias and significant variation in service utilization across ethnic groups raises concerns about ethnic disparities in access to care.

The Changing Demographic Profile of Eating Disorders

AN emerged into the public consciousness as a disorder associated with young women who were white and affluent. Hilde Bruch's early influential work drew attention to the unusual epidemiological footprint of AN at a time when psychiatric epidemiologists, medical anthropologists, and cultural psychiatrists were deeply engaged in intellectual debate over the culturally particular patterning of mental disorders relative to universal commonalities. Perhaps few other mental disorders in the DSM have excited as much academic interest in the sociocultural patterning of illness as the eating disorders. This interest, in turn, has arguably had substantial influence on the direction of scientific inquiry, as well as clinical and lay understandings of these disorders. Indeed, a previous iteration of the DSM had suggested that AN is uniquely culture-bound to the "West." This conceptual framing was later revisited, but not without some entrenchment of clinical stereotypes about the relation of ethnicity and culture to risk.

Indeed, much of the seminal literature on cultural differences emerged from studies on immigrant populations moving to high-income countries and examination of the impacts of encounters with cultural exposures in the setting of acculturation, assimilation, and intergenerational conflict. Although these impacts are by no means uniform, the aggregate data support an association between novel cultural encounters through acculturation and exposure to social norms characterizing modernity with greater risk of eating disturbance among young women. Despite previous documentation of the regional variation in eating disorders, epidemiological, ethnographic, and clinical reports also support their broadening global distribution and associated health burdens. These data also provide a counternarrative to prior assumptions about the limited geographical distribution and public health relevance of eating disorders in the Global South.

Diffusion of "Global Cultural" Exposures and Migration of Social Norms

The shifting global epidemiology of eating disorders, in turn, raises critical questions about whether wide diffusion of certain cultural exposures, including ideas, images, values, and commercial products—enabled by communications technologies as well as increasing global movement and transnational marketing—also broadly promote risk factors for eating disorders, such as body dissatisfaction and dieting. Major etiological models implicate the mass media, among other social-contextual influences, in promulgating valuation and internalization of a thin ideal and social comparison, leading to body dissatisfaction and eating disturbances in some vulnerable individuals. Taken together, cross-sectional and experimental studies support an association between media-based exposures and eating disturbance risk. Thus, the globalizing diffusion through the mass media and social media of particular ideas and values—many derived from historically Western cultures and capitalist societies—may propagate cultural exposures that bear on risk for body image and eating disturbance. These might particularly impact frequent users, including youth, who increasingly have new access to the Internet through mobile devices. Moreover, social media usage is rapidly impacting how young people socialize and position themselves within an increasingly remote community. Cultural critics argue that new capacities to post and edit photographs and, in turn, solicit and garner feedback from peers and strangers, potentially amplify effects of social comparison, with uncertain but concerning relevance to body dissatisfaction and eating disorder risk.

Implications of Social Factors for Care Delivery

In addition to implications for etiological and maintaining factors, the influence of social norms has relevance to preventive and therapeutic interventions. Clinicians should be aware that eating disorders can occur in individuals from all ethnic, cultural, and social backgrounds. That being said, there may be marked social diversity in help-seeking patterns for eating disorders, and individuals from certain ethnic/minority groups in the United States, previously thought to be at lower risk, appear to be at higher risk for nonreceipt of care. Clinicians should also be aware that social identity comprises multiple dimensions, including nationality, religion, gender, education, ethnicity, and region. Some individuals endorse plural and/or hybrid ethnic identities that may, in turn, emerge developmentally and in relation to their immediate and remote peer and social networks. Clinicians should avoid assuming that any particular ethnic or social group is "culturally protected" from an eating disorder, since this could result in clinical nondetection or adversely impact a patient's willingness to disclose symptoms.

Since body image and eating disturbances may draw some significance from their departure from local social norms, diagnostic assessment will be enhanced by familiarity with these norms and values. Given that comprehensive and up-to-date knowledge of the numerous ethnic, cultural, and social identifies within a multicultural setting may not always be possible, clinicians should understand how to engage clinically relevant social identity with a more generalizable and patient-centered approach, which can serve to elicit the relevant social context of the patient's symptoms and illness experience. Few existing data guide adaptations of therapeutic approaches, but dissonance-based eating disorder prevention may be uniformly effective across ethnically diverse participants. Additionally, the context of the patient's social environment governing family meals, weight expectations and autonomy, and valuation of body ideals will have clinical relevance to how therapeutic strategies are deployed. Patient adherence to treatment may also be influenced by stigma perceived in the clinical encounter.

Conclusions

Cross-cultural variation in eating disorder risk is consistent with major etiological models for eating disorders premised on links among body dissatisfaction, drive for thinness, dieting, and eating pathology. Various dimensions of body image and culturally sanctioned dietary and bodily practices are closely tied to local social norms, values, and constraints. Body shape ideals vary across cultures, as do the salient dimensions of body image and body satisfaction. Mass media and social media provide platforms for global diffusion and homogenization of images and ideas that may promote and reinforce unhealthful body ideals pertinent to eating disturbance risk. In addition, these platforms enable new opportunities for and experiences of social comparison. Evidence indicates that the footprint of eating disorders across world regions may be changing. Despite considerable diversity in the presentation and prevalence of eating disorders across a variety of social contexts, eating disorders now have broad global distribution, including in low- and middle-income countries.

Whereas numerous studies have drawn attention to ethnicity-based distinctions in body image and eating disorders risk, social identities are frequently plural, hybrid, and in flux. To the extent that risk factors for eating disorders—such as body dissatisfaction, internalization of a thin ideal, and dieting—may be increasingly diffuse and shared across culturally diverse communities, clinicians should be aware that individuals across cultural, ethnic, and social groups may present with body image disturbance or an eating disorder, and that social identity may also impact symptom presentation, help seeking, and therapeutic alliance.

Suggested Reading

Becker, A. E. (Ed.). (2004). New global perspectives on eating disorders [Special issue]. *Culture, Medicine and Psychiatry, 28*(4).—A collection of articles describing emerging evidence of eating disorders risk across a variety of cultural settings undergoing modernization and westernization, including Belize, Fiji, South Africa, and Japan.

Becker, A. E., Fay, K. E., Agnew-Blais, J., Khan, A. N., Striegel-Moore, R. H., & Gilman, S. E. (2011). Social network media exposure and adolescent eating pathology in Fiji. *British Journal of Psychiatry, 198*(1), 43–50.—Presents study findings linking Western cultural exposures and secondhand television exposure with greater risk of eating disturbance among adolescent *iTaukei* women in Fiji.

Grabe, S., Ward, L. M., & Hyde, J. S. (2008). The role of the media in body image concerns among women: A meta-analysis of experimental and correlational studies. *Psychological Bulletin, 134*, 460–476.—A meta-analysis demonstrating the association between mass media exposure and body image disturbance.

Lee, S., Ng, K. L., Kwok, K., & Fung, C. (2010). The changing profile of eating disorders at a tertiary psychiatric clinic in Hong Kong (1987–2007). *International Journal of Eating Disorders, 43*(4), 307–314.—Describes increases in the proportions of BN and fat-phobic presentations of AN in Hong Kong Chinese patients with eating disorders over two decades, emphasizing convergence with patterns seen in Western clinical settings.

Levine, M. P., & Murnen, S. K. (2009). "Everybody knows that mass media are/are not [pick one] a cause of eating disorders": A critical review of evidence for a causal link between media, negative body image, and disordered eating in females. *Journal of Social and Clinical Psychology, 28*(1), 9–42.—An erudite discussion of evidence for a model linking mass media exposure to risk for eating disorders.

Marques, L., Alegria, M., Becker, A. E., Chen, C. N., Fang, A., Chosak, A., et al. (2011). Comparative prevalence, correlates of impairment, and service utilization for eating disorders across US ethnic groups: Implications for reducing ethnic disparities in health care access for eating disorders. *International Journal of Eating Disorders, 44*(5), 412–420.—Presents an analysis of data drawn from the NIMH Collaborative Psychiatric Epidemiology Surveys, showing that the prevalence of AN and BED are similar across major U.S. ethnic groups, whereas utilization of mental health services among those with a lifetime history of an eating disorder was lower for ethnic/minority groups than for non-Latino whites.

Nasser, M., Katzman, M., & Gordon, R. A. (Eds.). (2001). *Eating disorders and cultures in transition*. Hove, UK: Psychology Press.—An edited volume examining how economic and social transition have had a local impact on eating disorders across diverse global settings.

Perloff, R. M. (2014). Social media effects on young women's body image concerns: Theoretical perspectives and an agenda for research. *Sex Roles, 71*(11–12), 363–377.—Discusses a framework for future investigation of the impact of social media on eating disturbance among young women.

Swami, V., Frederick, D. A., Aavik, T., Alcalay, L., Allik, J., Anderson, D., et al. (2010). The attractive female body weight and female body dissatisfaction in 26 countries across 10 world regions: Results of the International Body Project I. *Personality and Social Psychology Bulletin, 36*(3), 309–325.—Presents comparative data across 26 countries demonstrating cultural differences in body weight ideals and body satisfaction.

Van den Berg, P., Thompson, J. K., Obremski-Brandon, K., & Coovert, M. (2002). The Tripartite Influence model of body image and eating disturbance: A covariance structure modeling investigation testing the mediational role of appearance comparison. *Journal of Psychosomatic Research, 53*(5), 1007–1020.—Describes and presents support for a model relating social influences to body image and eating disturbances.

Stigma, Discrimination, and Obesity

REBECCA M. PUHL

Substantial evidence has documented stigma and discrimination against individuals with obesity. Weight-based inequities occur in multiple life domains, including employment, health care, education, the mass media, and close interpersonal relationships. Estimates from national studies indicate that weight discrimination has increased in recent decades and is the second most prevalent form of discrimination reported by women, and the third most common among men. Experiences of weight stigmatization can lead to a range of adverse consequences for the emotional and physical health of those who are affected, some of which may reinforce obesity and create barriers to improving weight-related health. Research has begun to examine policy remedies that could help reduce societal weight discrimination.

Weight Discrimination in Employment

Several decades of research indicate that the workplace is a common setting in which weight discrimination occurs. Employees who have obesity are vulnerable to multiple employment inequities because of their weight, such as being subjected to unfair hiring practices, lower wages, fewer promotion prospects, stigma from coworkers, and job termination. Experimental studies have consistently demonstrated that job applicants who appear to be obese are evaluated more negatively and are less likely to be hired than thinner applicants with identical qualifications. Weight stigmatization against job applicants with obesity has been shown to have a stronger negative effect on hiring practices than on any other performance outcomes.

Obesity wage penalties have been documented in population-based studies as a persistent form of weight discrimination in employment. Recent evidence indicates that among white women, compared to women with a body mass index (BMI) in the "normal" range, those whose BMIs indicate overweight or obese experienced 9 andr 15% decreases in wages, respectively. Among white men, an 11-unit increase in BMI has been documented to result in significant wage reductions (as much as 50%). Obesity wage penalties have also been documented in blacks and Hispanics, with recent evidence showing that overweight Hispanic men in some occupations have as much as a 17% reduction in hourly wages compared to thinner counterparts. Among multiple racial groups, wage reductions appear particularly pronounced for jobs that involve interpersonal and social interactions.

Reported experiences of weight discrimination in the workplace suggest that these inequities are indeed prevalent. Nationally representative studies of Americans show that compared to nonoverweight persons, individuals with obesity are 37 times more likely to report employment discrimination, and those with severe obesity are 100 times more likely to report these experiences. Research examining experiences of stigmatization among women with overweight or obesity found that 54% reported being subjected to weight bias from coworkers and 43% reported such bias from employers, with many indicating that these experiences had occurred multiple times.

Weight Stigmatization in Health Care

Medical professionals are not immune to societal weight bias, and recent comparisons indicate that expressions of weight bias are as prevalent among physicians as the general public. Research has consistently demonstrated negative weight-based stereotypes and bias by medical providers across a range of specialty areas, including primary care physicians, endocrinologists, cardiologists, nurses, dietitians, mental health professionals, and medical students. Common stereotypes include views that patients with obesity are lazy, lacking in discipline and willpower, noncompliant with treatment, less adherent to medications, and at fault for their weight. Recent evidence suggests that some negative weight biases have worsened, rather than improved, over time, even among researchers and health professionals who specialize in obesity.

Weight bias expressed by health care providers can interfere with health care delivery for patients with obesity. Physicians have reported less respect for patients with obesity and less desire to help these patients, and indicate that treating obesity is "more annoying" and a greater waste of their time than providing care to thinner patients. In addition, compared to interactions with thinner patients, some doctors spend less time in appointments, provide less education about health, and are more reluctant to perform certain procedures with patients who have obesity.

In line with these findings, some patients with obesity perceive that they have been stigmatized about their weight in the health care setting. These experiences include patient reports of lack of empathy from providers, negative judgment and/or blame for their weight by doctors, attribution of unrelated presenting problems to their weight, experiencing distress from comments that providers make about their weight, as well as physical barriers, such as lack of appropriate-size medical equipment that is functional for their body size (e.g., scales, blood pressure cuffs, patient gowns). Patients who perceive themselves as targets of weight stigma indicate reluctance to discuss their weight concerns, are more likely to switch doctors, and avoid future medical appointments. Reduced health care utilization as a result of weight bias (including avoidance of preventive health care services) has been particularly documented among women with obesity.

Weight Stigmatization in Education Settings

Youth with obesity are vulnerable to weight stigma in the form of pervasive teasing, bullying, and victimization. Research shows that peers are the most frequent perpetrators of weight-based bullying, and that school is the most frequent venue in which these incidents occur. Recent studies indicate that students, parents, and teachers perceive weight-based bullying as one of the most frequent forms of bullying that youth experience at school. In 2011, the National Education Association issued a nationwide survey of over 5,000 educators, showing that teachers considered weight-based bullying to be more problematic than bullying because of a student's gender, sexual orientation, or disability. Even among ethnic/minority students who experience race-based bullying, weight-based harassment has been reported as the most prevalent form of peer harassment experienced by girls, and the second most common form of harassment reported by boys.

Of concern, adolescents with obesity report that their classroom teachers and coaches are additional perpetrators of weight-based victimization in the school setting. Experimental research also indicates that educators have lower expectations for heavier students than for thinner students (despite being portrayed as having identical skills and abilities), including views that students with obesity have inferior reasoning, cooperation, and social skills compared to thinner peers. Weight stigma from educators may extend to postsecondary education, where graduate students may be less likely to be accepted to graduate programs after the in-person interview process if they are obese compared to thinner applicants, even after accounting for students' grade point averages and letters of recommendation.

Weight Stigma in the Media

Stigmatizing portrayals of individuals with obesity are common in television shows, movies, advertisements, news media, and even in youth programming. Characters who appear to be overweight or obese in television and film are often ridiculed, depicted as engaging in stereotypical behaviors (e.g., eating or bingeing), and less likely to have positive social interactions. In youth-targeted media, overweight characters are depicted as being aggressive, antisocial, evil, unattractive, unfriendly, disliked by others, and eating food compared to thinner characters, who are more often portrayed as sociable, kind, successful, popular, and attractive.

News media also reinforce weight bias and stereotypes. Research shows that obesity is frequently attributed to personal responsibility rather than to societal causes in news reports, and that remedies for obesity are more often framed as the responsibility of the individual rather than the need to change societal-level factors. Visual portrayals of obesity in the news media can additionally reinforce weight stigma beyond written news content. Research analyzing news reports about obesity have found that more than two-thirds of images accompanying news reports portrayed obese children and adults in a stigmatizing manner. Experimental studies additionally show that viewing these types of stigmatizing images leads to increased weight bias, regardless of the gender or race of the individual portrayed in the image. Furthermore, studies with youth have demonstrated that television viewing predicts negative weight stereotyping, and that media exposure is positively associated with stigmatizing attitudes toward obese youth. Taken together, this evidence indicates that the media is an influential source that can reinforce bias against people with obesity.

Health Consequences of Weight Stigma

Children and adults who experience weight stigma are vulnerable to numerous consequences affecting their psychological and physical health. Psychological consequences include increased risk of depression, anxiety, low self-esteem, poor body image, substance abuse, and suicidal thoughts and behaviors. Many of these outcomes persist even after accounting for factors such as BMI, obesity onset, gender, and age, indicating that negative psychological consequences emerge from stigmatizing experiences rather than from obesity per se.

Experiencing weight stigma also increases vulnerability to unhealthy behaviors that can contribute to weight gain and increase risk for obesity, including binge eating, maladaptive weight control practices, increased calorie intake, avoidance of exercise, and lower motivation for physical activity. Emerging evidence has additionally demonstrated heighted physiological reactivity in response to experiences of weight stigmatization, including heightened cortisol reactivity, C-reactive proteins, and blood pressure, as well as harmful effects of waist-to-hip ratio on glycemic control.

Recent longitudinal studies suggest that these health consequences of weight stigma may have more direct links to obesity and weight gain. In a nationally representative sample of over 6,000 adults from the Health and Retirement Study, those who reported weight discrimination (but not other forms of discrimination) were 2.5–3 times more likely to develop obesity or remain obese over time compared to individuals who did not experience weight discrimination, regardless of their baseline BMI. A study of 2,944 adults from the English Longitudinal Study of Aging similarly found that individuals who reported experiencing weight discrimination had greater odds of developing obesity and experienced significant increases in weight and waist circumference, regardless of baseline BMI.

Adverse health consequences resulting from experiences of weight stigma can reduce quality of life and create considerable obstacles in efforts to effectively prevent and treat obesity. This evidence suggests that weight stigma and discrimination represent a public health issue and should be prioritized alongside efforts to address this problem as a societal injustice.

Potential Legal and Policy Remedies

Given the pervasiveness of weight stigma and discrimination, legislative remedies may be necessary to help reduce societal weight discrimination. Currently no federal laws in the United States prohibit weight discrimination, and only one state (Michigan), and six U.S. localities currently have civil/human rights laws or municipal/police codes in place to protect individuals from discrimination due to weight. Despite the lack of legal options available to address weight discrimination, recent studies indicate increasing public support for policy strategies to prohibit weight discrimination. National studies show that 75% of Americans favor laws to prohibit weight discrimination in the workplace, and the majority also support extending disability protection for individuals with obesity and adding body weight as a protected class in existing state civil rights statutes. Public support for these measures has remained consistent, and in some cases has increased, in recent years.

Proposed policy strategies to address weight-based bullying in youth have also received considerable public support. Recent national estimates show consistent and high support from Americans (as much as 88%) to implement school-based antibullying policies that protect students from being bullied about their weight, and over 66% support strengthening existing state antibullying laws to include specific protections against weight-based bullying. Parental support for these measures remains high regardless of their child's body weight status, suggesting that there is widespread recognition that weight-based bullying is a problem in need of broad remedies.

This research evidence documenting substantial public support for policy-level solutions to address weight-based bullying and discrimination suggests that one of the key catalysts for motivating political will for policy change is sufficiently established. It will be important for policy research to continue in this area, to identify and determine legislative and policy measures that are most feasible to implement and likely to have the highest impact on reducing weight-based inequities.

Conclusions

Several decades of evidence indicate consistent stigma and discrimination against children and adults with obesity in major life areas of employment, medical care, education, and the mass media. Weight-based inequities and prejudice in these settings reinforce broader societal weight stigma and lead to numerous negative health consequences for those who are affected. These consequences can create significant obstacles in efforts to prevent and treat obesity. Taken together, existing evidence indicates that broad-scale efforts to implement stigma reduction strategies are warranted. This will not only require stigma reduction interventions targeted to different settings (e.g., education and training of medical professionals to reduce weight-based stigma in health care), but it may also necessitate broader policy initiatives to help prohibit systemic societal weight-based discrimination and prejudice that otherwise remain pervasive and impair quality of life for so many who are affected.

Suggested Reading

Andreyeva, T., Puhl, R. M., & Brownell, K. D. (2008). Changes in perceived weight discrimination among Americans, 1995–1996 through 2004–2006. *Obesity, 16*(5), 1129–1134.— Nationally representative study documenting increases in perceived weight discrimination.

Bucchianeri, M. M., Eisenberg, M. E., & Neumark-Sztainer, D. (2013). Weightism, racism, classism, and sexism: Shared forms of harassment in adolescents. *Journal of Adolescent Health, 53*(1), 47–53.—Weight-based harassment is reported to be among the most common forms of harassment among ethnic/minority youth.

Hatzenbuehler, M. L., Keyes, K. M., & Hasin, D. S. (2009). Associations between perceived weight discrimination and the prevalence of psychiatric disorders in the general population. *Obesity, 17*(11), 2033–2039.—Perceived weight discrimination associated with susbtantial psychiatric morbidiy and comorbidity in sample of 22,231 overweight and obese individuals.

Johar, M., & Katayama, H. (2012). Quantile regression analysis of body mass and wages. *Health Economics, 21,* 597–611.—Data from National Longitudinal Survey of Youth examining relationship between body mass and wages.

Puhl, R. M., & Suh, Y. (2015). Health consequences of weight stigma: Implications for obesity prevention and treatment. *Current Obesity Reports, 4*(2), 182–190.—Summarizes evidence in the past several years on links between perceived weight-based stigmatization and psychological and physical health indices.

Rudolph, C. W., Wells, C. L., Weller, M. D., & Baltes, B. B. (2009). A meta-analysis of empirical studies of weight-based bias in the workplace. *Journal of Vocational Behavior, 74*(1), 1–10.—Meta-analysis of 25 experimental studies examining effects of weight-based bias on evaluative workplace outcomes.

Sabin, J. A., Marini, M., & Nosek, B. A. (2012). Implicit and explicit anti-fat bias among a large sample of medical doctors by BMI, race/ethnicity and gender. *PLoS ONE, 7*(11), e48448.—Demonstrates that strong implicit and explicit weight-based bias is as pervasive among MDs as it is among members of the general public.

Suh, Y., Puhl, R. M., Liu, S., & Milici, F. F. (2014). Support for laws to prohibit weight discrimination in the United States: Public attitudes from 2011–2013. *Obesity, 22,* 1872–1879.—At least 75% of participants consistently favored laws prohibiting weight discrimination in the workplace. Individuals became increasingly supportive of extending disability protections for individuals with obesity and adding body weight as a protected class in civil rights statutes.

Sutin, A. R., & Terracciano, A. (2013). Perceived weight discrimination and obesity. *PLoS ONE, 8*(7), e70048.—Four-year, longitudinal study demonstrating that experiences of weight-based discrimination (but not other forms of discrimination) increases the risk for becoming and remaining obese.

Throop, E. M., Skinner A. C., Perrin, A. J., Steiner, M. J., Odulana, A., & Perrin, E. M. (2014). Pass the popcorn: "Obesogenic" behaviors and stigma in children's movies. *Obesity, 22,* 1694–1700.—Content analysis of top-grossing children's films documenting frequent weight stigmatization.

Body Image, Obesity, and Eating Disorders

J. KEVIN THOMPSON
LAUREN SCHAEFER

Although the term *body image* was once thought simply to describe a person's internal representation of his or her outer appearance, researchers increasingly conceptualize body image as a complex and multidimensional construct that comprises the perceptual, cognitive, emotional, and behavioral experiences associated with how a person views his or her body. In other words, *body image* refers to one's mental image of the body and physical sensations; thoughts about one's body; affective states associated with viewing or thinking about one's body; and actions in which one engages to modify, conceal, expose, or otherwise accommodate one's own appearance. The nature of these experiences and a person's relationship with his or her body may have a profound effect on his or her quality of life and lived experience. "Negative body image" (i.e., dissatisfaction with or shame about one's body, holding negative views of the body, engaging in unhealthy behaviors aimed at manipulating one's appearance, and acceptance and pursuit of unhealthy appearance ideals) may contribute to decreased self-esteem, negative affect, social withdrawal, feelings of worthlessness and incompetence, unhealthy weight control practices, and eating pathology.

In large-scale surveys, girls and women consistently report higher levels of negative body image compared with boys and men. In addition, males and females differ with regard to the specific aspects of appearance that are cited as being most relevant to their overall body image and the particular appearance ideals for which they strive. For women, body image concerns generally center on issues of weight and a desire for a thinness. Within Western culture, the predominant appearance ideal for women, termed the *thin ideal*, is a very slender frame with low body fat, a toned physique, and ample breasts. Body image concerns for men tend to center on a desire for leanness and increased muscularity. The male *muscular ideal* is lean but muscular, with well-developed and -defined upper body muscles, a V-shaped torso, and a slim waist and hips.

Assessment of Body Image

Numerous tools are available to assess the perceptual, cognitive, affective, and behavioral dimensions of body image. Perceptual measures of body image once flourished in investigations of body size distortion. However, considerable controversy in the last 40 years regarding the validity of these measures, combined with inconsistent findings, has led to a decline in their use. Modern approaches to the assessment of body image instead tend to focus on attitudinal components of body image.

Global subjective satisfaction measures broadly assess satisfaction with one's appearance. Figure rating scales present respondents with an array of numbered artist- or computer-generated images representing the human body in varying shapes, weights, and sizes. Respondents indicate the figure that best represents how they view their "real" physical appearance and the one that represents their "ideal" physical appearance. Body dissatisfaction scores are calculated as discrepancy scores (i.e., the difference between the two identified figures). Numerous self-report questionnaires have also been developed to assess overall body satisfaction and satisfaction with specific aspects of one's appearance (e.g., weight and shape).

A growing number of measures have been developed to assess additional dimensions of body image. For example, affective measures assess feelings such as anxiety, distress, and shame associated with one's body. Cognitive measures assess beliefs, thoughts, interpretations, and attributions related to one's appearance. Such scales may seek to assess beliefs about the importance of appearance to a respondent's overall self-image or the perceived impact of appearance on his or her relationships and opportunities. Increasingly, researchers are using measures to assess important behavioral manifestations of a person's body image attitudes. For example, measures may assess the frequency of body avoidance (e.g., avoidance of mirrors, nudity, or self-weighing) or body checking (e.g., pinching adipose tissue, increased use of mirrors or scales).

Body Image and Disordered Eating

Numerous etiological theories highlight the role of body image in the development and maintenance of disordered eating. Such theories suggest that individuals who are unhappy with their weight and shape may engage in dieting and unhealthy weight control practices in order to influence their appearance. In support of such theories, Stice's (2002) meta-analytic review of prospective and longitudinal studies suggests that body dissatisfaction is one of the most reliable risk and maintenance factors for eating pathology.

In addition to increasing risk for the development of disordered eating, body image disturbance is designated by the fifth edition of the *Diagnostic and Statistical Manual of Mental Disorders* (DSM-5) as a core feature of both anorexia nervosa (AN) and bulimia nervosa (BN). AN is marked by "intense fear of gaining weight or becoming fat, even though underweight" and "disturbance in the way in which one's body weight or shape is experienced, undue influence of body weight or shape on self-evaluation, or persistant lack of recognition of the seriousness of the current low body weight" (p. 339). Diagnostic criteria for BN similarly require that "self-evaluation is unduly influenced by body shape and weight" (p. 345).

The exact nature of the body image disturbance at the heart of disordered eating has been long debated, with most researchers investigating perceptual body size distortions and evaluative dissatisfaction. Given the puzzling clinical presentation in AN, in which emaciated clients may refer to their underweight bodies as "fat" and report an intense fear of gaining even a small amount of weight, clinicians and researchers have hypothesized a significant perceptual deficit in size estimation. Cash and Deagle's (1997) meta-analytic review examining perceptual distortions and body dissatisfaction in patients with AN and BN compared to controls suggests moderate differences in body size estimation. On average, patients with eating disorders exhibited greater size distortion (i.e., overestimation) than 73% of controls. Perceptual measures, however, did not distinguish between eating disorder groups. Results suggest that size overestimation is more prevalent among individuals with eating disorders, but it is not unique to eating disorders overall or to AN specifically. Results examining body dissatisfaction in patients with eating disorders and controls produced much larger effect sizes, with the average patient reporting levels of body dissatisfaction that exceeded 87% of controls. Body dissatisfaction also discriminated between individuals with BN and those experiencing AN; on both global and weight/shape specific attitudinal measures, individuals with BN reported higher levels of body dissatisfaction than individuals with AN.

In contrast to DSM-5 criteria for AN and BN, body image disturbance is not required for a diagnosis of binge eating disorder (BED). However, considerable debate exists within the field regarding the importance of body image in BED. Research so far has focused largely the degree of concern with shape and weight that is present in individuals with BED. These studies have found levels of shape and weight concerns comparable to those observed in individuals with AN and BN, but higher than those of normal weight and overweight controls without BED.

More recently, researchers have begun to examine overvaluation of shape and weight in BED. This aspect of body image focuses more acutely on the excessive influence that weight and shape may have on one's overall self-judgments or definitions of self-worth, and is required for a diagnosis of both AN and BN. Research suggests that a large subset of patients with BED experience clinical levels of weight/shape overvaluation. Compared to patients with subclinical levels of overvaluation, those with clinical overvaluation also report greater eating pathology, general psychopathology, psychological concerns, and interpersonal concerns. Moreover, patients with BED evidence higher average levels of overvaluation than overweight individuals without BED. Treatment studies also suggest the potential clinical importance of body image disturbance in BED, with increased shape/weight concerns and overvaluation at intake predicting poorer treatment outcomes. Based on accumulating evidence that overvaluation is a common and clinically significant feature of BED, researchers have suggested that overvaluation be included as a specifier or subtype in the diagnosis.

Body Image and Obesity

Given prominent and continuously reinforced societal ideals emphasizing thinness for women and leanness for men, as well as pervasive weight-based bias and stigma associating excess weight with laziness, gluttony, and a lack of self-discipline, it is frequently assumed that all individuals with obesity experience heightened body dissatisfaction. However, research indicates that although obesity is associated with poor body image, a substantial number of obese individuals do not report elevated body image disturbance.

Unfortunately, obese individuals who do experience higher levels of body dissatisfaction appear to be at increased risk for greater physical and psychosocial impairment.

Researchers have identified several risk factors for increased body image concerns among obese individuals, including demographic variables such as gender and ethnicity. Overweight women, who generally report greater weight-based discrimination than overweight men, are also more likely to classify themselves as overweight and to report greater body dissatisfaction than do overweight men. Ethnic group membership also appears to impact body image among obese individuals. Although higher rates of obesity are observed among black women compared with white women in the United States, obese black women report less weight and appearance dissatisfaction than their obese white peers. Such differences are likely due in part to variation in sociocultural ideals and acceptance of larger figures among different ethnic groups.

Experience of weight-based bias and stigma appear to strengthen the association between weight status and body image. Unfortunately, individuals with obesity (especially individuals with a BMI ≥ 40) face frequent and varying forms of weight stigmatization. Increased experiences of stigmatization are associated with poorer body image and psychosocial functioning, even when researchers control for weight. As discussed earlier in this chapter, the presence of BED also increases the likelihood of body image concerns among obese individuals. Obese individuals with BED report greater weight/shape dissatisfaction and lower appearance satisfaction than those without BED. Among obese individuals with BED, more frequent binging is associated with a more negative body image. Additional proposed risk factors for body image disturbance among individuals with elevated weight status include age of obesity onset and a history of weight cycling.

Although weight loss alone appears to have a positive impact on body image among obese individuals, these improvements are largely lost with subsequent weight gain. Studies suggest that the addition of a body image component in weight loss treatment does not substantially improve body image outcomes compared to weight loss treatment alone. However, researchers applying stand-alone body image treatment to obese populations have demonstrated significant improvements in body image and binge eating in the absence of significant weight loss.

Conclusions and Future Directions

Body image is a central feature of eating disorders, and body image disturbance has been linked to the onset and maintenance of these disorders. Additionally, body image problems occur at increased rates among individuals who are obese, which may be explained in part by experiences of pervasive societal weight-based bias. Management of both eating disorders and obesity should entail consideration of the assessment and treatment of body image issues.

Future work in this area is needed to further our understanding of specific dimensions of body image disturbances, especially for the relatively new BED. Prospective studies are also indicated, particularly in the area of weight-based bias and stigmatization to illustrate whether early experience of such incidents predicts poor health and psychological outcomes in the future. Future research should also consider how body image disturbances can best be addressed in individuals with eating disorders and obesity.

Suggested Reading

Burke, N. L., Schaefer, L. M., & Thompson, J. K. (2010). Body image. In V. S. Ramachandran (Ed.), *Encyclopedia of human behavior* (2nd ed.). San Diego, CA: Academic Press.—This chapter covers the nature, history, theoretical models, and assessment of body image.

Cash, T. F., & Deagle, E. A., III. (1997). The nature and extent of body-image disturbance in anorexia nervosa and bulimia nervosa: A meta-analysis. *International Journal of Eating Disorders, 22,* 107–125.—A meta-analysis examining perceptual and attitudinal dimensions of body image among individuals with AN and BN.

Crowther, J. H., & Williams, N. M. (2011). Body image and bulimia nervosa. In T. F. Cash & L. Smolak (Eds.), *Body image: A handbook of science, practice, and prevention* (2nd ed., pp. 288–295). New York: Guilford Press.—This chapter reviews the literature on the role of body image disturbance in BN.

Delinsky, S. S. (2011). Body image and anorexia nervosa. In T. F. Cash & L. Smolak (Eds.), *Body image: A handbook of science, practice, and prevention* (2nd ed., pp. 279–287). New York: Guilford Press.—This chapter reviews the literature on the role of body image disturbance in BN.

Grilo, C. M. (2013). Why no cognitive body image feature such as overvaluation of shape/weight in the binge eating disorder diagnosis? *International Journal of Eating Disorders, 46,* 208–211.—This review examines the relevance of body image disturbance in BED and argues for the inclusion of overvaluation of weight/shape as a diagnostic specifier.

Hrabosky, J. I. (2011). Body image and binge eating disorder. In T. F. Cash & L. Smolak (Eds.), *Body image: A handbook of science, practice, and prevention* (2nd ed., pp. 296–304). New York: Guilford Press.—This chapter reviews the literature on the role of body image disturbance in BED.

Hrabosky, J. I., Cash, T. F., Veale, D., Neziroglu, F., Soll, E. A., Garner, D. M., et al. (2009). Multidimensional body image comparisons among patients with eating disorders, body dysmorphic disorder, and clinical controls: A multisite study. *Body Image, 6,* 155–163.—This article examines various dimensions of body image among individuals with AN, BN, body dysmorphic disorder, and psychiatric controls drawn from 10 treatment centers in the United States.

Latner, J. D., & Wilson, R. E. (2011). Obesity and body image in adulthood. In T. F. Cash & L. Smolak (Eds.), *Body image: A handbook of science, practice, and prevention* (2nd ed., pp. 189–197). New York: Guilford Press.—This chapter examines the risk factors, manifestation, and treatment of body image disturbance in obesity.

Schwartz, M. B., & Brownell, K. B. (2004). Body image and obesity. *Body Image, 1,* 43–56.—This review examines the role of body image in obesity, including risk factors and treatment of body image disturbance in obese individuals.

Stice, E. (2002). Risk and maintenance factors for eating pathology: A meta-analytic review. *Psychological Bulletin, 128,* 825–848.—This meta-analysis reviews evidence for proposed risk factors of disordered eating from prospective and experimental studies.

23

Body Dysmorphic Disorder

KATHARINE A. PHILLIPS

Clinical Features

Core Diagnostic Features

Body dysmorphic disorder (BDD) is a common and often severe disorder in which individuals are preoccupied with one or more perceived defects or flaws in their appearance that are not observable or that appear only slight to others. The fifth edition of the *Diagnostic and Statistical Manual of Mental Disorders* (DSM-5) classifies BDD as an obsessive–compulsive and related disorder, but BDD shares some features with eating disorders, such as distorted body image and apparent abnormalities in processing visual information.

BDD preoccupations may focus on any body area, most often the skin (e.g., perceived scarring, acne, color), hair (e.g., excessive or insufficient head, facial, or body hair), and nose (e.g., size or shape). In one study, 30% of individuals with BDD were preoccupied with their weight, but only 4% reported weight as their primary concern, and none reported it as their sole concern. Persons with BDD typically describe the disliked body areas as "ugly" or "abnormal"; descriptions may range from "unattractive" to "monstrous." The appearance preoccupations occur, on average, for 3–8 hours a day. They are intrusive, unwanted, distressing, and difficult to resist or control.

These preoccupations/obsessions trigger negative emotions such as depressed mood, anxiety, distress, or shame. Emotions such as these, in turn, trigger excessive repetitive behaviors that are intended to (but often do not) alleviate the emotional distress. Virtually all individuals with BDD perform one or more of these repetitive behaviors at some point during the course of the disorder. The behaviors are performed, on average, for 3–8 hours a day; they are difficult to control and time-consuming. Common excessive behaviors include comparing with others, checking disliked body parts in reflecting surfaces or directly, excessive grooming (e.g., styling, cutting, or shaving hair), skin picking (to remove tiny blemishes), seeking reassurance or questioning others about the appearance of the disliked body areas, seeking and/or receiving cosmetic procedures, body touching, excessive clothes changing (e.g., to more effectively camouflage disliked areas), compulsive shopping (e.g., for makeup or skin or hair products), dieting, excessive exercising or weightlifting, compulsive tanning, and hair plucking/pulling. Most individuals with BDD attempt to camouflage their perceived flaws (e.g., with their hair, sunglasses, a hat, makeup, clothes, body position), which may be repetitive in nature (e.g., reapplying makeup 20 times a day).

DSM-5 requires that the appearance preoccupations cause clinically significant distress or impairment in social, occupational, or other important areas of functioning. DSM-5 diagnostic criteria also state that if the person's only appearance concerns involve excessive body fat or weight, and diagnostic criteria for an eating disorder are met, then the body fat/weight concerns should be diagnosed as an eating disorder rather than as BDD. However, eating disorders and BDD (with concerns that focus on other body areas) commonly co-occur.

DSM-5 added two new specifiers to the diagnostic criteria for BDD:

1. The *muscle dysmorphia specifier* identifies individuals (nearly always men) who are preoccupied with the idea that their body build is too small or insufficiently muscular. In reality, they appear normal or sometimes unusually muscular due to excessive weight lifting or anabolic-androgenic steroid use. It appears that some, but not all, patients with muscle dysmorphia have abnormal eating behavior (e.g., eating large amounts of food or high-protein meals).

2. The *insight specifier* indicates level of insight regarding BDD beliefs (e.g., "I look ugly"). Insight levels are (a) "with good or fair insight" (the person recognizes that his or her belief about appearance is definitely or probably not true, or that it may or may not be true); (b) "with poor insight" (the person thinks his or her BDD belief probably is true); and (c) "with absent insight/delusional beliefs" (the person is completely convinced that his or her BDD belief is true). Insight is usually poor or absent.

Associated Features

Common associated features include ideas or delusions of reference (the false belief that others take special notice of him or her in a negative way because of how he or she looks; e.g., they mock, talk about, or stare at him or her); high levels of social anxiety, social avoidance, anxiety, and depression; low self-esteem; and embarrassment and shame.

Course of Illness

BDD most often onsets in early adolescence; in two-thirds of individuals it onsets before age 18. BDD usually appears to be chronic. However, a majority of patients improve with evidence-based treatment (see below).

Psychosocial Functioning and Quality of Life

BDD is associated with markedly poor psychosocial functioning and quality of life. It is common for those with BDD to drop out of school, be housebound, and be psychiatrically hospitalized because of BDD symptoms.

Suicidality

Rates of suicidal ideation and suicide attempts are very high in youth and adults in both clinical and epidemiological samples. Although the rate of completed suicide has been only minimally studied, it appears markedly elevated.

Comorbidity

Major depressive disorder is the most common comorbid disorder; many patients attribute their depressive symptoms to BDD-induced distress. Other commonly comorbid disorders are substance use disorders, social anxiety disorder, obsessive–compulsive disorder (OCD), and eating disorders.

Gender, Youth, and Culture

BDD appears largely similar in females and males, although there are some differences, including more frequent preoccupation with weight and eating disorder comorbidity in women. BDD's features appear largely similar in youth and adults, although youth appear to have poorer BDD-related insight and a higher rate of suicide attempts. BDD characteristics also appear largely similar across countries and cultures (although cross-cultural comparison studies are lacking). Cultural preferences and values may shape symptom content to some degree, however.

Epidemiology

Five nationwide epidemiological studies of adults have consistently found that BDD's point prevalence is about 2% (1.7–2.9%). In a study of high school students, current BDD prevalence was 2.2%. BDD is far more common than this in clinical populations, for example, in mental health, dermatology, cosmetic surgery, and orthodontia settings. Compared to individuals without BDD, those with BDD are less likely to be married or employed. BDD appears to be slightly more common in females than in males.

Etiology and Pathophysiology

While data on BDD's etiology and pathophysiology are quite limited, the disorder likely results from multiple genetic and environmental risk factors. BDD appears to be familial and to have genetic overlap with OCD. BDD is associated with abnormal visual processing, which consists of a bias for encoding and analyzing details of faces and nonfacial objects, rather than use of holistic visual processing strategies (i.e., seeing "the big picture"). Preliminary data suggest abnormal early visual system functioning, which may contribute to perceptual distortions, in both BDD and anorexia nervosa. Preliminary data also suggest abnormalities in executive functioning in BDD. Small studies suggest that BDD may be characterized by compromised white-matter fibers (reduced organization) and inefficient connections—or poor integration of information—between different brain areas, which is associated with poorer BDD-related insight. One study found relative hyperactivity in the left orbitofrontal cortex and bilateral head of the caudate when subjects viewed their own faces, possibly reflecting obsessional preoccupation; this activation pattern is also characteristic of OCD. Individuals with BDD appear to have difficulty identifying emotional facial expressions and to have a bias toward interpreting neutral faces and scenarios as threatening. BDD may also be associated with a history of teasing and perceived childhood neglect and/or abuse.

Assessment and Differential Diagnosis

BDD usually goes undiagnosed. Many patients are reluctant to reveal their appearance concerns because they are embarrassed, they fear being misunderstood or considered vain, or they believe that their problem is physical rather than mental. Thus, to detect BDD, clinicians must inquire directly about BDD symptoms, using questions such as the following:

- *Appearance preoccupations:* "Are you very worried about your appearance in any way?" or "Are you unhappy with how you look?"
- *Repetitive behaviors:* "Is there anything you feel an urge to do over and over again in response to your appearance concerns?" Offer examples of repetitive behaviors.
- *Clinically significant distress or impairment in functioning:* "How much distress do your appearance concerns cause you?"; "Do these concerns interfere with your life in any way?"

Several measures, such as the Body Dysmorphic Disorder Questionnaire (BDDQ), are available to screen for, diagnose, and assess the severity of BDD and BDD-related insight.

BDD must be differentiated from other disorders with which it is commonly confused, such as OCD (diagnose BDD if obsessions focus on perceived appearance flaws) and social anxiety disorder or agoraphobia (diagnose BDD if avoidance is due to appearance concerns).

When compulsive skin picking or hair plucking/pulling is triggered by concerns about perceived flaws of the skin or hair, BDD should be diagnosed rather than excoriation (skin-picking) disorder or trichotillomania (hair-pulling disorder). BDD symptoms that are characterized by absent insight/delusional beliefs are diagnosed as BDD rather than a psychotic disorder.

Both BDD and eating disorders involve dissatisfaction with one's appearance and distorted body image; however, they differ in a number of ways, such as gender ratio, body areas of concern, and treatment response. Several studies found greater impairment in psychosocial functioning in BDD than in anorexia nervosa or bulimia nervosa. If appearance concerns focus only on being too fat/overweight and qualify for an eating disorder diagnosis, then an eating disorder rather than BDD is diagnosed. However, when eating disorders and BDD co-occur (with BDD typically focusing on skin, hair, or facial features), both disorders should be diagnosed.

Treatment

Pharmacotherapy and Other Somatic Treatments

Serotonin reuptake inhibitors (SRIs; or selective SRIs [SSRIs]) are currently considered first-line medications for BDD. Two blinded controlled trials (with fluoxetine and clomipramine) and four rigorous open-label studies indicate that SRIs usually decrease core BDD symptoms; intention-to-treat response rates are 53–83%. Depression, anxiety, anger–hostility, psychosocial functioning, and quality of life also significantly improve. SRIs may also protect against worsening of suicidality and decrease suicidal ideation in people with BDD. Although data are limited, SRIs appear more efficacious than non-SRI antidepressants or other types of psychotropic medication. An SRI, rather than antipsychotic monotherapy, is recommended for patients with absent insight/delusional BDD beliefs.

Effective SRI doses often appear to be substantially higher than those typically needed for disorders such as depression (although rigorous dose-finding studies are lacking). Patients may further improve when the maximum SRI dose recommended by the manufacturer is exceeded (although this approach is not advised for citalopram or clomipramine). The mean time to SRI response is 4–9 weeks, with occasional patients requiring 14 or even 16 weeks (while reaching a high enough dose) to improve substantially. Small open-label trials suggest that the serotonin–norepinephrine reuptake inhibitor (SNRI) venlafaxine and the antiepileptic levetiracetam may also improve BDD symptoms. Neuromodulation techniques and electroconvulsive therapy (ECT) have not been studied in BDD.

Cognitive-Behavioral Therapy

Cognitive-behavioral therapy (CBT) is currently considered the psychotherapy of choice for BDD. Only one study in a clinical setting has compared CBT to a treatment that controlled for therapist time and attention (anxiety management); all other studies used a waiting-list control. Four CBT studies and one metacognitive therapy study found that CBT was more efficacious than the comparison treatment or waiting list.

CBT must be tailored to BDD's unique symptoms; it is not advisable to use CBT for another disorder, such as OCD. Because BDD can be difficult to treat, use of a published treatment manual for BDD is recommended.

Recommended treatment includes laying essential groundwork (e.g., goal setting) and building an individualized cognitive-behavioral model of the patient's illness. Because poor or absent insight is so common, motivational interviewing techniques are often needed to engage and retain patients in treatment. Core treatment elements include cognitive restructuring, exposure (e.g., to avoided social situations) combined with behavioral experiments, and ritual (response) prevention (e.g., decreasing mirror checking). Other recommended elements include mindfulness/perceptual retraining with mirrors, cognitive approaches that target core beliefs (e.g., "I am worthless"), habit reversal for BDD-related skin picking or hair pulling/plucking, a focus on more severe depressive symptoms, and a desire for cosmetic treatment, if needed. Treatment ends with relapse prevention; booster sessions should be provided, if necessary. Most patients need at least 6 months of weekly, hourlong treatment, combined with daily structured homework assignments. CBT skills should continue to be practiced after treatment has ended.

Suicidal ideation must be carefully assessed and monitored, and hospitalization should be considered when necessary. More highly suicidal patients should receive an SRI and also be encouraged to participate in BDD-focused CBT. Incorporation of cognitive-behavioral approaches for suicidality into treatment is also recommended for higher-risk suicidal patients.

Suggested Reading

Buhlmann, U., Glaesmer, H., Mewes, R., Fama, J. M., Wilhelm, S., Brähler, E., et al. (2010). Updates on the prevalence of body dysmorphic disorder: A population-based survey. *Psychiatry Research, 178*(1), 171–175.—In this nationwide epidemiological study, the point prevalence of BDD was 1.8%. Individuals with BDD, relative to individuals without BDD, reported significantly more often a history of cosmetic surgery (15.6 vs. 3.0%), as well as higher rates of suicidal ideation (31.0 vs. 3.5%) and suicide attempts due to appearance concerns (22.2 vs. 2.1%).

Feusner, J. D., Moody, T., Hembacher, E., Townsend, J., McKinley, M., Moller, H., et al. (2010). Abnormalities of visual processing and frontostriatal systems in body dysmorphic disorder. *Archives of General Psychiatry, 67,* 197–205.—This functional magnetic resonance imaging study found abnormalities in visual processing and frontostriatal systems in BDD, including hypoactivation in the occipital cortex for low spatial frequency faces and frontostriatal hyperactivity.

Hrabosky, J. I., Cash, T. F., Veale, D., Neziroglu, F., Soll, E. A., Garner, D. M., et al. (2009). Multidimensional body image comparisons among patients with eating disorders, body dysmorphic disorder, and clinical controls: A multisite study. *Body Image: An International Journal of Research, 6,* 155–163.—The anorexia nervosa, bulimia nervosa, and BDD groups were all characterized by significantly elevated disturbances in most body image dimensions relative to their gender-matched clinical controls. However, there was variability among the three clinical groups, including foci of body dissatisfaction and greater body image impairment and poorer quality of life in those with BDD than in those in with an eating disorder.

Li, W., Lai, T. M., Bohon, C., Loo, S. K., McCurdy, D., Strober, M., et al. (2015). Anorexia nervosa and body dysmorphic disorder are associated with abnormalities in processing visual information. *Psychological Medicine, 45*(10), 2111–2122.—This study provides preliminary evidence of similar abnormal spatiotemporal activation in anorexia nervosa and BDD for configural/holistic information for appearance- and non-appearance-related stimuli. These findings suggest a common phenotype of abnormal early visual system functioning, which may contribute to perceptual distortions.

Phillips, K. A. (2009). *Understanding body dysmorphic disorder: An essential guide.* New York: Oxford University Press.—This book provides a clinically focused overview of BDD for professionals and the public.

Phillips, K. A., Albertini, R. S., & Rasmussen, S. A. (2002). A randomized placebo-controlled trial of fluoxetine in body dysmorphic disorder. *Archives of General Psychiatry, 59,* 381–388.—In this randomized controlled trial, the SRI fluoxetine was more efficacious for BDD and associated symptoms than placebo.

Phillips, K. A., Coles, M., Menard, W., Yen, S., Fay, C., & Weisberg, R. B. (2005). Suicidal ideation and suicide attempts in body dysmorphic disorder. *Journal of Clinical Psychiatry, 66,* 717–725.—Subjects had high rates of lifetime suicidal ideation (78.0%) and suicide attempts (27.5%). Suicidal ideation was significantly predicted by comorbid major depression and greater lifetime impairment due to BDD; suicide attempts were significantly predicted by comorbid posttraumatic stress disorder, a substance use disorder, and greater lifetime impairment due to BDD.

Phillips, K. A., Menard, W., Fay, C., & Weisberg, R. (2005). Demographic characteristics, phenomenology, comorbidity, and family history in 200 individuals with body dysmorphic disorder. *Psychosomatics, 46,* 317–332.—This report in the largest clinically assessed sample for whom a broad range of demographic and clinical features has been reported examines demographic features, phenomenology, comorbidity, and family history.

Veale, D., & Neziroglu, F. (2010). *Overcoming body dysmorphic disorder: A treatment manual.* West Sussex, UK: Wiley-Blackwell.—This is an empirically based CBT treatment manual for therapists to use when treating BDD.

Wilhelm, S., Phillips, K. A., & Steketee, G. (2013). *Cognitive-behavioral therapy for body dysmorphic disorder: A treatment manual.* New York: Guilford Press.—This is an empirically based CBT treatment manual for therapists to use when treating BDD.

Does Addressing Obesity Create Risk for Eating Disorders?

KENDRIN R. SONNEVILLE
S. BRYN AUSTIN

First, Do No Harm

The fundamental ethical principle of nonmaleficence reminds clinicians, researchers, and policymakers alike to consider the possible harm an intervention might do. Otherwise stated as "first, do no harm," nonmaleficence favors doing nothing over the risk of causing more harm than good. While the known health consequences of obesity compel us to action, efforts to address obesity can cause unintended harm, despite our having the best of intentions. Given the high prevalence and serious health consequences of eating disorders, and the paucity of evidence that considers both the intended effects and unintended consequences of strategies to address obesity, several pertinent ethical questions warrant consideration:

1. Do strategies to address obesity create risk for eating disorders in individuals with obesity?
2. Do strategies to address obesity create risk for eating disorders in individuals, irrespective of obesity status?
3. Do strategies to address obesity exacerbate risk for individuals with eating disorders or an eating disorder history?

The Intersection of Weight-Related Disorders

A large number of studies have demonstrated shared risk factors for disordered eating behaviors and obesity. For example, dieting, body dissatisfaction, and weight-related teasing are key risk factors for disordered eating behaviors and eating disorders that are also associated with excess weight gain. Given the many shared risk factors, there is much to be gained from using a combined approach that reduces risk for all. Primary prevention efforts to address obesity should be designed to protect against eating disorders and should avoid messages that may increase body dissatisfaction, dieting, use of unhealthy weight control practices, and weight stigma.

Co-occurrence of obesity and eating disorders is common. Data from 14 countries participating in the World Health Organization's World Mental Health Survey Initiative found that approximately 40% of respondents with bulimia nervosa or binge eating disorder in the past year also had obesity. Similarly, in a study of adolescents from Minnesota, about one-half of males and one-third of females who engaged in extreme weight control behaviors and/or binge eating were also overweight/obese. A recent study of adolescents conducted at a specialty eating disorder clinic found that more than one-third of patients with restrictive eating disorders had a history of being at a weight that would categorize them as either overweight or obese. These studies and a large body of observational research support the notion that individuals with obesity are vulnerable to disordered eating and eating disorders.

Recommendations

Health promotion strategies for obesity and eating disorders tend to be conducted separately, and very little research has been done to ascertain whether obesity prevention and treatment programs may be harmful in relation to eating disorders. Most studies that evaluate the long-term impact of strategies to address obesity do not systematically measure and evaluate the impact of those strategies on eating disorders. As such, the impact of obesity programs on eating disorders risk is not yet well understood. One review of 22 childhood obesity prevention programs found no evidence of unintended psychological harm, but it also noted that assessments of eating pathology in these students was not rigorously done. In the absence of best possible evidence, however, there is ample research on eating disorder risk factors to guide the development of practice guidelines that can be utilized across several obesity-related practice areas. Efforts to address obesity should be designed to protect against body image issues and eating disorders, and should avoid the following strategies, which may cause harm:

1. Promoting rigid or restrictive approaches to eating. Dieting is a known predictor of the onset of disordered eating symptoms. While reducing caloric intake or shifting energy balance is compulsory in obesity treatment, advice that is unduly restrictive is not sustainable and may cause harm. Unhealthy dieting or use of unhealthy weight control practices should be discouraged, and extreme language related to food or eating, or moralization of food should be avoided.

2. Increasing body dissatisfaction. Body dissatisfaction does not motivate people to lose weight or to maintain a healthy weight. In fact, young women with overweight/obesity who are dissatisfied with their bodies are far more likely to start binge eating regularly than those who are satisfied with their bodies. Avoid messages that may increase body dissatisfaction.

3. Reinforcing weight-based stigma. Antiobesity campaigns that utilize stigmatizing campaign messages may cause harm. Maladaptive eating behaviors are among the myriad consequences of weight-based stigma. Individuals who are subject to weight-based stigma are more likely to binge-eat, use unhealthy weight control practices, and cope

with stigma by eating more food. Avoid stigmatizing language, images, or assumptions that reinforce weight-based stigma.

4. Focusing narrowly on weight/body mass index (BMI). Weight is not a behavior; therefore, it is not an appropriate target for behavior modification. Emphasize health rather than weight, and target specific modifiable behaviors (e.g., family meals or TV viewing) rather than focusing on changing weight.

Recommendations to avoid strategies that promote rigid dieting, increase body dissatisfaction, reinforce weight-based stigma, or focus solely on weight can be applied to a range of obesity strategies and across practice settings.

Clinical Settings

Weight-based bias among health care professionals, including those who specialize in obesity, is well documented. Critical to averting the onset of eating disorders in individuals with obesity is avoiding weight-based stigma in a clinical encounter. The Rudd Center for Food Policy and Obesity has developed materials and guidelines for preventing weight-based bias in clinical practice. Best-practice recommendations include creating an accessible and comfortable office environment, using equipment (e.g., scales, blood pressure cuffs) that can accurately assess patients with obesity, and using neutral terms such as *weight* and *BMI* rather than *obesity* or *fat*. In addition, providers should evaluate their own assumptions and biases about weight and explore all causes of the patient's presenting problems, not just weight. While acknowledging the difficulty of making lifestyle changes and providing support, providers should emphasize behavior changes rather than focusing only on weight and avoid recommending extreme approaches to weight control.

Schools

Schools play a critical role in promoting the health of young people and, as such, are important stakeholders in addressing obesity. Schools provide education about nutrition and health, and are a major provider of meals to students. Furthermore, the school environment reinforces eating- and activity-related norms. Health promotion activities should focus on improving children's health and habits rather than reducing their weight. In addition, schools should rely on evidence-based approaches (e.g., Planet Health, a curriculum shown to reduce both obesity prevalence and eating disorder risk among middle school girls) rather than ad hoc activities such as teaching calorie counting in health classes or holding schoolwide "biggest loser" weight loss competitions. To prevent unintended negative consequences of health promotion activities, schools should treat weight-based bullying seriously and on par with other types of bullying.

Screening

Notifying youth with overweight or obesity of their elevated weight status is routinely done as part of clinical and school-based BMI screening. Several states require school-based BMI screening with parental notification ("BMI report cards") and the U.S. Preventive Services Task Force and the American Academy of Pediatrics recommend that clinicians screen children ages 6 years and older for obesity. Research evaluating the effectiveness of school-based and clinical BMI screening is lacking, and several ethical concerns of school-based screening have been raised. BMI is a measure of weight and not a direct measure of health. While BMI is highly correlated with adiposity at a population level, false positives and false negatives are expected when using BMI for individual screening. BMI screening could overemphasize weight as an indicator of health and worsen weight stigma, especially in school settings, where appropriate clinical counseling is not likely to be available and unstandardized weighing practices (e.g., use of untrained parent volunteers, lack of privacy during weighing) may be used.

Social Marketing

Drawing on the same research and planning principles used by commercial marketers, the public health community utilizes social marketing to promote behavior change and improve population health. Social marketing campaigns, which must grab the attention of their intended audience, often use shocking or controversial messages. Unfortunately, obesity campaigns that have generated public attention by shaming or stigmatizing people with obesity are all too common. For example, a childhood obesity campaign in the state of Georgia, which included a series of billboards, print ads, television ads, and social media featuring overweight children, talked about the negative social and health consequences of obesity. The program was criticized for reinforcing messages of body shame, normalizing bullying, and excluding overweight children, which can be unintended consequences of programs that are designed to increase awareness. Another public health campaign that targeted teens in Boston, Massachusetts, featured teens getting hit in the face by "blobs of fat" after drinking a soda, along with the tag line: "Don't get smacked by fat." This campaign, designed to reduce intake of sugar-sweetened beverages, inadvertently reinforced antifat messages while also sending an extreme message about diet that vilified sugar-sweetened beverages. Antiobesity campaigns that utilize stigmatizing campaign messages may cause harm and should be avoided. The Rudd Center discourages obesity campaigns that show headless images, use pejorative language, blame the individual, or communicate weight-biased stereotypes. Instead, campaigns should use respectful and full-person portrayals, and suggest specific actions when promoting health behaviors. The Rudd Center Media Gallery is a public resource for nonstigmatizing portrayals of individuals with obesity.

Workplace

Workplace wellness programs have become increasingly prevalent over the past two decades, and reduction in overweight is one of the most common targets in these initiatives. While, in theory, wellness programs might be a welcome addition to the workplace given the importance of environmental influences on health, in practice, these programs have fallen short of expectations. Many employers develop their own ad hoc programs or purchase the services of outside vendors, but these programs are rarely evidence based. Reviews of workplace overweight prevention and reduction programs in North America and Europe have found very modest to no sustained beneficial effects on weight, particularly when considering results from rigorously designed randomized controlled trials. In the U.S. market, the Department of Labor recently issued a comprehensive report indicating that these programs do not achieve health benefits for workers and do not even garner cost savings for employers. In addition, collection of biometric data such as BMI, as done in many workplace wellness programs, has led to federal lawsuits against companies suspected of using employees' data in discriminatory ways. Health promotion practitioners developing workplace wellness programs to address overweight have a professional responsibility to use strategies that are well documented in the scientific literature to be effective, and to ensure they are administered in ways that are not stigmatizing or discriminatory toward people with obesity, eating disorders, or other health conditions.

Conclusions

Clinicians, researchers, educators/schools, policymakers, activists, and other stakeholders engaged in strategies to address obesity should err on the side of doing no harm. Strategies to address obesity should be evidence based and avoid promoting rigid dieting, increasing body dissatisfaction, reinforcing weight-based stigma, or focusing solely on weight. Moving forward, all strategies to address obesity should be evaluated for both intended effects and unintended consequences to establish an evidence base of strategies that reduce obesity without increasing risk of eating disorders.

Acknowledgments

S. Bryn Austin is supported by the Ellen Feldberg Gordon Challenge Fund for Eating Disorders Research and by training grants (Nos. T71-MC-00009 and T76-MC-00001) from the Maternal and Child Health Bureau, Health Resources and Services Administration, U.S. Department of Health and Human Services.

Suggested Reading

Austin, S. B. (2011). The blind spot in the drive for childhood obesity prevention: Bringing eating disorders prevention into focus as a public health priority. *American Journal of Public Health, 101*(6), e1–e4.—Commonly held myths about eating disorders hinder public health efforts to address childhood obesity. These myths include the mistaken beliefs that eating disorders affect only white, affluent, underweight females; that focusing on eating disorders necessarily distracts from obesity prevention; and that the activities of the weight loss industry and the marketing and sale of its products are tangential to public health priorities.

Austin, S. B., Field, A. E., Wiecha, J., Peterson, K. E., & Gortmaker, S. L. (2005). The impact of a school-based obesity prevention trial on disordered weight-control behaviors in early adolescent girls. *Archives of Pediatrics and Adolescent Medicine, 159*(3), 225–230.—Planet Health, a randomized controlled trial of a behaviorally focused obesity prevention program delivered to middle school students in Massachusetts, reduced obesity prevalence among girls and also reduced eating disorder risk; girls in intervention compared to controls were half as likely to report use of purging or diet pills at follow-up (odds ratio [OR]: 0.41; 95% confidence interval [CI]: 0.22–0.75).

Carter, F. A., & Bulik, C. M. (2008). Childhood obesity prevention programs: How do they affect eating pathology and other psychological measures? *Psychosomatic Medicine, 70*(3), 363–371.—The existing evidence does not support the view that childhood obesity prevention programs are associated with unintended psychological harm; however, conclusions about the possible iatrogenic effects of these programs are premature. Among 22 studies of interventions designed to prevent obesity in childhood, symptoms of eating disorders were assessed by a minority of studies.

Haines, J., Neumark-Sztainer, D., Eisenberg, M. E., & Hannan, P. J. (2006). Weight teasing and disordered eating behaviors in adolescents: Longitudinal findings from Project EAT (Eating Among Teens). *Pediatrics, 117*(2), e209–e215.—This longitudinal study of male and female adolescents assessed whether weight-related teasing predicts the development of binge eating, unhealthy weight control behaviors, and frequent dieting. Boys who were teased about their weight were more likely than their peers to initiate binge eating with loss of control and unhealthy weight control behaviors 5 years later, whereas girls who were teased were more likely than their peers to become frequent dieters.

Lebow, J., Sim, L. A., & Kransdorf, L. N. (2015). Prevalence of a history of overweight and obesity in adolescents with restrictive eating disorders. *Journal of Adolescent Health, 56*(1), 19–24.—This retrospective cohort study was conducted on all new patients with a restrictive eating disorder seen in a specialty eating disorder clinic. Of 179 adolescents, 36.7% were found to have a BMI history above the 85th percentile. Findings suggest that adolescents with a history of overweight or obesity represent a substantial portion of treatment-seeking adolescents with restrictive eating disorders.

Neumark-Sztainer, D. R., Wall, M. M., Haines, J. I., Story, M. T., Sherwood, N. E., & van den Berg, P. A. (2007). Shared risk and protective factors for overweight and disordered eating in adolescents. *American Journal of Preventive Medicine, 33*(5), 359–369.—Weight-related problems, including obesity, eating disorders, and disordered eating, often co-occur. About 40% of girls with overweight/obesity and almost 20% of boys with overweight/obesity also engage in binge eating, extreme weight-control behaviors, or both. Weight-related problems share similar longitudinal risk factors, such as weight-related teasing, weight concerns and body dissatisfaction, and dieting and unhealthy weight-control behaviors.

Puhl, R. M., & King, K. M. (2013). Weight discrimination and bullying. *Best Practice and Research: Clinical Endocrinology and Metabolism, 27*(2), 117–127.—Among youth with obesity, weight stigmatization translates into pervasive victimization, teasing, and bullying. Multiple adverse outcomes are associated with exposure to weight stigmatization, including depression, anxiety, low self-esteem, body dissatisfaction, suicidal ideation, poor academic performance, lower physical activity, maladaptive eating behaviors, and avoidance of health care.

Puhl, R. M., Moss-Racusin, C. A., & Schwartz, M. B. (2007). Internalization of weight bias: Implications for binge eating and emotional well-being. *Obesity, 15*(1), 19–23.—Anorexia nervosa and body dysmorphic disorder are associated with abnormalities in processing visual information. This study examined the relationship between internalization of negative weight-based stereotypes and indices of eating behaviors and emotional well-being in a sample of women with overweight and obesity. Participants who believed that weight-based stereotypes were true reported more frequent binge eating in response to stigmatizing experiences than did those who reported stereotypes to be false.

Rudd Center for Food Policy and Obesity, University of Connecticut. (n.d.). Preventing weight bias: Helping without harming in clinical practice. Available at *http://biastoolkit.uconnruddcenter.org.*—This toolkit is designed to help clinicians across a variety of practice settings with easy-to-implement solutions and resources to improve delivery of care for patients with obesity. The resources are designed for busy professionals and customized for various practice settings.

Sonneville, K. R., Calzo, J. P., Horton, N. J., Haines, J., Austin, S. B., & Field, A. E. (2012). Body satisfaction, weight gain and binge eating among overweight adolescent girls. *International Journal of Obesity, 36*(7), 944–949.—This study examined the prospective association between body satisfaction and BMI change, and the onset of frequent binge eating among adolescent girls with overweight/obesity. Girls who reported being at least somewhat satisfied with their bodies made smaller BMI gains and had 61% lower odds of starting to binge-eat frequently (OR: 0.39; 95% CI: 0.24–0.64) than their less satisfied peers.

Part II

EATING DISORDERS

CLINICAL CHARACTERISTICS
OF EATING DISORDERS

The History of Eating Disorders

RICHARD A. GORDON

Although it is commonly assumed that most eating disorders are distinctly modern diseases, there is little question that phenomena similar to eating disorders have a long history. The explanation of this apparent contradiction has much to do with the framework through which eating disorders are interpreted. Whereas self-imposed fasting was typically described in spiritual terms in medieval times, and binge eating was described moralistically as demonic, or medically as being due to a gastrointenstinal disturbance, medical and psychiatric interpretations have been the leading paradigms (for the most part) since the late 19th century. And since the middle of the 20th century, a powerful new dimension has been associated with eating disorders: a preoccupation with body image, a "drive for thinness," and a fear of obesity. In this chapter we focus on the historical development of the modern conceptions of eating disorders, particularly as psychiatric diagnoses.

Anorexia Nervosa

Wherever there has been fasting, it would seem, abuse of the practice by some seems almost inevitable. This fact alone would suggest that anorexia nervosa (AN) must be historically and culturally pervasive. However, the first life stories for which there is enough detail to argue the presence of AN are those of the fasting female saints in late medieval Europe. The gender pattern, as well as the developmental and familial context, of these women have been the origin of detailed accounts of such "holy anorexia." Nevertheless, skepticism arose because of the radically different spiritual motivation of the saints, in contrast to the secular body image concerns of contemporary patients. Self-imposed starvation was also exhibited by the "miraculous maidens" of the 18th and 19th centuries, whose behavior often attracted much public and official attention.

AN received its first medical description in two brief but highly suggestive case histories by English physician Richard Morton, buried in his massive *Treatise on Consumption*, published in 1692. And whereas there were sporadic medical references to self-starvation for the next two centuries, the first formal descriptions of AN did not appear until 1873, in the writings of British physician Sir William Gull and French neurologist Charles Lasègue. Gull, who gave the syndrome its modern name, recognized the essentially psychiatric nature of food refusal, and gave special emphasis to behavioral characteristics such as excessive activity. Lasègue, who discovered the disease independently in Paris, wrote about many of the behavioral and attitudinal characteristics that are easily recognizable today and offered telling descriptions of the interactions of the sufferer with her family.

Was there a "first great wave" of AN, as historian Edward Shorter has suggested? The disease was also identified in the late 19th century in Italy, Russia, and Germany. Psychiatrists Dejerine and Gauckler, in a book published in 1911, suggested that the many kinds of anorexia were common. In light of their speculation, it is of great interest that references to AN radically declined from about 1915 to the early 1930s. The most likely reason for this was the identification in 1915 of an endocrine disease, Simmonds' pituitary cachexia, which undoubtedly led to the misdiagnosis of many cases of AN for about 15–20 years. By the 1930s, though, a number of observers, for example, Ryle in England and Sheldon in the United States, became acutely aware of the differences in the two illnesses and the distinctness of AN.

AN continued to be interest in the 1940s and 1950s in the United States, the United Kingdom, France, and Germany, and, as one observer put it, the literature was voluminous but repetitive. The illness was described in detail, and there were interesting suggestions about refeeding, but there were virtually no advances in understanding the etiology. This was also the heyday of psychoanalytic therapists, a small number of whom developed an influential but long-since-discarded theory of the disease that equated a fear of eating with anxiety about oral impregnation. The idea that physical factors, especially endocrine factors, were somehow intimately involved with the illness led to a temporary subsuming of AN under the broad category of "psychosomatic illness," a framework that became popular in both American and continental psychiatry in the 1940s and 1950s.

A key period in the emergence of modern concepts of AN was the 1960s and 1970s, an era during which incidence of the disorder appeared to have increased. Central to this period was the work of Hilde Bruch in the United States, whose concept of primary AN, in which an all-consuming drive for thinness was the central feature, exerted enormous subsequent influence. Bruch's work was paralleled and even anticipated by that of Italian psychiatrist Mara Selvini Palazzoli, whose book on self-starvation strongly emphasized developmental, familial, and cultural factors, such as the changing pressures on women following World War II. During the same two decades, psychiatrists Arthur Crisp and Gerald Russell led inpatient units in London, dedicated to the treatment of AN, and both formulated conceptions of the disorder in which the drive for thinness and the fear of fatness played a central role.

The modern concept of AN, then, revolves around the diagnostic centrality of the drive for thinness and associated anxiety about and distortions of body image, which have been central in the diagnosis of AN in many editions of the *Diagnostic and Statistical Manual of Mental Disorders,* from DSM-III (published in 1980) up to DSM-5 (published in 2013). It has been proposed by Habermas that body image and weight consciousness were always present in AN, beginning with the writings of Gull and Lasègue, but were overlooked or not well formulated by the early observers. This notion is controversial among historians of the disease, but it does offer an interesting formulation of why the disorder appeared rather suddenly in the late 19th century, after the appearance of the concern with obesity and the concept of dieting emerged in the middle of that century.

Bulimia Nervosa

Bulimia nervosa (BN), especially the terminology of the diagnosis, has a rather complex and somewhat confusing history. The term *bulimia* has ancient roots in the Greek word *boulimia,* derived from a combination of the words for "ox" (*bous*) and "hunger" (*limos*). Ziolko, a German psychiatrist, documented elaborate references to the term beginning in ancient times, including its appearance in American and French medical dictionaries in the 19th century. Ziolko argued that these data suggest that what we call BN is hardly new, and that the modern disorder represents an ancient pattern dressed in modern clothing. This argument is questionable, if only because the vast majority of instances reported by Ziolko are instance of binge eating not accompanied by compensatory purging in order to control body weight. The issue is made even more confusing by the fact that the first appearance of the modern diagnosis of BN in DSM-III in 1980 was really a diagnosis of binge eating disorder (see below) rather than BN. The latter did not appear until the publication of DSM-III-R in 1987.

Bulimic behavior was first noticed, beginning in the 1940s, in a number of case reports among anorectic patients, but the syndrome that we now call BN in normal-weight individuals was first described in the early 1960s by French psychiatrists, who reported a number of cases of binge eating followed by purging in a series of 15 women who had used diet pills. Ziolko also made note of a syndrome of binge eating and purging in the 1960s, which he dubbed "hyperorexia nervosa." By 1976, Ziolko had reported seeing over 70 such cases. In the 1970s, psychologist Marlene Boskind-White described a large number of women who secretly binged and purged at Cornell University in Ithaca, New York. Noting the similarity of these womens' concerns with those who had AN (particularly their drive for achievement coupled with their preoccupation with thinness), she dubbed the syndrome "bulimarexia." Credit for the modern diagnostic term of BN goes to English psychiatrist Gerald Russell, who also noted an increasing number of cases in the 1970s and published a definitive article that gave the syndrome its modern name in 1979. Like Boskind-White, he thought the pattern was closely akin to AN, but unlike Boskind-White, he felt that the prognosis for BN was far worse than that of AN (hence, the subtitle of his article: "An Ominous Variant of AN"). In light of later developments that showed BN to be relatively responsive to treatment, especially when compared with AN, Russell later retracted the "ominous variant" characterization.

BN began to be characterized as a "hidden epidemic" in the early 1980s after inquiries by Craig Johnson in the United States and Christopher Fairburn in England yielded responses from thousands of sufferers who had kept their disorder hidden for a number of years. Perhaps as a result of this and a sense of the urgent need for treatments, research on BN surged in the 1980s.

An important development in the 1980s was the design of effective treatments for the disorder. In a series of studies, Fairburn and colleagues showed that a model of cognitive-behavioral therapy that emphasized self-monitoring, the normalization of eating, and cognitive restructuring of body image distortions was significantly more effective than behavioral treatments that attempted to directly eliminate bingeing and purging activities. An unexpected by-product of Fairburn's work was that interpersonal therapy, which was originally used as a control, was of comparable effectiveness to CBT. Another direction in treatment was undertaken by investigators at Harvard and Columbia, who showed that antidepressants (at that time, the tricyclics and monoamine oxidase inhibitors [MAOIs]) were significantly effective in the treatment of BN.

Recent demographic trends in BN suggest that it is emerging at a somewhat younger age, and that its overall prevalence may have declined somewhat. This is possibly a reflection of the overestimation of the prevalence of the disorder in earlier studies that did not employ the more rigorous frequency requirements that became incorporated into diagnostic criteria in 1987.

Binge Eating Disorder

As noted earlier, historical reviews have suggested that binge eating disorder (BED) may have an even more extensive ancient history than AN and BN. A remarkable fact about the modern history of eating disorders is that by far the most common eating disorder (BED) was the one to be identified last in the modern diagnostic system. Possible explanations for this anomaly are the drama (and potential lethality) of self-starvation in a relatively affluent population, the visibility and fascination with self-induced vomiting symptoms in college populations in the 1980s, and the reluctance to associate a psychiatric disorder with obesity that permeated psychiatric thought in the 1970s and 1980s.

Albert J. Stunkard, a key figure in the discovery of binge eating problems, expressed amazement at this sequence of events. Stunkard himself had introduced the term *binge* in 1959 (it, in turn, had been suggested to him by a patient), and had been instrumental in formulating the criteria for what was called *bulimia* in DSM-III in 1980. He noted, in retrospect, that these were really criteria for what 14 years later became *binge eating disorder*. Somehow, the focus on binge eating and purging in middle- and upper-class college students led to a radical transformation of "bulimia" to "BN" in DSM-III-R, while BED, with its lack of compensatory behavior, at least temporarily was ignored.

In the early 1990s, however, led by Robert Spitzer, the architect of the 1980 DSM-III, a group that included Stunkard proposed the inclusion of a separate diagnosis for BED in DSM-IV (published in 1994). Validation research for the diagnosis included relatively large numbers of people currently in weight control programs, a nonpatient community sample, and a small group of patients with BN. The principal findings were that BED was more common among the subjects in weight control programs, and that it was more common than BN in the general population. Both of these findings held up in later studies (a recent Australian study found BED to be at least five times as common AN or BN). A significant percentage of subjects with BED are overweight and have a history of chronic dieting. Yet, unlike BN, for most with BED, the binge eating historically precedes dieting, rather than the opposite sequence.

DSM-IV included BED as a provisional diagnosis, a category that indicated it was in need of further study, but it became a diagnosis in its own right in DSM-5. Research since 1994 has corroborated the fact that BED is significantly more prevalent than AN or BN, that it manifests more frequently in older populations than the other two eating disorders, that it is more equally prevalent among men and women, and that it does not show the differential prevalence between European American and African American groups that seems evident in AN and BN.

Studies have shown that BED may be modified by both cognitive-behavioral and pharmacological treatments, although much needs to be learned about these interventions and how to improve them. BED may be particularly influenced by both nutritional and psychological and emotional triggers. It may well be, as David Kessler has suggested, that BED has become elevated in modern culture due to the omnipresence of particular types of appealing, calorie-rich, commercially prepared foods. We have much to learn about the interaction of possibly "addicting" foods with the cognitive and emotional antecedents of BED.

Suggested Reading

Note: This bibliography is centered on historical works, with the assumption that the numerous clinical writings referred to in the text can be readily located.

Bell, R. M. (1985). *Holy anorexia*. Chicago: University of Chicago Press.—The now classic but still controversial work hypothesizes, through detailed case studies, that medieval figures such as Catherine of Siena evidenced both behavior and underlying psychology that was strongly akin to AN.

Bliss, E. L., & Branch, C. H. H. (1960). *Anorexia nervosa*. New York: Hoeber.—This book, although dismissed by Hilde Bruch as being overly inclusive and amorphous in its diagnostic approach and theory of etiology, contains a wealth of forgotten references to studies of AN that took place in the first half of the 20th century, particularly from the late 1930s to 1960, after the psychiatric study of AN was revived.

Habermas, T. (1989). The psychiatric history of anorexia nervosa and bulimia nervosa: Weight concerns and bulimic symptoms in early case reports. *International Journal of Eating Disorders, 8,* 259–274.—Suggestions from early reports and various data from the international literature are marshaled to argue that body image and weight concerns have been central in AN nervosa since Gull and Lasègue, but were overlooked, owing in part to efforts on the part of patients to hide them.

Keel, P. K., & Klump, K. L. (2003). Are eating disorders culture-bound syndromes?: Implications for conceptualizing their etiology. *Psychological Review, 129,* 747–769.—The authors trace in detail the history of AN, including an attempt at a estimate of the frequency of cases before systematic epidemiological data were kept, and conclude that the incidences of AN have been more or less constant over many centuries, whereas BN is of relatively recent origin.

Russell, G. F. M. (1997). The history of bulimia. In D. M. Garner & P. E. Garfinkel (Eds.), *Handbook of treatment for eating disorders* (pp. 11–24). New York: Guilford Press.—This essential chapter by the originator of the BN diagnosis presents the case for the disorder being an essentially modern condition.

Russell, G. F. M., & Treasure, J. (1989). The modern history of anorexia nervosa: An interpretation of why the illness has changed. *Annals of the New York Academy of Sciences, 575,* 13–30.—The authors invoke the concept of "pathoplasticity" to account for how sociocultural influences operated to give rise to the modern form of AN, in which body image and fear of weight gain are central.

Stunkard, A. J. (1993). A history of binge eating. In C. G. Fairburn & G. T. Wilson (Eds.), *Binge eating: Nature, assessment and treatment* (pp. 15–34). New York: Guilford Press.—This review has many valuable insights into the discovery of binge eating problems, in which the author played a central role, and the confusion that arose in differentiating the diagnosis of BN from that of BED.

Vandereycken, W. (1994). Emergence of bulimia nervosa as a separate diagnostic entity: Review of the literature from 1960 to 1979. *International Journal of Eating Disorders, 16,* 105–116.—A detailed account of the evolution of the BN diagnosis, beginning with a number of untranslated French sources in the early 1960s to Russell's definitive article in 1979.

Vandereycken, W., & van Deth, R. (1994). *From fasting saints to anorexic girls: The history of self-starvation*. New York: New York University Press.—This meticulous work, which can be read along with Joan Brumberg's *Fasting Girls,* covers in depth the history of anorectic-like behavior and the emergence of AN in the 19th century.

Ziolko, H. U. (1996). Bulimia: A historical outline. *International Journal of Eating Disorders, 20,* 345–358.—An extensive documentation of descriptive and medical cases of binge eating.

Classification of Eating Disorders

B. TIMOTHY WALSH

A critical question to address before considering how eating disorders should be classified is, "What is the definition of an eating disorder?" It was suggested in the first edition of this book that the fundamental characteristic of an eating disorder is *a persistent disturbance of eating or eating-related behavior that results in the altered consumption or absorption of food and that significantly impairs physical health or psychosocial function.* This definition continues to comport well with the leading official diagnostic systems, the *Diagnostic and Statistical Manual of Mental Disorders* (DSM) of the American Psychiatric Association and the *International Classification of Diseases* (ICD) of the World Health Organization.

However, the number of formally recognized eating disorders has increased in recent years, and the category has been further expanded by encompassing problems previously considered "feeding disorders" confined largely to childhood. These changes were incorporated in DSM-5, published in 2013, and will likely also be included to a large degree in ICD-11, currently planned for publication in 2018. The conceptualizations and descriptions of the "classic" eating disorders, anorexia nervosa and bulimia nervosa, are largely unchanged. Binge eating disorder, relegated to an appendix in DSM-IV, is officially recognized in DSM-5. In DSM-IV, three diagnostic categories were described in a section entitled "Feeding and Eating Disorders of Infancy or Early Childhood": pica, rumination disorder, and feeding disorder of infancy or early childhood. In DSM-5, the last category was expanded and renamed avoidant/restrictive food intake disorder (ARFID), and these three disorders were included in the retitled DSM-5 chapter, "Feeding and Eating Disorders."

Anorexia Nervosa

The core characteristics of anorexia nervosa (AN) have not changed since the syndrome received its name over a century ago: relentless restriction of calorie intake in the successful pursuit of a substantially reduced body weight, accompanied by a minimization of the resulting psychological and physical impairment and by a distorted assessment of body shape and weight. The successive DSM and ICD editions have attempted to capture these characteristics in concise and interpretable criteria. Current DSM-5 criteria (Table 26.1) require that the individual's weight be "significantly low" but, unlike DSM-IV, which included the somewhat confusing example of "less than 85% of that expected," no specific weight is mentioned in the criteria. However, the accompanying DSM-5 text describes several guidelines to aid clinicians' judgment, such as the fact that a body mass index (BMI) of 18.5 kg/m^2 is frequently employed as the lower limit of normal for adults.

Two significant changes incorporated into DSM-5 criteria were made with the goal of making the definition slightly less restrictive. First, the DSM-IV criterion requiring amenorrhea was eliminated; however, the DSM-5 text emphasizes that serious medical complications such as amenorrhea are associated with AN, and that their presence supports the diagnosis. Second, Criterion B, requiring evidence of fear of gaining weight, now permits the clinician to judge this criterion to be satisfied on the basis of behavior to avoid weight gain, even if the individual does not explicitly acknowledge being afraid of gaining weight.

As have prior editions, DSM-5 suggests that individuals with AN be classified as having either the restricting or the binge eating/purging type at the time of their assessment. This distinction is clinically useful, since those with the binge eating/purging type are more likely to engage in other impulsive behaviors, such as drug abuse and suicide attempts. However, these subtypes are not fixed over time; at the time of onset, most individuals with AN are classified as having the restricting type, but, over time, about one-half meet criteria for the binge eating/purging type.

A new feature introduced in DSM-5 is severity ratings. DSM-5 suggests that the minimum level of severity of AN be based on the BMI, or, for children and adolescents who are still growing, on the BMI percentile. The level of severity may be increased to reflect other clinical features, such as the level of functional impairment or physical complications. Although of great potential utility for both clinicians and researchers, these metrics have not yet been extensively studied.

Bulimia Nervosa

The core features required for the diagnosis of bulimia nervosa (BN), a syndrome first clearly described by Gerald Russell in 1979, have changed little since that time. The key characteristics are repeated episodes of *binge eating* (the consumption of an unusually large amount of food in a brief period of time accompanied by a sense of loss of control) and repeated episodes of inappropriate behavior, most commonly self-induced vomiting to avoid weight gain. These behavioral characteristics are accompanied by an overconcern regarding shape and weight similar to that in AN. The sole modification introduced in DSM-5 (Table 26.2) is the reduction in the required minimum average frequency of binge eating and of inappropriate compensatory behaviors from twice weekly to once weekly. And, as in the case of AN, a severity rating scheme has been introduced in DSM-5, based primarily on the frequency of episodes of inappropriate compensatory behavior.

It is important to note that, although frequent binge eating and purging occur among a substantial subset of individuals with AN, by DSM-5 guidelines, they are not assigned the diagnosis of BN, but of AN, binge eating/purging type. This nosological distinction reflects the fact that the course, outcome, complications, and treatment responses of such

TABLE 26.1. DSM-5 Criteria for AN

A. Restriction of energy intake relative to requirements leading to a significantly low body weight in the context of age, sex, developmental trajectory, and physical health. Significantly low weight is defined as a weight that is less than minimally normal, or, for children and adolescents, less than that minimally expected.

B. Intense fear of gaining weight or becoming fat, or persistent behavior that interferes with weight gain, even though at a significantly low weight.

C. Disturbance in the way in which one's body weight or shape is experienced, undue influence of body shape or weight on self-evaluation, or persistent lack of recognition of the seriousness of current low body weight.

Note. Reprinted with permission from the *Diagnostic and Statistical Manual of Mental Disorders, Fifth Edition* (Copyright © 2013), American Psychiatric Association.

individuals have much more in common with those of individuals with the restricting type of AN than those of individuals with BN.

Binge Eating Disorder

The syndrome now known as *binge eating disorder (BED)*, described by Stunkard in 1959, did not receive significant attention until the process of developing DSM-IV was under way. Led by Robert Spitzer, a group of investigators proposed the name and a set of diagnostic criteria, and suggested that BED be officially recognized in DSM-IV. However, the limited data available concerning the characteristics of the disorder at that time led to its inclusion only in an appendix of DSM-IV. The almost 20 years between the publication of DSM-IV and DSM-5 witnessed a surge of interest in BED, presumably triggered by the availability of the criteria in DSM-IV and growing clinical recognition of the problem. The data accumulated since the publication of DSM-IV provided the

TABLE 26.2. DSM-5 Criteria for BN

A. Recurrent episodes of binge eating. An episode of binge eating is characterized by both of the following:
   1. Eating, in a discrete period of time (e.g., within any 2-hour period), an amount of food that is definitely larger than what most individuals would eat in a similar period of time under similar circumstances.
   2. A sense of lack of control over eating during the episode (e.g., a feeling that one cannot stop eating or control what or how much one is eating).

B. Recurrent inappropriate compensatory behaviors in order to prevent weight gain, such as self-induced vomiting; misuse of laxatives, diuretics, or other medications; fasting; or excessive exercise.

C. The binge eating and inappropriate compensatory behaviors both occur, on average, at least once a week for 3 months.

D. Self-evaluation is unduly influenced by body shape and weight.

E. The disturbance does not occur exclusively during episodes of anorexia nervosa.

Note. Reprinted with permission from the *Diagnostic and Statistical Manual of Mental Disorders, Fifth Edition* (Copyright © 2013), American Psychiatric Association.

foundation for the decision to formally recognize BED in DSM-5 (Table 26.3), with only minimal changes to the criteria provided in DSM-IV.

The hallmark of BED is a pattern of binge eating, defined as in BN, but without the inappropriate compensatory behaviors that characterize the latter disorder. Because it can be difficult to distinguish binge eating from "normal" overeating in the absence of clearly abnormal behaviors such as self-induced vomiting, Criteria B and C require that the individual endorse indicators of loss of control, such as eating alone because of embarrassment, and intense distress over the binge eating.

Individuals with BED are generally overweight or obese but report more symptoms of anxiety and depression than otherwise similar peers. There are indications that treatments aimed at weight reduction should be tailored to fit the needs of individuals with the disorder and that BED may be associated with increased risk of further weight gain.

Avoidant/Restrictive Food Intake Disorder

The redefinition and expansion of the DSM-IV category feeding disorder of infancy or early childhood into avoidant/restrictive food intake disorder (ARFID) were among the major changes introduced in the DSM-5 section "Feeding and Eating Disorders" (Table 26.4). The DSM-IV disorder had been introduced to capture presentations of children whose nutrition was inadequate because of feeding problems thought to be related to impaired interactions with primary caregivers. The category received little research attention or clinical use, so that, when DSM-5 was under development, there was little published information about the disorder. In addition, it had become clear that other presentations characterized by significantly reduced food intake were not captured within DSM-IV. The criteria for ARFID were developed to encompass not only presentations

---

TABLE 26.3. DSM-5 Criteria for BED

A. Recurrent episodes of binge eating. An episode of binge eating is characterized by both of the following:
   1. Eating, in a discrete period of time (e.g., within any 2-hour period), an amount of food that is definitely larger than what most individuals would eat in a similar period of time under similar circumstances.
   2. A sense of lack of control over eating during the episode (e.g., a feeling that one cannot stop eating or control what or how much one is eating).

B. The binge-eating episodes are associated with three (or more) of the following:
   1. Eating much more rapidly than normal.
   2. Eating until feeling uncomfortably full.
   3. Eating large amounts of food when not feeling physically hungry.
   4. Eating alone because of being embarrassed by how much one is eating.
   5. Feeling disgusted with oneself, depressed, or very guilty after overeating.

C. Marked distress regarding binge eating is present.

D. The binge eating occurs, on average, at least once a week for 3 months.

E. The binge eating is not associated with the recurrent use of inappropriate compensatory behavior as in bulimia nervosa and does not occur exclusively during the course of bulimia nervosa or anorexia nervosa.

Note. Reprinted with permission from the *Diagnostic and Statistical Manual of Mental Disorders, Fifth Edition* (Copyright © 2013), American Psychiatric Association.

TABLE 26.4. DSM-5 Criteria for ARFID

A. Eating or feeding disturbance (e.g., apparent lack of interest in eating or food; avoidance based on the sensory characteristics of food; concern about aversive consequences of eating) as manifested by persistent failure to meet appropriate nutritional and/or energy needs leading to one or more of the following:
  1. Significant weight loss (or failure to gain weight or faltering growth in children).
  2. Significant nutritional deficiency.
  3. Dependence on enteral feeding or oral nutritional supplements.
  4. Marked interference with psychosocial functioning.

B. The disturbance is not better explained by lack of available food or an associated culturally sanctioned practice.

C. The eating disturbance does not occur exclusively during the course of Anorexia Nervosa or Bulimia Nervosa, and there is no evidence of a disturbance in the way in which one's body weight or shape is experienced.

D. The eating disorder is not attributable to a concurrent medical condition or not better explained by another mental disorder. If the eating disturbance occurs in the context of another condition or disorder, the severity of the eating disturbance exceeds that routinely associated with the condition or disorder and warrants additional clinical attention.

Note. Reprinted with permission from the *Diagnostic and Statistical Manual of Mental Disorders, Fifth Edition* (Copyright © 2013), American Psychiatric Association.

meeting the criteria for feeding disorder of infancy or early childhood but also presentations with other characteristics, such as food avoidance related to sensory properties (e.g., refusal to eat foods with "lumps"). Although only limited data are currently available regarding the characteristics of individuals with ARFID, the DSM-5 criteria appear to capture the symptoms of a number of young individuals presenting to specialists in adolescent medicine and nutrition.

As with many disorders, the dividing line between ARFID and normality is not a sharp one. Many individuals, both children and adults, have idiosyncratic patterns of food choice and restrict their food intake for a variety of reasons, but they do not develop clinically significant problems; "picky eating" is not synonymous with ARFID. A critical judgment required in making a diagnosis of ARFID is that the resultant nutritional or psychosocial problems are substantial and require attention.

Pica and Rumination Disorders

Pica refers to the repeated ingestion of nonfood substances, such as dirt, and *rumination* to the repeated regurgitation of food that has been swallowed. Both disorders were described in DSM-IV in the section "Feeding and Eating Disorders of Infancy or Early Childhood." For DSM-5, the criteria were slightly revised for clarification and to recognize that the disorders can occur throughout the life cycle.

Other Eating Disorders

Although the disorders recognized by DSM-5 appear to describe a larger fraction of individuals presenting for treatment than did DSM-IV, a significant number of individuals with an eating disorder do not fulfill the criteria for any of the disorders formally defined in DSM-5. In an attempt to provide useful labels for some of these problems, DSM-5 includes a section on other specified feeding and eating disorders, with very brief descriptions of five presentations, such as purging disorder (purging to control shape or weight in the absence of binge eating). DSM-5 also includes the category unspecified feeding or eating disorder, for use if the clinician is unable to assess the specific features of the eating disorder.

Unresolved Issues

There is convincing evidence that the current, officially recognized feeding and eating disorders have clinical utility: These definitions provide clinicians with a nomenclature that conveys important information on the course and outcome of the disorders, and facilitates efficient and reliable communication for both clinical use and research. However, there are a number of significant problems.

A widely recognized nosological problem is that the DSM and ICD systems are categorical, whereas the phenomena they describe are, for the most part, continuous. Therefore, although the specific requirements to satisfy criteria, such as binge eating at least once weekly for 3 months, are reasonable, they are also arbitrary. A related problem is that, by design, the disorders are narrowly defined to yield very homogeneous groups, and do not provide a clear method of combining similar problems under broader rubrics. For example, both AN and ARFID are distinct disorders but with a similar core behavioral problem, the restriction of food intake; similarly, both BN and BED are characterized by binge eating.

Even more broadly, a large fraction of individuals with a feeding or eating disorder experience clinically significant problems with anxiety and depression, and meet diagnostic criteria for another mental disorder. The significance of such common comorbidity is unclear, and its existence is a source of confusion to patients, clinicians, and investigators. I hope that future research will address this and other problems surrounding how best to describe and classify human eating disorders.

Suggested Reading

Attia, E., Becker, A. E., Bryant-Waugh, R., Hoek, H. W., Kreipe, R. E., Marcus, M. D., et al. (2013). Feeding and eating disorders in DSM-5. *American Journal of Psychiatry, 170*(11), 1237–1239.—A very brief overview of the rationale for the changes incorporated in DSM-5.

Fisher, M. M., Rosen, D. S., Ornstein, R. M., Mammel, K. A., Katzman, D. K., Rome, E. S., et al. (2014). Characteristics of avoidant/restrictive food intake disorder in children and adolescents: A "new disorder" in DSM-5. *Journal of Adolescent Health, 55*(1), 49–52.—One of the first published descriptions of ARFID.

Keel, P. K., Brown, T. A., Holm-Denoma, J., & Bodell, L. P. (2011). Comparison of DSM-IV versus proposed DSM-5 diagnostic criteria for eating disorders: Reduction of eating disorder not otherwise specified and validity. *International Journal of Eating Disorders, 44*(6), 553–560.—A discussion of the impact of DSM-5 versus DSM-IV.

Smink, F. R., Hoeken, D., Oldehinkel, A. J., & Hoek, H. W. (2014). Prevalence and severity of DSM-5 eating disorders in a community cohort of adolescents. *International Journal of Eating Disorders, 47*(6), 610–619.—Frequency and severity of DSM-5 eating disorders in an adolescent sample.

Uher, R., & Rutter, M. (2012). Classification of feeding and eating disorders: Review of evidence and proposals for ICD-11. *World Psychiatry, 11,* 80–92.—Early considerations regarding feeding and eating disorders in ICD-11.

Walsh, B. T., & Sysko, R. (2009). Broad categories for the diagnosis of eating disorders (BCD-ED): An alternative system for classification. *International Journal of Eating Disorders, 42,* 754–764.—A description of a less restrictive classification system for eating disorders.

Wonderlich, S. A., Gordon, K. H., Mitchell, J. E., Crosby, R. D., & Engel, S. G. (2009). The validity and clinical utility of binge eating disorder. *International Journal of Eating Disorders, 42,* 687–705.—Summary of data supporting the inclusion of BED in DSM-5.

Anorexia Nervosa

EVELYN ATTIA

Anorexia nervosa (AN) is an eating disorder characterized by a relentless pursuit of thinness and a fear of gaining weight despite the presence of a significantly low body weight. AN, a serious psychiatric disorder, is associated with high rates of medical and psychiatric morbidity and a mortality rate as high as that associated with any psychiatric illness. AN is a persistent illness, first described in the medical literature in the 17th century, with very little change in its clinical presentation throughout the centuries that have followed. Despite its long history, AN remains a challenge to treat because its core behaviors often become entrenched and are difficult to reverse, especially for adult patients who have been ill for longer periods of time.

Historical Background

AN was first described in the medical literature in 1689 by Richard Morton, who described cases of extreme fasting and reported loss of appetite without evidence of an underlying physical cause. It is surmised that the medieval saints who refused food in order to achieve spiritual purity may have been earlier examples of individuals affected by the same illness. AN received its current name from Sir William Gull, one of Queen Victoria's physicians, who coined the term in the late 19th century in his report of a small case series of women with the disorder. AN was first included, and distinguished from bulimia, in the third edition of the American Psychiatric Association's *Diagnostic and Statistical Manual of Mental Disorders* (DSM-III), published in 1980.

Diagnosis and Clinical Features

The diagnosis of AN requires the presence of a significantly low weight in the context of an individual's age, sex, developmental trajectory, and/or physical health, achieved and maintained by restricting food intake relative to requirements. The illness generally includes an acknowledged fear of gaining weight or becoming fat, or persistent behaviors that interfere with weight gain. Individuals with AN demonstrate overconcern with body shape or weight, a disturbance in the way they experience their actual body weight or shape, or a lack of recognition of the seriousness of their low body weight. There are two subtypes of AN. The restricting type describes individuals who have not engaged in binge eating or purging behaviors in the last 3 months and whose low weight results solely from restricted food intake and/or exercise. The binge eating–purging type of AN describes those who, during the prior 3 months, have engaged in recurrent episodes of binge eating or purging behavior (e.g., self-induced vomiting, misuse of laxatives or diuretics).

Some individuals do not report fear of fat or of weight gain, likely resulting from their reluctance to describe the thinking associated with their disordered eating. It is also possible that, in different cultures, the rationale for food refusal is not expressed as a concern about weight gain. The inclusion of persistent behaviors to avoid weight gain in the diagnostic criterion for AN regarding fear of weight gain permits the inclusion of individuals who meet all other criteria for the illness but verbally deny fear of becoming fat as their motivation for the eating disturbance to receive the diagnosis of AN.

DSM-5 does not provide a specific definition of significantly low weight. However, body mass index (BMI; calculated as weight in kilograms/height in meters^2) is a useful measure in weight assessment. The World Health Organization (WHO) has suggested a BMI of 18.5 kg/m^2 as the lower limit of a normal weight for adults, while most individuals with AN weigh much less. In certain instances, an adult with a BMI at or above 18.5 kg/m^2 might be considered underweight if clinical factors or physiological disturbances support this conclusion. For children or adolescents, it is useful to calculate a BMI-for-age percentile, and to use an individual's growth trajectory in determining whether the current weight is low or less than expected.

AN is associated with a multitude of physical and psychological signs and symptoms, most of which result from the low-weight state that is the core feature of this illness. AN can affect every organ system, and physical signs may include changes to vital signs (e.g., bradycardia, hypothermia) and other physical features (e.g., thinning hair, lanugo), laboratory assessments (e.g., leukopenia, anemia, electrolyte disturbances, hepatic transaminitis), and physiological functioning (e.g., amenorrhea, osteoporosis). Many psychological disturbances develop or intensify in individuals with AN, including depression, anxiety, and obsessionality. The Minnesota Starvation Experiment performed during World War II documented the development of similar psychological changes associated with weight loss in otherwise healthy men, including obsessionality and ritualized behaviors, anxiety, anhedonia, and insomnia.

Individuals with AN often describe thinking about food from the moment they wake up in the morning, including obsessional thoughts about food calories, ingredients, and preparation. They often impose rigid rules for themselves regarding food intake, including the types and quantity of foods consumed, rituals around eating behavior (e.g., cutting, chopping, mixing of foods), and timing and rate of consumption. There may be periods of fasting during the day (e.g., no food before evening, or no food after 6:00 P.M.), and slowed rates of chewing or sipping of allowed foods. They may engage in obsessional weight monitoring and body checking (i.e., touching, pinching, and examining the body to assess their thinness). Additionally, individuals with AN may develop other behaviors that interfere with weight gain. For many of those with the binge eating–purging subtype, this includes behaviors that specifically aim to compensate for food consumed, such as self-induced vomiting, or use of laxative or diuretic medications. Many with AN engage in excessive physical activity, such as standing or walking for long periods, shaking or fidgeting, or varieties of formal exercise. Others insist on leaving food on their plates, eating in isolation, or using exceedingly small utensils to support restrictive food intake.

AN is a complex behavioral disorder and its etiology is multifactorial, including biological and environmental elements. Ample evidence supports biological and genetic contributions to the development of AN. Family studies have demonstrated that AN aggregates in families, and twin studies have identified that genetic factors contribute greatly to this aggregation. AN occurs in environments in which there is both adequate food supply and cultural elements that value thinness. The illness is known to occur throughout North America, Europe, and Australia, but it has also been identified in most countries in Asia and South America, and in several countries in Africa. Additionally, occupations that emphasize thinness and may include weight monitoring, such as ballet, modeling, and some sports, are associated with higher rates of AN. Identified risk factors are otherwise general, such as being female and adolescent, and do not explain more specifically who is at risk for developing AN.

Epidemiology, Course, and Outcome

Information regarding the numbers of individuals with AN is limited because AN is an uncommon illness and affected individuals often deny or diminish symptoms and do not pursue treatment. Studies assessing the incidence of AN (i.e., new cases per 100,000 persons per year) report far higher rates among adolescent samples than those among adults. Incidence rates identified from large European community samples range from 4.2–7.7 per 100,000 person-years, with far higher rates among adolescents 15–19 years of age, with an incidence rate of 109.2 per 100,000 person-years in one Dutch sample, and, in a sample from Finland, 270 per 100,000 person-years among female twins of the same age range. While there has been some debate about whether incidence rates of eating disorders are on the rise, several studies have concluded that incidence rates for AN have been stable in Europe and the United States since the 1970s. The lifetime prevalence of AN is estimated at 0.9% among females. Prevalence in males is far lower, commonly estimated as being one-tenth of the rates seen among females. Whereas in a sample in the United States researchers found a prevalence rate of 0.3% in male adolescents, researchers in several European countries found far lower rates.

Mortality rates are consistently high in AN. In fact, one meta-analysis of excess mortality found that AN was associated with the highest rate of mortality among all mental disorders. Weighted crude mortality rate (CMR), indicating the number of deaths within the study population over a specified period, has been identified for AN as 5.1 deaths per 1,000 person-years. Approximately 20% of deaths associated with AN are due to suicide. The standardized mortality ratio (SMR) for AN, describing the ratio of actual deaths to expected deaths for a given population, is approximately five in most studies, with the highest SMR for adolescents, since baseline mortality rates are very low for younger individuals.

AN generally presents in mid-to-late adolescence, not infrequently associated with a normal developmental stressor such as leaving home for the first time. The illness usually begins innocently, with dieting or an attempt to "eat healthy" that does not seem different from behaviors tried by other adolescents, most of whom do not develop AN. Some modest initial weight loss is commonly met by a compliment or other positive response from peers or adults, such as a teacher or a coach. Individuals who develop AN describe a powerful response, in turn, to the positive feelings associated with weight loss, or a tendency to attempt additional weight loss to cope with a negative feeling. Food restriction commonly worsens over time in AN as fewer foods, as well as smaller amounts, are consumed. Additionally, eating behaviors may become more disordered over time, with binge eating and/or compensatory behaviors that aim to interfere with weight gain, such as purging and excessive physical activity, eventually developing in more than 50% of individuals with AN.

The course of AN is variable. Younger patients with relatively short illness duration are the most responsive to treatment. They generally respond to interventions that emphasize weight restoration, including a family-based therapy that encourages parents to help refeed their malnourished child. Older patients, who may be more entrenched in their symptoms, may find it more difficult to achieve behavioral change. Weight restoration is the essential first step in a successful treatment for AN for patients of any age, and different treatment settings may be utilized to help individuals achieve this change. Intensive outpatient, residential, and inpatient settings afford opportunity for close clinical monitoring and meal supervision, and many adult patients with AN use these settings during their clinical course. Most follow-up studies report recovery rates of approximately one-third of patients evaluated over a period of several years, with adolescent patients achieving higher recovery rates than adults. Significant numbers of individuals with AN may relapse following an attempt at weight restoration; some reports indicate that close to 50% of adults who receive inpatient treatment for weight restoration may relapse within 1 year of discharge. Approximately 20–30% of individuals with clinically significant AN may develop an enduring variant of the illness. These individuals are seriously affected by the psychiatric and medical morbidity associated with AN, yet they may be reluctant to pursue treatments to stabilize or improve their clinical condition.

Treatments

AN is a challenge to treat, especially in adults, and empirical support is lacking for specific treatments. Many treatments have been considered for AN, but controlled trials are relatively few, and usually include small numbers of participants. Participants are reluctant to participate in treatment trials, and study completion rates are low. Symptom overlap with other psychiatric disorders, such as depression and anxiety, led to early examination of multiple antidepressant medications for AN. Surprisingly, no benefit to eating, weight, or other psychological symptoms has been associated with these medications compared to placebo. More recent interest in atypical antipsychotic medications for psychological improvement or weight gain has resulted from several small studies; a larger multisite study of olanzapine compared with placebo identified a small but statistically significant effect on weight gain associated with olanzapine. Several specific psychotherapies for AN have been studied in controlled trials. Behaviorally oriented approaches appear to be most helpful for acute AN, as behavioral change and weight restoration are the primary treatment goals. Family-based therapy for adolescents with AN, a treatment that empowers parents to refeed their underweight youngsters, has been highly effective in helping young patients restore weight and achieve recovery using an outpatient intervention. Behavioral programs conducted within treatment settings that provide supervision for meals and snacks (e.g., intensive outpatient, residential, and inpatient programs) are commonly used, especially for adult patients. Other structured psychotherapies, including cognitive-behavioral therapy (CBT), interpersonal therapy (IPT), and a supportive treatment named specialist supportive clinical management (SSCM) are all associated with modest treatment effects, including small amounts of weight.

Future Directions

Despite its long history, well-characterized presentation, and compelling clinical course in which young, previously healthy persons develop an illness with notably high rates of morbidity and mortality, AN remains an active problem in the 21st century, with alarmingly few empirically supported treatments. The eating disorders field has begun to turn for answers to cognitive neuroscience, a discipline that studies brain function by examining neural networks responsible for specific behaviors and behavioral disturbances. One hypothesis for the development of AN posits that the dieting behaviors become habitual, contributing to the difficulty in altering them. This hypothesis is consistent with the findings that early intervention and shorter illness duration are associated with better treatment outcomes, and that the subgroup of individuals who develop severe and enduring AN is particularly resistant to treatment. This new area of research suggests that, while the initial food restriction, and for some, associated physical activity, may begin as goal-oriented tasks that aim to achieve modest weight reduction, the behaviors are reinforced, become highly practiced, and develop into more automated habits. Research is needed to test this hypothesis. If confirmed, this model may facilitate the development of novel treatments to target neural networks implicated in the development and maintenance of this disorder.

Suggested Reading

Attia, E., & Walsh, B. T. (2007). Anorexia nervosa. *American Journal of Psychiatry, 164*(12), 1805–1810.—These authors begin with a hypothetical case and review current data on prevalence, diagnosis, pathophysiology, and treatment.

Attia, E., & Walsh, B. T. (2009). Behavioral management for anorexia nervosa. *New England Journal of Medicine, 360*(5), 500–506.—This article reviews principles of behavioral management commonly used in various treatment settings to achieve weight restoration and eating behavior change.

Bell, R. M. (2014). *Holy anorexia.* Chicago: University of Chicago Press.—This book examines early cases of documented food refusal and suggests that cases of food refusal associated with pursuit of spiritual purity in the Middle Ages represented AN, as we understand the syndrome today.

Schiele, B. C., & Brozek, J. (1948). "Experimental neurosis" resulting from semistarvation in man. *Psychosomatic Medicine, 10*(1), 31–50.—This landmark study describes the psychological and behavioral changes observed in 36 healthy male volunteers who participated in a study of food restriction and weight loss.

Smink, F. R., van Hoeken, D., & Hoek, H. W. (2012). Epidemiology of eating disorders: Incidence, prevalence and mortality rates. *Current Psychiatry Reports, 14*(4), 406–414.—This comprehensive review describes results from available studies, organized by eating disorder.

Steinglass, J., & Walsh, B. T. (2006). Habit learning and anorexia nervosa: A cognitive neuroscience hypothesis. *International Journal of Eating Disorders, 39*(4), 267–275.—This article reviews clinical neuropsychological and neuroimaging findings in both obsessive–compulsive disorder and AN relevant to understanding a potential mechanism of the perpetuation of AN.

Trace, S. E., Baker, J. H., Peñas-Lledó, E., & Bulik, C. M. (2013). The genetics of eating disorders. *Annual Review of Clinical Psychology, 9*, 589–620.—The authors of this review describe the literature on genetic factors that may contribute to eating disorders, including studies using twin registries.

Walsh, B. T. (2013). The enigmatic persistence of anorexia nervosa. *Perspectives, 170*(5), 477–484.—The author proposes that the core behaviors of AN become entrenched because habits develop, and suggests that cognitive neuroscience may help identify neural networks implicated in the maintenance of illness behaviors.

Watson, H. J., & Bulik, C. M. (2013). Update on the treatment of anorexia nervosa: Review of clinical trials, practice guidelines and emerging interventions. *Psychological Medicine, 43*(12), 2477–2500.—This review describes available data from randomized clinical trials for AN, including the nil or small effect sizes associated with many of the interventions studied.

Severe and Enduring Anorexia Nervosa

STEPHEN W. TOUYZ
PHILLIPA J. HAY

There is now a consensus that recovery from anorexia nervosa (AN) is often a lengthy process. The impact of severe malnutrition and medical instability can be addressed in a more timely fashion than in the past, but the persistent, unrelenting, and all-consuming ruminations pertaining to food, shape, and weight have proved to be barriers to successful treatment outcomes. As a result, clinicians find themselves in the position of having to treat patients with severe and enduring AN (SE-AN) without the "luxury" of an evidence base to inform them. Clinical judgment and intuition therefore come to the fore with the need to either adapt existing treatments or to consider redefining treatment goals, including the often vexing issue of the need to attain a healthy body weight. There is also the temptation to focus attention on comorbid complicating disorders rather than the eating pathology per se, or to turn to more supportive treatments on an ad hoc basis. If all else fails, the intensity of treatment is raised to higher levels of care, even when this has not been helpful in the past. What is perhaps most disconcerting of all is that many such patients fail to present themselves for treatment even when previously assessed, and go on to develop a persistent and unrelenting course. Such patients, especially those with repeated treatment failures, are a much neglected group and worthy of our attention.

Thinking "Outside the Square": Time for a Reconceptualization

In a comprehensive review of the literature including 119 studies of 5,590 patients with a follow-up period between 1 and 29 years, Steinhausen (2002) found that whereas a mean of 47% of patients recovered (range 0–92%) and a further 34% improved (range 0–75%), 5% died and 21% developed a persistent and chronic course (range 0–75%). The latter have often had multiple treatment failures and pose significant challenges to those clinicians who find themselves in a position of providing treatment for them. In the absence of evidence, opinions range from withholding treatment of those who fail to comply with traditional regimens to the imposition of involuntary treatment, or, at the extreme, palliative care. Such severe illness imposes a heavy burden on not only patients and their caregivers and mental health services but also emergency and medical departments. The personal cost is significant because such patients are often under- or unemployed and suffer from ongoing medical complications (e.g., renal, liver, and cardiovascular disease; osteoporosis). Caregivers and families struggle to understand the perceived irrationality of their loved one's behavior, but find themselves in the position of having to provide ongoing financial support, often in a highly emotionally charged environment.

The time has come to reconceptualize SE-AN both as an illness with major psychiatric and medical sequelae and also as one that is fraught with family, social, and occupational complications. In a series of qualitative studies, it was found that patients with severe and enduring eating disorders obtained similar scores on quality-of-life measures to scores of persons suffering from a severe depressive illness. However, of even greater concern was that the life skills scores were on par with scores of persons with schizophrenia. Such findings make a strong argument for the adoption of a rehabilitation model in which long-term follow-up, crisis intervention, specific psychological interventions, and attention to substance misuse become the hallmarks of effective treatment. These core strategies are further supplemented by attention to basic self-care needs, including nutrition, housing, financial issues, and recreational activities, as well as occupational needs.

A common explanation for the poorer outcomes of persons with a more persistent form of the illness is the extreme ambivalence of sufferers in accepting change, as well as an ego-syntonic attachment to the maintenance of a low weight. Others have proffered a biological explanation for the poorer therapeutic outcome reported in adolescents with a duration of illness over 3 years following both individual and family-based therapies. They attribute the poorer outcome to the combined effects of both starvation and stress on the developing brain. This occurs at an inopportune time because this is when both structural (dendrite pruning and myelination) and functional development needs to take place. As a result, prefrontal maturation, which is crucial for the development of executive function and emotional regulation, is impeded at this critical juncture of late adolescent development. In a not dissimilar vein, a neurobiological model has been proposed to explain the putative temperamental phenotypes so often observed in such patients. This model is also based on a neurodevelopmental perspective. Such phenotypes include an inclination toward worry and fearfulness, an ability to adapt to circumstances in which anxiety or discomfort is elevated, poor self-esteem, behavioral rigidity, and marked perseverance. One is struck by the absence of reward and of the ability to engage in self-soothing behaviors or seek pleasurable activities; such individuals leave the impression that these are, in fact, aversive and should be actively avoided. When one places this within a developmental framework, there are often signs of reduced emotional reactivity and heightened stress arousal with rigidity and compulsivity, which may indicate a "pathway of vulnerability" to AN. It is therefore perhaps not surprising that anxiety disorders are found more frequently in patients with AN than in the community at large. Such anxiety disorders predate the development of AN and may predispose an individual to developing an eating disorder.

The Heterogeneity of AN: A Need for Staging

AN is as a relatively homogenous disorder with two distinct subtypes: restricting and binge–purge subtypes. Although this classification has served us well for over 35 years, its utility, especially as it pertains to SE-AN, is being called into question. There is now an urgent need to develop a new classification system that takes into account the inherent phenomenological differences seen in patients with a more severe and persistent form of the illness. Few would argue that a 12-year-old girl who had lost weight for the first time would present in a markedly different fashion than a 40-year-old woman with a history of multiple treatment failures and unsuccessful inpatient care. Such negative treatment experiences are usually associated with a pervasive sense of hopelessness, despair, and extreme isolation. Families who were supportive at the onset of the illness eventually become exasperated and angry, defeated by an ongoing "madness" that they fail to understand fully. A staging system, such as the ones developed for burns or cancer, is better able to accommodate those with more persistent illness and would allow for not only better communication but also the development of more appropriate treatments for those with early-onset AN and for others with a more persistent form of the disorder.

Treatment Guidelines for SE-AN

Patients with SE-AN pose unique treatment challenges. Typically, they express little or no motivation to change and doubt that weight gain might contribute to a better outcome. The clinician is often faced with a never-ending litany of arguments that any weight gain would cause such despair and unhappiness that it cannot be contemplated. The frequency of such impasses reinforces the need for the development of new, innovative, enhanced strategies not only to engage such patients successfully but also to retain them in treatment in order to reduce their suffering and deliver hope, however small, of some improvement. Such patients have usually experienced multiple treatment failures and present with myriad mental health problems and significant socioeconomic handicaps.

The first task is to ensure medical safety, then to clearly elucidate the goals of therapy. The overall aim is to establish a strong and durable collaborative therapeutic relationship that will form the cornerstone from which any change will emanate. A significant challenge is to maintain symptom stability while fostering improvement in quality of life, but with the clear understanding of the necessity for firm limits regarding issues such as medical instability and suicidal intent. One would hope that the patient can be led to understand the concept of the clinician's duty of care and recognize that there may come a time, despite vehement pleas to the contrary, that an admission to hospital is needed. At such times, when the consent of the patient may not be forthcoming, the potential of infringement of civil liberties arises. The decision to proceed with an involuntary admission is rarely straightforward. Ethical waters become muddied in regard to the decision about whether the capacity to make autonomous choices no longer exists, or is sufficiently compromised to the extent that the clinician must override the patient's expressed wishes. It is certainly preferable if the patient can be persuaded to accept admission without having to resort to the courts or tribunal hearings.

For the first time, multidisciplinary national clinical practice guidelines (from the Royal Australian and New Zealand College of Psychiatrists) have specifically addressed management of SE-AN. These guidelines also had the advantage of being informed by findings from the first randomized controlled trial of patients with SE-AN. Development of the guidelines was based on the premise that any such treatment must occur in a collaborative manner and after the goals of treatment have been clearly discussed with the patient. In addition, where appropriate, these goals should to be discussed with significant others in the patient's life. It is essential that patients feel that their treatment is being conducted within a setting that provides both support and comfort, and affords the opportunity for gradual change to occur. These guidelines, with the inclusion of a protocol to treat SE-AN, should draw more attention to this underresearched group and, we hope, not only improve treatment but lead to the development of more innovative strategies as well.

Rethinking Recovery

It is our belief that a *sine qua non* for the effective treatment of patients with SE-AN is the establishment of a dignified, collaborative therapeutic relationship with the added vital elements of empowerment and individual responsibility. With this in mind, and taking into account the high levels of disability, low motivation to change, and high attrition rate, we have advocated a new paradigm in which symptom reduction is not designated as the primary outcome measure. We accordingly adapted two existing treatment manuals (CBT and SSCM) and prioritized how the goals of treatment would be presented to patients. Although we actively promoted weight gain, our primary outcome goal was improvement of quality of life, and we conveyed both of these aims to patients. Both treatment arms were successful in promoting change, but CBT was more successful in promoting social adjustment at the end of treatment. At the end of the 12-month follow-up period, those patients who were randomized to the CBT arm had fewer eating disorder symptoms, as well as greater readiness to recover than those randomized to the SSCM arm. This study was one of the first to show that patients with SE-AN are not only capable of responding to but may also benefit from psychological treatments that have been specifically adapted for their particular needs. The findings of this study should not only provide hope for those patients with SE-AN but also stimulate clinicians' interest in developing new, innovative psychosocial treatments.

Concluding Remarks

There can be no doubt that treatment of a chronically ill patient poses unique challenges and at times pushes against the frontiers of both medicine and the law. The therapist regularly feels frustrated by the incessant need of the patient to argue against any change, and treatment teams often become split by strong disagreements that arise relative to the appropriate course of action. Clinicians may experience the same sense of futility and hopelessness as patients do, which renders decision making impotent. At such times, review of well-considered clinical practice guidelines regarding the treatment of those with SE-AN may make this difficult therapeutic journey easier to navigate. Finally, one should never lose hope: Such patients sometimes turn the corner and make what can only be described as a miraculous recovery against very long odds. Such recoveries testify to what is possible and underscore the need to find a definitive cure for this devastating illness.

Suggested Reading

Kaye, W., & Strober, M. (2009). Biology of eating disorders. In A. F. Schatzberg & C. B. Nemeroff (Eds.), *The American Psychiatric Publishing textbook of psychopharmacology* (4th ed., pp. 1027–1045). Washington, DC: American Psychiatric Publishing.—The authors propose a neurobiological developmental model to better understand how AN begins and to explore some of the maintaining factors.

Maguire, S., Touyz, S., Surgenor, L., Lacey, H., & Le Grange, D. (2011). Why DSM V needs to consider a staging model for anorexia nervosa. In Y. Latzer, J. Merrick, & D. Stein (Eds.), *Understanding eating disorders: Integrating culture, psychology and biology* (pp. 15–27). Hauppauge, NY: Nova Science.—This chapter makes a cogent argument that a staging model of illness is needed for AN, like those developed for neoplasia and burns.

Robinson, P. (2009). *Severe and enduring eating disorder (SEED): Management of complex presentations of anorexia and bulimia nervosa.* Chichester, UK: Wiley.—This book makes a compelling argument as to why those patients with a severe and enduring eating disorder should be treated with a rehabilitation model.

Steinhausen, H. C. (2002). The outcome of anorexia nervosa in the 20th century. *American Journal of Psychiatry, 159*(8), 1284–1293.

Strober, M., Grilo, C. M., & Mitchell, J. E. (2010). The chronically ill patient with anorexia nervosa: Development, phenomenology, and therapeutic considerations. In C. M. Grilo & J. E. Mitchell (Eds.), *The treatment of eating disorders: A clinical handbook* (pp. 225–237). New York: Guilford Press.—Utilizing clinical vignettes, this chapter provides an in-depth description of the phenomenology of SE-AN and clear clinical guidelines as to how it is best treated.

Swinbourne, J. M., & Touyz, S. W. (2007). The co-morbidity of eating disorders and anxiety disorders: A review. *European Eating Disorders Review, 15*(4), 253–274.—Many patients presenting with an eating disorder and, in particular, AN have had an anxiety disorder diagnosed in childhood, particularly social anxiety.

Touyz, S., & Hay, P. (2015). Severe and enduring anorexia nervosa (SE-AN): In search of a new paradigm. *Journal of Eating Disorders, 3*, 26.—The complex presentation of SE-AN is explored, clinical practice guidelines are presented, and vexing issues such as involuntary treatment and palliative care are explored.

Touyz, S., Le Grange, D., Lacey, H., Hay, P., Smith, R., Maguire, S., et al. (2013). Treating severe and enduring anorexia nervosa: A randomized controlled trial. *Psychological Medicine, 43*(12), 2501–2511.—This groundbreaking randomized controlled trial is the first to explore specially adapted psychological treatments (CBT:SE-AN and SSCM:SE-AN) in a cohort of patients with severe and enduring AN.

Treasure, J., & Russell, G. (2011). The case for early intervention in anorexia nervosa: Theoretical exploration of maintaining factors. *British Journal of Psychiatry, 199*(1), 5–7.—It is now generally accepted that the factors that may contribute to the development of AN are not necessarily the same as the ones that maintain it; the authors propose a neurodevelopmental model to emphasise the importance of early intervention.

Wonderlich, S., Mitchell, J. E., Crosby, R. D., Myers, T. C., Kadlec, K., LaHaise, K., et al. (2012). Minimizing and treating chronicity in the eating disorders: A clinical overview. *International Journal of Eating Disorders, 45*(4), 467–475.—This article provides a comprehensive clinical overview as to what is known about severe and enduring AN.

Bulimia Nervosa

PAMELA K. KEEL

Bulimia nervosa (BN) involves recurrent binge eating episodes coupled with inappropriate compensatory behaviors to prevent the effects of food on weight or shape. To meet the criteria of the fifth edition of the *Diagnostic and Statistical Manual for Mental Disorders* (DSM-5), these episodes must occur, on average, at least once per week for a period of 3 months. In addition, BN is characterized by the undue influence of weight or shape on self-evaluation. Although approximately 30% of individuals with BN have a lifetime history of anorexia nervosa (AN), BN can only be diagnosed when it occurs outside of the context of AN.

Clinical Presentation

Binge eating differs from normal eating in two key ways. First, binge episodes are defined by consumption of a very large amount of food within a limited period of time. Feeding laboratory studies suggest that women with BN will consume an average of 3,600 kcal in less than 2 hours, representing approximately 2 days of caloric needs for the average woman. Second, binge episodes involve feeling a loss of control over eating. This may be experienced as an inability to control what or how much one is eating, an inability to stop the episode once it has started or to prevent the episode, or experiencing an episode as if it is happening to one rather than being a behavior in which one has agency. Individuals differ in their experience of loss of control, with some reporting that they have no control over their eating, and others endorsing ambivalence about the extent to which they control their eating. Some individuals have highly ritualized binge episodes that involve specific foods eaten in specific quantities, and in a specific order. These kinds of planned episodes may not be characterized by the same quality of loss of control as those that emerge more spontaneously. Some rituals around the content of binge episodes are designed to facilitate self-induced vomiting or the perceived effectiveness of vomiting. For example, patients have reported that ending a binge with ice cream or liquids makes vomiting easier, and starting an episode with vibrantly colored food provides a means for tracking when the beginning of a binge has been expelled. Knowledge that food will be purged also can impact patients' experience of control over their episodes. Although not part of the definition of binge eating, episodes often involve highly palatable foods that individuals with BN otherwise try to avoid. For example, binge episodes may include a large pizza followed by ice cream and cookies, or a box of sugary cereal with milk, or a bag of chips with dip and soda.

Inappropriate compensatory behaviors include self-induced vomiting, laxative abuse, diuretic abuse, fasting, and excessive exercising, as well as misuse of other medications, such as omission of insulin in type 1 diabetes. Of these, self-induced vomiting is the most common method used to compensate for binge eating in Western cultures. Within non-Western cultures, herbal laxative use is more commonly reported. Means involving the forceful evacuation of matter from the body (vomiting, laxatives, etc.) are considered purging methods. In contrast, nonpurging methods work with the body's metabolism to offset binge episodes by either not allowing calories into the body (fasting) or utilizing calories at a higher rate (excessive exercise). The distinction between purging and nonpurging does not impact whether or not a person is diagnosed with BN but it does impact identification of current subtypes for AN and the potential diagnosis of the other specified eating disorder, purging disorder (PD; discussed below). The use of multiple methods of compensation (e.g., self-induced vomiting *and* laxatives) has been associated with greater eating disorder severity, comorbidity, and suicide risk.

The minimum frequency of binge/compensatory episodes was lowered from twice per week in the DSM-IV to once per week in DSM-5, based on evidence that there are no differences in clinical significance or treatment response between these thresholds. In addition, lowering the threshold reduces the preponderance of eating disorder not otherwise specified diagnoses that plagued the DSM-IV system. An average frequency is used because it is common for individuals to report vacillating between "good" periods and "bad" periods. Among women not using hormonal contraceptives, these variations coincide with phases of the menstrual cycle, such that episode frequency increases when estrogen levels are low in relation to progesterone levels. It also is common for purging frequency to exceed the frequency of binge eating episodes because individuals may feel the need to get rid of food even when they have not consumed excessive quantities. This is particularly like to occur when the individual feels a loss of control over eating a forbidden food or feels physical discomfort despite having consumed a normal amount of food.

The undue influence of weight and shape on self-evaluation is both a defining feature of BN and a factor that contributes to illness risk and maintenance. Factors that influence how people evaluate themselves may include the quality of relationships with family, friends, and colleagues; performance at work or school; community service, sports, hobbies, or other leisure activities; as well as appearance, including weight and shape. Individuals with BN place weight and shape near the top of the list, if not at the top of the list, of factors that influence how they feel, judge, or evaluate themselves. Of note, this is not the same as what is important to them or their values. An individual with BN may genuinely feel that world peace is more important than whether she maintains her weight at 110 pounds; however, the absence of world peace would not impact her sense of personal value, whereas gaining 5 pounds would contribute to feelings of worthlessness. This is also different from body dissatisfaction because there may be no discrepancy between current and desired weight/shape as much as extreme investment in maintaining current weight/shape.

Severity

In DSM-5, illness severity is assessed by frequency of compensatory behaviors. Individuals who are compensating twice or more per day are considered to fall at the "extreme" end of severity; an average of more than once per day but less than twice per day is considered "severe"; four to seven episodes per week (up to once per day) is considered "moderate"; and one to three episodes per week falls at the "mild" end of severity. Importantly, the presence of other symptoms (e.g., use of multiple purging methods, extremity of binge episode size), associated medical complications (electrolyte imbalances), and functional disability also may be considered in determining current illness severity.

Changing Definitions

Definitions of BN have changed since "bulimia" was first included in DSM-III in 1980. In its original incarnation, bulimia was characterized by large binge episodes but was not necessarily defined by the use of inappropriate compensatory behaviors. Instead, DSM-III provided a list of associated features that accompanied binge episodes, from which a minimum number was needed for diagnosis. In addition, individuals could be diagnosed with bulimia in addition to receiving a diagnosis of AN. Thus, in DSM-III, bulimia could include those who would now be diagnosed with binge eating disorder or AN-binge–purge subtype. DSM-III-R and DSM-IV defined BN similarly to how the illness is defined today.

In contrast to the modest revisions made to diagnostic criteria for BN between the DSM-IV and DSM-5, the committee for the next edition of the *International Classification of Diseases* (ICD-11) is contemplating more substantive changes. The following is an excerpt from the online beta version:

> Bulimia Nervosa is characterized by frequent, recurrent episodes of binge eating (e.g., once a week or more over a period of at least one month). A binge eating episode is a distinct period of time during which the individual experiences a subjective loss of control over eating, eating notably more or differently than usual, and feels unable to stop eating or limit the type or amount of food eaten. Binge eating is accompanied by repeated inappropriate compensatory behaviours aimed at preventing weight gain (e.g., self-induced vomiting, misuse of laxatives or enemas, strenuous exercise). There [*sic*] individual is preoccupied with body shape or weight, which strongly influences self-evaluation. The individual is not significantly underweight and therefore does not meet the diagnostic requirements of Anorexia Nervosa.

This working definition differs from the DSM-5 definition in two ways. The duration of illness is 1 month instead of 3, and binge episodes do not necessarily involve a large amount of food. Instead, the individual may be eating "differently than usual," and feel unable to limit "the type" of food eaten. Thus, individuals who would receive a diagnosis of other specified feeding or eating disorder (OSFED) for subthreshold BN due to limited duration, or for PD due to the absence of objectively large binge episodes, are included in this proposed definition.

Arguably the duration of illness for diagnosing BN is arbitrary, and it is unclear whether a minimum duration of 1 month impacts clinical significance of BN. Duration of illness at presentation is one of the most reliable predictors of syndrome maintenance.

Thus, lowering this threshold could contribute to better treatment response and higher rates of spontaneous remission. Importantly, there is likely to be a meaningful difference between an individual who has engaged in some disordered eating behaviors and one who has an eating disorder. Whether that distinction falls between experiencing three and four episodes occurring over 4 weeks versus 11 or 12 episodes over 12 weeks is unknown.

Eliminating the requirement that binge episodes involve a large amount of food represents not only a departure from how BN is defined in DSM-5 but a departure from how it has been defined since its first appearance in the medical literature. Indeed, everything that is known about BN has been determined in those who have large binge episodes because "we study what we define." A related line of research that may illuminate the consequence of this change has examined those who purge following consumption of normal or even small amounts of food—a condition identified as PD.

Purging Disorder

Similar to BN, individuals with PD are not underweight but do endorse the undue influence of weight or shape on self-evaluation or express intense fear of gaining weight or becoming fat. Recommended research criteria for PD suggest a minimum threshold of purging once per week for 3 months. However, this was selected to match the frequency for DSM-5 BN, and some preliminary data, rather than being based on extensive studies into a meaningful threshold for diagnosis. Unlike BN, individuals with PD may or may not experience a loss of control over their eating. Frequency of loss of control over eating in PD has been associated with a host of indicators of distress and problems with impulse control. Overall, comparisons between women with PD and those with BN suggest that both are characterized by functional disability in major life roles, but that PD is associated with less distress than BN. Thus, the proposed ICD-11 definition would restrict the diagnosis of PD to those who do not experience loss of control over their eating by pulling those who do into a diagnosis of BN.

Aside from similarities and differences related to how PD has been defined, women with PD resemble women with BN on levels of dietary restraint and purging frequency but have reported less body image disturbance and overall severity of eating pathology, as measured by both global measures of eating pathology. In addition, individuals with PD endorse less hunger, less disinhibition around food, greater satiation, and greater postprandial fullness and stomach discomfort compared to women with BN. They also demonstrate a greater cholecystokinin response to food intake and higher levels of glucagon-like peptide 1 over the course of a test meal compared to women with BN—both of which may be linked to differences in food consumption prior to purging between groups. Finally, data from Germany support increased risk of mortality in PD compared to BN, with crude mortality estimates indicating that 1 in 20 women with PD had died by 5-year follow-up compared to 1 in 100 women with BN.

Summary

BN can be characterized as a binge–purge syndrome. What constitutes a binge has been debated and reasonably well studied. Thus, ongoing discussions do not reflect a lack of information as much as a lack of consensus on whether observed patterns are clinically relevant. Moreover, any clinical description of a syndrome glosses over differences among individuals in order to group them together—which of these differences matter versus which do not remains an open question. Clinical relevance is determined by factors that influence illness development, course, and treatment, as these directly inform prevention and treatment efforts. To the extent that we have no perfect prevention and no perfect treatment, efforts in these domains will continue. Parallel to these efforts, attention to differences in clinical presentation that impact outcomes could significantly advance our understanding of what BN is and what it is not.

Suggested Reading

Keel, P. K. (2015). *Eating disorders* (2nd ed.). New York: Oxford University Press.—Provides a research-based primer on eating disorders, including case studies for BN and the related OSFED, PD.

Keel, P. K., & Striegel-Moore, R. H. (2009). The validity and clinical utility of purging disorder. *International Journal of Eating Disorders, 42,* 706–719.—Presents evidence for the clinical significance and distinctiveness of PD, as well as recommended research criteria for future studies.

Koch, S., Quadflieg, N., & Ficther, M. (2013). Purging disorder: A comparison to established eating disorders with purging behavior. *European Eating Disorders Review, 21,* 265–275.—Demonstrated that PD demonstrates greater longitudinal stability of diagnosis than AN and higher risk of mortality compared to BN, supporting the clinical significance and distinctiveness of PD.

Russell, G. (1979). Bulimia nervosa: An ominous variant of anorexia nervosa. *Psychological Medicine, 9,* 429–448.—Presents first clinical description of BN as the syndrome currently recognized today.

Uher, R., & Rutter, M. (2012). Classification of feeding and eating disorders: Review of evidence and proposals for ICD-11. *World Psychiatry, 11,* 80–92.—Provides a review of limitations of the DSM-IV and ICD-10 definitions of eating disorders and includes rationale for proposed revisions to definition of BN to include subjective binge episodes and reduce duration of illness to 4 weeks.

Van Hoeken, D., Veling, W., Sinke, S., Mitchell, J. E., & Hoek, H. W. (2009). The validity and utility of subtyping bulimia nervosa. *International Journal of Eating Disorders, 42,* 595–602.—Reviews dearth of evidence supporting the distinction between purging and nonpurging BN due to relative infrequency of nonpurging BN.

Walsh, B. T., & Kahn, C. B. (1997). Diagnostic criteria for eating disorders: Current and concerns and future directions. *Psychopharmacology, 33,* 369–372.—Describes scientific and social factors that impact what and how disorders are defined within diagnostic systems.

Wilson, G. T., & Sysko, R. (2009). Frequency of binge eating episodes in bulimia nervosa and binge eating disorder: Diagnostic considerations. *International Journal of Eating Disorders, 42,* 603–610.—Reviews evidence that there is no meaningful difference in severity, course or outcome between those who experience episodes at least twice versus at least once per week over a 3-month period.

Wolfe, B. E., Baker, C. W., Smith, A. T., & Kelly-Weeder, S. (2009). Validity and utility of the current definition of binge eating. *International Journal of Eating Disorders, 42,* 674–686.—Reviews the literature considered by the DSM-5 Eating Disorders Workgroup prior to their decision to retain the definition of binge eating episodes utilized in DSM-IV.

World Health Organization. (2015). Beta draft for the ICD-11. Retrieved May 29, 2015, from *http://apps.who.int/classifications/icd11/browse/l-m/en.*—Presents beta draft for revisions under consideration for the definition of BN for ICD-11.

30

Binge Eating Disorder

MICHAEL J. DEVLIN

In 1993, shortly before publication of the fourth edition of the *Diagnostic and Statistical Manual of Mental Disorders* (DSM-IV), a coalition of researchers known for their work in eating disorders, obesity, and psychiatric nosology published a position paper arguing strenuously in favor of the inclusion of binge eating disorder (BED) as a psychiatric diagnosis. First recognized in the 1950s as a distinct eating pattern among obese individuals, binge eating reemerged in the 1980s as a phenomenon of interest not just in obesity research and treatment settings but also in eating disorders programs that recognized the pattern of uncontrolled consumption of large amounts of food in individuals across the weight spectrum. Such individuals did not meet criteria for bulimia nervosa (BN), because they used neither purging nor nonpurging methods to compensate for their binge episodes. At issue was the validity of the putative new diagnostic category, its distinctness from existing eating disorders, particularly nonpurging BN, and its utility for clinical practice. When DSM-IV was published in 1994, it included BED, not as an eating disorder diagnosis in its own right, but as an example of an eating disorder not otherwise specified and also as a set of criteria in Appendix B, "Criteria Sets and Axes Provided for Further Study."

Despite the lack of inclusion as an eating disorder diagnosis, the publication of the provisional diagnostic criteria sufficed to stimulate significant subsequent research, treatment development, and advocacy. Perhaps of equal importance, the bridge between the theretofore largely separate worlds of obesity and eating disorders continued to expand, to the benefit of both fields. Two decades later, the inclusion of BED in DSM-5 reflected the tremendous progress made in defining and characterizing BED, as well as understanding its treatment. This chapter provides an overview of BED, including what is known about its clinical characteristics, epidemiology, and medical significance, and what remains to be learned, largely concerning its etiology and psychobiology.

Diagnosis and Clinical Features

The core feature of BED is the occurrence, at least once a week, of *eating binges*, defined as the consumption of an objectively large amount of food in a discrete period of time, accompanied by a sense of loss of control, and without attempted compensation either through purging, fasting, or exercise. DSM-5 diagnostic criteria for BED (see Chapter 6), like DSM-IV criteria, also require marked distress regarding the binge eating and the presence of behavioral indicators of loss of control, such as eating past the point of fullness or feeling disgusted, depressed, or very guilty following an eating binge. The DSM-5 criteria set includes a severity rating of mild to extreme based on binge frequency, as well as specifiers for partial and full remission, although the period of abstinence required for remission is not defined. Of note, the diagnostic criteria do not require either overweight/ obesity or overconcern with shape and weight, although both are frequent concomitants of the disorder, particularly in clinical samples.

In the years between the initial proposal of BED as a diagnostic category in its own right and its inclusion in DSM-5, a number of studies examined the reliability and validity of the construct. These studies yielded several relatively firm conclusions and raised significant questions. BED can be reliably diagnosed in clinical and community samples using either self-report tools, such as the Questionnaire on Eating and Weight Patterns— Revised (QEWP-R), or structured interviews, such as the Eating Disorder Examination (EDE) and, more recently, the Eating Disorder Assessment for DSM-5 (EDA-5). Obese individuals with BED eat more than comparably obese individuals without BED in laboratory meals, whether instructed to binge-eat or to eat normally. A particularly robust finding, similar to that seen in other eating disorders, is that individuals with BED compared to individuals of similar weight without BED have higher rates of current and lifetime psychopathology, particularly depression, and more frequent dieting and weight fluctuation. It is common for individuals with BED to report periods of binge eating, during which weight increases, alternating with periods of strict control, during which weight decreases. Overreliance on shape and weight as determinants of self-worth, often seen as the core psychological feature of eating disorders, is a sufficiently prominent feature that, some have argued, should be included as a diagnostic criterion. While the phenomenology of BED is relatively well established, the ultimate measure of its validity as a construct awaits an as yet unattained understanding of its etiology and pathophysiology.

Epidemiology, Course, and Outcome

One of the key issues that initially arose with respect to the inclusion of BED as a psychiatric diagnosis was its prevalence. While the phenomenon of occasional overeating is much too common to merit serious consideration as a mental disorder, the number of individuals meeting full BED criteria, when carefully assessed, including significant distress regarding binge eating, is far fewer. It is this smaller group of individuals, particularly those presenting for treatment for either binge eating or obesity, that has been the focus of studies characterizing the nature and course of BED and its impact on individuals, families, and the community.

In considering prevalence, course, and outcome, it is important to distinguish between community and clinical samples. In the community, a landmark study, the National Comorbidity Survey Replication, estimated the lifetime prevalence of BED as

3.5% among women and 2.0% among men. In a recently published overview of studies, the 12-month prevalence of BED in the United States is estimated at 1.7% for women and 0.8% for men. Interestingly, the reduction in the binge frequency from two binge days per week for the past 6 months in DSM-IV to one binge episode per week for the past 3 months in DSM-5 had minimal impact on prevalence. Outside the United States, across upper-middle- and high-income countries, the prevalence of BED is variable but comparable overall, and consistently higher than that of BN.

Unfortunately, very little information is available regarding the course and outcome of BED among adults in the community. However, there is clearly a cross-sectional association between binge eating and obesity, and some evidence suggests that BED confers increased risk for subsequent overweight and obesity. The existing studies of course and outcome for BED in the community are somewhat stronger with regard to adolescents. One large-scale longitudinal cohort study in adolescents found that BED is associated with increased risk both for subsequent overweight or obesity and for depression. Another study that followed participants for 8 years found that 3% of teenage girls developed DSM-5 BED, but had an impressively high 1-year remission rate of 93%, underscoring the relapsing and remitting nature of the disorder.

Clinical studies provide additional information regarding the subset of individuals with BED who seek treatment. One key distinction between community and clinical samples relates to the overlap with obesity. While almost half of individuals in the community who meet criteria for BED are not overweight or obese, nearly all clinical studies of BED have been conducted in obese or overweight individuals. Looking at the overlap between obesity and BED from the other direction, it was initially estimated that as many as 20–30% of individuals in obesity treatment samples suffered from BED. However, subsequent studies using more rigorous diagnostic methods have yielded somewhat lower figures, even in severely obese samples, such as individuals presenting for bariatric surgery. In the large-scale multicenter Longitudinal Assessment of Bariatric Surgery (LABS) study, 15.7% of severely obese individuals met BED criteria. As detailed in other chapters, the short-term treatment response rate with regard to binge eating across treatment modalities and even including pill placebo is quite high, suggesting that binge eating may remit with relatively minimal intervention. Whether this represents stable and long-lasting remission is a more difficult question, as is the question of spontaneous remission outside of a treatment setting in adults with well-established binge eating.

Considering all sources of information, it is reasonable to conclude that in the community, BED is a fairly common problem that, for many individuals, follows an unstable course and at least in some, can have an impact on subsequent health and well-being.

Medical and Psychological Comorbidity

A key indicator of the utility of BED as a diagnosis relates to its association with medical and psychological disorders, independent of weight status. Of most relevance to clinicians is the question of whether the index of suspicion for comorbid psychological or medical conditions ought to be raised in an overweight or obese individual with BED compared to an individual of comparable body mass index without binge eating. The answer is clear with regard to psychological comorbidity. Numerous studies have reported elevated rates of psychopathology and psychiatric disorders, with anywhere from a substantial minority to a large majority of research participants with BED presenting with at least one additional diagnosis. Mood disorders, anxiety disorders, and. in some studies, substance use disorders are most frequently associated with BED. Moreover, it is clear that this association holds true even when weight status is controlled (i.e., when the association is specifically with binge eating and not with severity of obesity). Elevated rates of personality disorders have also been noted, although the question of whether these rates differ between those with and without BED in treatment-seeking samples of obese individuals is not resolved. Notably, this elevated psychological comorbidity is also characteristic of other eating disorders, including anorexia nervosa and BN, and, as is also true for these disorders, the psychopathology is often intertwined with dissatisfaction with body shape and weight-related distress. There are some indications that comorbid psychopathology in patients with BED predicts poorer prognosis, as indicated by treatment dropout or binge relapse following treatment. In a somewhat more recent line of research, both BED and severe obesity have been found to be associated with childhood maltreatment and psychological trauma. However, the specificity of the relationship between trauma and binge eating is not well established. While it is possible that a history of trauma may be associated with comorbid psychopathology and poor treatment response in BED, further studies are needed.

The relationship between binge eating, independent of weight, and medical comorbidity is much less clearly understood. Studies controlling for psychiatric comorbidity have suggested that individuals with BED more frequently report health problems and disability. In addition studies controlling for weight report more new diagnoses of metabolic syndrome components, including dyslipidemia and type 2 diabetes mellitus, in individuals with BED. However, studies that rely on self-report are inconclusive in that they are subject to reporting bias (i.e., the possibility that individuals with BED may be more aware of or more likely to report comorbid medical conditions). The aforementioned LABS study, controlling for potential confounders, including body mass index, reported that severely overweight individuals with BED were more likely to have impaired glucose levels and high triglycerides. This provides at least a preliminary suggestion that binge eating may indeed have adverse medical consequences apart from those attributable purely to obesity. With regard to health outcomes, for the significant and growing proportion of severely obese individuals who undergo bariatric surgery, binge eating or loss-of-control eating following surgery appears to be associated with poorer weight outcome. Further research is very much needed to expand and clarify these putative associations which, if confirmed, would certainly underscore the health benefits of preventing and treating BED.

Frontiers in BED Research

As is clear from this brief review, what is most lacking with regard to BED is a clear understanding of its etiology and mechanisms, including the genetic and environmental risk factors for its onset, as well as the psychobiological and neurocognitive drivers and sequelae of binge eating. A more complete knowledge is needed of the interrelationships among the behavior of binge eating; the psychological features of shape and weight overconcern, often with concomitant depression and/or anxiety; and the somatic phenomena of weight fluctuation, weight gain, and obesity. Investigators have approached this challenge by characterizing the behavior of binge eaters; by considering potential analogies with other disorders, such as addictions; and most recently, by attempting to apply neurocognitive frameworks, such as the Research Domain Criteria (RDoC) to eating disorders, including BED.

Although a thorough discussion of this work is beyond the scope of this chapter, a few key findings and challenges are worth highlighting here. One key question relates to eating and energy balance in individuals with BED. While laboratory studies of binge eating have demonstrated that individuals with BED eat more than those without BED, whether instructed to binge-eat or to eat normally, reported total daily energy consumption in individuals with BED typically exceeds that of obese control participants on binge days only. In one study using a metabolic chamber, intake of BED participants was more variable than, but did not exceed, that of control participants, and resting metabolic rate was similar between the two groups. Related to this is the interesting observation that binge cessation, in the context of successful response to treatment, is often not associated with significant weight loss. Thus, the specific causal relationship between binge eating and obesity is as yet an unresolved issue of tremendous importance, from both a mechanistic and a clinical standpoint.

Possibly the most active area of mechanistic inquiry with regard to obesity in general, and BED in particular, is the overlap with addictive disorders. Based on what many see as a phenomenological resemblance, with addiction-like craving, tolerance, and binge escalation over time, much animal and human research has examined the role of reward systems in the nonhomeostatic overeating, either binge eating or other forms of overeating, that leads to weight gain and obesity. While there have been several findings that suggest individuals with severe obesity differ from the nonobese in their reward sensitivity, as gauged by questionnaire response, and in their neural reactivity to palatable food cues, as gauged by functional imaging of various neural systems, the meaning of these findings with respect to the overall similarities between severe obesity (and/or BED) and addictive disorders remains to be clarified. The implications for treatment are, of course, complicated by the fact that abstinence from the abused substance is far from straightforward when the substance in question is food.

In summary, since it was first proposed as a psychiatric diagnosis, a great deal of progress has been made in defining the BED construct, characterizing its features, elucidating its prevalence in the community, and understanding its impact on health. BED has largely passed the tests of validity and clinical utility. Ultimately, however, the integrity of BED as a well-defined psychiatric diagnosis and the development of theory-based prevention and treatment strategies will require an increasingly deep and detailed understanding of its etiology and pathophysiological mechanisms.

Suggested Reading

Engel, S. G., Kahler, K. A., Lystad, C. M., Crosby, R. D., Simonich, H. K., Wonderlich, S. A., et al. (2009). Eating behavior in obese BED, obese non-BED, and non-obese control participants: A naturalistic study. *Behaviour Research and Therapy, 47*(10), 897–900.—Usefully reviews and extends findings regarding eating behavior in BED, supporting the validity of BED.

Field, A. E., Sonneville, K. R., Micali, N., Crosby, R. D., Swanson, S. A., Laird, N. M., et al. (2012). Prospective association of common eating disorders and adverse outcomes. *Pediatrics, 130*(2), e289–e295.—Prospective study demonstrating association of BED with later development of depression and overweight.

Hudson, J. I., Hiripi, E., Pope, H. G., & Kessler, R. C. (2007). The prevalence and correlates of eating disorders in the National Comorbidity Survey Replication. *Biological Psychiatry,*

61(3), 348–358.—Large-scale epidemiological study establishing the relatively high prevalence of BED in the community.

Mitchell, J. E., King, W. C., Pories, W., Wolfe, B., Flum, D. R., Spaniolas, K., et al. (2015). Binge eating disorder and medical comorbidities in bariatric surgery candidates. *International Journal of Eating Disorders, 48*(5), 471–476.—Demonstrates association of BED with measured medical comorbidities, independent of weight.

Schreiber, L., Odlaug, B., & Grant, J. (2013). The overlap between binge eating disorder and substance use disorders: Diagnosis and neurobiology. *Journal of Behavioral Addictions, 2*(4), 191–198.—Reviews the literature on BED as an addictive disorder, spanning several levels of analysis.

Smink, F. R., van Hoeken, D., & Hoek, H. W. (2013). Epidemiology, course, and outcome of eating disorders. *Current Opinion in Psychiatry, 26*(6), 543–548.—Recent summary of epidemiological data on BED and other eating disorders.

Spitzer, R. L., Stunkard, A., Yanovski, S., Marcus, M. D., Wadden, T., Wing, R., et al. (1993). Binge eating disorder should be included in DSM-IV: A reply to Fairburn et al.'s "The classification of recurrent overeating: The binge eating disorder proposal." *International Journal of Eating Disorders, 13*(2), 161–169.—Of historical interest, this position piece made the case for including BED in DSM-IV.

Stice, E., Marti, C. N., & Rohde, P. (2013). Prevalence, incidence, impairment, and course of the proposed DSM-5 eating disorder diagnoses in an 8-year prospective community study of young women. *Journal of Abnormal Psychology, 122*(2), 445–457.—Provides useful data regarding the relapsing and remitting course of BED.

Tanofsky-Kraff, M., Bulik, C. M., Marcus, M. D., Striegel, R. H., Wilfley, D. E., Wonderlich, S. A., et al. (2013). Binge eating disorder: The next generation of research. *International Journal of Eating Disorders, 46*(3), 193–207.—Summary of a recent expert consensus conference with useful lists of key citations.

Wonderlich, S. A., Gordon, K. H., Mitchell, J. E., Crosby, R. D., & Engel, S. G. (2009). The validity and clinical utility of binge eating disorder. *International Journal of Eating Disorders, 42*(8), 687–705.—Summary of the evidence that led to the inclusion of BED in DSM-5.

Avoidant/Restrictive Food Intake Disorder

RACHEL BRYANT-WAUGH

This chapter provides an overview of the current status of avoidant/restrictive food intake disorder (ARFID), a relatively newly introduced term. ARFID is a diagnosis covering specific clinically significant presentations of restricted eating occurring across the lifespan. This chapter describes the background to the introduction of ARFID and covers the main diagnostic features. Current knowledge about the demographics and clinical characteristics of ARFID is summarized, with emerging assessment and treatment guidance. Relatively few data exist on clinical course, prognosis, and outcome of ARFID, but preliminary statements are possible and are set out here. The chapter closes with suggested priorities for future study.

Diagnosis and Classification

ARFID first appeared as a diagnostic category in 2013. Its inclusion as one of the feeding and eating disorders in DSM-5 was justified on the basis of a growing body of evidence suggesting that there are specific presentations characterized by restricted eating behavior that are clearly distinct from anorexia nervosa and bulimia nervosa. In line with DSM-5's emphasis on understanding psychopathology throughout the lifespan, ARFID is a diagnosis that is applicable to children, adolescents, and adults alike. Despite developmental differences in expression, the core features remain the same.

The characteristic symptom of ARFID is limited food intake, either in relation to range of foods eaten or overall quantity, and in some cases both. Food intake is restricted, typically, with a clear avoidant component to the presentation. Such behavior may be related to a number of underlying features and may have a range of consequences. The most common contributory factors are those related to the appearance or sensory characteristics of food (e.g., texture, color); fear of the consequences of eating (e.g., vomiting or choking); and lack of interest in food or eating, not explained by any other medical or psychiatric condition. Such factors can occur singly or in combination in different individuals. The most common physical consequences of ARFID include weight loss, nutritional compromise, and growth delay and disruption of physical development in younger patients. Some individuals who may require nutritional interventions such as sip or enteral feeding to ensure adequacy of intake may in some instances become dependent on these. Others may need to supplement their intake on an ongoing basis with multivitamin and mineral preparations to avoid symptoms of nutritional deficiency. Individuals with ARFID may present with low weight, normal weight, or above normal weight. Aside from adverse physical consequences, the behavioral disturbances of ARFID can lead to significant impairment in psychosocial development and functioning. Depending on the age of the individual, this can include difficulties maintaining intimate relationships, avoidance of social situations, difficulties spending time away from home, and stress at family mealtimes. Overall quality of life can be markedly diminished.

Demographics and Clinical Characteristics

Because ARFID is a newly introduced diagnosis, robust data on demographics and clinical characteristics are limited, with epidemiological studies largely absent. So-called "picky eating" is relatively common in early childhood, with up to 50% of children in population samples having been described as picky eaters at some stage. The majority of children progress in terms of their acceptance of a wider range of foods without undue difficulty or the need for clinical attention. However, the differentiation between those likely to develop a persisting problem that may reach clinical significance in the form of ARFID and those who are going through a normal developmental stage remains hampered by a lack of both well-evaluated assessment tools and longitudinal research studies. Incidence data relating to distribution of age of onset of ARFID and cross-sectional prevalence data for different ages are also scarce, again due to a combination of a dearth of reliable screening and assessment measures, and the recent introduction of formal diagnostic criteria for ARFID. A number of centers are currently working to address this, with both population screening tools and clinical assessment measures in development. At this stage, early studies suggest that it is possible to identify features of ARFID in late childhood/early adolescent community samples and to differentiate these from features of other eating disorders. So far, evidence suggests that ARFID features identified in the community tend to be associated with low weight. In addition, early findings from screening other clinical populations of patients with medical conditions in which eating problems might be expected (e.g., gastroenterological conditions), suggest that rates of ARFID are low. This is reassuring in that it suggests that the diagnostic criteria are not overinclusive.

Most information relating to clinical populations is based on previous studies involving individuals who had originally been assigned other diagnoses or terms to describe their eating behavior. This includes studies of early childhood feeding disorders and other restrictive eating disorders in children and adolescents, some of which formed the evidence base for the introduction of ARFID as a diagnosis. Further information is emerging from studies involving patients who have retrospectively been assigned a diagnosis of ARFID, mostly having previously received a diagnosis of eating disorder not otherwise specified or atypical eating disorder. Almost all the work summarized below has been conducted with child and adolescent populations.

Among existing clinic populations of young people with eating disorders, up to 20% have been reported to meet diagnostic criteria for ARFID. The relatively consistent picture that is emerging suggests that there are a number of significant demographic and clinical characteristics that differentiate young people with ARFID from those with anorexia nervosa, bulimia nervosa, and related eating disorders. In particular, a uniform finding is that there is a greater preponderance of males in the ARFID population than in other eating disorders. Furthermore, patients with ARFID are likely to present at a younger age and have a longer duration of illness prior to presentation. In terms of clinical characteristics, in intensive treatment settings (e.g., day programs), patients with ARFID have been identified as being significantly underweight, with similar degrees of weight loss and malnutrition to those of persons with anorexia nervosa. Compared to those with anorexia nervosa, a lower, but nevertheless significant, fraction of ARFID patients have been found to require hospital admission for medical instability. Patients with ARFID have also been identified as having higher rates of comorbid medical and/or psychiatric difficulties than do patients with other eating disorders, in particular, with anxiety disorders. Findings so far suggest that patients with ARFID may be less likely to have comorbid mood disorders than those with anorexia nervosa or bulimia nervosa. Comorbidity with pervasive developmental disorders (e.g., autism spectrum disorder) and learning disability/disorder has also been noted. Emerging data therefore support the introduction of ARFID as a valid diagnostic category, with evidence of potential for differentiation between ARFID presentations and normality, other medical conditions, and other eating disorders.

Assessment and Treatment

The aim of a number of assessment measures currently in development is to enable standardized, reliable measurement of the features and severity of ARFID. In the meantime, clinical guidance that has emerged regarding assessment suggests that a number of domains are considered in line with diagnostic criteria. Key domains relating to the patient's history include early development, medical history, feeding and eating history, and the presence of any significant events that may have had an impact on willingness to eat. In relation to the ARFID presentation, clinicians have been advised to assess current eating behavior and food intake, cognitions related to food and eating, the presence of any weight or shape concerns such as those found in anorexia nervosa or bulimia nervosa (which would mean ARFID is unlikely to be an appropriate diagnosis), current mental state, impact of eating difficulties on day-to-day functioning, and current physical state. Main areas of risk are physical, psychological, and developmental.

Treatment research is also very limited. Formal eating disorder treatment guidance published after the introduction of ARFID as diagnostic category has tended not to specify recommended treatment approaches because there have been no trials to guide practice. Suggestions based on the clinical experience of centers familiar with ARFID presentations, again, mostly child and adolescent clinics, are broadly consistent. In general, a multimodal approach to treatment is recommended, which comprises medical and nutritional intervention (with ongoing physical monitoring and monitoring of the nutritional adequacy of intake through treatment); individual cognitive and behavioral psychological interventions targeting eating behavior and/or anxiety; parenting interventions; and family interventions predominantly related to mealtime management. Specific treatment recommendations for ARFID in adults include mostly treatment suggestions similar to those in phobias.

Prognosis and Outcome

While there are some data on the longer-term outcome of childhood feeding disorders and restrictive eating disorders other than anorexia nervosa, there is very little information on outcome in patients originally diagnosed with ARFID. This situation is likely to change over time; in the interim, only very general statements can be made. It is well documented that some presentations of restricted eating behavior, present since early childhood, can persist until adulthood. It has also been shown that untreated early childhood eating difficulties tend to persist, with problems related to eating behavior and emotional adjustment extending into later childhood. The literature investigating the presence of an association between restricted eating behaviors in childhood and later eating disorders is much harder to interpret. In part this is due to inconsistent use of definitions relating to early eating difficulties, and in part due to the very limited number of studies that have used an adequate study design. As a consequence, findings tend to be conflicting or unreplicated. Some authors have suggested that a proportion of ARFID patients may warrant a diagnosis of anorexia nervosa as treatment progresses, but this may be due as much to diagnostic difficulties as to progression of the eating disorder.

Conclusion and Recommendations

It is evident from the preceding discussion that there is a great need for further research in relation to ARFID. This is unsurprising given its recent introduction to the diagnostic lexicon. The number of publications relating to this clinical presentation is growing, with authors highlighting specific areas requiring further study. First and foremost is the need for more research related to characterization of ARFID, which covers a number of previously described presentations and is in some respects quite broadly specified. Particular examples include reference to psychosocial and nutritional impairment without objective definitions of the meaning of these terms in this context. It is also unclear at this stage whether distinct subgroups will emerge. Current diagnostic criteria include examples of three main associated features in the form of lack of interest in food and eating, avoidance related to the sensory aspects of food, and avoidance related to the feared consequences of eating. It seems unlikely that these will form separate subgroups as it is evident from clinical experience, plus some related routinely collected data, that patients commonly present with at least two of these features. Further research investigating the clinical validity and utility of the phrasing of the existing diagnostic criteria is also needed. Some difficulties have been encountered in distinguishing between some presentations of anorexia nervosa and ARFID, and between some anxiety disorders and ARFID. Likewise, a current exclusion criterion stipulates that the eating restriction should not be primarily accounted for by any other medical or psychiatric condition. In some potentially comorbid situations, this can be a difficult judgement to make, yet interrater reliability is an important aspect of diagnostic validity. Clarification of thresholds of clinical significance still need to be established.

Research is needed on all aspects of identification, assessment, and treatment. This includes the development of reliable screening and assessment measures, studies investigating incidence and prevalence in a range of clinical and nonclinical populations across the lifespan, and robust treatment trials. It will be important to include patient perspectives on areas to target in treatment, as well as in the development of meaningful outcome measures. Properly conducted longitudinal studies, in both clinical and nonclinical populations, will be essential to improve knowledge about risk factors, prognostic indicators, course, and outcome.

Finally, due to the potential for both short- and long-term risk associated with ARFID relative to physical and psychological health and well-being, research into preventive strategies is indicated. The focus of such research is likely to be on secondary and tertiary prevention, at least initially. It is my hope that moving forward in relation to improving identification and developing protocols for effective interventions, as outlined earlier, will enable swifter access to treatments that work. It is imperative that ARFID be fully embraced by both researchers and clinicians working with people of all ages who present with eating disturbances, in order to ensure the field moves forward.

Suggested Reading

Bryant-Waugh, R. (2013). Avoidant restrictive food intake disorder: An illustrative case example. *International Journal of Eating Disorders, 46,* 420–423.—Clinical guide to making a diagnosis of ARFID and planning treatment.

Eddy, K. T., Thomas, J. J., Hastings, E., Edkins, K., Lamont, E., Nevins, C. M., et al. (2015). Prevalence of DSM-5 avoidant/restrictive food intake disorder in a pediatric gastroenterology health care network. *International Journal of Eating Disorders, 48*(5), 464–470.—Study suggesting discriminant validity of ARFID diagnostic criteria.

Fisher, M. M., Rosen, D. S., Ornstein, R. M., Mammel, K. A., Katzman, D. K., Rome, E. S., et al. (2014). Characteristics of avoidant/restrictive food intake disorder in children and adolescents: A "new disorder" in DSM-5. *Journal of Adolescent Health, 55*(1), 49–52.—Comparison of ARFID patients with those with anorexia nervosa and bulimia nervosa.

Forman, S. F., McKenzie, N., Hehn, R., Monge, M. C., Kapphahn, C. J., Mammel, K. A., et al. (2014). Predictors of outcome at 1 year in adolescents with DSM-5 restrictive eating disorders: Report of the national eating disorders quality improvement collaborative. *Journal of Adolescent Health, 55*(6), 750–756.—A retrospective study, including investigation of the demographics of ARFID and predictors of weight restoration.

Kurz, S., Van Dyck, Z., Dremmel, D., Munsch, S., & Hilbert, A. (2015). Early-onset restrictive eating disturbances in primary school boys and girls. *European Child and Adolescent Psychiatry, 24*(7), 779–785.—General population study using a new ARFID screening measure.

Nicely, T. A., Lane-Loney, S., Masciulli, E., Hollenbeak, C. S., & Ornstein, R. M. (2014). Prevalence and characteristics of avoidant/restrictive food intake disorder in a cohort of young patients in day treatment for eating disorders. *Journal of Eating Disorders, 2*(1), 21.—Study of patients with a range of eating disorders demonstrating significant clinical severity in ARFID.

Norris, M. L., Robinson, A., Obeid, N., Harrison, M., Spettigue, W., & Henderson, K. (2014). Exploring avoidant/restrictive food intake disorder in eating disordered patients: A descriptive study. *International Journal of Eating Disorders, 47*(5), 495–499.—Comparison of adolescent ARFID and anorexia nervosa to confirm characteristic differences.

Night Eating Syndrome

KELLY C. ALLISON

Many people snack after dinner to wind down, to satisfy a craving, or as part of a social situation. However, for about 1.5% of members of the general population who meet diagnostic criteria for night eating syndrome (NES), such eating becomes a more habitual, distressing, and shameful behavior. The prevalence of NES rises with increased body mass index (BMI), with a range of 5–15% of individuals seeking nonsurgical weight loss interventions, bariatric surgery, or psychiatric treatment meeting criteria.

Diagnostic Criteria and Clinical Characteristics

NES was first described by Stunkard and colleagues in the 1950s as a pattern of eating among individuals who were having difficulty losing weight. Morning anorexia, evening hyperphagia, and insomnia were identified as the three core features. Over time, these symptoms have been described in more detail, and, in 2013, NES was included in the fifth edition of the *Diagnostic and Statistical Manual of Mental Disorders* (DSM-5) under the category other specified feeding or eating disorders. In DSM-5, NES is described briefly either as eating after awakening from sleep or as eating excessively after the evening meal. Awareness of the episodes is required to differentiate the disorder from a sleep-related eating disorder (SRED). Distress and impairment in functioning must also be present, and the pattern of intake should not be better accounted for by another medical or mental disorder.

Research studies have used various criteria to diagnose NES. To unify the field, research criteria were proposed at the International Night Eating Symposium in 2008 (Table 32.1). These criteria specify a delayed pattern of intake, such that at least one-fourth of one's daily intake is consumed after dinner and/or that an individual awakens to eat at least twice per week. Awareness of the nocturnal eating is also required by these criteria. Although morning anorexia was originally considered a core diagnostic feature, studies have found that, while it is common among those with NES, it is not specific to

TABLE 32.1. Proposed Research Diagnostic Criteria for NES

A. The daily pattern of eating demonstrates a significantly increased intake in the evening and/or nighttime, as manifested by one or both of the following:
1. At least 25% of food intake is consumed after the evening meal
2. At least two episodes of nocturnal eating per week

B. Awareness and recall of evening and nocturnal eating episodes are present.

C. The clinical picture is characterized by at least three of the following features:
1. Lack of desire to eat in the morning and/or breakfast is omitted on four or more mornings per week
2. Presence of a strong urge to eat between dinner and sleep onset and/or during the night
3. Sleep onset and/or sleep maintenance insomnia are present four or more nights per week
4. Presence of a belief that one must eat in order to initiate or return to sleep
5. Mood is frequently depressed and/or mood worsens in the evening

D. The disorder is associated with significant distress and/or impairment in functioning.

E. The disordered pattern of eating has been maintained for at least 3 months.

F. The disorder is not secondary to substance abuse or dependence, medical disorder, medication, or another psychiatric disorder.

Note. From Allison et al. (2010). Copyright © 2010 John Wiley and Sons, Inc. Reprinted by permission.

NES. It is now included as one of five possible features of NES, at least three of which are required for diagnosis.

One of the features described in the criteria, the belief that one must eat to fall asleep initially or to resume sleep after awakening during the night, appears to be relatively specific to NES because it does not occur commonly in other eating disorders, including binge-eating disorder (BED). In addition, nocturnal ingestions—episodes of eating after awakening—are not typically as objectively large as binge episodes, although 15–20% of persons with NES also meet criteria for BED. In general, food is used in the evening and/or nighttime as a way of soothing anxiety, ridding oneself of a persistent craving, or as an effective sleep aid. In fact, persons with NES who are prescribed sleep medications such as zolpidem still tend to rise from bed and seek food, but they are more likely to be in a drowsy, sleepwalking state and may be at a higher risk for harming themselves while seeking or preparing food; for this reason, sleep medications are not recommended for the treatment of NES.

NES has been linked to weight gain prospectively in the Swedish Twin Registry, the Danish MONICA study, and in laboratory studies with long-term follow-up assessment. Furthermore, diabetic patients with night eating tend to have higher hemoglobin A1c levels and less overall control of their diabetic symptoms than similar patients without NES. Thus, the syndrome appears to be linked with deleterious physical effects.

While food intake is significantly delayed, the timing of the sleep period is not. However, studies comparing the circadian rhythms of hormones related to eating, weight regulation, sleep, and stress, including insulin, glucose, leptin, ghrelin, and cortisol, were found to be phase-delayed, with the exception of ghrelin, which was phase-advanced, among women with NES compared to similar controls.

Despite NES being linked to an increased risk of weight gain and obesity, research has shown that persons with NES who are of normal weight tend to have a more severely delayed pattern of eating than those with NES who are overweight or obese. It seems that normal-weight persons with NES are more likely to restrict their intake purposefully during the day, such that they often do not start eating until late afternoon. This pattern then pushes the percentage of total daily intake consumed after the evening meal to be higher—at about 50% of the total intake in one study as compared to about 35% in overweight persons with NES. Normal-weight persons with NES also tend to have more frequent nocturnal ingestions than persons with NES who are overweight, with one study averaging 11 per week versus eight per week among the normal-weight and overweight persons with NES, respectively. In addition to the more deliberate daytime eating restriction, normal-weight persons with NES tend to exercise to compensate for their evening and nocturnal ingestions. Thus, the more extreme NES symptoms among normal-weight individuals might be explained by a more intense biological pressure to eat given their more extreme fasting and exercise behaviors.

The prevalence of night eating among those with anorexia nervosa (AN) and particularly bulimia nervosa (BN) also tends to be higher than the prevalence found in the general population, with one study of inpatients indicating that 25% of patients met criteria. As the relationship of night eating to the other symptoms of AN and BN has not been well studied, it is recommended to treat the symptoms of AN or BN while also addressing the night eating, but not to assign a diagnosis of NES until it is clear that the eating pattern is not better understood as a manifestation of AN and BN. No studies exist on the crossover from other eating disorders to NES, although, clinically, I have observed this phenomenon.

Assessment Methods

Three tools have been developed to aid the assessment of NES and have potential utility. The most widely validated screening instrument for NES is the Night Eating Questionnaire (NEQ), a 14-item survey using 0- to 4-point Likert responses, which was normed using a large Internet survey sample of self-identified persons with NES and a sample of bariatric surgery candidates. The items assess the core features and associated symptoms of NES, including lack of morning appetite (two items), loss of control, and degree of cravings over eating before bedtime and during the night (four items), initial and middle insomnia (three items), mood disturbance (two items), frequency of eating during the night, belief that one needs to eat to sleep, and level of awareness over these eating episodes. The item assessing awareness does not count toward the final score; it is used to distinguish NES from SRED. Scores may range from 0 to 52.

In an obese population, the positive predictive power of the NEQ is a relatively low 40.7% using a cutoff score of 25, but rises to 72.7% using a score of 30. The NEQ does not identify persons with NES who only have evening hyperphagia (no nocturnal ingestions), as there are stop points built into the survey, such that the survey ends if individuals do not report awakening, or awakening and eating. Therefore, persons without nocturnal ingestions who are consuming large amounts of their daily intake after dinner will not be identified with this survey. The NEQ has been translated into many different languages, including published studies in Spanish (Spain), Portuguese (Brazil), Italian, French (Canada), German, Hebrew, Arabic (Egypt), and Korean. It is available for free use by researchers.

The Night Eating Syndrome History and Inventory (NESHI) is a semistructured interview that incorporates the NEQ items and allows the interviewer to gather more details about the average weekly frequency of nocturnal ingestions. The NESHI also includes a recall of one's typical daily intake, which helps the interviewer estimate the proportion of food an individual consumes, on average, after the evening meal. One of the most difficult parts of assessing NES is obtaining an accurate appraisal of the proportion of food eaten after the evening meal because people who are seeking help for night eating, except those who restrict purposefully during the day, as described earlier, tend to underestimate the amount of food they eat before that time. This may inflate the percentage of intake that they estimate consuming after the evening meal. For example, one study showed that participants reported consuming at least half of their intake after dinner by self-report, but, by food diaries, the intake was approximately 35% of daily caloric intake. A careful review of food intake over a typical 24-hour period, including the use of food records, is needed to make a rigorous assessment of evening hyperphagia. The NESHI also assesses impairment in functioning and distress associated with NES symptoms, the history of the disorder, and related psychosocial factors (e.g., shift work and life stress), and the presence of inappropriate compensatory behaviors (to aid in ruling out other eating disorders).

The Night Eating Diagnostic Questionnaire, a self-report instrument, has also been developed to assess NES. Unlike the NEQ, it is not formatted with Likert responses, but instead asks for specific values for the presence and frequency of night eating-related symptoms and behaviors related to the proposed diagnostic criteria. No validation study has yet been published for this measure, but it has face validity based on the NES symptoms assessed.

Treatment

Stunkard first described NES in persons struggling to lose weight in an obesity treatment program. He tried the predominant therapeutic approach of his time, psychodynamic therapy, but noted no significant response. In the 1980s and 1990s, some behavioral therapy case reports suggested mixed treatment effects for NES. At this point, researchers began to test pharmacological approaches, first with a few case series using serotonergic agents, with some success.

The first clinical trials with selective serotonin reuptake inhibitors (SSRIs) used sertraline. Two open-label trials showed reductions in percent of food consumed after the evening meal and number of nocturnal ingestions per week. The first double-blind, randomized controlled trial studied 34 participants over 8 weeks. The number of awakenings per week was reduced by 74 versus 14% in the sertraline and placebo groups, respectively; the number of nocturnal ingestions per week was reduced by 81 versus 14%, respectively; and the percentage of calories consumed after dinner was reduced by 68 versus 47%. Additionally, participants who were overweight or obese lost 2.9 kg versus 0.3 kg on sertraline and placebo, respectively, a significant difference over the 8 weeks. Overall, there was a low placebo response rate, with only 18% of those on placebo being judged "much improved" or "very much improved" on the Clinical Global Impression Improvement scale compared to 71% of those on sertraline, including 41% in remission.

Two studies have been published testing the efficacy of escitalopram, another SSRI, for NES. One was an open-label trial that tested escitalopram among 31 participants with NES over 12 weeks. Significant decreases were found in the number of awakenings (8.1 to 2.7) and nocturnal ingestions (5.8 to 1.2) per week, and the percentage of intake consumed after dinner (46 to 17%). Weight also decreased slightly from 90.2 to 88.6 kg, which was statistically significant.

The other study using escitalopram was a double-blind placebo-controlled trial among 40 participants. This study also noted decreases across NES symptoms, but the placebo response rate of 35% on the Clinical Global Impression Improvement scale was higher than that reported in the previous sertraline trial, making the comparison between the drug and placebo groups nonsignificant. Additionally, African American participants did not respond as well to escitalopram as did European American participants.

Case studies with topiramate and bright light therapy have also shown promise in treating NES, but larger, controlled trials are needed to test their efficacy.

Two randomized controlled trials testing the efficacy of progressive muscle relaxation (PMR) for NES have also been conducted. This approach focused on the presumed stress-related nature of the night eating behavior, and aimed to aid sleep and reduce the need to eat to initiate or resume sleep. The first, small study of 20 participants found decreases in perceived stress, depressed mood, anxiety, and hunger among the active PMR group compared to the control group, but no significant decreases in specific NES symptoms. A more recent study of 44 participants participating in a PMR intervention, a PMR plus exercise intervention, or an education-only group found reductions in stress, depressive, anxiety, and NES symptoms across all of the groups. The only significant difference in NES specific symptoms was for evening overeating in the PMR group compared to the education-only group.

Finally, a 12-session/14-week open trial of cognitive-behavioral therapy (CBT) for 25 participants with NES has been reported. CBT for NES includes aspects of CBT treatments that have been established for BED, insomnia, and depression. Additionally, because many of the participants were seeking treatment for NES due to increasing weight, structured behavioral weight management was included in the intervention for overweight and obese participants. Structured eating across the day was a core intervention for all participants, along with logging of sleep, awakenings, and food intake across the 24 hours. Significant reductions in total caloric intake after dinner (35 to 24%), number of nocturnal ingestions (8.7 to 2.6 per week), and weight (82.5 to 79.4 kg) were found at the end of the 14 weeks. Randomized controlled trials are needed to confirm these findings.

Suggested Reading

Allison, K. C. (2012). Cognitive-behavioral therapy manual for night eating syndrome. In J. D. Lundgren, K. C. Allison, & A. J. Stunkard (Eds.), *Night eating syndrome: Research, assessment, and treatment* (pp. 246–265). New York: Guilford Press.—This chapter contains the CBT treatment manual for NES.

Allison, K. C., Lundgren, J. D., O'Reardon, J. P., Geliebter, A., Gluck, M. E., Vinai, P., et al. (2010). Proposed diagnostic criteria for night eating syndrome. *International Journal of Eating Disorders, 43*(3), 241–247.—This article provides a description and the reasoning behind the proposed diagnostic criteria for NES.

Allison, K. C., Lundgren, J. D., O'Reardon, J. P., Martino, N. S., Sarwer, D. B., Wadden, T. A., et al. (2008). The Night Eating Questionnaire (NEQ): Psychometric properties of a measure of severity of the Night Eating Syndrome. *Eating Behaviors, 9*(1), 62–72.—This study validated the use of the NEQ to screen for NES, with an alpha of 0.70 for the full scale.

Goel, N., Stunkard, A. J., Rogers, N. L., Van Dongen, H. P., Allison, K. C., O'Reardon, J. P., et al. (2009). Circadian rhythm profiles in women with night eating syndrome. *Journal of Biological Rhythms, 24*(1), 85–94.—This article showed the delay in not only eating but also the circadian regulation of insulin, glucose, leptin, ghrelin, melatonin, and cortisol.

Lundgren, J. D., Allison, K. C., O'Reardon, J. P., & Stunkard, A. J. (2008). A descriptive study of non-obese persons with night eating syndrome and a weight-matched comparison group. *Eating Behaviors, 9*(3), 343–351.—The first article to describe more pronounced delayed pattern of eating and daytime compensatory behaviors among persons of normal weight with night eating.

Lundgren, J. D., Allison, K. C., Vinai, P., & Gluck, M. E. (2012). Assessment instruments for night eating syndrome. In J. D. Lundgren, K. C. Allison, & A. J. Stunkard (Eds.), *Night eating syndrome: Research, assessment, and treatment* (pp. 197–217). New York: Guilford Press.—This book contains the NESHI and NEDQ assessment measures.

O'Reardon, J. P., Allison, K. C., Martino, N. S., Lundgren, J. D., Heo, M., & Stunkard, A. J. (2006). A randomized, placebo-controlled trial of sertraline in the treatment of night eating syndrome. *American Journal of Psychiatry, 163*(5), 893–898.—The first randomized controlled trial for NES, showing significant reductions in all of the core NES symptoms, including proportion of calories consumed after dinner and number of nocturnal ingestions.

Root, T. L., Thornton, L. M., Lindroos, A. K., Stunkard, A. J., Lichtenstein, P., Pedersen, N. L., et al. (2010). Shared and unique genetic and environmental influences on binge eating and night eating: A Swedish twin study. *Eating Behaviors, 11*(2), 92–98.—This study showed that although there is overlap in heritability between binge eating and night eating, they are related but not identical disorders.

Vander Wal, J. S., Gang, C. H., Griffing, G. T., & Gadde, K. M. (2012). Escitalopram for treatment of night eating syndrome: A 12-week, randomized, placebo-controlled trial. *Journal of Clinical Psychopharmacology, 32*(3), 341–345.—This randomized controlled trial showed significant decreases in night eating symptoms in both the active and placebo groups, but no significant difference between escitalopram and placebo.

33

Eating Disorders in Males

THEODORE E. WELTZIN

Males currently make up approximately 10% of patients with anorexia nervosa (AN) and bulimia nervosa (BN) and 30–40% of patients with binge eating disorder (BED). Data suggest that rates of eating disorders among males are increasing, with some studies reporting that as many as 25% of patients with AN are male. We anticipate that, moving forward, it is likely that one-fourth to one-third of patients presenting for treatment of all eating disorders will be males. This chapter highlights features of clinical presentation and symptoms expressed more commonly in males than in females that inform the treatment process. These characteristics include body image concerns, most commonly an increase desire for muscularity in males, and excessive exercise as a core behavioral manifestation of the eating disorder. Other factors that may increase the risk of developing an eating disorder in males include mood disorders, a history of childhood adversity, alcohol abuse, and psychotic disorders. It is important to underscore that males with mental illnesses, including eating disorders, are less likely to recognize that they have a problem, less likely to be diagnosed or identified as having a problem by professionals, less likely to seek treatment, and less likely to be referred for specialty care. Males with eating disorders who seek treatment services also tend to receive a shorter duration of treatment than females.

Body Image

Men with eating disorders are as concerned about body image as are women when assessed using instruments to systematically rate body image concerns and perceptions. Men with AN and BN perceived themselves as almost twice as "fat" as they actually were, indicating that body distortion in addition to body dissatisfaction—a core symptom of eating disorders in women—also occurs in males. Notably, men with eating disorders most commonly endorse a muscular body image ideal and/or overvalue increased muscle definition, especially in the abdominal region. Several factors that contribute to an abnormal desired or "idealized" body and to body image distortion in males include the media, cultural changes leading to unrealistic expectations of male body image and muscularity, and bodybuilding. Men engage in activities that increase their muscularity because they believe that greater muscularity will enhance feelings of masculinity and confidence, and improve their attractiveness.

Exercise

Males with eating disorders may be more likely than females to engage in problematic exercise; one study indicated that as many as 84% of affected males have a lifetime prevalence of problematic exercise. Signs of excessive exercise include highly structured and repetitive routines (commonly running) that tend to focus on physical endurance. Patients may engage in exercise rather than spend time with family, attend school, or work. Furthermore, as do some females, males with eating disorders may continue to engage in exercise when injured, while underweight and in treatment, and against the recommendations of the treatment team, and they frequently exhibit emotional distress when exercise is limited.

Males with eating disorders who engage in excessive exercise typically describe two behavioral patterns that may have increased their risk of developing an eating disorder. First, they reduced food intake incrementally over time, to a very low caloric intake, and avoided fats and carbohydrates. Second, exercise activities are not aimed at maintaining strength and muscle mass; rather, there is an increase in time spent in calorie-burning activities. Both patterns can accelerate inadequate nutritional intake and weight loss, and promote changes in muscle definition through reduced body fat rather than increased muscle mass.

Sexual Orientation

While the majority of males with eating disorders are heterosexual, the frequency of homosexuality among males presenting for treatment of an eating disorder appears greater than that in the general population. Reasons for this include an increased concentration on body image and higher scores on rating of eating psychopathology and body image concerns, media influence on idealized body image, and body-image-related anxiety in homosexual males as compared to heterosexual males. Second, homosexual males also report higher levels of peer pressure to maintain a particular body type than do heterosexual males. Finally, higher levels of body dissatisfaction may account for higher levels of disordered eating and, for younger gay men, be related to a history of being overweight.

Treatment

Among the obstacles for males seeking treatment for an eating disorder is the misconception that eating disorders exclusively affect females. Especially for men, stigma about eating disorders is a significant factor that negatively influences illness identification, public awareness, and treatment accessibility; for example, eating disorders are viewed more negatively by the public than other mental illnesses, such as depression. Males also report less support from family, friends, school, coaches, and employers.

Patients often report feeling forced into treatment. Engaging the male patient in treatment can be facilitated by using all-male treatment groups, which allow patients to see other males discussing eating disorder symptoms that typically have been viewed as "female" problems, and appropriately expressing emotion in a manner that is identified as demonstrating strength rather than weakness.

Given the stigma associated with mental illness and eating disorders, particularly for males, it is essential from the first treatment encounter to focus on establishing and maintaining a positive therapeutic alliance because this can enhance the chances of a positive treatment outcome. Once engaged in treatment, males benefit from treatment being delivered by a comprehensive and cohesive treatment team focusing on several essential goals, including (1) accurate diagnosis of the eating disorder and of co-occurring psychiatric illnesses, as well as identification of symptoms that do not rise to the level of diagnosis but will likely influence treatment; (2) a comprehensive medical assessment; (3) identification of nutritional goals that are realistic and support normalization of eating behavior and weight/nutritional status; (4) delivery of evidence-based psychotherapy (individual, group, and family) that takes into account specific patient characteristics; (5) education of and collaboration with the patient's family and support system; (6) support of the patient and family in adapting to any changes in the treatment team; and (7) when necessary, provision of continuity across multiple levels of care. For severely affected individuals, treatment usually requires at least 6 to 12 months, but it may require several years or even decades.

Clinical experience suggests that cognitive-behavioral therapy (CBT) is a useful treatment tool for working with males with an eating disorder. CBT gives patients a framework with which to work on not only eating disorder symptoms but also on anxiety and affective disorders. Males tend to externalize emotional distress and, in general, are less likely to be comfortable talking about their feelings, negative experiences, or life events. Our experience working with men is that CBT provides an understandable and structured approach that both addresses externalizing tendencies and facilitates a positive exploration of thoughts and feelings. In addition, CBT helps to identify and challenge errors in thinking concerning food, weight, body image, and the drive to exercise, along with the many different triggers, thoughts, and feelings associated with eating disorder behaviors.

The techniques of CBT for eating disorders, especially as described in generally available preprinted materials, have been developed with a focus on the treatment of girls and women. Among the differences in employing CBT with males is that there are fewer consistent and predictable overvalued beliefs concerning food, weight, and shape. While women frequently report feeling overweight, even when at a normal or low weight, men may not report such feelings, even while continuing to experience severe anxiety and distress concerning eating, fullness, and weight gain. It is often helpful to individualize treatment by identifying struggles that may not fit the classic model of CBT for women with eating disorders. The therapist's recognition that males may utilize externalized coping skills and exhibit anger when depressed may facilitate expression of thoughts and feelings as an alternative to less helpful coping skills. For boys, family therapy is essential to permit appropriate and productive emotional expressions of emotion and of conflict, rather than using eating disordered behaviors as the main mechanism for emotional regulation. Experiential therapy programs that include art therapy, movement, and recreation therapy are particularly useful for work on body image and healthy nonverbal expression, team building, problem solving, and exercise issues.

For males with eating disorders, treatment of problematic exercise can be particularly challenging. It is essential to understand underlying issues associated with the initiation or maintenance of problematic exercise; for example, a past history of obesity or anxiety about acceptance in social situations may be linked to excessive exercise behaviors. Interventions should first identify important behavioral manifestations of problematic exercise, including the frequency, intensity, and duration of physical activity; medical conditions that directly result from problematic exercise, including physical injuries resulting from overuse and/or abuse; and the psychosocial impact on time management, job performance, and personal relationships. Anyone with an eating disorder, regardless of weight status, can exhibit excessive exercise as a symptom akin to food restriction, binge eating, or purging. Therefore, an appropriate treatment goal is the cessation of problematic exercise, in parallel with the goal of extinction of other eating disordered behaviors such as food restriction, binge eating, and purging. Throughout treatment and recovery, the amount of exercise should be monitored, and if an individual returns to a significant level of problematic exercise, this may constitute a relapse. Excessive exercise behaviors often need to be addressed as part of treatment, and individualization of therapy should be based on an assessment of the patient's fitness beliefs and behaviors. Obtaining collateral information from family and coaches is recommended because patients typically minimize these behaviors and are often reluctant to identify exercise behaviors as dysfunctional.

As mentioned previously, sexuality is a common theme in the psychotherapy of males with eating disorders. However, simply assuming that sexuality is a core issue, without establishing a therapeutic alliance with the patient and exploring the broad range of potential psychological stressors, can lead to frustration on the part of the patient. Treatment in a group setting with other males may be beneficial, and focusing on group cohesiveness and trust, and reviewing past episodes of victimization, be they related to being teased or bullied about weight or about sexuality, can create common themes.

Finally, the team needs to be adaptive because, for a variety of reasons, team members change over the course of treatment for an individual. Effective and integrated communication, generated within a team-based plan, encourages patients, family members, and caregivers to experience treatment as continuous, cohesive, and collaborative. Thus, disruption of progress should be minimized if there are changes in therapists, physicians, or dietitians. Past treatment experiences, both positive and negative, should be assessed because it is important for the current treatment team to take previous treatments into account when planning treatment and preparing the patient for a team member change.

Outcome

Outcome research specific to males with eating disorders is very limited. Studies suggest that men benefit from early diagnosis and treatment, have a similar response to treatment as women, and have a similar duration of illness prior to seeking treatment. As for women, prognosis after discharge from treatment is improved by positive social supports, and effective coping and problem-solving skills. Other protective factors for both males and females with eating disorders are the amount weight gain (for underweight patients), positive self-esteem, emotional stability, school achievement, and family connectedness.

While the data are limited, it is likely that the majority of males who are diagnosed with AN recover from their illness. On the other hand, roughly 25% of males with AN go on to develop enduring eating disorder symptoms. Furthermore, mortality rates and the incidence of medical complications appear to be similar for males and females with eating disorders.

Summary

In summary, it is likely that rates of eating disorders in males will continue to increase. While differences exist in risk factors and symptom expression in males with eating disorders, a growing body of evidence suggests that males respond well to treatment. However, treatment needs to be individualized for the male patient, ideally in a setting with other males and with staff experienced in working with males. Obstacles to treatment include a lack of awareness that males are at risk for eating disorders and the stigma males often perceive on receiving a diagnosis.

Suggested Reading

Andersen, A. E., & Holman, J. E. (1997). Males with eating disorders: Challenges for treatment and research. *Psychopharmacological Bulletin, 33*(3), 391–397.—An early description of the problem of eating disorders in males.

Bean, P., Loomis, C. C., Timmel, P., Hallinan, P., Moore, S., Mammel, J., et al. (2004). Outcome variables for anorexic males and females one year after discharge from residential treatment. *Journal of Addictive Diseases, 23*(2), 83–94.—An article reviewing similarities and differences between males and females in terms of symptom presentation, treatment reponse, and outcome 1 year after intensive treatment.

Boisvert, J., & Harrell, W. A. (2009). Homosexuality as a risk factor for eating disorder symptomology in men. *Journal of Men's Studies, 17,* 210–225.—A review of the relationship between sexual orientation and risk for eating disorders.

Fichter, M., & Krenn, H. (2003). Eating disorders in males. In J. Treasure, U. Schmidt, & E. van Furth (Eds.), *Handbook of eating disorders* (2nd ed., pp. 369–383). West Sussex, UK: Wiley.—A comprehensive review of eating disorders in males including risk factors, presentation, and treatment.

Hausenblas, H. A., Campbell, A., Menzel, J. E., Doughty, J., Levine, M., & Thompson, J. K. (2013). Media effects of experimental presentation of the ideal physique on eating disorder symptoms: A meta-analysis of laboratory studies. *Clinical Psychology Review, 33*(1), 168–181.—Review of the impact on males of cultural expectations in terms of body image.

Hudson, J. I., Hiripi, E., Pope, H. G., Jr., & Kessler, R. C. (2007). The prevalence and correlates of eating disorders in the National Comorbidity Survey Replication. *Biological Psychiatry, 61*(3), 348–358.—A population-based survey of eating disorder prevalence.

Strober, M., Freeman, R., Lampert, C., Diamond, J., Teplinsky, C., & DeAntonio, M. (2006). Are there gender differences in core symptoms, temperament, and short-term prospective outcome in anorexia nervosa? *International Journal of Eating Disorders, 39*(7), 570–575.—A look at gender difference and treatment reponse for males and females with AN.

Medical Complications of Anorexia Nervosa

PHILIP S. MEHLER

In contrast to other psychiatric disorders, such as schizophrenia, bipolar illness, and depression, which are not associated with frequent serious physical problems, anorexia nervosa (AN) has a litany of medical complications that are directly attributable and inextricably connected to this eating disorder. No body system is spared from the ravages of AN, especially as the symptoms become more chronic and severe. Herein these complications and their treatments are described.

Overview of Medical Complications

In AN, the medical complications are due to weight loss and malnutrition. It is well documented that the mortality rate in AN greatly exceeds that of all other psychiatric disorders. A significant portion of this excess mortality rate is directly attributable to the medical complications found in AN. There is a direct correlation between the incidence of the medical complications with both the duration of AN and its severity. While there is no universally accepted severity grading system for the medical complications, it is generally accepted that severe AN is defined by a body mass index (BMI) less than 15 kg/m^2 or by a weight less than 70% of ideal body weight (IBW).

General Signs and Symptoms

Patients with AN may complain of fatigue, irritability, and cold intolerance. They often have growth of fine downy hair, called *lanugo,* on the sides of their faces and along their spines, which is not a sign of verilization, but more likely represents a heat-conserving mechanism. It quickly fades away with weight restoration. Easy bruisability, brittle nails, thinning of scalp hair, and excessive pruritus–xerosis are also present. Acrocyanosis may be noted as weight loss progress. Lagophthalmos and patulous eustachian tube dysfunction are two issues related to the eyes and ears, respectively. The former refers to the inability of the eyelids to completely cover the eye when sleeping, resulting in a complaint that the eyes feel irritated by a foreign-body sensation likely due to corneal abrasions from the incomplete covering of the eye. This is treated by taping the eyelids shut at night until some weight gain is accomplished. Eustachian tube dysfunction manifests with the sensation of speaking into a hollow tube, and its cause has not been elucidated.

Gastrointestinal Symptoms

With more severe degrees of weight loss, there is development of dysphagia, which can interfere with the ability of the patient to engage in oral feeding. This is due to pharyngeal muscle weakness. Enlisting the services of a speech therapist, temporary dietary modifications, and avoidance of straws are useful early in refeeding. These patients may complain of coughing during meals or have a history of aspiration pneumonia. A large percentage of patients with AN have gastroparesis and delayed gastric emptying. This also worsens with greater amounts of weight loss. Symptoms include bloating, left-upper-quadrant abdominal pain, and early satiety. A good history alone will lead to the correct diagnosis; confirmatory proof can be obtained with a nuclear medicine gastric emptying study, but this is rarely needed. Expert dietitian input to institute small particle-size diets with soft and liquid foods is often all that is necessary to treat this temporary problem; however, on occasion, judicious use of low-dose metoclopramide before meals and/or erythromycin may be temporarily necessary early in the refeeding process. Similarly, there is prolonged transit time through the colon in patients with AN due to reflex hypofunctioning of the colon. Thus, constipation is a common complaint, even among those who have never abused stimulant laxatives. Fiber should be avoided as a treatment because of its propensity to cause bloating and distention. Rather, an osmotic-type laxative, such as polyethylene glycol, is more useful. Less commonly, these patients may complain of diarrhea early on in the refeeding process. This is likely due to intestinal villous atrophy, with resultant malabsorption. Diamine oxidase activity is reduced as a result and may serve as a surrogate serum marker of this transient complication of weight loss. One additional, fairly rare cause of abdominal pain in AN is the superior mesenteric artery (SMA) syndrome. Normally the SMA is cushioned by a fat pad that keeps it from compressing the lumen of the duodenum as it passes between the SMA and the aorta. With weight loss, there is atrophy of this fat pad, which causes the SMA to shift medially and obstruct the lumen of the third portion of the duodenum, basically resulting in a mechanical small bowel obstruction. Symptoms include upper-quadrant abdominal pain, distention, and early satiety. Diagnosis is made by computed tomography (CT) scan of the abdomen, and treatment is some weight restoration to reestablish the fat pad. This can be accomplished with a liquid oral diet or the insertion of a nasojejunal tube, or a tube placed percutaneously.

Hepatic Symptoms

As malnutrition and weight loss worsen, there ensues a process of programmed cell death of hepatocytes, referred to as *apoptosis*. This is manifested by progressive elevations of hepatic transaminases (aspartate [AST] and alanine [ALT]). Bilirubin and alkaline phosphatase are not generally abnormally elevated in AN. The ALT is generally disproportionately elevated compared with the AST. As refeeding ensues, these typically revert back to normal over the course of a few weeks, with the ALT lagging behind the AST. Less commonly, these transaminases are elevated due to the actual refeeding process in a mechanism akin to the steatosis of obesity. Treatment involves dietary modification to reduce the carbohydrate and fat content of the diet. A right-upper-quadrant ultrasound can help differentiate steatosis from apoptosis-induced transaminitis. Refeeding pancreatitis has been rarely described in AN with a similar presentation to more common causes of pancreatitis.

Cardiac Symptoms

Sudden cardiac death is a root cause for the impressively high mortality rate of AN. This is not due to obstructive atherosclerotic coronary artery disease. Rather, it is likely attributable to the confluence of multiple cardiac structural and functional changes. Patients have an attenuated blood pressure response to exercise, bradycardia, and hypotension. National guidelines recommend hospitalization for heart rates less than 40 beats/minute or systolic blood pressures less than 70 mmHg. These cardiac changes appear to resolve with sustained and significant weight gain. The bradycardia is due to excessive vagal tone, and the blood pressure changes are due to a reduction in left ventricular mass and cardiac output. The sinus bradycardia can degenerate into a junctional escape rhythm that is transient and extinguishes with exercise.

In the past, QT prolongation was felt to be an inherent high-risk conduction abnormality in AN. However, more recently, there is increasing evidence that QT prolongation is not inherent to AN but rather, when present, likely represents the effects of electrolyte abnormalities or a medication effect. Also, reduced heart rate variability has been recently noted in AN, along with increased QT dispersion. Both of these are indicative of increased ventricular irritability and a propensity toward fatal ventricular arrhythmias, such as ventricular tachycardia.

In addition to the aforementioned reduction in the size of the cardiac muscle, there are also increasingly noted pericardial effusions seen on echocardiograms. The etiology of these is not clear, nor is their natural history. Coronary artery fibrosis has also recently been reported by coronary magnetic resonance imaging (MRI) angiography.

Pulmonary Symptoms

Relative to other body systems, the lungs are not often affected in AN. However, spontaneous pneumothorax and pneumomediastinum have been described. They are difficult to heal once they develop. Abnormal pulmonary function testing, with changes consistent with obstructive lung disease, have been rarely reported. Aspiration pneumonia due to weakened pharyngeal muscles and dysphagia may also occur.

Hematological Symptoms

Trilinear hypoplasia as a result of malnutrition is commonly seen. Anemia, leukopenia, and thrombocytopenia occur in decreasing frequency. The anemia is typically normocytic and generally not due to vitamin or iron deficiency. Frank neutropenia may occur with more severe degrees of AN but does not appear to be associated with a heightened risk of infections. However, increased vigilance is indicated because the other typical signs of infection, such as fever and elevated erythrocyte sedimentation rate, are generally absent. All of these complications are due to serous fat atrophy in the bone marrow, with replacement of normal marrow fat with a gelatinous mucopolysaccharide that interferes with progenitor heme cell formation. This is also reversible with weight restoration; hence, usage of growth factors is not indicated.

Endocrine Symptoms

Pituitary-induced hypogonadism is the rule as AN worsens. Thus, males present with decreased libido and erectile dysfunction, and the vast majority of females are hypoestrogenemic and amenorrheic. Fertility is unlikely to be permanently impaired. There is an increased risk of preterm deliveries and miscarriages in patients with AN, as well as that for unplanned pregnancies. Cortisol levels tend to be elevated due to increased adrenal production and decreased renal clearance. The significance of this remains elusive. Growth hormone levels are also increased, but insulin-like growth factor 1 levels are low, consistent with a state of growth hormone resistance. Leptin levels are reduced in AN and may be a marker of recovery as they revert to normal. Resumption of natural menses, also a sign of recovery, generally occurs when weight gain exceeds 90–95% of ideal body weight. There appears to some association between type 1 diabetes and AN, but the exact nature of the connection has not been defined.

As a direct result of some of the aforementioned endocrine complications of AN, a substantial proportion of these patients have osteopenia and even osteoporosis, notwithstanding their typically young age. Loss of bone density begins early in the course of this illness, and the expert recommendations are to obtain a screening bone density (dual X-ray absorptiometry [DXA]) after 9–12 months of amenorrhea in females or within 1 year of diagnosis in males. In fact, the degree of osteoporosis in males with AN may be worse than that in their female counterparts. This exuberant loss of bone density in AN results in a heightened lifetime risk of fragility fractures, even in adolescents. Moreover, this diminished bone density may never be recoverable, especially in those with more protracted courses of their illness. This fact underscores the need for the core treatment of AN, namely, weight restoration and resumption of menses. As bridge therapy, it is worthwhile to offer treatment with calcium and vitamin D. In addition, there is emerging evidence in support of judicious consideration of bisphosphonate therapy for both males and females or of teriparatide injections. Testosterone replacement therapy for males might be considered as first-line treatment if there are documented low serum testosterone levels and hypogonadal symptoms. Oral contraceptives do not have a primary role for the treatment of osteoporosis in females with AN. Transdermal estrogen may be of utility.

Neurological Symptoms

Musculoskeletal weakness and deconditioning ensue as the disease becomes more severe and chronic. This is reversible with thoughtful strengthening exercises following the recommendations of a physical therapist. Cortical brain atrophy affecting both gray and white matter has been consistently reported. While this appears likely to normalize over time with overall recovery, there may remain irreversible neurocognitive deficiencies that hamper higher brain functions.

Glucose and Electrolyte Levels

For those patients with restricting AN, serum electrolyte levels are typically normal. Thus, the finding of hypokalemia or acid–base abnormalities in these patients may be evidence of covert purging behaviors. The two most commonly abnormal serum chemistry values in AN are glucose and sodium levels. Hypoglycemia is a bad prognostic sign because it is consistent with depleted hepatic glycogen stores and reduced gluconeogenic substrate, reflecting a more severe degree of malnutrition. Hyponatremia is occasionally noted in patients with restricting type AN. This is not due to syndrome of inappropriate antidiuretic hormone production (SIADH). Rather, it is due to an inherent inability to clear free water due to diminished solute load in the kidney. Thus, these patients need to be cautioned about excessive water consumption to avoid severe hyponatremia and its dangers. Diabetes insipidus has also been rarely described in AN.

Conclusion

In summary, AN is a highly lethal illness, with a significant proportion of deaths due to the inherent medical complications. No body system is protected from the malnutrition associated with this disease. However, most of the medical complications are reversible with effective and timely interventions.

Suggested Reading

Fazeli, P. K., & Klibanski, A. (2014). Anorexia nervosa and bone metabolism. *Bone, 66,* 39–45.—Article concerning the deleterious effects of AN on bone density.

Fonville, L., Giampietro, V., Williams, S. C. R., Simmons, A., & Tchanturia, K. (2014). Alterations in brain structure in adults with anorexia nervosa and the impact of illness duration. *Psychological Medicine, 44*(9), 1965–1975.—Article concerning brain changes associated with AN.

Gaudiani, J. L., Sabel, A. L., Mascolo, M., & Mehler, P. S. (2012). Severe anorexia nervosa: Outcomes from a medical stabilization unit. *International Journal of Eating Disorders, 45*(1), 85–92.—Article on common complications of AN.

Mehler, P. S. (2001). Diagnosis and care of patients with anorexia nervosa in primary care settings. *Annals of Internal Medicine, 134*(11), 1048–1059.—Describes basic medical care for a patient with AN.

Mehler, P. S., Cleary, B. S., & Gaudiani, J. L. (2011). Osteoporosis in anorexia nervosa. *Eating Disorders, 19*(2), 194–202.—Documents a high prevalence of loss of bone density in AN.

Miller, K. K., Grinspoon, S. K., Ciampa, J., Hier, J., Herzog, D., & Klibanski, A. (2005). Medical findings in outpatients with anorexia nervosa. *Archives of Internal Medicine, 165*(5), 561–566.—Article on common lab abnormalities in AN.

Olivares, J. L., Vázquez, M., Fleta, J., Moreno, L. A., Pérez-González, J. M., & Bueno, M. (2005). Cardiac findings in adolescents with anorexia nervosa at diagnosis and after weight restoration. *European Journal of Pediatrics, 164*(6), 383–386.—Cardiac structure is often affected during the course of AN.

Sabel, A. L., Gaudiani, J. L., Statland, B., & Mehler, P. S. (2013). Hematological abnormalities in severe anorexia nervosa. *Annals of Hematology, 92*(5), 605–613.—Article on heme changes from AN.

Smith, R. W., Kornenblum, C., Tracker, K., Bonifacio, H. J., Gonska, T., & Katzman, D. K. (2013). Severely elevated transaminases in anorexia nervosa. *International of Journal Eating Disorders, 46,* 751–754.—Article about hepatic complications of AN.

Strumia, R. (2013). Eating disorders and the skin. *Clinics in Dermatology, 31*(1), 80–85.—Describes multiple different dermatological complications of AN.

Medical Complications of Bulimia Nervosa

PHILIP S. MEHLER

Like anorexia nervosa, bulimia nervosa (BN) is associated with an increased mortality rate, largely due to the medical complications related to the mode and frequency of purging behaviors. This chapter focuses on the complications associated with self-induced vomiting and laxative abuse, and offers some additional comments about the complications of diuretic abuse.

Self-Induced Vomiting

Self-induced vomiting is the most common mode of purging in patients with BN. The medical complications that emanate from self-induced vomiting can be divided into those caused by the local effects of excessive vomiting and those related to the fluid, electrolyte, and acid–base abnormalities that occur as a result of this form of purging.

Local Complications

As a result of excessive self-induced vomiting, there is progressive weakening of the lower esophageal sphincter and a breach in the natural mechanics keeping gastric acid contained in the stomach. Therefore, ultimately, there is free flux of caustic gastric acid into the esophagus, and gastric esophageal reflux disease (GERD) ensues with attendant substernal burning pain and sour taste in the mouth. In addition, chronic regurgitation of acid causes inflammation of the esophageal mucosal lining, which in turn may result in esophageal strictures and resultant dysphagia. Even more concerning is the possibility of developing Barrett's esophagus, a precancerous change in the esophageal mucosa. Esophageal carcinoma has been described in patients with BN as a result of long-standing esophageal reflux disease. Hematemesis (vomiting blood) is usually due to self-limited Mallory-Weiss tears.

The aforementioned acid reflux is treated as it is when not associated with BN, with proton pump inhibitors and lifestyle changes. An upper gastrointestinal endoscopy should be considered if there is suspicion of Barrett's esophagus.

Other potential adverse effects of chronic self-induced vomiting include *perimyolysis*, which refers to erosion of the enamel on the lingual surfaces of the teeth from acid exposure. Patients also have excess dental caries. *Cheilosis*, inflammation at the corners of the mouth, may develop as a result of poor oral hygiene associated with vomiting. *Sialadenosis* refers to bilateral parotid and salivary gland hypertrophy, which gives the appearance of having the mumps and occurs in some patients who induce vomiting; it may also develop 3–4 days after the abrupt cessation of excessive vomiting. Tissue examination of these parotid glands reveals large acini with prominent zymogen granules without other pathology.

Perimyolysis can be mitigated by gentle brushing and use of a fluorinated mouthwash. Sialadenosis can be preempted or easily treated with the use of sialagogues, such as lemon drops, plus nonsteroidal anti-inflammatory medications and the frequent application of warm packs to the affected sides of the face for 1–2 weeks. Rarely, oral pilocarpine is required to decompress the swollen glands in refractory cases.

Other rare complications of the retching associated with self-induced vomiting include epistaxis (nosebleeds), subconjunctival hemorrhages, esophageal perforation (Boerhaave syndrome) and pneumomediastinum.

Fluid and Electrolyte Levels

Excessive vomiting will predictably result in loss of gastric acid leading to a metabolic alkalosis. Chronic dehydration also stimulates excess adrenal aldosterone production to prevent hypotension via increased renal sodium reabsorption and acid secretion in the urine. This further exacerbates the metabolic alkalosis. In fact, because of the dual mechanisms causing acid loss, the metabolic alkalosis resulting from self-induced vomiting is more severe than that associated with other modes of purging; serum bicarbonate levels greater than 38 meq/L are a specific indicator of purging via self-induced vomiting. The other common electrolyte abnormality found with self-induced vomiting is hypokalemia. Indeed, the finding of unexplained hypokalemia in a young patient is highly suggestive of covert BN.

The aforementioned elevated aldosterone levels, in response to a state of chronic dehydration, produce a constellation of changes that can make it difficult to abruptly desist from this purging behavior. The elevated aldosterone levels caused by dehydration take several weeks to return to normal. Therefore, there is a propensity toward edema formation upon abrupt cessation of purging behaviors due to an imbalance between sodium retention and the absence of excessive sodium loss once purging ceases. This phenomenon is known as pseudo-Bartter syndrome, and may lead to severe edema formation if a patient with BN receives intravenous saline too quickly. Such edema can be prevented with the judicious use of spironolactone (50–200 mg/day). Spironolactone should be continued for 2–3 weeks after the purging ceases until aldosterone levels return to normal. When a patient presents to emergency department for symptoms of dizziness or paresthesias secondary to fluid and electrolyte abnormalities, and intravenous fluids are necessary, they should be given over 12–24 hours, not as rapidly as they are typically given for acute states of dehydration.

Most patients with BN use a finger or a utensil to induce vomiting, or they learn to induce vomiting voluntarily. However, some use syrup of ipecac to induce vomiting. The active ingredient in ipecac is emetine, which is toxic to cardiac muscle. Each bottle of ipecac contains 30 mg of emetine, and when the cumulative dose exceeds 1,250 mg over a short period of time, an irreversible cardiomyopathy may ensue, leading to congestive heart failure.

Diuretic Abuse

The excessive abuse of diuretics, especially those available only by prescription, causes the same electrolyte abnormalities seen with self-induced vomiting. This mode of purging may be utilized, in particular, by health care professionals who have ready access to such medications. Thus, a state of hypokalemic metabolic alkalosis, albeit less severe than seen with self-induced vomiting, ensues. Similarly, such patients are chronically dehydrated and develop elevated aldosterone levels as part of pseudo-Bartter syndrome. Spironolactone has utility for this group of patients when they present for care and are ready to cease abuse of diuretics.

Laxative Abuse

There are two major classes of laxatives, the osmotic type and the stimulant type. Osmotic laxatives work by drawing water into the colonic lumen, thereby promoting defecation. In general, they are safe, difficult to abuse, and do not cause dependence. In contrast, stimulant laxatives contain senna, cascara, or bisacodyl. They are associated with significant harm if abused and taken in excess for extended periods of time. As with self-induced vomiting, the medical complications are due either to local adverse effects on the colon or to the fluid, electrolyte, and acid–base disturbances that result from the large amounts of diarrhea they cause.

Historically, there have been concerns that the active ingredients of stimulant laxatives, when abused in excess, might damage the myenteric plexus (*Auerbach's plexus*), which provides motor innervation of the gut. It was thought that, at the extreme, damage would result in the colon becoming an inert tube, incapable of propagating fecal material, with resultant progressively severe constipation and obstipation (*cathartic colon*). However, in recent years, such concerns have diminished. Nonetheless, because of the other problems associated with laxative abuse, patients should be urged and aided to cease their use of stimulant laxatives.

Local adverse effects of stimulant laxatives include rectal prolapse due frequent straining and long periods of time sitting on the toilet. Hematochezia (blood per rectum) can also occur due to excessive defecation, rectal irritation along with hemorrhoids, and anal fissures. *Melanosis coli* refers to a dark black discoloration of the colonic mucosa due to abuse of anthraquinone-type stimulant laxatives (e.g., cascara); it is noted during colonoscopic procedures and is likely a benign finding of no known clinical import. There has long been a debate whether stimulant laxative abuse is associated with an increased risk of colorectal carcinoma; currently, there is no definitive evidence of a causal relationship.

Fluid and Electrolyte Levels

Again, similar to self-induced vomiting and diuretic abuse, laxative abuse results in significant hypokalemia. However, in contrast to the other two modes of purging, laxative abuse initially causes a hyperchloremic metabolic acidosis (non-anion gap acidosis).

Ultimately, with prolonged excessive laxative abuse and resultant dehydration, a metabolic alkalosis ensues due to the aforementioned elevated serum aldosterone levels as a defense mechanism to prevent hypotension and syncope from dehydration as a result of ongoing fluid losses.

Conclusion

BN, just like anorexia nervosa, is associated with a number of medical complications. These complications are a direct result of the mode and frequency of purging behaviors. There are two main types of medical complications: those due to the resultant fluid, electrolyte, and acid–base aberrations, and those due to the local adverse effects of the mode of purging utilized. Judicious and informed medical care is critical to identifying such adverse effects and definitively treating them.

Suggested Reading

Bahia, A., Mascolo, M., Gaudiani, J. L., & Mehler, P. S. (2012). PseudoBartter syndrome in eating disorders. *International Journal of Eating Disorders, 45*(1), 150–153.—Defines the pathophysiology of this complication from bulimia.

Brown, C. A., & Mehler, P. S. (2012). Successful "detoxing" from commonly utilized modes of purging in bulimia nervosa. *Eating Disorders, 20*(4), 312–320.—Defines caveats that may arise when purging behaviors are ceased.

Brown, C. A., & Mehler, P. S. (2013). Medical complications of self-induced vomiting. *Eating Disorders, 21*(4), 287–294.—Article on the medical complications of purging.

Bryant-Waugh, R., Turner, H., East, P., Gamble, C., & Mehta, R. (2006). Misuse of laxatives among adult outpatients with eating disorders: Prevalence and profiles. *International Journal of Eating Disorders, 39*(5), 404–409.—Describes the medical complications of laxative abuse.

Denholm, M., & Jankowski, J. (2011). Gastroesophageal reflux disease and bulimia nervosa—a review of the literature. *Diseases of the Esophagus, 24*(2), 79–85.—Common complication from the self-induced vomiting of BN.

Mascolo, M., Trent, S., Colwell, C., & Mehler, P. S. (2012). What the emergency department needs to know when caring for your patients with eating disorders. *International Journal of Eating Disorders, 45*(8), 977–981.—Useful resource for emergency department staff who are asked to treat patients with BN.

Mehler, P. S. (2003). Bulimia nervosa. *New England Journal of Medicine, 349*(9), 875–881.—Review article on the medical complications of bulimia.

Mehler, P. S. (2011). Medical complications of bulimia nervosa and their treatments. *International Journal of Eating Disorders, 44*(2), 95–104.—Discusses the medical complications of BN.

Mignogna, M. D., Fedele, S., & Lo Russo, L. (2004). Anorexia/bulimia-related sialadenosis of palatal minor salivary glands. *Journal of Oral Pathology and Medicine, 33*(7), 441–442.—Article on the oral complications of purging.

Trent, S. A., Moreira, M. E., Colwell, C. B., & Mehler, P. S. (2013). ED management of patients with eating disorders. *American Journal of Emergency Medicine, 31*(5), 859–865.—Focuses on emergency management of eating disorders.

Medical Complications of Eating Disorders in Children and Adolescents

NEVILLE H. GOLDEN

Medical complications of eating disorders in children and adolescents develop either as a result of adaptive responses to malnutrition or secondary to unhealthy weight control practices such as self-induced vomiting or the use of laxatives, diuretics, or diet pills. The body's adaptive responses to malnutrition are initially protective but with continued dietary restriction and weight loss, they can become life threatening. In general, medical complications in children and adolescents are similar to those seen in adults with eating disorders, with two important exceptions. First, because of limited nutritional reserves and increased metabolic demands for growth and development, children and adolescents can become medically compromised more rapidly than adults or after relatively small amounts of weight loss. Second, because of their immature skeletons and incompletely developed brains, children and adolescents are at risk for potentially irreversible complications. Consequently, it is important to recognize and treat the medical complications early in their course to prevent long-term morbidity.

Medical complications can affect every organ system and are usually correlated with the degree of malnutrition. Most, but not all, of the complications are reversible with nutritional rehabilitation, weight restoration, and treatment of the underlying eating disorder. Some complications, such as growth retardation or reduced bone mass, may not be entirely reversible. Shorter duration of illness and early intervention have been shown to improve outcome.

Medical Complications by Organ System

Fluid and Electrolyte Disturbances

Dehydration and electrolyte disturbances may occur with fluid restriction or purging behaviors. Potassium, the main intracellular cation in the body, is important for cardiac contractility. Even small changes in serum potassium levels can rapidly lead to cardiac arrhythmias. The most frequently encountered electrolyte abnormality in children and adolescents with eating disorders is hypokalemia, usually as a result of vomiting or abuse of laxatives or diuretics. Loss of hydrogen and chloride in vomitus results in a metabolic alkalosis, accompanied by a high urine pH. Hyponatremia can develop in those who drink large amounts of water, either to suppress hunger urges or to fake weight gain. Severe hyponatremia can lead to seizures, coma, and death. Phosphorus and magnesium are necessary for cardiac and neuromuscular function. Patients may have low serum phosphorus levels (hypophosphatemia) on presentation but more frequently, serum phosphorus levels are normal on presentation but drop as phosphorus is utilized to produce energy during refeeding. Hypophosphatemia is thought to play a role in development of *refeeding syndrome,* a potentially lethal condition characterized by cardiac, respiratory, and hepatic failure; delirium, coma, and seizures; and, in some cases, death. Refeeding hypophosphatemia occurs in approximately 14% of hospitalized adolescents with anorexia nervosa and is associated with degree of malnutrition more than energy intake. Hypomagnesemia occurs later in the course of refeeding than hypophosphatemia and is more prevalent in those who purge. Fortunately, refeeding syndrome is rare and can be prevented by careful monitoring of electrolytes and cardiac function during refeeding, especially in those who are severely malnourished.

Cardiovascular Complications

Resting heart rates can be as low as 30–40 beats per minute, and both systolic and diastolic blood pressures can be low. Postural changes in pulse and blood pressure indicate medical instability if the pulse increases more than 20 beats per minute from lying to standing or if the blood pressure drops more than 20 mmHg systolic or 10 mmHg diastolic from lying to standing. These orthostatic changes can cause dizziness, palpitations, and syncope. In anorexia nervosa, both cardiac structure and function are affected. Heart size is reduced, exercise capacity is diminished, and heart rate variability is increased, but cardiac output and left ventricular function are usually preserved. Electrocardiographic abnormalities include sinus bradycardia, low voltage complexes, a prolonged corrected QT interval (QTc), first- and second-degree heart block, and various atrial and ventricular arrhythmias. Findings on echocardiography confirm not only decreased cardiac size and reduced left ventricular wall thickness but also may reveal mitral valve prolapse and a pericardial effusion that usually is asymptomatic. Mitral valve prolapse is thought to be the result of an apparent redundancy of the mitral valve. Congestive heart failure does not usually occur during the starvation phase, but it can occur during refeeding. Adolescents with bulimia nervosa may also develop bradycardia and orthostasis secondary to dietary restriction. Purging behaviors typical of this syndrome can cause electrolyte abnormalities and cardiac arrhythmias.

Gastrointestinal Complications

Bloating and constipation are frequent complaints of patients with eating disorders and reflect delayed gastric emptying and decreased intestinal motility. Severe weight loss can lead to loss of the fat pad between the superior mesenteric artery and the aorta, resulting in external compression of the duodenum by the superior mesenteric artery and causing pain and vomiting after eating, so-called "superior mesenteric artery (SMA) syndrome." Elevated liver enzymes are found in approximately 40% of adolescents with anorexia nervosa. The elevations are usually mild, most frequently are present before refeeding has been initiated, and are associated with the degree of malnutrition. In the majority of patients, elevated liver enzymes improve with refeeding. In a minority of patients, a transient increase in liver enzymes may be associated with refeeding. Rapid weight loss can be associated with gallstone formation.

Recurrent vomiting can lead to parotid and submandibular gland enlargement, loss of the gag reflex, dental enamel erosion, gastroesophageal reflux, esophagitis, elevations in serum amylase, and Mallory–Weiss tears. Esophageal or gastric rupture can occur but is rare. Prolonged vomiting causes Barrett's esophagus, precancerous changes in the epithelium of the distal esophagus caused by recurrent exposure to acid stomach contents. Laxative abuse can be accompanied by profuse bloody diarrhea and rectal prolapse. In contrast to other forms of malnutrition seen in children and adolescents, serum albumin levels are usually normal. Serum cholesterol levels may be elevated and tend to improve with nutritional rehabilitation.

Endocrine Complications

In children and adolescents who develop an eating disorder before completion of growth, growth retardation and short stature can occur. Boys are at particular risk because their growth spurt occurs late in puberty and they grow, on average, 2 years longer than girls. In contrast, in girls, the growth spurt occurs early in puberty, and most growth is complete by menarche. Catch-up growth can occur with nutritional rehabilitation, but final adult height may still be lower than genetic potential. Interruption of puberty can occur in those who develop an eating disorder prior to completion of puberty. In girls, primary or secondary amenorrhea is common and usually follows weight loss, but it precedes it in 20% of cases. The hypothalamic–pituitary–gonadal axis is suppressed, causing low estrogen levels in girls and low testosterone levels in boys. In girls with anorexia nervosa, the ovaries and uterus regress to prepubertal size. Girls with bulimia nervosa usually have regular menses, but menses can also become irregular during cycles of dietary restriction.

In anorexia nervosa, in addition to amenorrhea and menstrual irregularities, hypothalamic dysregulation is evidenced by disturbances in satiety, difficulties with temperature regulation, and inability to concentrate urine. The hypothalamic–adrenal axis is activated with high levels of serum cortisol, and the hypothalamic–thyroid axis is suppressed. Serum levels of triiodothyronine (T3), the most active thyroid hormone, are low; so-called "low T3 syndrome," or "sick euthyroid syndrome," is caused by preferential peripheral conversion of thyroxine to reverse T3, the inactive optical isomer of T3, instead of conversion to the active form of T3, as an adaptive response to starvation. Thyroid function disturbances correct with nutritional rehabilitation and should not be treated with thyroid replacement hormone.

Musculoskeletal Complications

Between 40 and 60% of adult bone mass is accrued during the adolescent years, and peak bone mass is only achieved toward the end of the second decade of life. An episode of anorexia nervosa during adolescence can compromise peak bone mass acquisition, resulting in reduced bone mass and increased fracture risk. Reduced bone mineral density (BMD) for age has been identified in both adolescent boys and girls with anorexia nervosa, and low BMD has been shown to persist in adults 20 years after recovering from adolescent-onset anorexia nervosa. A past history of anorexia nervosa results in a two- to threefold increase in fracture risk in adults. Adolescent girls who develop anorexia nervosa before menarche have lower BMD than those who develop it after menarche. Studies utilizing markers of bone turnover in adolescents have identified evidence of reduced bone formation, as well accelerated bone resorption. Prospective observational studies have shown that compared with healthy girls, adolescent girls with anorexia nervosa do not increase BMD, whereas heathy girls continue to accrue bone. Patients with bulimia nervosa may also have reductions in BMD, especially if they were previously amenorrheic or had low weight. Contributing factors include low body weight; dietary deficiencies of calcium, vitamin D, and protein; and hormonal alterations, including hypogonadism, hypercortisolism, and low levels of insulin-like growth factor 1.

The optimal treatment of low bone mass in anorexia nervosa is not known. Weight gain and resumption of menses is accompanied by some improvements in BMD, but weight gain without resumption of menses is not accompanied by significant increases in BMD. Oral contraceptives have not been shown to be effective in adolescents with anorexia nervosa. One study found that a patch containing physiological doses of estrogen with oral cyclic oral progesterone increased BMD of the spine and hip in adolescent girls with anorexia nervosa compared to controls. Pilot studies of the use bisphosphonates in adolescents and young adults have demonstrated some benefits, but the effect has been modest; because of concerns about potential side effects, their use is not recommended. Current recommendations include weight restoration with resumption of spontaneous menses, optimal calcium (1,300 mg/day of elemental calcium) and vitamin D (600 IU units/day) intake, and treatment of vitamin D deficiency.

Hematological Complications

Suppression of the bone marrow causes low white blood cell, red blood cell, and platelet counts. A low white blood cell count has been reported in approximately one-third of patients with anorexia nervosa but does not appear to be associated with an increased risk of infection. Anemia may be caused by bone marrow suppression, but it may also be secondary to nutritional deficiencies of vitamin B_{12}, folate, or iron. Bruising of the lower extremities is not infrequently seen in anorexia nervosa and may be secondary to a combination of low platelet counts and increased capillary fragility. The erythrocyte sedimentation rate (ESR) is usually low in malnourished patients, and any elevation of the ESR should raise suspicion of another diagnosis. All hematological abnormalities improve with nutritional rehabilitation.

Neurological Complications

The major neurological complications of eating disorders in children and adolescents are syncope, seizures (secondary to electrolyte disturbances), and structural brain changes noted on neuroimaging studies. Muscle weakness and a peripheral neuropathy may also occur. Volume deficits of both gray and white matter have been identified in low-weight patients with anorexia nervosa, and neuropsychological testing has demonstrated impairment of attention, concentration, and memory, with deficits in visuospatial ability. These abnormalities improve substantially with weight restoration. Functional MRI studies have identified abnormalities in the ventral limbic system, in particular the insula, regions involved in appetite regulation and harm avoidance.

Key Issues and Future Directions

In children and adolescents with eating disorders, medical complications develop early in the course of the illness and can have long-lasting effects on linear growth, bone health, and brain development. Some of the complications, such as electrolyte abnormalities and cardiac problems, can be life threatening. Others improve or resolve with weight restoration and treatment of the eating disorder. However, some of the complications may not be entirely reversible, and their long-term consequences remain unknown.

Because of the importance of these complications, medical assessment and ongoing monitoring are important at each level of care (outpatient, partial hospitalization, and inpatient treatment). Priorities for future research include the identification of optimal rates of refeeding to safely promote weight restoration, without increasing risk for refeeding syndrome, and finding an effective treatment for low bone mass. In the past, most treatments for osteoporosis have focused on reducing bone resorption. For adolescents, the ideal agent would increase bone formation to potentiate peak bone mass acquisition. Teriparatide (recombinant human parathyroid hormone) is an anabolic agent that has recently been approved to treat osteoporosis in adults. Preliminary results in adults with anorexia nervosa are encouraging, but this medication has not been studied in adolescents. Furthermore it requires daily subcutaneous injection and has been associated with osteosarcomas in rats. Future research should focus on discovering a safe oral anabolic agent that is effective in promoting bone formation and increasing bone mass in adolescents with anorexia nervosa.

Suggested Reading

Golden, N. H., Katzman, D. K., Sawyer, S. M., Ornstein, R. M., Rome, E. S., Garber, A. K., et al. (2015). Update on the medical management of eating disorders in adolescents. *Journal of Adolescent Health, 56*, 370–375.—This article updates the practitioner on the role of the medical provider in diagnosis and treatment of eating disorders, newer methods of assessing the degree of malnutrition, and current approaches to refeeding.

Katzman, D. K. (2005). Medical complications in adolescents with anorexia nervosa: A review of the literature. *International Journal of Eating Disorders, 37*(Suppl.), S52–S59; discussion, S87–S89.—An excellent overview of the medical complications of eating disorders in adolescents.

Misra, M., Katzman, D., Miller, K. K., Mendes, N., Snelgrove, D., Russell, M., et al. (2011). Physiologic estrogen replacement increases bone density in adolescent girls with anorexia nervosa. *Journal of Bone and Mineral Research, 26*(10), 2430–2438.—In this placebo-controlled trial, adolescent girls randomized to receive transdermal estrogen with cyclic oral progesterone increased bone mass more than did healthy-weight controls, but bone mass did not normalize.

Misra, M., Prabhakaran, R., Miller, K. K., Goldstein, M. A., Mickley, D., Clauss, L., et al. (2008). Weight gain and restoration of menses as predictors of bone mineral density change in adolescent girls with anorexia nervosa-1. *Journal of Clinical Endocrinology and Metabolism, 93*(4), 1231–1237.—This prospective observational study demonstrates that weight gain with spontaneous resumption of menses is associated with significant improvement in bone mass in adolescents with anorexia nervosa, but girls who gain weight but do not resume menses continue to have low bone mass.

Nagata, J. M., Park, K. T., Colditz, K., & Golden, N. H. (2015). Associations of elevated liver enzymes among hospitalized adolescents with anorexia nervosa. *Journal of Pediatrics, 166*(2), 439–443.—In this retrospective observational study of 356 adolescents hospitalized with anorexia nervosa, elevated liver function tests were found on admission in 37%, and an additional 5.1% developed elevated liver function tests during refeeding, suggesting that, in most cases, elevated liver function tests are secondary to malnutrition and not refeeding.

O'Connor, G., & Nicholls, D. (2013). Refeeding hypophosphatemia in adolescents with anorexia nervosa: A systematic review. *Nutrition in Clinical Practice, 28*(3), 358–364.—This systematic review found that the average incidence rate of refeeding hypophosphatemia in hospitalized adolescents with anorexia nervosa was 14%, suggesting that severity of malnutrition is a marker for development of refeeding hypophosphatemia more than total energy intake.

Rosen, D. S. (2010). Identification and management of eating disorders in children and adolescents. *Pediatrics, 126*(6), 1240–1253.—Guidelines for the pediatrician regarding evaluation and management of children and adolescents with eating disorders.

Society for Adolescent Health and Medicine. (2014). Refeeding hypophosphatemia in hospitalized adolescents with anorexia nervosa: A position statement of the Society for Adolescent Health and Medicine. *Journal of Adolescent Health, 55*(3), 455–457.—This position statement of the Society for Adolescent Health and Medicine reviews the evidence showing that refeeding hypophosphatemia is correlated with the degree of malnutrition and stresses the importance of heightened awareness of refeeding hypophosphatemia when initiating nutritional rehabilitation in severely malnourished patients with anorexia nervosa.

Vestergaard, P., Emborg, C., Støving, R. K., Hagen, C., Mosekilde, L., & Brixen, K. (2002). Fractures in patients with anorexia nervosa, bulimia nervosa, and other eating disorders—a nationwide register study. *International Journal of Eating Disorders, 32*(3), 301–308.—In this population-based cohort from Denmark, a past history of anorexia nervosa was associated with a twofold increased risk of fracture; fracture rate was also increased in those with a past history of bulimia nervosa.

Connections between Eating Disorders and Obesity

MARSHA D. MARCUS

Accumulating evidence documents a strong association between obesity and eating disorders, including bulimia nervosa (BN) and binge eating disorder (BED), and to a lesser extent, anorexia nervosa (AN), although there is not a definitive understanding the nature of the relationship. This chapter reviews data documenting the links between obesity and eating disorders, briefly considers several lines of research that have begun to elucidate the complex interactions among varying levels of explanatory factors, and examines implications for treatment.

Epidemiology of Obesity and Eating Disorders

Obesity refers to excess adiposity, widely defined using body mass index (BMI), a ratio of weight to height, because of its strong association with obesity-related medical complications. A BMI of 30 kg/m^2 or greater defines the threshold for obesity. According to the World Health Organization, global rates of obesity have doubled since 1980, and there now are more than 600 million individuals with obesity. Obesity is associated with multiple complications, including but not limited to diabetes mellitus, cardiovascular disease, pulmonary problems, musculoskeletal problems, and certain cancers. Given the resulting health burden and medical costs, there is widespread consensus on the imperative to prevent and treat obesity.

Eating disorders are characterized by regular and persistent disturbances in eating or eating-related behaviors, with associated distress and dysfunction. AN is characterized by severe dietary restriction and unusually low weight, while BN and BED are characterized by persistent binge eating (the episodic intake of large amounts of food with an associated sense of loss of control), with or without regular compensatory behaviors designed to undo the effects of binge eating. Evidence from epidemiological studies has documented that eating disorders are uncommon relative to obesity, with lifetime prevalence rates of 0.6, 1.0, and 2.8% for AN, BN, and BED, respectively, as reported in the U.S. National Comorbidity Survey Replication (NCS-R) study. Nevertheless, prevalence rates have increased in more recent cohorts, and eating disorders are strongly associated with other psychiatric disorders and impairment.

Epidemiological studies have documented strong correlations between disorders characterized by binge eating, that is BN and BED, and obesity. For example, data from the NCS-R showed that 31.3% of individuals with BN and 42.4% of those with BED were obese. In contrast, AN was associated with a lower prevalence of obesity and a higher prevalence of low BMI. A multinational study reporting data from the World Health Organization World Mental Health Surveys also reported elevated rates of obesity among individuals with lifetime BN or BED (38.1 and 41.7%, respectively). Given increases in the prevalence of obesity (e.g., 68.3% of U.S. adults are overweight or obese), it is unclear whether the high rates of obesity among individuals with BN and BED reflect shifts in population BMI, shared or overlapping causal factors, or both.

The etiologies of both obesity and eating disorders are complex and involve an intricate and variable interplay of diverse factors, ranging from genes to the environment; thus, pathways are multifactorial in the development of both problems. Nevertheless, there is substantial evidence that changes in eating behavior, particularly increased consumption of widely available, highly palatable food, are a salient factor in the increases in obesity. Aberrant overeating of palatable food also is characteristic of binge eating, so the idea of shared risk for obesity and eating disorders has considerable face validity.

What Explains the Relation between Disordered Eating and Obesity?

We know that not all individuals with obesity have disordered eating, and that not all people with eating disorders are obese. Nevertheless, eating disorder risk factor studies have implicated obesity in the pathogenesis of eating disorders; conversely, binge eating may be a risk factor for weight gain and obesity. Well-conducted retrospective case–control studies designed to identify risk factors for AN, BN, and BED have found that parental obesity, childhood obesity, and cultural, family, and individual factors that increase the likelihood of dieting and obesity are risk factors for BN and BED. Other data have suggested that loss-of-control eating (the sense that one cannot control how much one is eating), which is one of the required components of binge eating, as well as persistent binge eating, predict excess weight gain in community samples. Thus, available data are consistent with the notion that obesity and eating disorders have a bidirectional relationship, but the mechanisms responsible for the relationship have not been characterized completely.

For example, the link between eating disorders and obesity may be explained in part by an overlapping risk for psychiatric disorder, particularly depression. Obesity is associated with depression, which has been linked prospectively with the onset of obesity. Conversely, BN and BED are highly comorbid with depression. Thus, it may be that a diathesis for depression predisposes a subset of individuals to develop eating problems and obesity. Similarly, numerous studies have linked symptoms of attention-deficit/hyperactivity disorder (ADHD) with binge eating and obesity; thus, patterns of impulsivity associated with ADHD also may partially explain the overlap between eating and weight problems.

One complication in understanding the relation between obesity and eating disorders and how vulnerability or exposure to other potential risk factors, such as psychiatric disturbance, may contribute to the observed connection between them is that these phenomena are variable. That is, obesity, eating disorders, and psychiatric status can change during the course of development and adult life, and thus establishing the temporal relationship among these phenomena and causal risk is not feasible. Moreover, as noted, there is a consensus that biological, environmental, and sociocultural factors are involved in the pathogenesis of obesity and disordered eating. Research integrating multiple factors in prospective investigations will be necessary to understand patterns of risk.

Current understanding of the etiology of complex conditions has led to additional research strategies that may clarify the ways in which the causes of obesity and disordered eating may interact. For example, recent studies of psychopathology reflect decreased reliance on the traditional syndrome-based psychiatric nomenclature and increased emphasis on the study of neurobiologically relevant domains of functioning across multiple units of analysis, as exemplified by the Research Domain Criteria (RDoC) initiative. There also is emphasis on understanding how the varying dimensions and units of analysis develop over time to elucidate causal pathways leading to symptoms seen across disorders. The RDoC initiative has been criticized for emphasizing biological factors at the expense of social and cultural factors involved in the expression of psychiatric disorders, but it provides an example of how research can incorporate the inherent complexity of these disorders to elucidate small, but specific, aspects of causal pathways that contribute to overall understanding. A review of the rapidly growing literature relevant to the relationship between obesity and eating disorders is beyond the scope of this chapter, but examples of neurobiologically informed research at different levels of analysis are provided to illustrate the breadth and depth of ongoing work.

For example, genetic research has shown that both obesity and eating disorders aggregate in families. Twin studies have shown that there is substantial heritability for obesity, moderate heritability for binge eating, and a small genetic overlap between obesity and binge eating. Genomewide association studies have identified many genetic loci affecting obesity, with the multiple loci each yielding small effects on BMI. One of the first identified loci with a robust relation with obesity was a variant of the fat mass and obesity-related (*FTO*) gene. Interestingly, recent work has shown that this single-nucleotide polymorphism (SNP) in the *FTO* gene also is relevant for AN (unexpectedly) and BN. Another gene that has been linked repeatedly with obesity is the melanocortin 4 receptor (*MC4R*) gene, and emerging data suggest that its effects on obesity may be mediated by its relation with emotional eating and food cravings, which, of course, also are seen in disordered eating. These findings regarding two of the many genetic loci implicated in obesity and disordered eating merely exemplify a rapidly expanding literature and illustrate how genetic research will promote elucidation of causal pathways.

The overlap between obesity and eating disorders also may reflect shared risk factors at the molecular level given that serotonin, dopamine, and other neurotransmitters all have been implicated in the regulation of feeding behavior and appetite. Leptin, a hormone released by white adipose tissue, provides the brain with information on peripheral fat stores and is critically involved in the regulation of food intake, body weight, and energy metabolism. Leptin is associated with obesity, but it also plays an important role in neurocognitive processes and is thought to play a role in mood and anxiety disorders. For example, leptin levels are inversely related with depression symptoms in women, independent of BMI. Other work has confirmed derangement in leptin levels among individuals with AN and BN that cannot be explained by variations in body weight. Research focusing on molecular overlaps in energy and mood regulation, and their interactions with other facets of risk will contribute to explication of shared and distinct pathways.

There has been a spate of research focusing on the circuitry implicated in feeding and eating behavior, with particular emphasis on homeostatic and reward systems. For example, dysfunction (hypo- or hyperactivity) of the hypothalamic–pituitary–adrenal axis, which is crucial for homeostasis, plays a role in the regulation of feeding behavior and is thought to be involved the development of obesity, psychiatric, and inflammatory disorders in vulnerable individuals. Similarly, there has been substantial work focusing on reward neurocircuitry in the development of obesity. Research has demonstrated differences in neural activation between obese and lean individuals in response to palatable food cues, and the observation that there are parallels between overeating palatable foods and responses to addictive substances has led to the hypothesis that particular forms of overeating are types of food addiction. The integration of findings across neurocircuits and including different units of analysis will play an important role in understanding eating disorder and obesity phenotypes.

Finally, there is interest in how environmental factors interact with other units of analysis to promote the expression of obesity and eating disorders. There is substantial interest in gene–environment interactions that may promote the expression of obesity and disordered eating. For example, maternal stress and nutrition during pregnancy may impact fetal development and adversely affect child health outcomes. At a different level of analysis, changes in the global food system that drive the production of dense, highly palatable food appear to interact with individual-level vulnerability to overeating and the development of excess adiposity. Similarly, the actions of genes associated with disordered eating probably exert their effects in the context of environmental exposures that promote the idealization of thinness and body dissatisfaction.

In summary, connections between obesity and eating disorders are not completely understood, and they are stunningly complex. Ultimately, the elucidation of the manifold pathways that underlie vulnerability to these problems will lead to understanding various obesity and eating disorder phenotypes and identifying new treatment targets. In the meantime, given the high rates of obesity among individuals with eating disorders, there already are clear implications for clinicians.

Implications for Treatment

Clinicians treating patients with BN and BED increasingly will be dealing with patients with overweight and obesity, and it is crucial to understand and consider the relevance of obesity to treatment. Clinicians treating patients with eating disorders need to be familiar with obesity-related medical morbidity (e.g., cardiovascular and metabolic risk) and be prepared to make appropriate referrals for assessment and treatment. Obesity also has important implications for treatment of eating disorders per se. Clinicians are encouraged to reflect on their own attitudes related to obesity and to understand the importance of weight-related stigma. Exposure to stigma and body shaming has strong negative effects; indeed, patients with eating disorders with obesity report high levels of body shame and dissatisfaction, which in turn contribute to a strong desire to lose weight. Available data suggest that although weight loss programs may not be contraindicated for individuals with BED, it may be desirable to address binge eating problems before consideration of pursuing weight loss. If patients with obesity and disordered eating want to pursue weight loss, there is evidence that participation in comprehensive behavioral lifestyle programs is not associated with exacerbation of eating disorder or other psychiatric symptoms, despite persisting beliefs that dietary restriction of any kind is contraindicated for all individuals with disordered eating.

Conclusion

Individuals with eating disorders, like other people, have high rates of obesity. The nascent understanding of the development of complex phenomena such as obesity and disordered eating is evolving rapidly, and identification of shared and overlapping risk factors may lead to more focused and powerful treatment and prevention programs. In the meantime, it is critically important for professionals to be aware of the clinical implications of co-occurring eating disorders and obesity.

Suggested Reading

Campbell, I. C., Mill, J., Uher, R., & Schmidt, U. (2011). Eating disorders, gene–environment interactions and epigenetics. *Neuroscience and Biobehavioral Reviews, 35*(3), 784–793.— This article examined how gene–environment interactions may be involved in the development and maintenance of eating disorders and obesity; for example, environmental factors leading to epigenetic changes in the stress system or those that affect peripheral cells, such as adipocytes, may be related to obesity and disordered eating.

Fairburn, C. G., Doll, H. A., Welch, S. L., Hay, P. J., Davies, B. A., & O'Connor, M. E. (1998). Risk factors for binge eating disorder: A community-based, case–control study. *Archives of General Psychiatry, 55*(5), 425–432.—In this carefully conducted, community-based retrospective case–control study the investigators found that BED is associated with exposure to risk factors for obesity and psychiatric disorder.

Farr, O. M., Tsoukas, M. A., & Mantzoros, C. S. (2015). Leptin and the brain: Influences on brain development, cognitive functioning and psychiatric disorders. *Metabolism, 64*(1), 114–130.—This article considers leptin, which has a well-documented role in the regulation of energy intake and expenditure, in influencing brain processes and the development psychiatric disorders, as well as obesity.

Hudson, J. I., Hiripi, E., Pope, H. G., & Kessler, R. C. (2007). The prevalence and correlates of eating disorders in the National Comorbidity Survey Replication. *Biological Psychiatry, 61*(3), 348–358.—This study presents data on the prevalence of eating disorders using a nationally representative sample of 9,282 and documents a strong association between BN and BED, and obesity.

Hudson, J. I., Lalonde, J. K., Berry, J. M., Pindyck, L. J., Bulik, C. M., Crow, S. J., et al. (2006). Binge eating disorder as a distinct familial phenotype in obese individuals. *Archives of General Psychiatry, 63*(3), 313–319.—In this study, the authors evaluated the familial aggregation of BED independent of obesity, and found that BED aggregated strongly in families independent of obesity, but that relatives of probands with BED had a significantly higher prevalence of severe obesity.

Kessler, R. C., Berglund, P. A., Chiu, W. T., Deitz, A. C., Hudson, J. I., Shahly, V., et al. (2013). The prevalence and correlates of binge eating disorder in the World Health Organization World Mental Health Surveys. *Biological Psychiatry, 73*(9), 904–914.—This study of 24,124 adult respondents in 14 countries using the World Health Organization Composite International Diagnostic Interview documented the lifetime prevalence of eating disorders and associated comorbidities, including obesity.

Marcus, M. D., & Wildes, J. E. (2009). Obesity: Is it a mental disorder? *International Journal of Eating Disorders, 42*(8), 739–753.—This review evaluates the evidence for and against the proposition that obesity is a mental disorder and reviews data examining overlapping and distinct factors associated with obesity and eating disorders.

Muller, T. D., Greene, B. H., Bellodi, L., Cavallini, M. C., Cellini, E., Di Bella, D., et al. (2012). Fat mass and obesity-associated gene (FTO) in eating disorders: Evidence for association of the rs9939609 obesity risk allele with bulimia nervosa and anorexia nervosa. *Obesity Facts, 5*(3), 408–419.—This study examined the association of the obesity-promoting *FTO* allele in a large sample of eating disorder patients and controls, and suggested that this allele was salient for eating disorders as well as obesity.

Striegel-Moore, R. H., & Bulik, C. M. (2007). Risk factors for eating disorders. *American Psychologist, 62*(3), 181–198.—This article presents a comprehensive review of risk factors for eating disorders and considers how to move the field forward by incorporating more sophisticated conceptualizations of risk and causal pathways.

Trace, S. E., Baker, J. H., Peñas-Lledó, E., & Bulik, C. M. (2013). The genetics of eating disorders. *Annual Review of Clinical Psychology, 9,* 589–620.—This article reviews the literature on genetic factors that influence eating pathology, including those that are implicated in the development of obesity and psychiatric disorder, given that 40–60% of the liability for eating disorders is accounted for by additive genetic influences.

EPIDEMIOLOGY AND ETIOLOGY OF EATING DISORDERS

38

Epidemiology of Eating Disorders

HANS W. HOEK

This chapter provides an overview of the epidemiology of the eating disorders anorexia nervosa (AN), bulimia nervosa (BN), and binge eating disorder (BED). In the fifth edition of the *Diagnostic and Statistical Manual of Mental Disorders* (DSM-5) classification, not only AN, BN, and BED, but also pica, rumination disorder, and avoidant/restrictive food intake disorder (ARFID) are included in the combined DSM-5 category "Feeding and Eating Disorders." However, little is known about the epidemiology of the last three disorders. Probably the most common feeding disorder, ARFID, is a new disorder, redefining the rarely used DSM-IV diagnosis feeding disorder of infancy or early childhood. There are also few data on the epidemiology of pica and rumination disorder, although both disorders are more commonly reported among individuals with intellectual disability.

Researchers in epidemiology study the occurrence of disorders and try to determine the factors associated with vulnerability to their development. Incidence and prevalence are the two principal measures of the distribution of a disorder. The *incidence rate* is defined as the number of *new* cases in the population per year. Incidence rate differences between groups are better clues to the etiology than prevalence rates. The *point-prevalence* is defined as the number of actual cases in a population at a certain point in time. Another frequently used measure is the 1-year-period prevalence rate, which is calculated by adding the point prevalence and the annual incidence. One-year prevalence rates are useful measures for describing morbidity at different levels of health care. Another measure is the lifetime prevalence, which refers to the proportion of a population that at some point in life (up to the time of assessment) has experienced an eating disorder. Prevalence and incidence for eating disorders are commonly expressed as the rate per 100,000 population (male and female persons of all ages).

In epidemiological research on eating disorders, prevalence studies vastly outnumber incidence studies. Prevalence studies of eating disorders are often conducted in high-risk populations, such as schoolgirls or female college students. A two-stage screening strategy has been widely used. The first stage involves screening a large number of individuals for suspected cases by means of an easily administered questionnaire. The second stage involves (semistructured) interviews with the persons who are likely to have an eating disorder, based on their answers to the questionnaire. Also interviewed are a number of randomly selected persons who—on the basis of their questionnaires—do not appear to suffer from a disorder, to confirm that they are not cases. Two-stage surveys using strict diagnostic criteria reveal much lower prevalence rates than the early surveys conducted in the previous century that relied exclusively on questionnaires.

Anorexia Nervosa

AN—usually considered as the prototype of an eating disorder, but a relatively rare disorder in the general population—was included in DSM-I in 1952. Most epidemiological studies on eating disorders, however, have been conducted after the introduction of the DSM-III in 1980.

Incidence

Because the incidence of eating disorders is relatively low, few studies have examined their incidence in the general population. It is impossible to screen a sufficiently large population, for instance, 100,000 people, for several years. Therefore, incidence rates have often been based on detected cases in hospital records and case registers of inpatients and outpatients in mental health care facilities. Although different strategies have been used in these studies, the results suggest an increase in the incidence of AN between 1930 and 1970. Since the 1970s into the 21st century, the incidence of AN in mental health care facilities in the Netherlands has been stable at around 5 per 100,000 population per year (see Figure 38.1).

The incidence of AN has also been studied in primary care facilities. General practitioners in the United Kingdom and the Netherlands, using criteria based on DSM-III-R and DSM-IV, have studied the incidence of eating disorders in large representative samples. The figures obtained were 4–8 per 100,000 population per year.

Prevalence

The prevalence has mostly been studied in the high-risk group of young females. Table 38.1 presents estimates of the 1-year-period prevalence rates per 100,000 young females at three levels of health care. The first level ("Community") represents the number of young females with AN in the community, whether or not they are receiving treatment. The data are calculated with the findings of two-stage surveys of the point prevalence of eating disorders, combined with estimates of the yearly incidence based on primary care studies. The next level ("Primary care") comprises those patients whom primary care physicians consider to have an eating disorder. The third level ("Mental health care") represents patients with eating disorders who are receiving treatment from outpatient or inpatient mental health care services, based on case register studies and referral rates from Dutch studies of general practitioners' patients. On the basis of the data presented in Table 38.1, it seems that around 40% of community cases of AN are detected by general practitioners, and most of these detected patients are referred for mental health care.

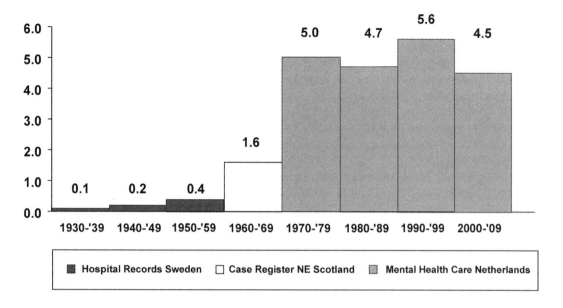

FIGURE 38.1. Registered incidence of AN per year (pooled data from different studies).

Bulimia Nervosa

BN first entered the DSM system in DSM-III in 1980.

Incidence

Screening medical records for BN or related symptoms, researchers in Minnesota found an incidence of 13.5 per 100,000 population per year during 1980–1990. General practitioners in the Netherlands, using DSM criteria, have studied the incidence of BN in a large representative sample of the Dutch population. They found the incidence of BN in primary care settings to be 11 per 100,000 population per year during the period 1985–1989, but significantly lower incidence rates were found in the period 1995–1999 and in the 21st century. Incidence rates found in health care systems can serve only as a minimum estimate of the true incidence rate in the community because of the secrecy that accompanies BN and its effect on treatment seeking and the greater difficulty detecting cases compared with AN cases.

TABLE 38.1. One-Year-Period Prevalence Rates per 100,000 Young Females

Level of health care	AN	Bulimia nervosa
Community	400	1,000
Primary care	160	120
Mental health care	130	60

Prevalence

An apparent "epidemic" of BN appeared in Western countries at the end of the last century. The first surveys using questionnaires suggested that up to 19% of female students reported bulimic symptoms. However, recent studies using strict criteria and more sophisticated methods showed much lower prevalence rates of around 1% among the high-risk group of young females.

The prevalence of BN is mostly studied in young females. Table 38.1 presents some estimates of the 1-year-period prevalence rates per 100,000 young females at three levels of health care. The first level represents the estimated rate of young females with BN in the community; the estimates are calculated in the same fashion as described previously for AN. Only a small proportion (12%) of the community cases of BN are detected in primary care, and, of these, only half are referred for specialist treatment. Movement from the community to the primary care level depends on the "illness behavior" of the patient and the ability of the general practitioner to detect the disorder. Several studies have shown that general practitioners have difficulty detecting eating disorders, particularly cases of BN.

Binge Eating Disorder

In DSM-IV, BED was classified under the residual category eating disorder not otherwise specified (EDNOS) and described with research criteria in an appendix providing criteria sets for further study. In DSM-5, BED has been recognized as a specified eating disorder. For a diagnosis of BED according to DSM-5 criteria, recurrent episodes of binge eating must occur, on average, at least once per week for 3 months; this threshold for the frequency criterion was lowered compared to the research criteria for BED in DSM-IV, which required recurrent episodes of binge eating to occur, on average, at least 2 days a week for 6 months. Because of the lack of an official classification of BED other than the broad residual category EDNOS in medical registration systems, there are no real incidence studies of BED yet.

The estimated 1-year prevalence rate of BED among U.S. adult women is 1.6%. Several population studies among adults found only very small increases in the prevalence rates of BED using DSM-5 criteria compared to the stricter DSM-IV research criteria for BED. A cross-national community survey including low-, middle-, and high-income countries found an average lifetime prevalence of 1.9% for BED. Lifetime prevalence estimates ranged from less than 1% in several European countries to 2.6% in the United States, and 4.7% in one urbanized area in Brazil (São Paulo).

Nontypical Groups

Throughout DSM-5, the influence of development, sex, and culture on the presentation of psychiatric disorders has been given more weight than in previous DSM editions, which may facilitate the classification of eating disorders not only among males and older females but also among people in non-Western countries. Most studies on the epidemiology of eating disorders have focused on young females in Western countries, the high-risk group for the development of eating disorders. However, eating disorders do occur in older women and in men, as well as in persons in non-Western countries.

In clinical samples, only 5–10% of patients with an eating disorder are males. However, epidemiological studies report smaller differences in rate ratios of lifetime prevalence in males vs. females: for AN, 1:3–1:12 and for BN, 1:3–1:18; in BED the gender ratio is far less skewed and the male:female rate ratio is estimated at 1:2–1:6. The lifetime prevalence among men for AN is estimated as 0.16–0.3%, for BN as 0.1–0.5% and for BED as 1–3%.

Recent epidemiological studies suggest that pathological eating behaviors and frank eating disorders, and associated body image disturbances are surprisingly common in older women. In a community study of middle-aged (40–60 years) Austrian women, no cases of AN were detected, but 4.6% of the women reported other eating disorders, as defined by DSM-IV criteria (BN, BED, and EDNOS) and another 4.8% reported subthreshold eating disorders. On many indices of disordered eating and body image, older women with eating pathology resemble younger women with similar conditions, although older women exhibit certain unique concerns, such as dealing with menopause and with aging.

Recent studies show increasing rates of eating disorders—especially for disorders other than AN—in non-Western countries such as Asia, Latin America, Africa, and the Arab region, and in Hispanic and African American minority groups in North America. A study in Curaçao showed that the overall incidence rate of AN was much lower than in the United States and Western Europe. The incidence of AN among the majority black population was nil, while the incidence among the minority mixed and white population of Curaçao was similar to that of the United States and the Netherlands.

Future Directions

To date, most of the epidemiological research on eating disorders has been descriptive in character. There is a need for more analytic epidemiological studies focused on the determinants of eating disorders. Such research is increasing, as shown, for example, by genetic–epidemiological studies and risk factor research.

Suggested Reading

Hoek, H. W. (2016). Review of the worldwide epidemiology of eating disorders. *Current Opinion in Psychiatry, 29*(6), 336–339.—A review of the epidemiology of eating disorders across different continents with a list of recent references.

Hoek, H. W, Van Harten, P. N., Hermans, K. M. E., Katzman, M. A., Matroos, G. E., Susser, E. S. (2005). The incidence of anorexia nervosa on Curaçao. *American Journal of Psychiatry, 162*(4), 748–752.—A study of the incidence of AN, comparing different ethnic groups.

Kessler, R. C., Berglund, P. A., Chiu, W. T., Deitz, A. C., Hudson, J. I., Shahly, V., et al. (2013). The prevalence and correlates of binge eating disorder in the World Health Organization World Mental Health Surveys. *Biological Psychiatry, 73*(9), 904–914.—Provides prevalence estimates for BED across several countries and is not restricted to only high-income countries.

Mangweth-Matzek, B., Hoek, H. W., Rupp, C. I., Lackner-Seifert, K., Frey, N., Whitworth, A. B., et al. (2014). Prevalence of eating disorders in middle-aged women. *International Journal of Eating Disorders, 47*(3), 320–324.—This community study assessed eating disorders and subthreshold eating disorders in middle-aged women.

Raevuori, A., Keski-Rahkonen, A., & Hoek, H. W. (2014). A review of eating disorders in males. *Current Opinion in Psychiatry, 27*(6), 426–430.—A recent review of the epidemiology of eating disorders in males.

Smink, F. R., van Hoeken, D., Donker, G. A., Susser, E. S., Oldehinkel, A. J., & Hoek, H. W. (2016). Three decades of eating disorders in Dutch primary care: Decreasing incidence of bulimia nervosa but not of anorexia nervosa. *Psychological Medicine, 46*(6), 1189–1196.—A recent study on the occurrence of eating disorders over three decades.

Smink, F. R., van Hoeken, D., & Hoek, H. W. (2013). Epidemiology, course, and outcome of eating disorders. *Current Opinion in Psychiatry, 26*(6), 543–548.—A review of the epidemiology of eating disorders, including studies applying DSM-5 criteria.

Global Mental Health and Priorities for Eating Disorders

KATHLEEN M. PIKE

Mental illness is the leading cause of disability in the world, and the momentum is growing for greater inclusion of mental health in the global health agenda. The field of eating disorders will benefit from understanding the global context of mental health and development, and developing effective classification systems, strategic partnerships, and integration with the larger global health community.

The modern study of eating disorders started with a narrow focus on a small segment of the world's geography (western Europe and North America) and within that region, only half the population (women), and among women, only a limited cross-section developmentally (adolescence and early adulthood). From this point of departure, we now understand that eating disorders are much more widespread in terms of geography, gender, and development than once thought, and our increased awareness of eating disorders globally parallels expanded recognition of all mental and behavioral disorders as common, serious, and global—and ruthlessly indiscriminate. Four pioneering initiatives over the course of the past 15 years provide essential context and direction in terms of the field of global mental health, and in turn, eating disorders.

The Millennium Development Goals

In 2000, the United Nations adopted the Millennium Development Goals (MDGs), which represented bold leadership by setting for the first time an explicit global agenda for development for all 194 member nations. The MDGs included eight specific targets—eradication of extreme poverty and hunger; universal primary education; gender equality and empowerment of women; reduced child mortality; improved maternal health; eradication of HIV/AIDS, malaria, and other diseases; sustainability; and enhanced global partnerships—to be achieved by 2015. The result was a coalescence of national and international economic, health, and societal development programs, multinational funding, and enormous human capital directed at these eight targets. By most evaluations, the MDGs have been lauded as the most successful global development campaign in modern history. All this is good news—except that the MDGs did not mention mental health anywhere. Not only was that unfortunate in terms of improving mental health, but the omission of mental health in the MDGs also hampered progress on many of the stated goals given the indissoluble connections that link these targets and mental health.

The 2010 Global Burden of Disease Study

The conspicuous omission of mental health was amplified by the Global Burden of Disease (GBD) publications documenting morbidity and mortality data for all health conditions worldwide. The 2010 GBD data indicate that approximately 20% of individuals around the world will experience a mental disorder over the course of their lifetime regardless of race, ethnicity, religion, geography, or economic status. Given advances in preventing and treating infectious and communicable diseases around the world, the relative burden of mental and behavioral disorders has grown to represent a greater public health burden across low-, middle-, and high-income countries alike. The result is that mental and behavioral disorders account for 7.4% of the global burden of disease and constitute the leading cause of disability worldwide. In the specific case of eating disorders, the burden of disease increased by 65% from 1990 to 2010, reflecting the greatest escalation of burden for any of the mental disorders.

The 2011 World Health Organization Mental Health Atlas

While the GBD data indicate that mental and behavioral disorders represent a significant disease burden globally, the 2011 Mental Health Atlas, based on information from 183 countries covering 99.3% of the world's population, lays bare how woefully underfunded and ill-prepared health systems are to address this burden. This is true everywhere, but as would be expected, the gaps are most pronounced in low- and middle-income countries (LMICs). Forty percent of countries are lacking dedicated mental health policy, and the median mental health expenditure per capita is $1.63, ranging from $0.20 in low-income countries to $44.84 in high-income countries. This represents less than 1% of total health care budgets in low-income countries and barely 5% in high-income countries. With fewer than two mental health professionals (psychologists, nurses, psychiatrists, community health workers combined) per 100,000 people in LMICs, more than 75% of people with severe mental disorders never receive treatment, and even in high-income countries, 35–50% of such individuals never receive care.

The Sustainable Development Goals

The GBD findings, the WHO Atlas data, and the success of the MDGs have synergistically converged to garner increased support for greater integration of mental health in the global health agenda. Global mental health advocacy efforts achieved a recent victory in this regard, such that mental health is included in the United Nations 2030 Agenda for Sustainable Development, adopted on September 25, 2015, by the United Nations General

Assembly. This agenda is the successor to the MDGs, and although the inclusion of mental health is limited in scope, it reflects a fundamental and dramatic step in the direction of greater recognition and integration of mental health as a global health priority.

What all this means for the field of eating disorders is yet to be determined. The eating disorders field stands at a critical juncture in terms of advancing knowledge, impacting policy, and disseminating evidence-based treatments; to be maximally effective, the field needs to expand its reach and engage with a wider community of researchers, health care providers, and institutional partners. The significant burden of disease associated with eating disorders in high-income, Western countries is well established, and as research on prevalence of eating disorders extends across the globe, virtually every study indicates that when we look, we find eating disturbances and eating disorders also increasing in LMICs. Although different countries and regions may report particular and nuanced expressions of eating disorders, this is more likely in addition to, not instead of, the eating disorders recognized by the WHO's *International Classification of Diseases* (ICD) and the American Psychiatric Association's *Diagnostic and Statistical Manual of Mental Disorders* (DSM).

Global Mental Health and Eating Disorders

In the global mental health literature, eating disorders are rarely mentioned. Even within the mental health professional community, the bias exists that eating disorders are problems of affluence that do not matter much in LMICs. It is true that eating disorders tend to increase with economic prosperity and related environmental and social changes, but so do heart disease, cancer, and obesity, and no one has relegated these health conditions to a back seat. The relatively scant attention paid to eating disorders exists in spite of the rising prevalence of eating disorders over the past 10 years, widespread documentation of eating and weight dysregulation across virtually all populations studied, and the fact that anorexia nervosa is associated with serious morbidity and the highest mortality rate of any psychiatric illness. Expanding global understanding, prevention and treatment of eating disorders will be advanced by three strategic priorities: (1) improved diagnostic clarity; (2) effective partnerships with related fields; and (3) consensus and collaboration on the research agenda.

Improving Diagnostic Clarity

The WHO is constitutionally mandated to administer the ICD, a classification system for all health conditions for its 194 member states. Given that the existing ICD-10 was adopted in 1990, the development of the ICD-11, which is currently under way, provides a historic opportunity to improve communication about eating disorders by expanding clinical descriptions to capture more fully the range of presentations of eating disturbances globally. This has been, and continues to be, a dynamic time in terms of research and treatment advances for eating disorders, and the ICD-11 has the opportunity to incorporate advances in the field of eating disorders that have occurred over the past 25+ years. Under the auspices of the WHO, the development of the ICD-11 intentionally includes researchers and mental health specialists from low-, middle- and high-income countries from all regions of the world to ensure the development of a culturally sensitive and representative system that will speak to and be relevant for individuals in practice around the globe. The effectiveness of the ICD-11 to advance identification of and mental health care for individuals with eating disorders depends on the field taking an active role in contributing to the development process, which is facilitated by joining the Global Clinical Practice Network for Mental Health (*https://gcp.network*), an online platform open to clinicians from around the world.

Forging Effective Partnerships with Related Fields and Disciplines

As is the case across all mental and behavioral disorders, there is a yawning abyss between the need for services and the service capacity for eating disorders, especially in light of the precipitous rise in prevalence of eating disorders globally. Given this reality, three approaches for forging partnerships may enhance our capacity to improve access to care in the field.

First, worldwide rates of overweight and obesity have nearly doubled since 1980, with current data estimating that around the globe approximately 1 billion individuals are obese, and another 850 million are overweight. The environmental factors of increased sedentary lifestyle coupled with the nutritional transformation associated with industrialization and economic prosperity increase risk for both weight dysregulation and body image dissatisfaction. The additional factors of changing gender roles for women in societies in transition, particularly when societal beauty ideals promote extreme thinness, only compound the risk of increasing rates of obesity and eating disorders. Thus, around the world, eating disorders are rising in tandem with what has been called the "global epidemic of obesity," and while eating disorders may still be largely hidden or stigmatized when they come into view, the public health consequences of obesity are widely recognized, and health ministries are mobilized to intervene. This creates an opportune partnership for advancing treatment of eating disorders globally. Rather than repeat the history of previous decades in which eating disorders and obesity research and treatment were addressed as two completely distinct fields and health conditions, to the extent that the eating disorders and obesity experts pursue partnerships across the spectrum of interventions from broad-based population health programs to targeted treatments, limited resources have the potential to be extended efficiently to improve overall health and nutrition, reduce risk for both obesity and eating disorders, and expand delivery of care.

A second strategy for expanding mental health care overall, and eating disorders specifically, is the pursuit of integration of mental health services with primary care. The vast majority of individuals with eating disorders will never see a specialist in the field. Integration of screening and treatment for eating disorders into primary care has the potential to reduce stigma and provide health services that are centralized and patient-centered, which in turn, should optimize both mental and physical health outcomes and strengthen the overall health system.

Integration of mental health services into primary care has gained substantial support on the part of the global mental health community; however, it is unclear whether already overburdened primary care providers are equally enthusiastic. Thus, a third strategy that the field of eating disorders has yet to exploit is greater engagement of individuals who have experienced mental health problems themselves, as well as training of nonprofessionals in basic eating disorders treatments. There are several creative and innovative strategies taking place within the field of global mental health for disseminating evidence-based treatments in low-resource communities. Strategies whereby individuals within a community are trained in the delivery of culturally relevant and sensitive adaptations of either cognitive-behavioral therapy (CBT) or interpersonal psychotherapy (IPT) for depression have demonstrated impressive efficacy, with the vast majority of individuals no longer meeting criteria for major depression at the end of either IPT or CBT treatment. These demonstration studies indicate that evidence-based treatments can be adapted for different cultural and regional contexts, and individuals within the cultural context with limited mental health training can learn to deliver and disseminate treatments effectively. Given that CBT and IPT both have demonstrated efficacy for eating disorders, engaging individuals with personal experience of eating disorders and/or general community members may be a viable strategy to extend our capacity as a field to reach those in need of care.

Consensus and Collaboration to Advance the Eating Disorders Research Agenda

With some exceptions, research in the field of eating disorders is dominated by studies conducted at single sites with a limited number of individuals, typically from Western and high-income countries. This model has multiple inherent limitations, and given the computing and networking potential available today, we have the opportunity, and perhaps the mandate, to move toward more large-scale, dynamic, and permeable collaborative research models. Small, independent studies may still contribute to generative and pilot research of new ideas or be most appropriate for the study of localized issues, but major advances in eating disorders globally will require more global engagement. The technologies available today make it possible to establish research platforms that amass large and sophisticated data sets. Such efforts can increase the potential for LMICs to contribute to the empirical knowledge base, which will increase the diversity, breadth, and depth of our knowledge of eating disorders globally.

Summary

Eating disorders are widespread and increasing around the globe. Understanding the rise of eating disorders in the context of global mental health illuminates some of the shared priorities, challenges, and opportunities for improving our eating disorders knowledge base, research efforts, and interventions.

Suggested Reading

Kakuma, R., Minas, H., van Ginneken, N., Dal Poz, M. R., Desiraju, K., Morris, J. E., et al. (2011). Human resources for mental health care: Current situation and strategies for action. *Lancet, 378,* 1654–1663.—The authors discuss the fact that the need for mental health services exceeds what mental health professionals provide, particularly in LMICs, and therefore recommend innovative strategies to close the gap.

Pike, K. M., Hoek, H. W., & Dunne, P. E. (2014). Cultural trends and eating disorders. *Current Opinion in Psychiatry, 27*(6), 436–442.—This article provides highlights of global trends in eating disorders.

Pike, K., Susser, E., Galea, S., & Pincus, H. (2013). Towards a healthier 2020: Advancing mental health as a global health priority. *Public Health Reviews, 35*(1), 1.—This article provides an overview of mental health in the global health agenda, the rationale for advancing mental health on a global scale, and key priorities.

Prince, M., Patel, V., Saxena, S., Maj, M., Maselko, J., Phillips, M. R., et al. (2007). No health without mental health. *Lancet, 370,* 859–877.—This article provides an overview of the indissoluble relationship between mental health and other priority health conditions and heralded a new era in global health that better integrates mental health.

Rahman, A., Malik, A., Sikander, S., Roberts, C., & Creed, F. (2008). Cognitive behaviour therapy-based intervention by community health workers for mothers with depression and their infants in rural Pakistan: A cluster-randomised controlled trial. *Lancet, 372,* 902–909.—This landmark study documented the success of task-sharing, such that nonprofessional community members who were trained in CBT were effective in reducing depression among perinatal women in rural Pakistan.

Reed, G. M., Rebello, T. J., Pike, K. M., Medina-Mora, M. E., Gureje, O., Zhao, M., et al. (2015). WHO's Global Clinical Practice Network for mental health. *Lancet Psychiatry, 2*(5), 379–380.—This commentary provides a brief overview of the platform that has been established for clinical research evaluating the ICD-11 recommendations and the transition of this platform to expand training and educational opportunities.

Saxena, S., Thornicroft, G., Knapp, M., & Whiteford, H. (2007). Resources for mental health: Scarcity, inequity, and inefficiency. *Lancet, 370,* 878–889.—This article highlights the limited resources allocated for mental health.

U.N. General Assembly. (September 25, 2015). Transforming our world: The 2030 agenda for sustainable development. Retrieved from *https://sustainabledevelopment.un.org/post2015/transformingourworld.*—This is the official declaration from the United Nations General Assembly articulating the primary targets that were adopted for the 2030 SDGs with elaborated context and rationale.

U.N. General Assembly, 55th Session. (September 18, 2000). Resolution (2000) United Nations Millennium Declaration. Retrieved from *www.unmillenniumproject.org/documents/ares552e.pdf.*—This landmark initiative is often lauded as the driving force that launched an era of the greatest economic, social, and health goals in modern history.

World Health Organization. (2011). Project Atlas: Resources for mental health and neurological disorders (2011). Retrieved from *www.who.int/mental_health/evidence/atlas/en.*— Based on data from 93% of the world population, the WHO 2011 Atlas Project has served as a global reference for the deficiencies in funding and capacity for mental health services around the globe, and particularly in LMICs.

The Genetics of Eating Disorders

CYNTHIA M. BULIK
GEROME BREEN

Family, twin, and molecular genetic studies have contributed to contemporary understanding of the role that genetic factors play in anorexia nervosa (AN), bulimia nervosa (BN), and binge eating disorder (BED), although progress in the field varies widely across disorders, with research on AN being most mature.

Familial Transmission

Eating disorders are familial. First-degree relatives of individuals with AN, BN, and BED are significantly more likely to report lifetime AN, BN, and BED than relatives of individuals without an eating disorder. Considerable coaggregation of eating disorders in families occurs (especially AN with BN), suggesting a broad spectrum of eating-related psychopathology represented in affected families. This pattern is consistent with what we know about the clinical course of eating disorders, namely, that considerable diagnostic flux across subtypes occurs throughout the course of illness.

Family studies of AN have been most extensive and reveal that AN is strongly familial. A comprehensive population register-based study in Denmark revealed that AN recurrence risk in relatives of patients with AN is significantly elevated. In terms of specific familial transmission patterns, mothers of those with AN were six times more likely to have AN than mothers of controls; siblings of those with AN, four times; and offspring of women with AN were five times more likely to have AN. All of these were significant elevations, underscoring the familiality of the disorder. BN also aggregates in families, and individuals who have a relative with AN or BN are at elevated risk for developing either disorder, indicating a potential genetic correlation between AN and BN. The familial transmission of BED has been less extensively studied; however, the disorder does appear to aggregate strongly in families, independent of obesity.

Although these studies have been an important starting point, family studies are unable to address fully the extent to which the observed aggregation is due to shared genetic factors or environmental influences. Moreover, not all cases of eating disorders are familial. Sporadic cases also occur that may be new presentations in a previously unaffected family, or simply the first detected case—which can be a function of generation, location, and availability of services.

Twin Studies

Twin studies provide an advantage over family studies by being able to parse out differential effects of genetic and environmental factors. In its most basic form, a twin study compares monozygotic (MZ, or identical) twins, who, for most intents and purposes, share 100% of their segregating genes, and dizygotic (DZ, or fraternal) twins, who share, on average, 50% of their genes. If, on average, both members of MZ twin pairs are more likely to be "concordant" (i.e., both have the disorder) than both members of DZ twin pairs, then the influence of inherited factors (highly probably genetic) that influence risk can be assumed. More sophisticated analyses of concordance patterns enable estimates of the contribution of genetic factors, shared environmental factors (factors that serve to make twins more similar), and unique environmental factors (factors that serve to make twins dissimilar) to the observed phenotypes. Importantly, heritability estimates are not specific; rather, they describe the maximum proportion of the variation between people that can be due to genetic variation for a specific population at a specific point in time.

Many twin studies have been conducted on eating disorders primarily in large European-ancestry populations. As such, a caution is warranted: These findings, although consistent, may not be universally applicable to more diverse populations. Reported heritability estimates range from 33 to 84% for AN, from 28 to 83% for BN, and from 41 to 57% for BED, with the remaining variance in liability typically attributable to unique environmental factors. In most twin models, shared environment did not contribute significantly to liability to these disorders.

Studies employing a more rigorous definition of AN (i.e., restricting analysis to individuals who meet all diagnostic criteria for the disorder) yielded higher heritability estimates than analyses that included more broadly defined cases. Twin studies have also shed light on possible mechanisms underlying the commonly observed diagnostic flux across AN and BN by identifying the genetic correlation between AN and BN to be .79, suggesting shared genetic factors across the disorders.

Molecular Genetics Studies

The field of medical molecular genetics has been transformed considerably over the last decade, moving beyond candidate gene and linkage approaches to more fruitful discovery-based genomewide association studies (GWAS) and similar approaches, such as whole-genome sequencing and exome sequencing. Because much of this earlier work failed to replicate findings of etiological significance, we focus our discussion in this section on contemporary approaches and directions for research in eating disorders.

Genomewide Association Studies

Modern GWAS include a broad scan of the entire genome in the absence of a priori hypotheses or guesses as to which genes might be implicated in a disorder or trait. A case–control approach, GWAS compares DNA from large samples of individuals with a trait or disorder to that of individuals without the trait, and scans the genome for differences. Rigorous standards for statistical significance are applied to account for multiple testing.

Two GWAS have been conducted for AN. Advances in the field confirm that the sample sizes for both studies were smaller than would be expected to yield significant results. The first GWAS included 1,033 AN cases and 3,733 controls and, as expected in retrospect, yielded no genomewide significant loci. The second, conducted by the Wellcome Trust Case–Control Consortium 3 and the Genetic Consortium for Anorexia Nervosa, included 2,907 AN cases with European ancestry in the discovery meta-analysis and 14,860 ancestry-matched female controls. The initial GWAS of the discovery meta-analysis yielded no genomewide significant findings; however, in a sign test comparing the results from the discovery meta-analysis and replication data sets, 76% of 72 independent markers with the lowest p-values yielded results in the same direction. This test strongly implies that analyzing larger sample sizes will yield genetic variants implicated in AN and has fueled our efforts to boost sample size worldwide.

GWAS are also able to reveal genetic variants that may influence the expression of several phenotypes and reveal mechanisms of comorbidity. We tested how well a type of genetic risk score (GRS) called a *polygenic risk score (PRS)*, derived from genomewide data of other psychiatric disorders, can predict AN status. A PRS is a single measure that quantifies the number of risk alleles an individual has for a particular disorder, adjusting for the effect size at each location in the genome. We found evidence of overlap in genetic risk between AN and autism spectrum disorder, major depressive disorder, schizophrenia, and bipolar disorder.

A newer approach, *linkage disequilibrium (LD) score regression*, allows calculation of genetic correlations across GWAS using only summary statistics (i.e., not individual-level data). This has allowed the creation of an atlas of the genetic correlations among 20 metabolic, somatic, and psychiatric phenotypes, which has shown, even in the absence of genomewide significant hits, that important information is emerging from the available AN GWAS data. In this atlas, AN was significantly negatively correlated with obesity and significantly positively correlated with schizophrenia and obsessive–compulsive disorder (OCD). Hints at negative correlations were also observed between AN and other metabolic traits such as triglycerides, fasting glucose, and type 2 diabetes. These observations encourage further inquiry into metabolic aspects of AN and suggest that genetic factors influencing normal variation in body mass may also influence the extreme dysregulation of body mass seen in AN. The positive correlation with OCD comes as no surprise given the frequency with which the two disorders co-occur, but it does suggest that this co-occurrence has genetic underpinnings. The positive correlation with schizophrenia also points toward new areas of inquiry. Typically, the distorted thinking and profound lack of insight associated with AN are not labeled as manifestations of a psychotic process, and schizophrenia is not ranked among commonly reported comorbid conditions. This correlation encourages a deeper inquiry into factors that may unite AN and schizophrenia etiologically.

Rare Variants

New and more affordable methods for detecting rare variants (minor allele frequency of less than 1%) are continually emerging. An investigation that combined linkage analysis, exome sequencing, and whole-genome sequencing in two densely affected eating disorder pedigrees revealed a missense mutation in estrogen-related receptor alpha (*ESRRA*) in the first pedigree, and a potentially deleterious mutation in histone deacetylase 4 (*HDAC4*) in the second. Further study of *ESRRA* in the mouse shows that it is expressed in the brain, regulated by energy reserves, and loss of expression of *ESRRA* is associated with behavioral phenotypes that are relevant to AN, such as operant response to high-fat diet, compulsivity, and social dominance deficits. Although intriguing, especially given the involvement of the estrogen system, these studies require replication and deeper inquiry.

Conclusions

Sample size augmentation for AN is under way globally. BN and BED initiatives lag woefully behind. The trajectory of results and the intriguing cross-disorder findings suggest that we will observe similar successes in AN to what have been observed in other psychiatric disorders, such as schizophrenia, in which GWAS has yielded over 108 loci associated with the disease. With increases in sample size, other approaches also become more powerful, such as the ability to identify biological pathways that harbor an increased number of risk variants, thereby unlocking new potential drug targets. Advances in genomic science will facilitate the identification of genes and pathways that reveal the neurobiology of eating disorder and inform the development and testing of new and novel treatments that target the core biology of the illness.

Acknowledgments

Cynthia M. Bulik is a consultant and grant recipient for Shire Pharmaceuticals. This work was supported in part by the Anorexia Nervosa Genetics Initiative, an initiative of the Klarman Family Foundation and in part by the Swedish Research Council. Gerome Breen is a consultant and grant recipient for Eli Lilly Ltd. For Dr. Breen, this review represents independent research, funded in part by the National Institute for Health Research (NIHR) Biomedical Research Centre at South London and Maudsley NHS Foundation Trust and King's College London. The views expressed are those of the authors and not necessarily those of the U.K. National Health Service, the NIHR, or the Department of Health.

Suggested Reading

Boraska, V., Franklin, C. S., Floyd, J. A., Thornton, L. M., Huckins, L. M., Southam, L., et al. (2014). A genome-wide association study of anorexia nervosa. *Molecular Psychiatry, 19*(10), 1085–1094.—Largest GWAS for AN reported to date by the Wellcome Trust Case–Control Consortium 3.

Bulik, C. M., Thornton, L. M., Root, T., Pisetsky, E., Lichtenstein, P., Pedersen, N. L. (2010) Understanding the relation between anorexia nervosa and bulimia nervosa in a Swedish national twin sample. *Biological Psychiatry, 67*, 71–77.—Using a Swedish twin sample, authors report genetic corelation between AN and BN to be .79.

Bulik-Sullivan, B., Finucane, H. K., Anttila, V., Gusev, A., Day, F. R., Perry, J. R., et al. (2015). An atlas of genetic correlations across human diseases and traits. *Nature Genetics, 47*(11), 1236–1241.—Presents results of genetic correlations across metabolic, psychiatric, and somatic traits calculated with LD score regression.

Bulik-Sullivan, B. K., Loh, P. R., Finucane, H. K., Ripke, S., Yang, J., Patterson, N., et al. (2015). LD score regression distinguishes confounding from polygenicity in genome-wide association studies. *Nature Genetics, 47*(3), 291–295.—Description of methodology underlying LD score regression approach.

Cui, H., Lu, Y., Khan, M. Z., Anderson, R. M., McDaniel, L., Wilson, H. E., et al. (2015). Behavioral disturbances in estrogen-related receptor alpha-null mice. *Cell Reports, 11*(3), 344–350.—Exploration of the effect of *ESRRA* expression in the mouse brain.

Cui, H., Moore, J., Ashimi, S. S., Mason, B. L., Drawbridge, J. N., Han, S., et al. (2013). Eating disorder predisposition is associated with *ESRRA* and *HDAC4* mutations. *Journal of Clinical Investigation, 123*(11), 4706–4713.—Using DNA from two large families affected by eating disorders, mutations segregating with illness were identified by whole-genome sequencing following linkage mapping or by whole-exome sequencing.

Schizophrenia Working Group of the Psychiatric Genomics Consortium. (2014). Biological insights from 108 schizophrenia-associated genetic loci. *Nature, 511*, 421–427.—Report of significant GWAS findings from schizophrenia, with sample size of 34,000 cases.

Wang, K., Zhang, H., Bloss, C. S., Duvvuri, V., Kaye, W., Schork, N. J., et al. (2011). A genome-wide association study on common SNPs and rare CNVs in anorexia nervosa. *Molecular Psychiatry, 16*(9), 949–959.—First GWAS for AN.

Yilmaz, Z., Hardaway, A., & Bulik, C. (2015). Genetics and epigenetics of eating disorders. *Advances in Genomics and Genetics, 5*, 131–150.—Comprehensive and detailed review of the genetics of eating disorders.

Risk Factors for Eating Disorders

KARINA L. ALLEN
ULRIKE SCHMIDT

The causation of eating disorders is widely thought to be "multifactorial," a term so broad that it is rendered useless without further qualification. Myriad individual risk factors have been studied. As in other areas of research, there are definite fashions here. During the 1960s and 1970s, an "anorexogenic family environment" was thought to be crucial for the development of anorexia nervosa, and during the 1980s and 1990s, childhood trauma, in particular, childhood sexual abuse, was promoted as causally important, mainly for bulimia nervosa. There has been a recent revival of interest in biological factors, prompted by the availability of new technologies, such as molecular biology and neuroimaging, as well as genetic and epigenetic studies. Several important classes of risk factors are discussed in detail elsewhere in this book (e.g., genetic factors in Chapter 40; other biological factors in Chapters 43 and 44; sociocultural factors in Chapter 21). The foci of this chapter are threefold: some of the methodological issues affecting this kind of research; research that attempts to integrate knowledge about the relative contribution of different risk factors to different eating disorders; and some of the newer lines of investigation in this area.

Methodological Issues

A *risk factor* is defined as a factor that is associated with a disorder, and that precedes the development of that disorder. There must also be some evidence to suggest a causal relationship. Causality may be demonstrated by (1) the risk factor being consistently associated with the disorder across multiple studies; (2) the risk factor being associated with one disorder only; and (3) an experimental intervention that eliminates the risk factor being found also to eliminate the disorder. Only when (3) is demonstrated may a risk factor be called a *causal risk factor*. Risk factors that predict disorder onset but are not modifiable, such as sex, are typically referred to as *fixed markers*. Fixed markers can help to identify groups most at risk of a disorder developing, whereas causal risk factors can be targeted directly in prevention programs.

It is relatively easy to identify an association between a purported risk factor and one or more of the eating disorders. However, many studies struggle to satisfy the requirement of precedence (i.e., that the risk factor clearly precedes eating disorder onset). This difficulty applies to cross-sectional studies, as well as to retrospective studies that do not clearly define and date the timing of the risk factor relative to the onset of the eating disorder. Even when onset of a clinical eating disorder is determined, it can be harder to establish accurately the onset and duration of earlier subthreshold symptoms.

Traditionally, two main types of study have been used to investigate risk factors: the case–control study (retrospective) and the cohort study (prospective). The main advantage of case–control studies is that they are valuable when the condition of interest is relatively rare, as with anorexia nervosa. The disadvantages relate to the many potential biases in the comparison of cases and controls. Recall bias and inaccurate retrospective data are common problems. The use of semistructured interviews that help patients to remember information in relation to autobiographic anchor points, and that use multiple probes to allow detailed description and encourage behavioral examples, can reduce these challenges. However, important considerations also include how cases and controls are selected and whether the two groups are matched on variables that might confuse the comparison.

Seminal case–control studies include the population-based case–control study of adolescent anorexia nervosa by Rastam and Gillberg (1992) and the Oxford risk factor studies by Fairburn and colleagues (1997, 1998, 1999). The Oxford Risk Factor Interview has informed a number of more recent studies, including a 2014 study by Hilbert and colleagues that used a case–control design to consider risk factors for anorexia nervosa, bulimia nervosa, and binge eating disorder.

Prospective cohort studies allow careful control of the nature and quality of the data recorded, as well as accurate information on the relative timing of risk factors and eating disorder onset. Given the relative rarity of eating disorders, these studies can require extremely large numbers and may need to be very long-term in order to detect associations of interest. One of the key disadvantages is that large samples may then result in assessment via self-report measures instead of semistructured interviews. This gives uncertain reliability in the measurement of both risk factors and eating disorders. Another major problem can be loss to follow-up, especially if participants are lost for reasons that are related to the outcomes being studied. Individuals with anorexia nervosa do actively avoid detection and have been found to be overrepresented among nonparticipants in population-based studies.

In recent years, cohort studies have become increasingly sophisticated, and these methodological concerns are often addressed. Examples with a specific focus on adolescence include the American cohort studies by Field and colleagues (2008; adolescent males and females followed over 7 years as part of the Growing Up Today Study) and Stice, Marti, and Durant (2011; adolescent females followed over 8 years). Both made use of frequent assessment points, as well as structured eating disorder measures, although assessment was via self-report in the Field and colleagues research. There are also a growing number of cohort studies beginning at or before birth, some of which incorporate a nested case–control design. In the Avon Longitudinal Study of Parents and Children (ALSPAC), Micali, Stahl, Treasure, and Simonoff (2014) studied the effects of a maternal eating disorder in pregnancy on later child development and eating behavior. In the

Western Australian Pregnancy Cohort (Raine) Study, Allen, Byrne, Oddy, Schmidt, and Crosby (2014) considered prenatal, early life, and childhood risk factors for eating disorders in adolescents and young adults. Both of these cohort studies make use of regular assessment points but do depend on self-report data.

Large, intergenerational studies allow for consideration of risk factors over even longer periods of time. Centralized, total-population medical research registers in Scandinavia have allowed for investigation of links between pregnancy and birth variables and family characteristics (including sociodemographic status and psychiatric history) and later onset of an eating disorder. These studies benefit from extremely large samples and populationwide data, although, given that they rely on medical records, they miss undiagnosed eating disorders.

The strength of current cohort research is that there are enough studies being conducted to allow for comparison of results across cohorts and research designs. This helps to offset the methodological limitations associated with individual studies and lends support to those findings that do emerge across multiple projects.

Risk Factors for Different Types of Eating Disorders

Female sex, internalization of the "thin ideal," body dissatisfaction, dieting, low self-esteem, negative affect, social problems, and behavioral problems have been found to predict eating disorders in multiple case–control and cohort studies. However, not all of these predictors may be considered specific risk factors for eating disorders because many also predict onset of general psychiatric disorders. In addition, many studies have considered eating disorders as a single outcome group, without attention to diagnostic differences. There is evidence to support overlap between risk factors for bulimia nervosa, binge eating disorder, and other binge–purge-type eating disorders (e.g., "purging disorder"), but anorexia nervosa may have different etiological pathways.

Research specific to each eating disorder type is outlined below. It is worth noting, however, that there is also an increasing focus on eating disorder phenotypes and dimensional, biologically based approaches to symptom classification. The National Institute of Mental Health's Research Domain Criteria (RDoC) is an example of this approach and may inform more studies on phenotypes and symptom clusters, as well as traditional diagnostic categories.

Anorexia Nervosa

There is a sizable genetic contribution to anorexia nervosa (AN), although it is not yet known precisely what is inherited or how genetic and environmental factors interact. Possibilities for what is inherited include a predisposition to leanness and/or the personality traits of perfectionism, obsessionality, negative self-evaluation, and extreme compliance.

Obsessive–compulsive symptoms and perfectionism appear to be specific environmental risk factors for AN. Unlike binge–purge-type eating disorders, dieting and body dissatisfaction may not be so important once other variables have been taken into account.

Perinatal factors have also been linked to AN and may be a specific risk factor for this disorder. There have been suggestions that perinatal complications may result in subtle brain damage, which may directly contribute to AN or do so via early feeding difficulties, poor infant attachment, or an altered stress response (hypothalamic–pituitary–adrenal axis functioning). There are also data to support a possible interaction between perinatal complications and childhood abuse in the prediction of AN.

Bulimia Nervosa

There is a sizable genetic contribution also to bulimia nervosa (BN), although it is not known precisely what is inherited or how genetic and environmental factors interact. Possibilities for what is inherited include a predisposition to obesity and/or the personality traits of impulsivity, emotional instability, and negative affect.

There are also clear environmental risk factors for BN. Evidence from case–control and cohort studies converges to suggest that risk increases as a result of exposure to (1) dieting and factors that increase the likelihood of dieting (including premorbid and parental obesity, critical comments from others about weight/shape, and body dissatisfaction), and (2) general risk factors for psychiatric disorders (especially alcohol/substance misuse, adverse childhood events, and family conflict). Both classes of risk factors contribute independently to risk.

Binge Eating Disorder

The genetic contribution to binge eating disorder (BED) is less well established than that AN and BN, but there is still clear support for a genetic component to the disorder. A predisposition to obesity appears to be relevant, but more research is needed to elucidate other possible mechanisms for the genetic contributions to BED.

As with BN, two classes of environmental risk factors have been identified: dieting and factors that increase the likelihood of dieting, and general risk factors for psychiatric disorders. There is evidence to suggest that degree of exposure to these risk factors is less in BED than in BN, but that the same pathways to risk may apply.

Interactions between Risk Factors

Several prospective cohort studies have considered how environmental risk factors may interact to predict eating disorder onset. This allows for a better understanding of risk moderators, mediators, and mechanisms. To date, body dissatisfaction has been found to interact with both depressive symptoms and negative comments from others about weight in the prediction of binge–purge-type eating disorders in females. Risk is greatest when high body dissatisfaction is combined with one of these additional exposures. In contrast, when body dissatisfaction is moderate or low, emotional eating and acting-out behavior (impulsivity) have emerged as risk factors for binge–purge-type eating disorders in females. One study also found dieting to be a stronger predictor of risk when body dissatisfaction was moderate than when it was high, possibly because dieting in the absence of marked body dissatisfaction is a less common behavior. These sorts of results allow for sophisticated predictions about who is most at risk of eating pathology, but more research is needed to determine whether results will generalize consistently across samples.

There is also a growing emphasis on identifying gene × environment interactions and epigenetic processes relevant to eating disorders. *Epigenetic processes* refer to environmental influences on gene expression, which produce changes in gene function by modifying DNA. There are likely to be developmentally sensitive periods, mostly likely prenatally or in early life, when epigenetic processes occur. These periods may account for some of the links identified between perinatal factors and risk for AN. It is also possible that peripubertal epigenetic changes contribute to the increased risk of eating disorders in women compared to men.

Outlook for the Future

There is a need for further research on how risk factors interact to increase risk. This includes interactions among environmental risk factors, as well as those between genetic and environmental influences. The challenge for the future is to also think about neurobiological risk factors (neuroendophenotypes) and how these may relate to both genetics and environmental exposures. The European IMAGEN study provides an example of this type of research and has already provided evidence for a compulsivity spectrum that links eating disorders and obsessive–compulsive disorders, and which relates to specific personality traits (e.g., neuroticism) and structural brain changes. These sorts of studies link risk factors from different domains and, over time, will allow for complex prediction models.

Suggested Reading

Allen, K. L., Byrne, S. M., Oddy, W. H., Schmidt, U., & Crosby, R. (2014). Risk factors for binge eating and purging eating disorders: Differences based on age of onset. *International Journal of Eating Disorders, 47,* 802–812.—A comparison of risk factors for eating disorders that develop in early versus later adolescence, using 20 years of population-based data from the Western Australian Pregnancy Cohort (Raine) Study.

Campbell, I. C., Mill, J., Uher, R., & Schmidt, U. (2011). Eating disorders, gene–environment interactions and epigenetics. *Neuroscience and Biobehavioral Reviews, 35,* 784–793.—A thorough review of epigenetic processes and gene × environment interactions, and how these may contribute to onset of an eating disorder.

Fairburn, C. G., Welch, S. L., Doll, H. A., Davies, B. A., O'Connor, M. E. (1997). Risk factors for bulimia nervosa. *Archives of General Psychiatry, 54,* 509–517.—One of the seminal case-control risk factor studies by the Oxford eating disorder group.

Fairburn, C. G., Doll, H. A., Welch, S. L., Hay, P. J., Davies, B. A., & O'Connor, M. E. (1998). Risk factors for binge eating disorder. *Archives of General Psychiatry, 55,* 425–432.—One of the seminal case-control risk factor studies by the Oxford eating disorder group.

Fairburn, C. G., Cooper, Z., Doll, H. A., & Welch, S. (1999). Risk factors for anorexia nervosa. *Archives of General Psychiatry, 56,* 468–476.—One of the seminal case-control risk factor studies by the Oxford eating disorder group.

Favaro, A., Tenconi, E., & Santonastaso, P. (2010). The interaction between perinatal factors and childhood abuse in the risk of developing anorexia nervosa. *Psychological Medicine, 40,* 657–665.—An Italian study providing evidence for an interaction between neonatal dysmaturity and childhood abuse in risk for AN.

Field, A. E., Javaras, K. M., Aneja, P., Kitos, N., Camargo, C. A., Taylor, B., et al. (2008). Family, peer and media predictors of becoming eating disordered. *Archives of Pediatric and Adolescent Medicine, 162,* 574–579.—The American Growing Up Today Study (GUTS) followed 6,916 girls and 5,618 boys over a 7-year period and identified sex- and age-specific predictors of eating disorders.

Hilbert, A., Pike, K. M., Goldschmidt, A. B., Wilfley, D. E., Fairburn, C. G., Dohm, F. A., et al. (2014). Risk factors across the eating disorders. *Psychiatry Research, 220,* 500–506.—A recent application of the Oxford Risk Factor Interview, which showed distinct risk factors for AN compared to BED, with some overlap between risk factors for each of these disorders and BN.

Jacobi, C., Hayward, C., de Zwaan, M., Kraemer, H. C., & Agras, W. S. (2004). Coming to terms with risk factors for eating disorders: Application of risk terminology and suggestions for a general taxonomy. *Psychological Bulletin, 130,* 19–65.—An excellent review of eating disorder risk factor research up to 2004, with a comprehensive summary of risk factor terminology and directions for future research.

Micali, N., Stahl, D., Treasure, J., & Simonoff, E. (2014). Childhood psychopathology in children of women with eating disorders: Understanding risk mechanisms. *Journal of Child Psychology and Psychiatry, 55,* 124–134.—A case–control study nested within the ALSPAC, showing that anxiety and depression during pregnancy may mediate the effects of a maternal eating disorder on later child psychopathology.

Montigny, C., Castellanos-Ryan, N., Whelan, R., Banaschewski, T., Barker, G. J., Büchel, C., et al. (2013). A phenotypic structure and neural correlates of compulsive behaviors in adolescents. *PLoS ONE, 8*(11), e80151.—The European IMAGEN study provides evidence for a compulsivity spectrum that links eating disorders and obsessive–compulsive disorders, with reference to personality traits and structural brain changes.

Rastam, M., & Gillberg, C. (1992). Background factors in anorexia nervosa: A controlled study of 51 teenage cases including a population sample. *European Child and Adolescent Psychiatry, 1,* 54–64.—One of the seminal case-control risk factor studies for anorexia nervosa.

Steinhausen, H. C., Jakobsen, H., Helenius, D., Munk-Jørgensen, P., & Strober, M. (2015). A nation-wide study of the family aggregation and risk factors in anorexia nervosa over three generations. *International Journal of Eating Disorders, 48*(1), 1–8.—An application of Danish Psychiatric Central Research Register data to show nationwide associations between a family history of AN or affective disorders, as well as year of birth, and risk for AN.

Stice, E., Marti, C. N., & Durant, S. (2011). Risk factors for onset of eating disorders: Evidence of multiple risk pathways from an 8-year prospective study. *Behaviour Research and Therapy, 49*(10), 622–627.—Evidence for a three-way interaction among body dissatisfaction, depression, and dieting in the prediction of eating disorders in population-based adolescent females.

Emotion Regulation and Eating Disorders

STEPHEN A. WONDERLICH
JASON M. LAVENDER

Although several new theories and treatment approaches for eating disorders have begun to emerge in recent years, cognitive-behavioral models and treatments have been, and arguably continue to be, the dominant approach utilized in the field. Variations of Beck's original cognitive-behavioral approach for the treatment of depression have been developed for anorexia nervosa, bulimia nervosa, and binge eating disorder. Furthermore, cognitive-behavioral treatments have been shown to be some of the most effective interventions available for individuals with eating disorders. However, despite the acknowledged significance of cognitive-behavioral models and associated treatments, these approaches have been criticized. For example, David Clark criticized cognitive-behavioral therapy on the grounds that it has a limited view of interpersonal factors, ignores the therapeutic alliance, overemphasizes conscious controlled processing, and, of particular relevance, offers a discounted view of emotion. Similarly, emotional processes have not received significant attention in cognitive-behavioral models of eating disorder psychopathology. For example, in Fairburn and colleagues' original cognitive behavior therapy manual for the treatment of bulimia nervosa, there are essentially no references to emotion-related processes. However, recent evidence implies that individuals with eating disorders have significant deficits in emotion regulation, and that eating disorder behaviors may temporarily reduce negative affect in a manner that is highly reinforcing. These findings have led clinicians and researchers to consider more seriously emotion-related constructs in eating disorder theories and treatments. In this chapter, we summarize recent theoretical developments regarding emotion and eating disorders, provide a synopsis of the empirical literature regarding emotion regulation processes in individuals with eating disorders, and also offer a brief overview of emerging emotion-focused eating disorder treatments.

Emotion-Based Theories of Eating Disorders

A number of emotion-related theories of eating disorder psychopathology have emerged in the literature. The specific foci of these theories vary to some degree, but each posits that emotion-based processes are important underlying factors related to eating disorder symptoms. For example, the dual-pathway model of bulimia nervosa suggests that one mechanism by which body image concerns are associated with bulimia nervosa is via the development of bulimic symptoms as maladaptive efforts to regulate negative affective states associated with body dissatisfaction. The escape theory of binge eating also includes an important role for negative emotional experiences, such that the process of binge eating functions as a way to escape from aversive aspects of self-awareness. With regard to anorexia nervosa, the cognitive–interpersonal maintenance model emphasizes cognitive rigidity, experiential avoidance, pro-anorectic beliefs, and the response of close others as important factors that may help to maintain the disorder over time. Furthermore, and of particular relevance to this chapter, the transactional emotion dysregulation model of anorexia nervosa emphasizes the functional role of eating disorder behaviors in relation to emotional arousal, as well as the exacerbating effects of eating disorder symptoms and interpersonal deficits in relation to emotional vulnerability. Although a full review of emotion-related theories of eating disorder psychopathology is beyond the scope of this chapter, it should be noted that additional theories have also been proposed, emphasizing various emotion-based processes such as fear conditioning, emotional avoidance, and distress intolerance.

Evidence of Disturbances in Emotional Functioning in Eating Disorders

Several lines of evidence support the existence of disturbances in emotional functioning in persons with eating disorders. For instance, a number of studies with both population-based samples and clinical samples have found high rates of co-occurring psychiatric disorders that are indicative of elevated or extreme negative emotional states (i.e., mood disorders, anxiety disorders, certain personality disorders) in both anorexia nervosa and bulimia nervosa. Also, individuals with eating disorders are commonly found to display elevated levels of negative emotion on dimensional measures, such as those assessing symptoms of depression and anxiety. Furthermore, higher levels of broadly defined negative affect, as well as specific negative affective states (e.g., anger, guilt, hostility), commonly characterize those with eating disorders. Relatedly, individuals with eating disorders tend to report higher scores on measures of emotion-relevant personality traits (e.g., obsessive–compulsiveness, neuroticism, negative emotionality, affective lability) that are indicative of difficulties in emotional functioning. In summary, evidence from these interrelated areas of research support the notion that individuals with eating disorders display disturbances in the experience of emotion, characterized by more frequent and more intense negative affective experiences, and that, in many cases, these disturbances may be substantial and impairing enough to warrant an additional co-occurring diagnosis.

Evidence of Emotion Dysregulation in Eating Disorders

In addition to accounting for the generation and experience of emotions, how one regulates emotional experiences is also an important consideration. *Emotion regulation* has been variously defined, but it can be broadly conceptualized as the process of modulating emotional experiences or responses, or any strategies of responding to one's emotions, regardless of their intensity or reactivity. From this perspective, eating disorder behaviors may be viewed as efforts to avoid or reduce negative emotions and in that regard may be seen to function as maladaptive strategies for regulating affective experiences.

In a recent review, one clinically informed conceptualization of emotion dysregulation, Gratz and Roemer's multidimensional model, was used as a framework for reviewing emotion regulation difficulties in anorexia nervosa and bulimia nervosa. The multidimensional model, characterized by four dimensions, emphasizes adaptive responding to emotional distress rather than efforts to suppress or control emotional arousal. The first dimension focuses on the flexible use of situationally appropriate strategies to adaptively and effectively modulate duration or intensity of emotions. The second dimension emphasizes the ability to inhibit impulsive behavior and to maintain goal-directed behavior in the context of emotional distress, which overlaps with the construct of *negative urgency*, defined as the tendency to act rashly in the face of negative affect. The third dimension focuses on awareness, clarity, and acceptance of emotions, including processes such as attention to and awareness of emotional states, ability to discern and distinguish between emotions, and accepting emotions without judgment or experiencing negative secondary reactions. Finally, the fourth dimension focuses on an individual's willingness to tolerate emotional distress in the context of pursuing activities that are important or meaningful for him or her, as opposed to engaging in avoidance behaviors. Within this framework, deficits in one or more of the dimensions are viewed as being indicative of emotion dysregulation. The major findings from the review addressing emotion dysregulation in anorexia nervosa and bulimia nervosa using the Gratz and Roemer conceptualization as a framework are briefly summarized below.

Findings reported in the review suggest that both anorexia nervosa and bulimia nervosa are characterized by emotion dysregulation across multiple dimensions. First, existing evidence suggests that those with anorexia nervosa and those with bulimia nervosa tend to report global difficulties with effectively regulating their emotional experiences, and tend to utilize more maladaptive emotion regulation strategies, while underutilizing adaptive skills. Second, a reduced capacity for tolerating distress and a tendency to exhibit behavioral control deficits in the context of heightened negative emotional arousal appear to characterize both anorexia nervosa and bulimia nervosa. Relatedly, negative emotional states frequently precede eating disorder behaviors, and there is some evidence that such behaviors may be followed by reductions in negative affect. Third, there is evidence to support the presence of reduced emotional awareness and clarity, and greater emotion suppression and nonacceptance of emotions, in anorexia nervosa and bulimia nervosa, although evidence of deficits in the ability to recognize emotions in others appears to be stronger for anorexia nervosa than for bulimia nervosa. Fourth, evidence indicates that individuals with anorexia nervosa and bulimia nervosa display elevated punishment sensitivity and a tendency to avoid situations that may elicit a negative emotional response, whereas individuals with the restricting subtype of anorexia nervosa appear to be characterized by relative insensitivity to reward, and those with bulimia nervosa and the binge–purge subtype of anorexia nervosa appear to be characterized by heightened sensitivity to reward.

Two other recent reviews provide further information regarding the nature of emotion dysregulation in eating disorders. One review focused on emotion generation and regulation in anorexia nervosa using Gross's process model of emotion regulation as a framework. Within this model, emotion regulation includes a variety of processes that can influence multiple aspects of an emotional experience, including the type of emotion experienced, when the emotion is experienced, and how the emotion is experienced and expressed. Emotion regulatory processes are broadly classified into antecedent-focused and response-focused strategies. Consistent with findings from the review we described earlier, this review reported poorer emotional awareness and clarity in anorexia nervosa, greater use of maladaptive emotion regulation strategies, and less use of adaptive emotion regulation skills. Another recent review focused on emotion regulation in binge eating disorder, based on studies that used experimental paradigms. Findings from this review suggested that negative emotions commonly function as triggers for binge eating in binge eating disorder, and that food intake appears to be associated with a short-term improvement in mood.

Eating Disorder Treatments Related to Emotion Regulation

Along with the recent theoretical and empirical interest in the role of emotion dysregulation in eating disorders, there has been a parallel increase in novel clinical interventions for eating disorders that target emotion-related constructs. These clinical developments have been significantly influenced by empirical findings suggesting that emotional states and eating disorder behaviors are functionally related; that is, emotional states serve as antecedents of eating disorder behavior, and eating disorder behaviors influence, or regulate, emotional states. Furthermore, contemporary emotion-oriented treatments for eating disorders cut across diagnostic boundaries. For example, emotion acceptance behavior therapy (EABT) and the Maudsley model of anorexia nervosa treatment for adults (MANTRA) are both emotion-oriented treatments for individuals with anorexia nervosa. Similarly, integrative cognitive–affective therapy (ICAT) and a modified form of dialectical behavior therapy (DBT) are emotion-oriented treatments that have been developed for individuals who binge-eat, including those with bulimia nervosa and binge eating disorder. Also, it is notable that enhanced cognitive behavior therapy (CBT-E), based on the transdiagnostic model of eating disorders, has evolved from the original version of CBT for bulimia nervosa and now includes a module addressing mood intolerance, reflecting a greater emphasis on the role of emotion, and, in particular, reactions to emotion, in the treatment of eating disorders. In summary, there are a growing number of emergent clinical strategies for the treatment of individuals with eating disorders that more directly consider and target emotional processes. Further empirical data collected via randomized controlled trials will help to clarify whether these interventions offer significant advances in the treatment of eating disorders.

Conclusion

Taken together, empirical evidence supports the notion that emotion dysregulation is a common characteristic among individuals with eating disorders. The apparent presence of broad deficits in adaptive emotion regulation is consistent with theoretical models positing that eating disorder behaviors may function as maladaptive methods for regulating aversive emotional states. Further research utilizing prospective designs will be needed to clarify the extent to which such emotion regulation skills deficits function as risk versus maintenance factors in eating disorders. However, whether emotion dysregulation is a predisposing factor or is more strongly implicated in the maintenance of eating disorder psychopathology, there is likely utility in the application of eating disorder interventions that seek to help patients develop more adaptive and effective emotion regulation strategies.

Suggested Reading

Cromwell, H. C., & Panksepp, J. (2011). Rethinking the cognitive revolution from a neural perspective: How overuse/misuse of the term "cognition" and the neglect of affective controls in behavioral neuroscience could be delaying progress in understanding the BrainMind. *Neuroscience and Biobehavioral Reviews, 35,* 2026–2035.—The authors address the importance of considering affective processes in addition to cognitive processes in behavioral neuroscience research.

Gratz, K. L., & Roemer, L. (2004). Multidimensional assessment of emotion regulation and dysregulation: Development, factor structure, and initial validation of the difficulties in emotion regulation scale. *Journal of Psychopathology and Behavioral Assessment, 26,* 41–54.—The authors describe the multidimensional model of emotion regulation, as well as the development of a measure assessing emotion regulation difficulties based on this conceptualization.

Gross, J. J. (1998). The emerging field of emotion regulation: An integrative review. *Review of General Psychology, 2,* 271–299.—The author describes the process model of emotion regulation.

Haedt-Matt, A. A., & Keel, P. K. (2011). Revisiting the affect regulation model of binge eating: A meta-analysis of studies using ecological momentary assessment. *Psychological Bulletin, 137,* 660–681.—This meta-analysis addresses evidence regarding affective antecedents and consequences of binge eating based on data collected from studies that utilized ecological momentary assessment.

Haynos, A. F., & Fruzzetti, A. E. (2011). Anorexia nervosa as a disorder of emotion dysregulation: Evidence and treatment implications. *Clinical Psychology: Science and Practice, 18,* 183–202.—The authors propose a model of anorexia nervosa based on a transactional emotion regulation framework.

Lavender, J. M., Wonderlich, S. A., Engel, S. G., Gordon, K., Kaye, W. H., & Mitchell, J. E. (2015). Dimensions of emotion dysregulation in anorexia nervosa and bulimia nervosa: A conceptual review of the empirical literature. *Clinical Psychology Review, 40,* 111–122.—This review summarizes evidence regarding emotion regulation difficulties in anorexia nervosa and bulimia nervosa based on the multidimensional model of emotion regulation.

Leehr, E. J., Krohmer, K., Schag, K., Dresler, T., Zipfel, S., & Giela, K. R. (2015). Emotion regulation model in binge eating disorder and obesity: A systematic review. *Neuroscience and Biobehavioral Reviews, 49,* 125–134.—This review summarizes evidence about the emotion regulation model of binge eating, based on studies using experimental paradigms.

Oldershaw, A., Lavender, T., Sallis, H., Stahl, D., & Schmidt, U. (2015). Emotion generation and regulation in anorexia nervosa: A systematic review and meta-analysis of self-report data. *Clinical Psychology Review, 39,* 83–95.—This review summarizes evidence regarding emotion dysregulation in anorexia nervosa based on the process model of emotion regulation.

Pearson, C. M., Wonderlich, S. A., & Smith, G. T. (2015). A risk and maintenance model for bulimia nervosa: From impulsive action to compulsive behavior. *Psychological Review, 122*(3), 516–535.—The authors propose a model for bulimia nervosa that addresses the transition from an initial impulsive nature of bulimic behaviors to a compulsive nature of the symptoms.

Schmidt, U., & Treasure, J. (2006). Anorexia nervosa: Valued and visible: A cognitive interpersonal maintenance model and its implications for research and practice. *British Journal of Clinical Psychology, 45,* 343–366.—Authors describe a model of anorexia nervosa that integrates cognitive, interpersonal, and affective factors.

Disturbances of the Central Nervous System in Anorexia Nervosa and Bulimia Nervosa

LAURA A. BERNER
WALTER H. KAYE

Eating disorders are characterized by unique symptoms including body image distortion and often denial of the seriousness of the illness; however, perhaps the primary defining characteristic of these disorders is abnormal extremes of food consumption. Advances in our understanding of disturbances in neural circuits associated with eating disorders are beginning to raise the possibility that the behavioral extremes characteristic of these disorders may be better understood based on a continuum of interacting neurocognitive constructs—reward and inhibition. While a relatively novel idea for understanding eating disorders, this perspective is consistent with the obesity and addiction literature. These fields have made substantial advances in delineating the circuitry that makes drugs and food rewarding, and that underlie the self-control mechanisms that may inhibit their use. These advances may serve as models to develop a mechanistic understanding of eating disorders.

This chapter focuses on how the symptoms of anorexia nervosa (AN) and bulimia nervosa (BN) may be related to an altered balance between reward, inhibition, and saliency. We focus primarily on the potential relevance of ventral and dorsal corticostriatal circuits. Ventral corticostriatal and corticolimbic neural circuits, which include the rostral anterior cingulate cortex (ACC), the ventromedial prefrontal cortex (PFC), and the anterior ventral striatum, evaluate rewarding or emotionally significant stimuli and generate affective responses to these stimuli. A dorsal cognitive neural circuit, which modulates self-regulatory control functions, including action inhibition, planning, effortful regulation of affective states, and decision making, includes the dorsal caudate, the dorsal ACC, the ventrolateral PFC (VLPFC) and dorsolateral PFC (DLPFC), the insula, and the parietal cortex.

Self-Regulatory Control

The spectrum of symptoms across eating disorders may reflect a range of self-regulatory control capacities, ranging from behavioral dysregulation in BN to exaggerated control in AN. Clinically, individuals with BN have difficulty resisting urges to purge and terminating eating during binge episodes, defined by a sense of "loss of control" over eating. In addition, they are prone to engage in other, co-occurring impulsive behaviors, including nonsuicidal self-injurious behavior, risky sexual behaviors, and substance use. Behavioral data on the inhibitory control capacities of individuals with BN, as measured by performance on neurocognitive tasks, are somewhat mixed, but the majority of findings are consistent with the clinical characteristics of BN and indicate motor inhibitory control impairments, which are even more pronounced when food or body-related stimuli are used instead of neutral pictures or words. Relatively few imaging studies have focused on BN; however, existing results suggest that the binge eating and purging behaviors characteristic of BN may result from brain-based functional impairments associated with deficits in the ability to inhibit behavioral responses. Most extant inhibitory control task-based imaging findings in BN suggest that individuals with this disorder have either reduced activation or deactivation in the PFC and striatal regions that are essential for self-regulation during inhibition tasks. Furthermore, reduced PFC volume and reduced gray matter in the striatum of individuals with BN compared with healthy control participants may explain the reduced neural activation observed. VLPFC volume reductions in BN in have been found to correlate inversely with symptom severity, inhibitory control task performance, and illness duration, and participants with BN demonstrate reduced activation in inhibitory lateral PFC regions in response to images of food, suggesting that aberrant structure and function of these regions in BN may contribute to dysregulated eating behavior.

Results of neuroimaging studies of self-regulatory control in AN have been mixed. On tasks assessing the ability to change behavioral responses flexibly with a new set of goals or rules (i.e., set shifting) or delay gratification for monetary rewards, both of which require self-regulation, individuals with AN show greater activation in the DLPFC than do controls, which may reflect inefficient, excessive brain activation in control-related regions; however, during tasks that require action inhibition, both participants with AN and those recovered from the disorder perform as well as control participants but demonstrate reduced PFC activation compared with controls as trials become increasingly difficult. Though further research is needed, existing results suggest increased neural efficiency when behavioral control is required, and that increased recruitment of control-related regions during the delay of gratification may underlie the extreme dietary restriction characteristic of AN.

Reward Processing

Imaging studies support the possibility that altered discrimination of reward and punishment may be a transdiagnostic trait across eating disorders. Individuals with BN tend to have increased sensitivity to reward, but findings are mixed in AN. Typically, healthy, normal-weight individuals tend to have a more robust response to positive relative to negative feedback within the ventral striatum and dorsal caudate, suggesting that they are more sensitive to reward than to punishment. Using a monetary choice task, several studies have shown that participants with AN and BN fail to differentiate reward and punishment in ventral striatal regions the way controls do. This may indicate a failure to bind, scale, or discriminate responses to salient stimuli appropriately, suggesting that individuals with these disorders share a difficulty in precisely identifying and/or modulating reward in response to salient stimuli. Poor context separation may interfere with motivation or ability to learn from experience, and lack of insight, which may contribute to treatment refractoriness.

Biobehavioral research on obesity and addiction highlights the importance of distinguishing between consummatory food reward and the anticipation of that reward. In fact, reward anticipated from food is a more robust determinant of intake than the reward experienced when the food is actually consumed. A growing body of evidence suggests individuals with AN demonstrate increased and anxious anticipatory responses in insula, striatum, and PFC regions to visually presented food cues and reduced responses in insula and striatum to tastes of palatable foods. Increased anxiety in anticipation of food stimuli and diminished reward after its receipt may underlie the extreme dietary restriction that progresses to starvation in AN. In contrast, individuals with BN may demonstrate the opposite processing pattern. It is possible that a failure to anticipate the consequences of stimuli appropriately, or exaggerated response to receipt of salient stimuli, contributes to poor impulse control in BN.

Imaging studies have also investigated the neural correlates of the high trait anxiety that is well established in both AN and BN. This research has examined limbic response—particularly in the amygdala, a region involved in both fear and emotion processing—to high-calorie or high-fat food stimuli or emotionally salient stimuli. Some studies indicate that, compared with controls, both ill and recovered persons with AN show hyperactivation of amygdala and insula in response to food images and body images. In addition, some results suggest increased amygdalar activation in underweight, fasting individuals with AN compared with controls in response to actual food taste stimuli; however, results to date are mixed, and no studies have suggested aberrant fear circuit activation in response to non-food-related but emotionally salient stimuli (e.g., emotional faces) in individuals with AN. In individuals with BN, some evidence suggests reduced activation compared with controls in the amygdala in response to the unexpected omission or receipt of palatable taste stimuli, and findings of increased activation in individuals with BN compared with controls in response to food images in PFC, ACC, occipital cortex, and insula have been interpreted as an "anxious" BN response to food stimuli. Overall, patients with AN may demonstrate an elevated anxiety response to anticipated food cues, whereas those with BN demonstrate a blunted response to unanticipated food cues.

Summary

Behavioral, cognitive, and neuroimaging evidence suggests that an altered balance of reward, inhibition, and salience contributes to disordered food consumption in eating disorders. Restricted eating in AN may emerge from excessive inhibition and/or anticipatory anxiety paired with diminished valuation of reward or salience. In contrast, the combination of dysregulated control and salience networks and excessive reward sensitivity may lead to a pattern of under- and overconsumption that is characteristic of BN and the binge eating–purging subtype of AN. Viewing eating pathology from the perspective of an altered balance of self-regulatory control and salience or reward processing provides a foundation for developing more specific and effective interventions for these debilitating disorders.

Confounding Factors and Directions for Future Research

Despite significant advances over the last decade in our understanding of brain-based factors that may contribute to AN and BN, the wide array of tasks that have been used in functional imaging studies and disparate participant characteristics make direct comparison of findings across studies challenging. For example, the study of participants who are actively ill may result in confounding effects of malnutrition. It is controversial whether findings in participants who are recovered reflect traits that constitute a vulnerability to develop an eating disorder or reflect scars of having the disorder. The study of individuals prior to their development of AN or BN is challenging given the relatively low prevalence of eating disorders. Large-scale, longitudinal studies are needed to better disentangle illness risk factors from state and trait alterations associated with AN and BN. In addition, further research is needed on subthreshold and other eating disorders to provide a foundation for understanding disordered eating behaviors along a continuum. For example, obese individuals with binge eating disorder (BED), compared both with lean and obese controls, demonstrate deficient activation in the PFC and insula when engaging inhibitory control and reduced bilateral ventral striatal activation during the anticipation of monetary reward or loss. Compared with controls and individuals with BN, individuals with BED also show increased medial orbitofrontal cortex activation in response to food cues. These initial findings indicate that BED may be characterized by alterations in reward responsivity even more exaggerated than in BN, and brain-based deficits in inhibitory control similar to those seen in BN.

Furthermore, hunger, satiety, menstrual status, sex, age, and stage of brain development at the time participants are scanned may all influence neuroimaging results but often are not assessed or reported. Whether our paradigms should be designed to capture the neural response associated with receipt or anticipation of food stimuli, or whether one is more relevant to one disorder over another remains unclear. In addition, some evidence suggests that studies assessing brain activation in response to rewards should include both random and expected stimuli, as unpredictable stimuli may reveal an underlying biological reward sensitivity rather than potentially increased cognitive inhibition as stimuli become increasingly predictable.

At the level of results interpretation, it is still unclear whether increased blood-oxygen-level-dependent (BOLD) responses measured by functional magnetic resonance imaging (fMRI) actually indicate increased brain activation, and whether decreased activation indicates greater efficiency or a deficiency. Finally, although several well-validated tasks exist to study concepts of self-regulation and reward, both constructs are highly complex, and single tasks cannot tap all aspects of these processes and abilities relevant to real-world behavior.

No neuroimaging technique is comprehensive, but new imaging data that incorporate multiple modalities (e.g., positron emission tomography with simultaneous fMRI) and integrate our understanding of neuropeptide function with neural function by, for example, administering neuropeptides to participants before scanning, may add to our understanding of eating disorders.

Conclusion

Despite some problematic, confounding factors in existing neuroimaging data, overall, results suggest disturbances in corticostriatal and corticolimbic pathways across eating disorders. These disturbances may relate to imbalances in self-regulation and reward processing and, in turn, alter experienced anticipation of eating and actual consummatory behavior, as well as general cognitive and behavioral abilities and symptoms (e.g., general impulsivity, anxiety, cognitive inflexibility) that may contribute to treatment resistance. Although evidence suggests a potential imbalance of reward and inhibition in eating disorders, no studies have reported on the functioning and potential interaction of both systems within the same sample. Longitudinal imaging of the neural circuits that supports self-regulatory control and reward will permit identification of neurodevelopmental trajectories within these circuits in both AN and BN. In addition, we do not yet know how the structure and function of these circuits may change with treatment, and imaging before and after treatment and at follow-up assessments would help identify mechanisms of treatment response and prognostic indicators to inform treatment development efforts.

Suggested Reading

Avena, N. M., & Bocarsly, M. E. (2012). Dysregulation of brain reward systems in eating disorders: Neurochemical information from animal models of binge eating, bulimia nervosa, and anorexia nervosa. *Neuropharmacology, 63*(1), 87–96.—This article comprehensively reviews findings from animal models of eating disorders implicating neurochemical alterations in reward circuitry in association with eating disorder behaviors.

Berner, L. A., & Marsh, R. (2014). Frontostriatal circuits and the development of bulimia nervosa. *Frontiers in Behavioral Neuroscience, 8*, 395.—The authors of this review describe the normal development of the circuits that support self-regulatory control, reward processing, and reward-based learning; review structural and functional imaging data from adolescents and adults with BN, indicating abnormalities within these circuits; and present a pathophysiological model of BN development within the context of frontostriatal circuit maturation.

Frank, G. K. W. (2013). Altered brain reward circuits in eating disorders: Chicken or egg? *Current Psychiatry Reports, 15*(10), 396.—This article provides a thorough review of reward circuit structure and function alterations in both ill and recovered AN and BN and posits that alterations in those circuits relate to eating disorder development and maintenance.

Friederich, H. C., Wu, M., Simon, J. J., & Herzog, W. (2013). Neurocircuit function in eating disorders. *International Journal of Eating Disorders, 46*(5), 425–432.—This review highlights functional imaging results indicating abnormal neural activation in AN and BN related to fear and anxiety, reward, and executive functions.

Lipsman, N., Woodside, D. B., & Lozano, A. M. (2015). Neurocircuitry of limbic dysfunction in anorexia nervosa. *Cortex, 62*, 109–118.—This review focuses on evidence for emotion processing-related brain abnormalities in AN, which are not reviewed in detail in this chapter.

O'Hara, C. B., Campbell, I. C., & Schmidt, U. (2015). A reward-centred model of anorexia nervosa: A focused narrative review of the neurological and psychophysiological literature. *Neuroscience and Biobehavioral Reviews, 52*, 131–152.—This comprehensive review of reward circuit alterations in AN proposes that the disorder is related to reward-based learning abnormalities, emphasizing an important role for the striatum.

Titova, O. E., Hjorth, O. C., Schioth, H. B., & Brooks, S. J. (2013). Anorexia nervosa is linked to reduced brain structure in reward and somatosensory regions: A meta-analysis of VBM studies. *BMC Psychiatry, 13,* 110.—This meta-analysis, including results from 228 participants with AN and 240 matched control participants, indicates that AN is characterized by global reductions in gray and white matter, and regional reductions in left hypothalamus, left inferior parietal lobe, left lentiform nucleus, and right caudate—all of which are regions relevant to somatosensory and appetitive functions.

Wierenga, C. E., Ely, A., Bischoff-Grethe, A., Bailer, U. F., Simmons, A. N., & Kaye, W. H. (2014). Are extremes of consumption in eating disorders related to an altered balance between reward and inhibition? *Frontiers in Behavioral Neuroscience, 8,* 410.—This article provides a more in-depth review, including detailed results of individual studies, of the concepts presented in this chapter.

Cognitive Neuroscience and Eating Disorders

JOANNA E. STEINGLASS

Eating disorders present a complex picture of cognitive functioning. Individuals are often high functioning, with generally intact intellectual function and normal IQ. Yet a closer look at cognition shows a pattern of cognitive deficits that appear potentially related to clinical features of the disorders. In anorexia nervosa (AN), the primary disturbances include attentional and executive function deficits with relatively preserved verbal functioning. In bulimia nervosa (BN), neuropsychological studies have identified impairments in the domains of impulsivity and decision making. As the study of the healthy brain has advanced, neural systems mediating cognitive functions have been identified. And, more recently, links have been made between cognition, behavior, and neural circuitry. These advances are derived from cognitive neuroscience, which provides a variety of methodological and experimental techniques that are beginning to be applied to understand psychiatric illnesses. As eating disorders are defined by disturbances in behavior, cognitive neuroscience techniques will necessarily focus on the neural mechanisms that mediate core behavioral phenomena (i.e., disturbances in eating). This chapter provides a discussion of neuropsychological and neural circuit data underlying executive function domains in eating disorders, and how approaches based on cognitive neuroscience may further our understanding of the neural underpinnings of the characteristic maladaptive behaviors.

Cognitive Dysfunction in AN

Clinical descriptions of individuals with AN have long noted that cognition is affected by the illness, especially in the malnourished state. Although results are not entirely consistent, the available data indicate that attention and visuospatial processing are significantly impaired in the acute state of AN (i.e., when underweight); attentional deficits tend to improve with weight restoration. *Executive function,* the higher-order processing involved in integrating information and creating responses, may be impaired, and some studies have used neuropsychological tasks to directly examine cognitive domains with apparent relevance to clinical features.

Set shifting is a measure of cognitive flexibility that tests the individual's capacity to change responses as the environmental contingencies (i.e., the rules of the task) change. A series of studies has used cognitive and perceptual tasks to assess set shifting across different populations of patients with AN: underweight, acutely weight-restored, and longer-term recovered individuals. Across studies, individuals with AN make more errors—specifically perseverative errors—than do healthy controls. Among adolescents, however, this deficit is not always present. It may be that the tendency to perseverate is related in some way to chronicity of illness. Attention to detail can be studied through neuropsychological tasks (e.g., the Rey–Osterrieth Complex Figure Test) that measure local versus global processing, and yield a measure of *central coherence,* the ability to see the bigger picture and not focus excessively on details. These studies have found that individuals with AN tend to focus on minute details at the expense of processing the whole figure. Studies of decision making have used tasks such as the Iowa Gambling Task that test an individual's ability to learn through incremental feedback. These studies have often found that individuals with AN show performance deficits, such that they persist in making disadvantageous choices.

There is sufficient variability in presentation that it has been difficult to discern what components of abnormal cognitive functioning are attributable to starvation alone, and what may be considered core features of AN. The ways in which malnourishment affects cognition and decision making may have a large impact on the individual's clinical status and course. Collectively, the neuropsychological findings in AN indicate subtle impairments that are suggestive of underlying neural circuit abnormalities.

Cognitive Dysfunction in BN

Disturbances in cognition are less pronounced in individuals with BN. Neuropsychological studies tend to show unimpaired global functioning. Attention and memory are largely normal—though some studies have found deficits in attention among a subset of individuals. Impairments have been noted in executive functioning, when information needs to be integrated for the purpose of problem solving. Similar to results described in AN, some studies of cognitive flexibility have detected set shifting deficits among individuals with BN. And, in studies using the Iowa Gambling Task to assess decision making, individuals with BN, like those with AN, have demonstrated poor performance, with excessive disadvantageous (or risky) choices.

Individuals with BN consistently show executive functioning abnormalities that indicate impulsivity, as might be expected from the behavioral disturbances characteristic of BN. The go/no-go task instructs participants to refrain from responding to particular stimuli and serves as a measure of motor impulsivity; individuals with BN show difficulty inhibiting responses. Some have suggested that these neuropsychological deficits relate to maladaptive impulsive behaviors. These findings have been incorporated into the development of models of the neural mechanisms of illness that suggest the need to examine the brain more directly.

Neural Circuits and Cognition

Cognitive activation probes are tasks that measure specific cognitive functions and can be used with concurrent neuroimaging to examine associated neural activity. Some cognitive processes have been well studied in healthy individuals, and the underlying neural mechanisms have been identified. These may be useful in testing models of brain pathophysiology in eating disorders. Examples of this approach in eating disorders have included the study of impulsivity, temporal discounting, and reward processing.

Impulsivity/Inhibition

Impulsivity refers to the inability to inhibit responding to a stimulus. On self-report measures, impulsivity is often rated higher by individuals with BN than by healthy controls. Behaviorally, impulsivity is measured through tasks that ask the participant to respond to one cue and inhibit responding to another, or in tasks that ask the participant to override instinctive responses. Across different types of cognitive tasks, individuals with BN have shown significantly greater impulsive responding than healthy participants. In one paradigm, called the Simon spatial incompatibility task, participants are asked to indicate whether an arrow is located on the left side of the screen or the right side of the screen. If the arrow is pointing to the left while situated on the right, the participant must inhibit the automatic tendency to indicate the direction in which the arrow is pointed in order to correctly identify its placement on the screen. During functional magnetic resonance imaging (fMRI), patients with BN showed the expected impulsive performance (increased errors on incongruent trials). This was associated with less neural activity in frontostriatal circuits compared with healthy peers. These findings have been interpreted to suggest deficits in cognitive control circuitry among patients with BN.

Temporal Discounting

Temporal, or *delay, discounting* refers to the tendency to value a reward that is available immediately more than the same reward that is available after a time delay. This behavioral characteristic has been well studied in the field of neuroeconomics, where it has been shown that people's tendency to select a delayed reward is mediated by dorsolateral prefrontal cortex activity, whereas the tendency to prefer the immediate reward is associated with ventromedial prefrontal cortex activity. While findings have not been entirely consistent across studies, individuals with AN, in the acutely ill state, have shown a preference for the delayed, larger reward that differentiates them from healthy peers, and may suggest greater self-control. However, the behavioral tendency to wait for the larger, later reward was *not* associated with dorsolateral prefrontal cortex activity, as expected on the basis of studies of healthy controls. Rather, it was associated with an unexpected decrease in striatal activity. Findings in these studies, and in studies like them, suggest frontostriatal circuit abnormalities among individuals with AN, which may relate to maladaptive behavior.

Reward Processing

Reward processing can be studied from many angles, using both disease salient (e.g., food) and disease neutral (e.g., money) stimuli. Much of the neuroimaging literature has investigated reward by measuring neural activity with passive viewing of food or body image stimuli. These studies have identified differences in neural activation among individuals with eating disorders compared to controls. But in passive viewing tasks, it is difficult to determine whether the neural activation differences represent an underlying abnormality in neurobiology or reflect a neural correlate of a behavioral abnormality. For example, when viewing images of food versus images of neutral items, individuals with AN and BN show increased activity in the insula. This may represent a fundamental abnormality in the insula, or it may represent an appropriate change in insula activity in response to the complex affective responses to food experienced by individuals with eating disorders. Such studies may therefore be difficult to interpret.

One paradigm designed to assess disease salient reward processes using a cognitive activation probe involves a reward conditioning task. In this task, the individual is trained to associate a geometric stimulus with the receipt of a taste reward, and neural activation in response to anticipation of the reward is then assessed by examining the response to the geometric stimulus. Individuals with AN showed heightened activity in loops linking the cortex, striatum, and thalamus. Furthermore, obese individuals showed an inverse response pattern. This type of study provides support for neural models of AN that hypothesize underlying abnormalities in brain pathways of reward that contribute to the persistence and development of the eating disorder.

Linking Brain and Behavior

Cognitive activation probes have yielded advances in characterizing neural abnormalities among individuals with eating disorders. However, studies to date have not demonstrated clear and consistent links between these cognitive probes and the disturbances in eating behavior that define eating disorders. Behavior can be viewed as the expression of choice based on learning and memory processes, and research on the underpinnings of eating disorders may be able to leverage growing knowledge of the neural basis of making choices. For example, in healthy individuals, decisions about what food to eat engage ventromedial and dorsolateral sections of the prefrontal cortex, which have been shown to relate to the valuation of food and the modulation of behavior, respectively.

Eating behavior is multifaceted, with psychological, social, and biological components. Much is understood regarding appetitive and inhibitory control of *normal* eating, and roles for reward circuitry (ventral striatum, anterior cingulate, insula) and limbic regions (hippocampus and amygdala) have been established. Yet neural mechanisms of disturbances in eating—including restrictive intake, loss-of-control eating, and compensatory behaviors—have only recently been examined. One new direction attempts to adapt an established paradigm that has been used to measure value-based choices in healthy individuals to examine restrictive intake in eating disorders.

It is common to conceptualize restrictive food choice in AN as a manifestation of exceptional self-control. Yet, paradoxically, individuals with AN seem to have limited ability to modify or control their restrictive eating behavior. It is possible that this pathological behavior is mediated by different neural processes than those employed by healthy individuals. In the food choice task, individuals are asked to rate the value of images of food along two different value systems (health and taste, separately). A food rated by the individual as neutral on both health and taste is selected as a reference item, and the participant then indicates how strongly he or she prefers the reference item versus each of the other foods. Performance on this task has been shown to correlate with actual caloric intake, suggesting that it is a valid model of the restrictive food choice seen in AN. Using this paradigm during fMRI, we have begun to examine the neural circuits underlying active food choice in AN, and found that individuals with AN engage the dorsal striatum more than do controls when they are making decisions about what to eat. Because the experimental paradigm directly examines salient disease symptoms, the choice of what to eat, the results may eventually lead to the identification of new targets for treatment. Furthermore, this paradigm allows for an examination of the neural mechanism by which emotion affects eating behavior and how such mechanisms may change with treatment.

By using experimental methods drawn from cognitive neuroscience, we are able to model clinically significant behavioral disturbances and examine their neural underpinnings. Emerging findings suggest a new direction for understanding the persistence of AN. More broadly, building on advances in cognitive neuroscience, experimental paradigms and new computational and neuroimaging approaches can be used to examine the brain mechanisms that underlie the behavioral disturbances that define eating disorders.

Suggested Reading

Daw, N. D., & Shohamy, D. (2008). The cognitive neuroscience of motivation and learning. *Social Cognition, 26*(5), 593–620.—This article reviews the role of the dopamine midbrain system in the cognitive neuroscience of motivation and learning.

Decker, J. H., Figner, B., & Steinglass, J. E. (2015). On weight and waiting: Delay discounting in anorexia nervosa pretreatment and posttreatment. *Biological Psychiatry, 78*(9), 606–614.—Patients with AN show less temporal discounting than healthy peers, and but did not show increased activity in the dorsolateral prefrontal cortex with delayed reward.

Foerde, K., Steinglass, J. E., Shohamy, D., & Walsh, B. T. (2015). Neural mechanisms supporting maladaptive food choices in anorexia nervosa. *Nature Neuroscience, 18*(11), 1571–1573.—This study linked brain and behavior in AN using a task that assesses active food choice during fMRI scanning; activity in the dorsal striatum was greater among individuals with AN than that in healthy peers during food choice and correlated with subsequent caloric intake, suggesting that dorsal frontostriatal circuits play a significant role in this disorder.

Frank, G. K., Reynolds, J. R., Shott, M. E., Jappe, L., Yang, T. T., Tregellas, J. R., et al. (2012). Anorexia nervosa and obesity are associated with opposite brain reward response. *Neuropsychopharmacology, 37*(9), 2031–2046.—This fMRI study of reward processing used taste as a conditioned reward and found increased neural activity in reward circuits among individuals with AN for unexpected reward receipt and omission, as well as the opposite pattern among obese individuals.

Kanakam, N., Raoult, C., Collier, D., & Treasure, J. (2013). Set shifting and central coherence as neurocognitive endophenotypes in eating disorders: A preliminary investigation in twins. *World Journal of Biological Psychiatry, 14*(6), 464–475.—Provides a review of set shifting, central coherence, reward and emotion processing across eating disorders.

Marsh, R., Steinglass, J. E., Gerber, A. J., O'Leary, K. G., Wang, Z., Murphy, D., et al. (2009). Deficient activity in the neural systems that mediate self-regulatory control in bulimia nervosa. *Archives of General Psychiatry, 66*(1), 51–63.—This fMRI study of impulsivity using the Simon spatial incompatibility task showed that individuals with BN responded more impulsively on the task compared with healthy controls; individuals with BN also showed differences in neural activity in frontostriatal regions during task performance.

O'Hara, C. B., Campbell, I. C., & Schmidt, U. (2015). A reward-centred model of anorexia nervosa: A focussed narrative review of the neurological and psychophysiological literature. *Neuroscience and Biobehavioral Reviews, 52,* 131–152.—A comprehensive review of research in AN using food- or body-image-relevant stimuli.

Steinglass, J. E., & Glasofer, D. R. (2011). Neuropsychology. In B. Lask & I. Frampton (Eds.), *Eating disorders and the brain* (pp. 106–121). West Sussex, UK: Wiley.—This chapter reviews the findings from neuropsychological studies of AN and BN.

TREATMENT AND PREVENTION
OF EATING DISORDERS

Assessment of Feeding and Eating Disorders

JENNIFER J. THOMAS

Valid and reliable measurement of eating disorder psychopathology is critical to conferring diagnoses, planning treatment, conducting research, and informing public policy. The eating disorder field currently enjoys several high-quality measures, including both clinical interviews and self-report questionnaires. However, because no single measure is ideal for all possible applications, selecting the appropriate assessment for a specific clinical or research encounter requires weighing key trade-offs. These include interview versus self-report formats, brevity versus comprehensiveness of content, current versus lifetime assessment, and established versus newer measures. To address these trade-offs, exciting new developments in the assessment field include the creation of new measures to assess the specific psychopathology of feeding disorders, and the growth of technology-assisted assessments.

Current Assessments

In 2015, the U.S. National Human Genome Research Institute and the National Institutes of Health sought input from the scientific community to compile a list of recommended measures of eating disorder psychopathology as part of its consensus measures for the Phenotypes and eXposures (PhenX) project. PhenX measures are meant to be well-established, high-quality, low-burden assessments that biomedical, epidemiological, and genomic researchers can utilize to facilitate cross-study comparisons and analyses. The following measures represent the subset of PhenX eating disorder measures that are most widely used and have the strongest psychometric properties.

Interview Assessments

Structured clinical interviews are ideal for establishing eating disorder diagnoses. Three publicly available interviews that focus specifically on eating disorders and have well-established reliability and validity are the Eating Disorder Examination (EDE-17.0D), the

Structured Interview for Anorexic and Bulimic Syndromes for Expert Rating (SIAB-EX), and the Eating Disorder Assessment for DSM-5 (EDA-5).

The EDE, now in its 17th edition (i.e., 17.0D) is the oldest and most widely used eating disorder interview. It evaluates the presence and severity of eating disorder symptoms over the previous 4 weeks. Items can be used to confer specific DSM-5 diagnoses for eating disorders (i.e., anorexia nervosa, bulimia nervosa, binge eating disorder, and all forms of other specified feeding or eating disorder), but not feeding disorders (i.e., avoidant/restrictive food intake disorder, pica, or rumination disorder). Furthermore, the assessor rates the frequency and severity of eating disorder features on a 7-point Likert scale to produce subscales, including Restraint, Eating Concern, Shape Concern, and Weight Concern, as well as a Global Score. Advantages of the EDE include its widespread use, which enables assessors to compare their findings across studies, and relatively comprehensive coverage of eating disorder psychopathology. However, disadvantages include the focus on concepts most relevant to cognitive-behavioral therapy, the length of time required for assessment (approximately 1 hour), and the lack of psychometric support for the factor structure of the four subscales.

Another interview measure, the SIAB-EX, which can also be used to derive eating disorder diagnoses, has the additional advantage of evaluating lifetime as well as current symptoms. In addition to conferring diagnoses, the SIAB-EX contains six subscales that provide dimensional measures of eating disorder-specific psychopathology (Body Image and Slimness Ideal, Bulimic Symptoms, Measures to Counteract Weight Gain, Fasting, and Atypical Binges), as well as other features commonly associated with disordered eating (General Psychopathology, Sexuality and Social Integration, and Substance Abuse). Advantages of the SIAB-EX include the evaluation of lifetime symptoms, as well as the assessment of both DSM-IV and ICD-10 diagnoses. Disadvantages include the lack of update for DSM-5 diagnoses, the inability to assess feeding disorders (i.e., avoidant/restrictive food intake disorder, pica, rumination disorder), and the assessment of some concepts (e.g., internal achievement motivation, grazing, substance use) that may not be a priority in all settings.

Last, the EDA-5, a relatively new measure, was designed specifically to confer DSM-5 feeding and eating disorder diagnoses. The EDA-5 features a series of open-ended questions for which the assessor uses clinical judgment to ascertain whether a diagnostic criterion is present or absent. The "app" version of the EDA-5 follows a diagnostic algorithm with skip-out criteria that guide the assessor through the diagnostic processes and ensure that relevant questions are asked, whereas potentially irrelevant items are skipped. In terms of advantages, the EDA-5 is quite brief to administer (just 15 minutes) and is currently the only interview that assesses all DSM-5 feeding and eating disorders, including anorexia nervosa, bulimia nervosa, binge eating disorder, avoidant/restrictive food intake disorder (ARFID), pica, rumination disorder, and all presentations of other specified feeding or eating disorder. In terms of disadvantages, the EDA-5 provides minimal dimensional assessment beyond body mass index and frequency of binge eating and purging, and the skip-out rules that enable brevity may lead to some clinical features being missed.

Self-Report Assessments

Whereas interviews are ideal for diagnostic evaluation, the strength of self-report questionnaires is their ability to provide continuous measures of eating disorder severity without the need for an expert assessor. Widely used self-report questionnaires highlighted in the PhenX initiative include the Eating Disorder Examination-Questionnaire (EDE-Q 6.0), Eating Disorder Inventory–3 (EDI-3), and Eating Pathology Symptoms Inventory (EPSI).

The EDE-Q is the self-report version of the EDE interview. Like the EDE, the EDE-Q evaluates symptom frequency and severity on a 7-point Likert scale and provides scores on the Restraint, Eating Concern, Shape Concern, and Weight Concern subscales, which can be combined to produce a Global Score. Advantages include the tight focus on eating disorder psychopathology and the high concordance with the EDE interview. However, the EDE-Q is not ideal for conferring eating disorder diagnoses because, unlike the interview version, which queries about the frequency of diagnostic items over the preceding 3 months, the EDE-Q focuses only on the preceding 4 weeks. Another disadvantage is the lack of support for the hypothesized factor structure of the measure.

The EDI-3, a 91-item questionnaire, comprises not only three eating disorder risk subscales (i.e., Drive for Thinness, Bulimia, Body Dissatisfaction), but also nine subscales measuring associated psychopathology and factors of potential etiological significance (i.e., Low Self-Esteem, Personal Alienation, Interpersonal Insecurity, Interpersonal Alienation, Interoceptive Deficits, Emotional Dysregulation, Perfectionism, Asceticism, and Maturity Fears). An advantage of the EDI-3 is the extensive support for the factor structure of the measure. A key feature of the EDI-3—the comprehensive coverage of both specific and general psychopathology—is both an advantage, because of the richness of data that can be obtained, and a disadvantage, because of the length of time the measure requires. Another disadvantage is the cost (unlike the EDE-Q and EPSI, the EDE-3 is not freely available and must be purchased—see Suggested Reading).

Last, the EPSI, a 45-item self-report measure, was recently developed using modern scale construction methods, including exploratory, confirmatory, and multigroup factor analysis. Respondents answer EPSI items on a 5-point Likert scale, which produces subscale scores for Body Dissatisfaction, Binge Eating, Cognitive Restraint, Purging, Muscle Building, Restricting, Excessive Exercise, and Negative Attitudes toward Obesity. Advantages of the EPSI are support for the proposed factor structure and the assessment of symptoms relevant to males (i.e., Muscle Building). The differential assessment of Cognitive Restraint (i.e., subjective attempts to reduce caloric intake) versus Restriction (i.e., objectively low caloric intake) is another attractive feature that distinguishes the EPSI from the EDE-Q and EDI-3. Disadvantages are the inability to confer diagnoses or calculate a global score.

Considerations When Selecting an Assessment

When selecting a measure for a specific application, clinicians and researchers must weigh the trade-offs between interview versus self-report format, brevity versus comprehensiveness of content, current versus lifetime assessment, and established versus newer measures. For example, interviews (i.e., EDE-Q, SIAB, EDA-5), which allow for expert clinical judgment, may provide more valid assessment of complex constructs, such as persistent behavior that interferes with weight gain and loss of control over eating. In contrast, self-reports (i.e., EDE-Q, EDI-3, EPSI) reduce assessor burden and provide for greater anonymity, which may enhance self-disclosure. Similarly, while brief interviews (i.e., EDA-5) and self-reports (i.e., EDE-Q, EPSI) reduce burden on both assessors and respondents, lengthier interviews (i.e., EDE-17.0D, SIAB) and self-reports (i.e., EDI-3) provide richer and more detailed clinical data. In terms of time frame, longitudinal assessments that provide lifetime data (i.e., SIAB) may be ideal for genetic studies, whereas snapshot measures that evaluate current (typically the past month) symptoms (i.e., EDE, EDA-5, EDE-Q, EDI-3, EPSI) may be ideal for treatment planning. Last, whereas using established measures (i.e., EDE, SIAB, EDE-Q, EDI-3) increases opportunities to compare findings across previous studies, newer measures provide more comprehensive coverage of novel diagnostic constructs (i.e., EDA-5) and may have greater validity with special populations such as males and ethnic/minority individuals (i.e., EPSI).

Future Directions in Assessment

New developments in the assessment field have been designed, in part, to address these trade-offs. Specifically, the development of a new measure to assess the specific psychopathology of feeding disorders will increase comprehensiveness of coverage, and the growth of technology-assisted assessments may reduce both assessor and respondent burden while pioneering the evaluation of novel constructs.

Currently, no existing measure provides a continuous measure of feeding disorder severity. Thus the Pica, ARFID, and Rumination Disorder Interview (PARDI) is a new clinical measure designed to assess the presence and severity of disorders involving the consumption of non-nutritive/nonfood substances, avoidant/restrictive eating, and persistent regurgitation. Importantly, the PARDI includes subscales evaluating Sensory Features, Lack of Interest in Eating, and Fear of Aversive Consequences, which enable the assessor to create a profile of ARFID symptoms that captures the clinical heterogeneity of the disorder. The PARDI is currently being pilot-tested for validity and reliability in an international multisite trial, after which it will be made publicly available.

The development of technology-assisted assessments is increasing our ability to characterize feeding and eating disorder symptoms while reducing assessor and respondent burden. For example, the EDA-5 is conveniently designed as an "app" in which the assessor inputs responses and the "app" guides the assessor toward the appropriate feeding or eating disorder diagnosis. Other innovative uses of technology completely obviate the need for an assessor while collecting novel data that cannot be captured in a traditional interview or self-report. For example, ecological momentary assessment paradigms (in which respondents report symptoms in their natural environment via smartphone) can be used to test hypotheses about momentary relationships between symptoms. Furthermore, implicit association tests (in which reaction time to paired words or images may reveal underlying but disavowed associations between relevant constructs, e.g., fear and weight gain) could help confer diagnoses (e.g., anorexia nervosa) among individuals who lack insight into their symptoms. In the longer-term, emerging differences in neural circuitry across feeding and eating disorder phenotypes suggest that brain imaging may be a future tool to confer diagnoses, predict course and outcome, and select appropriate treatments.

Suggested Reading

Bryant-Waugh, R., Thomas, J. J., Eddy, K. T., Micali, N., Melhuish, L., & Cresswell, L. (2016, October). *The development of the Pica, ARFID, and Rumination Disorder Interview (PARDI)*. Poster session at the annual conference of the Eating Disorders Research Society, New York.—The PARDI, a clinical interview assessing the presence and severity of pica, ARFID (including subscales for sensory features, lack of interest in eating, and fear of aversive consequences) and rumination disorder, is currently being pilot-tested for validity and reliability in an international multisite trial.

Fairburn, C. G., & Beglin, S. (2008). Eating Disorder Examination Questionnaire (EDE-Q 6.0). In C. G. Fairburn (Ed.), *Cognitive behavior therapy and eating disorders* (pp. 309–314). New York: Guilford Press.—Measure is freely available online at *www.credo-oxford. com/7.2.html*. The EDE-Q is a brief self-report version of the EDE interview.

Fairburn, C. G., Cooper, Z., & O'Connor, M. (2014). *Eating Disorder Examination, Edition 17.0D*. Oxford, UK: Center for Research on Dissemination at Oxford.—Measure is available online at *www.credo-oxford.com/7.2.html*. The EDE 17.0 is freely available online and confers DSM-5 eating disorder diagnoses, a global severity score, and subscale scores indexing Restraint, Eating Concern, Weight Concern, and Shape Concern.

Fichter, M. M., Herpertz, S., Quadflieg, N., & Herpertz-Dahlmann, B. (1998). Structured Interview for Anorexic and Bulimic disorders for DSM-IV and ICD-10: Updated (third) revision. *International Journal of Eating Disorders, 24*(3), 227–249.—Measure is available online at *www.klinikum.uni-muenchen.de/klinik-und-poliklinik-fuer-psychiatrie-und-psychother-apie/en/forschung/epidemiologie*. The SIAB-EX confers both current and lifetime eating-disorder diagnoses based on DSM-IV and ICD-10.

Forbush, K. T., Wildes, J. E., Pollack, L. O., Dunbar, D., Luo, J., Patterson, K., et al. (2013). Development and validation of the Eating Pathology Symptoms Inventory (EPSI). *Psychological Assessment, 25*, 859–878. Measure available online at *https://psych.ku.edu/sites/ psych.ku.edu/files/docs/cv/epsi.pdf*.—The EPSI, which is freely available online, is a 45-item self-report questionnaire measuring Body Dissatisfaction, Binge Eating, Cognitive Restraint, Purging, Muscle Building, Restricting, Excessive Exercise, and Negative Attitudes toward Obesity.

Garner, D. M. (2004). *Eating Disorder Inventory–3 professional manual*. Lutz, FL: Psychological Assessment Resources.—The EDI-3 provides a continuous measure of eating disorder severity in the domains of eating disorder risk (i.e., drive for thinness, bulimia, and body dissatisfaction), as well as co-occurring psychopathology (i.e., low self-esteem, personal alienation, interpersonal insecurity, interpersonal alienation, interoceptive deficits, emotional dysregulation, perfectionism, asceticism, and maturity fears); to obtain a copy, contact Psychological Assessment Resources, Inc., at *www.parinc.com*.

PhenX Toolkit. (2016). Consensus measures for Phenotypes and eXposures (PhenX). Retrieved August 21, 2015, from *www.phenx.org*.—Funded by the National Human Genome Research Institute with cofunding by the National Institute of Health, the PhenX Toolkit uses a consensus process and considers input from the scientific community on proposed measures.

Sysko, R., Glasofer, D. R., Hildebrandt, T., Klimek, P., Mitchell, J. E., Berg, K. C., et al. (2015). The Eating Disorder Assessment for DSM-5 (EDA-5): Development and validation of a structured interview for feeding and eating disorders. *International Journal of Eating Disorders, 48*(5), 452–463.—The EDA-5 is a semistructured interview meant to assist clinicians in the assessment of a feeding or eating disorders according to DSM-5 criteria, and is freely available online at *https://modeleda5.wordpress.com*.

Thomas, J. J., Roberto, C. A., & Berg, K. A. (2014). The Eating Disorder Examination: A semistructured interview for the assessment of the specific psychopathology of eating disorders. *Advances in Eating Disorders: Theory, Research and Practice, 2*(2), 190–203.—The authors review the innovations and limitations of this "gold standard" assessment and highlight directions for future research in eating disorder assessment.

Thomas, J. J., Roberto, C. A., & Berg, K. A. (2015). Assessment measures, then and now—A look back at seminal measures and a look forward to the brave new world. In B. T. Walsh, R. Sysko, D. Glasofer, & E. Attia (Eds.), *Handbook of assessment and treatment of eating disorders* (pp. 137–156). Arlington, VA: American Psychiatric Association.—This chapter provides a comprehensive review of the reliability, validity, strengths, and weaknesses of evidence-based interview measures of eating disorder psychopathology.

Cognitive Behavior Therapy and Eating Disorders

CHRISTOPHER G. FAIRBURN

ognitive behavior therapy (CBT) is the term for a class of theory-driven psychological treatments. These treatments share the premise that cognitive change is needed to overcome certain mental health problems. Accordingly, cognitive change is a central goal of the CBTs.

CBT was developed in the 1960s by Beck and colleagues as a short-term outpatient treatment for depression. It has evolved considerably since, with there now being distinct forms of CBT for a variety of disorders. These differ from each other and from Beck's CBT for depression, which remains largely unchanged. The leading indications for CBT are most anxiety disorders, depression, and the eating disorders. What is not widely appreciated is that the eating disorders provide the strongest indication for CBT.

CBT and eating disorders have been described as a "perfect match." One of the most distinctive features of the great majority of eating disorders—that is, anorexia nervosa (AN), bulimia nervosa (BN) and their variants—is the overevaluation of shape, weight, and control over eating. As this psychopathology is cognitive in nature, and most eating disorder features appear to stem directly or indirectly from it, this psychopathology is a natural target of treatment. Hence, it is the central target of CBT for eating disorders.

CBT for BN

CBT for eating disorders has its origins in the late 1970s, when CBTs for AN and BN began to be developed. The treatment for BN attracted particular attention because the disorder had just been identified and described as "intractable." The treatment focuses on the normalization of eating habits, the reduction of concerns about shape and weight, and the maintenance of change. It involves about 20 individual outpatient treatment sessions over 5 months.

Between 1981 and 2000, CBT for BN (CBT-BN) was the subject of numerous randomized controlled trials (RCTs) in which it was compared with waiting-list control conditions, other psychological treatments, dismantled versions of CBT-BN, and various forms of medication. The results were consistent. About 40% of patients who entered treatment ceased to binge and purge, an effect that was well maintained over the following year, the period of greatest risk of relapse. This response was as great or greater than that seen with all the other treatments. As a result, CBT-BN has been endorsed by most national clinical guidelines as the leading empirically supported treatment for BN.

CBT for Binge Eating Disorder

In the 1990s, CBT-BN was adapted to make it suitable for the treatment of binge eating disorder (BED). This mainly necessitated simplifying the treatment because there is less eating disorder psychopathology to address in BED than in BN. In common with the other leading treatments for BED—interpersonal psychotherapy (IPT) and guided self-help—about 60% of patients stop binge eating in response to CBT for BED (CBT-BED).

Self-Help Forms of CBT

Also in the 1990s, CBT-BN was converted into a self-help format, so that it could be made more widely available. This required that the treatment be "program-led" rather than "therapist-led." Several cognitive behavioral self-help programs for binge eating problems have been developed and published as books. They are all designed to be used either on their own or with support from a nonspecialist guide (guided self-help). Both approaches have been evaluated, although more is known about the effectiveness of the guided form of treatment delivery. Guided self-help is remarkably potent as a treatment for BED but much less so as a treatment for BN.

Transdiagnostic CBT

At the turn of the 21st century, CBT-BN was reconceptualized. Instead of being viewed as a treatment for BN, it was realized that it was a treatment for the psychopathology present in BN; that is, binge eating, extreme weight control behavior (strict dieting, purging, overexercising, etc.), overconcern about shape and weight, and the tendency to use eating to modulate mood or to cope with difficult circumstances. Because this psychopathology exists across the eating disorders (i.e., also in AN and the variants of AN and BN), it was therefore predicted that the therapeutic strategies and procedures that were proving successful in addressing the psychopathology of BN should also be capable of addressing the same psychopathology when it is seen in these other eating disorders. Accordingly, CBT-BN was adjusted so that it could be used with any form of eating disorder; that is, it was converted to being "transdiagnostic" in its clinical range. At the same time, aspects of CBT-BN were modified in an attempt to make it more effective overall. In particular, there was increased emphasis on engaging and retaining patients; a new strategy was developed for addressing the mechanisms that maintain the patient's eating disorder psychopathology, and in particular the disturbance of body image; and metacognitive strategies were introduced to minimize the risk of relapse. The resulting treatment was termed "enhanced CBT," or CBT-E. Figure 46.1 illustrates the structure

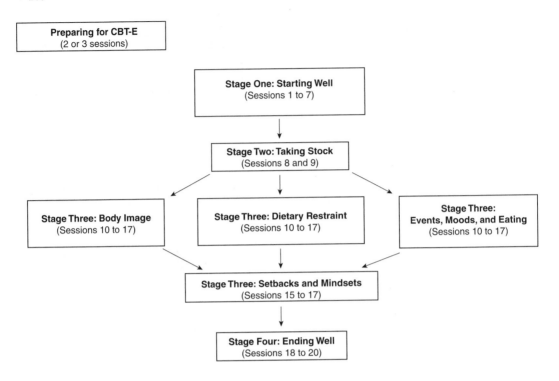

FIGURE 46.1. The "CBT-E map" illustrating the structure of CBT-E (focused, 20-session version). From the Web-Centred Training Programme in CBT-E (*credo-oxford.com*). Copyright © 2014 Christopher G. Fairburn.

of the treatment, and Figure 46.2 shows the transdiagnostic theory from which each patient's treatment is derived.

There are two forms of CBT-E, a "focused" form and a "broad" form. The focused form is the default version, and it designed for the majority of patients. It focuses exclusively on the modification of the patient's eating disorder psychopathology. The broad version is intended for a subgroup of patients in whom certain specific difficulties, distinct from the eating disorder, contribute to its persistence. These difficulties are extreme perfectionism, marked low self-esteem, and severe interpersonal problems. If one or more of these difficulties is present, and appears to be maintaining the eating disorder, then the broad version of CBT-E is designed to be used because it addresses both the eating disorder psychopathology and the external difficulty at the same time.

CBT-E also exists in two lengths. There is a 20-session version (over 20 weeks) for patients who are not underweight and an extended version for patients who need to regain weight. This is typically 30–40 sessions long (over 30–40 weeks); the increase in length is needed to address the reluctance of these patients to regain weight and the time it takes for them to do so.

The first report on CBT-E was published in 2003; the treatment guide (manual) was published in 2008; and the results of the first RCT were published in 2009. Since then, there have been numerous further studies of the treatment. These have confirmed that CBT-E is transdiagnostic in its clinical range. There is evidence supporting its use with

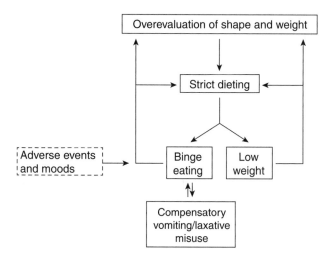

FIGURE 46.2. The transdiagnostic theory of the maintenance of eating disorder psychopathology. From the Web-Centred Training Programme in CBT-E (*credo-oxford.com*). Copyright © 2014 Christopher G. Fairburn.

patients with AN, BN, BED, and the many other eating disorder presentations. It can also be used with adolescents (age 12 or over) with only minor modifications.

The main research findings are as follows:

1. In adult patients who are not underweight (body mass index [BMI] > 17.5 kg/m²), it has been found that two-thirds make a full response by the end of treatment (intent-to-treat findings). This response is well maintained over the following year (CBT-E data from two RCTs conducted at two centers; $N = 219$). In such patients the focused form of CBT-E appears to be as effective as the broad form, but there is the suggestion of a moderator effect, with patients who have severe perfectionism, low self-esteem, or interpersonal difficulties responding better to the broad version. This finding needs to be replicated.

2. In adult patients who are underweight (BMI = 15.0–17.5 kg/m²), the response rate is lower than that of patients who are not underweight, with about 40% regaining a healthy weight by the end of treatment (intent-to-treat findings). This figure drops slightly over the following year (data from three independent cohorts from three centers; $N = 99$). The response of underweight adolescent patients appears to be better and faster than that of adults, and similar to that obtained with family-based treatment (cohort from one center; $N = 49$).

3. CBT-E has been compared with two other psychological treatments. With all patients who are not underweight, it has been found to be more effective than 20 sessions of IPT, and, with patients with BN, it has been found to be markedly superior to 100 sessions of psychoanalytic psychotherapy.

CBT-E has been adapted for use in inpatient and day patient settings. The results are promising (two cohorts from one center; $N = 107$). There have also been reports of its effectiveness in routine clinical settings. Data from three "real-world" clinics (three independent cohorts; $N = 600$) indicate that the outcome of patients who complete CBT-E or a CBT-E-like treatment is similar to that obtained in the main RCTs, but the completion rates are substantially lower.

Looking Forward

CBT for eating disorders has come a long way over the past 30 or so years. What was once a treatment for adults with BN is now a treatment for adolescents and adults, and for most eating disorder presentations. Its effectiveness and broad clinical range make CBT an attractive first-line treatment for use in many clinical settings, and it is already being recommended by national clinical guidelines.

All treatment innovations take a long time to be accepted and widely used. CBT for eating disorders is no exception. There are many reasons for this. One barrier to its dissemination may have been overcome, however. This is therapist training. The huge demand for training in CBT-E stimulated the development of a new, scalable form of training, so-called "Web-centered" training. This is now freely available worldwide.

There are obvious next steps for CBT-E. It needs to be made more efficient and more effective. This will require identifying the mediators of its effects, so that the active ingredients can be enhanced and the redundant elements discarded. The broad form of CBT-E in particular merits further study. CBT-E also needs to be compared with family-based treatment for adolescents in the hope that moderators of response will be identified, so that patients can to allocated to the treatment that best suits them. The use of CBT-E in routine clinical settings also needs further study; a major goal is to increase the treatment completion rate. Last, CBT-E needs to be made directly available to patients with eating disorders.

Acknowledgments

Christopher G. Fairburn's research on eating disorders has been supported by a succession of program grants from the Wellcome Trust (046386). Dr. Fairburn himself is supported by a Principal Research Fellowship from the Wellcome Trust (046386).

Suggested Reading

Cooper, Z., & Bailey-Straebler, S. (2015). Disseminating evidence-based psychological treatments for eating disorders. *Current Psychiatry Reports, 17*(3), 12.—An analysis of the barriers to the dissemination and implementation of evidence-based psychological treatments and a description of potential solutions.

Dalle Grave, R. (2011). *Intensive cognitive behavior therapy for eating disorders.* Hauppauge, NY: Nova Science.—An account of how inpatient and day patient settings may implement CBT-E.

Dalle Grave, R., Calugi, S., Doll, H. A., & Fairburn, C. G. (2013). Enhanced cognitive behaviour therapy for adolescents with anorexia nervosa: An alternative to family therapy? *Behaviour Research and Therapy, 51*, R9–R12.—A report on the effects of CBT-E in adolescents with AN.

Fairburn, C. G. (2008). *Cognitive behavior therapy and eating disorders.* New York: Guilford Press.—A detailed guide to the theory and practice of CBT-E.

Fairburn, C. G., Bailey-Straebler, S., Basden, S., Doll, H. A., Jones, R., Murphy, R., et al. (2015). A transdiagnostic comparison of enhanced cognitive behaviour therapy (CBT-E) and interpersonal psychotherapy in the treatment of eating disorders. *Behaviour Research and Therapy, 70*, 64–71.—The second transdiagnostic RCT to evaluate the effectiveness of CBT-E with patients who are not underweight.

Fairburn, C. G., Cooper, Z., Doll, H. A., O'Connor, M. E., Palmer, R. L., & Dalle Grave, R. (2013). Enhanced cognitive behaviour therapy for adults with anorexia nervosa: A UK–Italy study. *Behaviour Research and Therapy, 51*, R2–R8.—A report on the effects of CBT-E in adults with AN.

Tabri, N., Murray, H. B., Thomas, J. J., Franko, D. L., Herzog, D. B., & Eddy, K. T. (2015). Overvaluation of body shape/weight and engagement in non-compensatory weight-control behaviors in eating disorders: Is there a reciprocal relationship? *Psychological Medicine, 45*(14), 2951–2958.—A test of key aspects of the transdiagnostic theory of eating disorders.

Turner, H., Marshall, E., Stopa, L., & Waller, G. (2015). Cognitive-behavioural therapy for outpatients with eating disorders: Effectiveness for a transdiagnostic group in a routine clinical setting. *Behaviour Research and Therapy, 68*, 70–75.—A report on the effectiveness of CBT in a routine clinical setting.

Waller, G., Cordery, H., Corstorphine, E., Hinrichsen, H., Lawson, R., Mountford, V., et al. (2007). *Cognitive behavioral therapy for eating disorders*. Cambridge, UK: Cambridge University Press.—A guide to the use of a more generic form of CBT than CBT-E.

Wilson, G. T., & Zandberg, L. J. (2012). Cognitive-behavioral guided self-help for eating disorders: Effectiveness and scalability. *Clinical Psychology Review, 32*, 343–357.—A narrative review of the effectiveness and utility of guided cognitive-behavioral self-help.

47

Interpersonal Psychotherapy

DENISE E. WILFLEY
DAWN M. EICHEN

Interpersonal psychotherapy (IPT), developed as a short-term, outpatient therapy for depression by Klerman and colleagues (1984), has been successful in treating bulimia nervosa (BN) and binge eating disorder (BED). IPT is based on the tenet that problems in interpersonal functioning contribute to the development and maintenance of psychiatric symptoms. IPT aims to identify problematic interpersonal patterns associated with the onset and maintenance of symptoms, and to develop goals and strategies to change maladaptive interpersonal functioning to improve symptoms. This chapter reviews the link between interpersonal functioning and eating disorders, provides an overview of IPT treatment and evidence in support of its use for eating disorders, and concludes with a discussion of future directions.

Interpersonal Functioning in Eating Disorders

Impaired interpersonal functioning is a known risk factor for eating disorders. Theoretical models for the use of IPT with these disorders posit that problems in interpersonal functioning lead to negative affect and low self-esteem, which then result in disordered eating behaviors as a coping mechanism. These symptoms are then thought to exacerbate interpersonal problems, perpetuating the cycle. IPT works to disrupt this cycle by supporting changes in interpersonal functioning, thus reducing negative affect and, in turn, symptoms.

Research support for the role of problems in interpersonal functioning in eating disorders includes findings that negative affect mediates social functioning and symptoms of eating disorders, and that greater interpersonal problems are associated with an earlier onset of binge eating; specific problems include difficulties with interpersonal flexibility and ineffective interpersonal styles, such as being too dominant or too submissive. Laboratory findings have shown that when individuals are told whether they are rejected or accepted by a group, those who are rejected eat more than those who are not; among those rejected, higher negative affect was related to consuming more food. Therefore, research supports an interpersonal model for eating disorders.

Treatment Description

IPT is typically delivered across 15–20 sessions over 4–5 months, divided into three phases: initial, intermediate, and termination. The *initial phase* (up to five sessions) begins with a thorough psychiatric history and diagnostic evaluation of the presenting symptoms. The therapist then explains the diagnosis of the eating disorder and treatment expectations, so the client can understand that his or her symptoms are part of a known, treatable condition, thereby normalizing the condition and instilling optimism for recovery. A specialized semistructured assessment of the current and past social functioning of the client is then conducted. This evaluation is known as the interpersonal inventory (IPI), which sets the framework for IPT.

During the IPI, the therapist, in collaboration with the client, explores current and past social functioning and relationships, paying close attention to patterns and potential changes that occurred prior to the onset of symptoms. The IPI also allows for a thorough understanding of the important relationships in the client's life and the quality of these relationships. Throughout the IPI, the therapist and client make connections between interpersonal functioning and symptoms of the eating disorder. These connections are fundamental to the creation of the interpersonal formulation whereby the symptoms are related to at least one of the problem areas central to IPT: grief, interpersonal role disputes, role transitions, and interpersonal deficits. The identification of a problem area is a collaborative process, through which the therapist and client establish appropriate goals and strategies to practice over the course of the intervention. The collaborative nature of the IPI is impactful for clients, allowing them to understand the connection between their interpersonal functioning and their symptoms, and how working in IPT will help to alleviate their symptoms. Thus, the client feels invested in treatment from the outset and can progress quickly once the therapeutic work begins in the next phase of IPT.

In the *intermediate phase* (8–10 sessions), the therapist employs strategies based on the agreed-upon problem area. For a client experiencing grief, the therapist facilitates the mourning process, assisting the client in developing new relationships and activities to offset the loss. *Interpersonal role disputes* are defined as conflict with a significant relationship (e.g., roommate, spouse, family member), that typically involves differential expectations of roles in the relationship. The therapist aids in understanding the nature of the dispute and generating options for resolution. If resolution is not possible, the therapist assists the client in ending the relationship and coping with its termination. *Role transitions* involve difficulties dealing with a change in life status, such as getting a new job or moving away from home. The therapist helps process the positive and negative aspects of the new role and how to achieve a sense of mastery within the new role. Last, for *interpersonal deficits,* which are identified by chronic or long-standing difficulties in creating or sustaining relationships, the therapist may use the therapist–client relationship to help develop skills to improve the client's existing relationships or to help him or her build new ones.

IPT sessions in the intermediate phase focus on the present, and the therapist consistently links symptom presentation and changes in symptoms with changes in interpersonal functioning. The therapist remains active but not directive, which helps the client focus on generating his or her own solutions to the identified problem area(s).

In the *termination phase* (the last four or five sessions, sometimes biweekly), clients are encouraged to summarize the gains they have made, making sure they elucidate the connection between symptom improvements and improvements in their interpersonal functioning. The therapist helps the client address feelings associated with termination, creating plans to maintain positive changes, detailing continued areas for improvement and identifying and addressing signs of relapse.

Group IPT

IPT can be effectively administered in a group format and might potentially have added benefits over individual treatment as long as sufficient attention is paid to the development of an individualized goal or goals based on the client's identified problem area. The group setting allows the therapist to view clients' *in vivo* social interactions with other group members and provides a context to work on interpersonal skills. Therapists remain active in the group by encouraging appropriate disclosure, fostering cohesiveness, and helping to maintain the focus on each individual's problem areas and goals. It is essential that the therapist meet individually with each group member prior to beginning a course of group IPT, to conduct an IPI to establish individual problem areas and goals. This allows the group leader to ensure that each individual group member is staying on target by working on his or her individual goals. Individual meetings should occur again at midtreatment to assess progress and refine treatment goals, and again at the end of treatment to review progress and evaluate what future work may be needed to maintain or improve upon gains made during treatment.

Research on IPT for Eating Disorders

Bulimia Nervosa

IPT is the only treatment that has demonstrated long-term outcomes for BN comparable to those of cognitive-behavioral therapy (CBT), making IPT a viable alternative to CBT. Although studies have shown that CBT results in higher rates of binge eating abstinence and lower rates of purging at completion of treatment, effects of IPT and CBT are indistinguishable at 8 and 12 months following treatment. However, the studies that indicated differential rates of improvement between CBT and IPT early in treatment utilized a less potent form of IPT, one that did not include the therapist linking changes in eating disorder symptoms to changes in interpersonal functioning.

Binge Eating Disorder

IPT has demonstrated effectiveness for adults with BED in both group and individual formats. In a randomized controlled trial (RCT) examining comparative efficacy of group IPT and group CBT, both IPT and CBT demonstrated significant and comparable recovery from binge eating in individuals at posttreatment of 73 and 79%, respectively, with significant effects sustained at 1-year follow-up. A long-term follow-up study of a subset of these participants showed that both treatments demonstrated continued efficacy 4 years following treatment cessation. A multisite trial comparing IPT to CBT guided self-help (CBTgsh) and to behavioral weight loss treatment (BWL) showed that IPT and CBTgsh were both significantly more effective at reducing binge eating than BWL. Exploration of moderators showed that IPT was more effective than both CBTgsh and BWL for individuals with lower self-esteem and higher initial eating pathology. Furthermore, IPT resulted in the fewest dropouts. IPT was also found to be equally efficacious for individuals who responded rapidly to treatment and for those who were slower to respond. However, the same pattern did not hold true for rapid versus nonrapid responders to CBTgsh; rapid responders had better treatment outcomes than nonrapid responders to CBTgsh.

Anorexia Nervosa

Efficacy data of IPT for anorexia nervosa (AN) are limited. One study demonstrated that no differences between IPT, CBT, and a control condition called specialist supportive clinical management (SSCM) were found at long-term follow-up (at least 5 years posttreatment), although SSCM had better outcomes than IPT at the immediate posttreatment assessment time point. Given the overlap in psychopathology seen in AN and BN, and evidence that interpersonal factors serve as a risk factor in the development of AN, it is likely that IPT can be of some benefit to individuals with AN. However, due to the severity of AN, IPT might be most effective in conjunction with other therapies or be most effective in helping to maintain treatment gains or prevent relapse. Future research is needed to better understand IPT's potential role in the treatment for AN.

Prevention of Excess Weight Gain

Loss-of-control (LOC) eating, a known risk factor for the development of BED and obesity, is a potential early target of preventive interventions. A modified form of IPT has been developed and tested for the prevention of excess weight gain (IPT-WG) in adolescents at risk for excessive weight gain and BED due to the presence of LOC eating. Results from a pilot study that compared IPT-WG to a standard health education program demonstrated that IPT-WG was a feasible intervention, as adolescents in the IPT group were more likely to experience reductions in LOC eating and less-than-expected weight gain. A subsequent RCT revealed that girls in both groups experienced reductions in LOC eating and less-than-expected weight gain. However, moderator analyses suggested that IPT may be a better treatment for ethnic/minority adolescents because it resulted in greater decreases of LOC eating than the health education program for these participants. Additional study is needed to understand the full impact of IPT-WG, especially over a longer period of follow-up.

Future Developments

Briefer Forms of IPT for Eating Disorders

This chapter has focused on IPT for eating disorders, adapted from the original IPT developed for depression, which has traditionally been administered over 12–20 sessions. However, a brief form of IPT (5–10 sessions) has demonstrated effectiveness for some forms of depression and a brief 10-session format for BN that has been pilot-tested led to improvements in eating disorder symptoms compared to a waiting-list control. We and our colleagues are currently testing a brief form of IPT for the treatment of eating disorders on college campuses. College counseling centers, where many individuals present for treatment of eating disorders, often have strict session limits and are in high demand to deliver services to numerous students. A brief form of IPT could be very effective in this setting, especially given how interpersonal functioning is such an essential part of a college student's life.

Training in IPT for Eating Disorders

In addition to its effectiveness for eating disorders, IPT's broader applicability to comorbid conditions such as depression, and more recently for posttraumatic stress disorder, make it a valuable treatment for clinicians to master. Furthermore, IPT for eating disorders, although viewed as a specialist treatment, can easily be learned by experienced clinicians because it involves the application of general therapeutic skills in a focused manner within a specific interpersonal framework. Unfortunately, despite these advantages, IPT is not widely used by practitioners. Accordingly, it is important that training in IPT be incorporated into educational curricula and made available to practitioners who may not have had the opportunity to learn IPT during their graduate training. An unfortunate by-product of the unavailability of training in IPT for eating disorders is that, currently, only a limited number of individuals are qualified to train others and to supervise their delivery of IPT for eating disorders. To meet this need, ourselves and our colleagues are currently evaluating the effectiveness of two methods for training providers. Additionally, it will be important for future research to help determine how best to harness technology as a cost-effective way to train larger numbers of individuals.

Acknowledgment

Denise E. Wilfley and Dawn M. Eichen are supported by National Research Service Grant No. T32HL007456.

Suggested Reading

Agras, W. S., Walsh, B. T., Fairburn, C. G., Wilson, G. T., & Kraemer, H. C. (2000). A multicenter comparison of cognitive-behavioral therapy and interpersonal psychotherapy for bulimia nervosa. *Archives of General Psychiatry, 57,* 459–466.—A replication study on the original comparison study of CBT and IPT conducted by Fairburn and colleagues.

Fairburn, C. G. (1997). Interpersonal psychotherapy for bulimia nervosa. In D. M. Garner & P. E. Garfinkel (Eds.), *Handbook of treatment for eating disorders* (pp. 278–294). New York: Guilford Press.—A treatment description of using IPT for BN.

Hilbert, A., Hildebrandt, T., Agras, W. S., Wilfley, D. E, & Wilson, G. T. (2015). Rapid response in psychological treatments for binge eating disorder. *Journal of Consulting and Clinical Psychology, 83,* 649–654.—An analysis of short- and long-term effects of rapid response across three different treatments, including IPT, for BED.

Klerman, G. L., Weissman, M. M., Rounsaville, B. J., & Chevron, E. S. (1984). *Interpersonal psychotherapy of depression.* New York: Basic Books.—The original manual for IPT.

Markowitz, J. C., Petkova, E., Neria, Y., Van Meter, P. E., Zhao, Y., Hembree, E., et al. (2015). Is exposure necessary?: A randomized clinical trial of interpersonal psychotherapy for PTSD. *American Journal of Psychiatry, 172,* 430–440.—Evidence for IPT's similar efficacy to CBT in the treatment of posttraumatic stress disorder akin to earlier research comparing IPT and CBT for the treatment of BN.

Rieger, E., Van Buren, D. J., Bishop, M., Tanofsky-Kraff, M., Welch, R., & Wilfley, D. E. (2010). An eating disorder-specific model of interpersonal psychotherapy (IPT-ED): Causal pathways and treatment implications. *Clinical Psychology Review, 30*, 400–410.—A theoretical model of how IPT works for individuals with eating disorders.

Tanofsky-Kraff, M., Shomaker, L. B., Wilfley, D. E., Young, J. F., Sbrocco, T., Stephens, M., et al. (2014). Targeted prevention of excess weight gain and eating disorders in high-risk adolescent girls: A randomized controlled trial. *American Journal of Clinical Nutrition, 100*, 1010–1018.—A study comparing IPT-WG to a health education program.

Wilfley, D. E., Iacavino, J. M., & Van Buren, D. J. (2012) Interpersonal psychotherapy for eating disorders. In J. C. Markowitz & M. M. Weissman (Eds.), *Casebook of interpersonal psychotherapy* (pp. 125–148). New York: Oxford University Press.—A clinical description of the use of IPT to treat eating disorders, including a case example.

Wilfley, D. E., MacKenzie, K. R., Welch, R. R., Ayres., V. E., & Weissman, M. M. (2000). *Interpersonal psychotherapy for group*. New York: Basic Books.—A description of group IPT.

Wilfley, D. E., Welch, R. R., Stein, R. I., Spurrell, E. B., Cohen, L. R., Saelens, B. E., et al. (2002). A randomized comparison of group cognitive-behavioral therapy and group interpersonal psychotherapy for the treatment of overweight individuals with binge eating disorder. *Archives of General Psychiatry, 59*(8), 713–721.—A study comparing group IPT and CBT.

Wilson, G. T., Wilfley, D. E., Agras, W. S., & Bryson, S. W. (2010). Psychological treatments of binge eating disorder. *Archives of General Psychiatry, 67*(1), 94–101.—A study comparing individual IPT to CBTgsh and BWL.

Family Therapy and Eating Disorders

DANIEL LE GRANGE
IVAN EISLER

The earliest clinical descriptions of anorexia nervosa (AN) were made by William Gull and Charles Lasègue in the late 19th century and assigned considerable responsibility for the development of this disorder to the parents or families of the sufferer. Accounts by these and other clinicians at the time described the influence of parents in the case of AN as "particularly pernicious" and recommended that patients should be separated from their families if there was any hope for success in treatment. Holding parents responsible for the development of an eating disorder, as advocated by these clinicians who first described AN, heralded an era of excluding parents from treatment (also referred to as "parentectomy"). While this strategy is now seldom pursued, excluding parents from therapy is still widespread today, with clinicians in several centers around the world considering such an approach as the current *modus operandi*.

It was not until the 1960s that families were brought back into the treatment fold through the work promoted by Salvador Minuchin and Mara Selvini-Palazzoli. While Minuchin and Selvini-Palazzoli's respective views of families with an eating disordered offspring were perhaps not quite as stridently negative as that of Gull, Lasègue, and their contemporaries, these clinicians viewed eating disorders as an expression of an underlying dysfunctional family system, although Minuchin also emphasized that there also needed to be a vulnerability in the child for an eating disorder to develop. Therefore, families were considered important *in* treatment *because* of the need to normalize family functioning in order for the eating disorder to lose its role in the family system. While we cannot overlook the possibility that some family factors may increase the risk or contribute to the maintenance of the disorder, there is no consistent empirical evidence for the existence of specific family factors having an etiological role in the development of eating disorders. On the other hand, there is a growing body of evidence that highlights the crucial role parents can play in the recovery of their offspring. Such a stance poses a challenge to the perhaps fading orthodoxy of excluding parents from treatment.

Systematic Research in Family Therapy for Eating Disorders

Systematic research, in the form of controlled treatment studies utilizing family therapy for eating disorders, was relatively late to appear, but despite this rather slow start to methodologically rigorous inquiry, there now are more than a dozen randomized clinical trials (RCTs) in eating disorders that have compared either family therapy with one or two other treatment modalities, or different formats of family therapy for this patient population.

Family Therapy for Adolescent Eating Disorders

Anorexia Nervosa

The initial RCTs in eating disorders evaluated the relative efficacy of family therapy and individual supportive psychotherapy, as well as different formats of family therapy, for adolescents with anorexia nervosa (AN). These studies were conducted at the Maudsley Hospital in London, starting in the 1980s, and although somewhat underpowered, they largely support family therapy as an initial treatment for this patient population. Building on earlier family therapy approaches, this early research helped shape the treatment into a distinct form of family therapy with a specific focus on managing the eating disorder. More recent research has used manualized versions of this treatment (variously referred to as family-based treatment [FBT], Maudsley family therapy, or anorexia-focused family therapy [FT-AN]), and several published RCTs have broadened the evidence base for family involvement in supporting the ill adolescent with AN. Chief among these are four recent treatment studies that underscore the utility of the parents' role in their child's recovery.

First, setting out to test the relative efficacy of family therapy and individual adolescent-focused therapy, a two-site study conducted at Chicago and Stanford demonstrated that family therapy was superior to individual therapy at 6-month and 12-month follow-up in terms of remission. In this study, *remission* was defined as achieving at least 95% of expected body weight, in addition to the absence of eating disordered thoughts (as measured by the Eating Disorder Examination; EDE). Some advances have been made in terms of potential predictors and moderators of treatment and *how* family therapy actually works. In terms of predictors of outcome, this study, in addition to a few others, clearly confirms that early weight gain in family therapy (about 2 kg by the fourth treatment session) strongly predicts weight recovery (above 95% of expected body weight) at the end of treatment. We have also learned that weight recovery at end of treatment is the best predictor of weight recovery at follow-up. As for moderators, both baseline eating disorder psychopathology and obsessions and compulsions related to the eating disorder moderate treatment effect on outcome. That is, family therapy is especially suitable for patients with high levels of eating disorder psychopathology when compared to individual therapy. It would appear that the early focus on changing the eating behaviors, which is a key aspect of this family therapy approach, enables parents to better support their severely unwell offspring, compared to an individually focused therapy. In addition, it has been shown that one potentially potent mechanism of action in this treatment is its capacity to enhance parental empowerment; that is, the more parents feel they have mastered the task of supporting their child in the refeeding process, the more effective family therapy turns out to be. It has also been demonstrated that remission in family therapy at the end of treatment is sustained over 3- to 5-year follow-up.

The second recent RCT was conducted at Westmead Children's Hospital in Sydney, Australia. While not comparing family therapy with another form of treatment, in this study, medically unstable patients with AN were randomized to one of two groups: medical stabilization with family therapy or weight restoration with family therapy. That is, patients in the medical stabilization group were admitted to hospital, but once they were medically stable, they were discharged to outpatient family therapy. For those randomized to weight restoration, patients were admitted, but once they were medically stable, they remained in hospital until they reached 90% of expected body weight. It was only at this point that they were discharged to outpatient family therapy. Remission was defined in terms of weight *and* EDE recovery. As hypothesized, there were no differences in terms of clinical status between these two groups at 12-month follow-up, bringing into question the need for hospitalization beyond the point of medical stability, provided that the parents are encouraged to support their child posthospitalization. This study underscores the positive role played by parents when they are supported through family therapy to help their offspring overcome this disorder.

The third RCT set out to test a hypothesis: whether the effectiveness of family therapy in the treatment of these patients is due to bringing families to work together per se, as is the case in systemic family therapy, or whether it is the specific way in which parents are coached and encouraged to support their adolescent with AN that is, at least in part, central to the effectiveness of family therapy. In this randomized design, patients and their families received either FT-AN (using the FBT manual) or a more generic family therapy (using the Leeds systemic family therapy manual), then followed up 12-months posttreatment. Remission was defined in terms of weight recovery. At this time point, there were no significant differences in percent expected body weight, eating disorder symptoms, or comorbid psychiatric symptoms. However, FBT did bring about faster weight gain early in treatment, with fewer hospital days for those requiring hospital admission. FBT was also more cost-effective, with lower mean treatment costs per patient (FBT = $9,000 vs. systemic family therapy = $18,000). The response to the two family therapies was moderated by obsessive–compulsive disorder (OCD) symptoms, with those with higher in obsessive–compulsive ratings responding better to systemic family therapy.

A fourth RCT was conducted at the Royal Children's Hospital in Melbourne, Australia. This study compared conjoint family therapy (using the FBT manual) to a separated version of this treatment (referred to as parent-focused therapy, or PFT). In this separated version of family therapy, a nurse monitors the adolescent patient, while the clinician works exclusively with the parents. Patients received 6 months of therapy and were followed up at 6 and 12 months. At posttreatment, the separated model of family therapy was superior to the conjoint model in terms of remission (defined in terms of weight *and* EDE recovery) (43 vs. 22%, respectively), but this difference was no longer statistically significant at 6- and 12-months posttreatment (39 vs. 22% and 37 vs. 29%). This study highlights the utility of a separated format of family therapy that might, in some ways, be less burdensome on the family.

In addition to these RCTs, several other efforts at adaptations of family therapy for adolescents with AN have been pursued. These studies vary in terms of their scope, but foremost among these are multifamily therapy, more intensive or higher level of care family therapy, telemedicine for family therapy, and family therapy for transition-age youth, among others. Taken together, a considerable body of evidence has accumulated, demonstrating the efficacy of family therapy as the initial treatment for adolescents with AN who are sufficiently medically stable for outpatient treatment. The mechanism(s) by which this treatment gains its efficacy, while still not fully elucidated, has become clearer. Yet there remains considerable work to be done to allow the identification of who is most likely to respond to family therapy. Similarly, it would be useful to determine how treatment should be modified for those who do not respond to family therapy, or whether alternative treatments with potential efficacy, such as cognitive-behavioral therapy (CBT) or interpersonal psychotherapy (IPT), should be employed.

Bulimia Nervosa

Compared to the strong support for the involvement of families in the treatment of adolescents with AN, less work has been conducted for adolescents with bulimia nervosa (BN). Only three RCTs have been published, and all three compared family therapy with an individual approach. The first of these studies comes from the London group at the Maudsley Hospital and compares family therapy with CBT guided self-care (CBT). *Remission,* defined as no binge eating and purging, was achieved in about 40% of participants 6 months posttreatment. There were no significant differences between the two groups in terms of abstinence rates, but in terms of secondary outcomes, CBT guided self-care produced a more rapid reduction of binge eating, lower cost, and greater acceptability among adolescents with BN.

The second published RCT was conducted at the same time and comes from the Chicago group. In this study, adolescents with BN were randomized to either family therapy or individual supportive psychotherapy. Defining remission as above, the family therapy was statistically and clinically superior to supportive therapy at the end of treatment (40 vs. 20% abstinence, respectively), as well as at 6-month follow-up (30 vs. 10% abstinence, respectively).

The third and, to date, the largest RCT was conducted at Chicago and Stanford. In this multisite study, adolescents with BN were randomized to either family therapy or CBT. Participants received treatment for 6 months and were followed up at 6- and 12-months posttreatment, and remission was defined in the same manner as the first two RCTs. At the end of treatment (39 vs. 20%) and at 6-month follow-up (44 vs. 25%), abstinence in family therapy was statistically and clinically superior to CBT. However, there was no difference in abstinence between these groups at the 12-month follow-up (49 vs. 32%).

None of these studies has been able to provide follow-up for these patients beyond 12-months posttreatment, and it therefore remains unclear whether the benefits derived from either family therapy or CBT were sustained beyond 1 or 2 years posttreatment. Given these three published RCTs, and notwithstanding the limited available data, family therapy shows great promise for this patient population, while CBT remains a viable alternative.

Family Therapy for Adult Eating Disorders

Family therapy for adults with eating disorders received some attention in the 1980s and early 1990s with two published studies from the London group. These two studies compared family therapy to individual supportive or individual psychodynamic therapy. Findings from both RCTs were equivocal, with the first study (with patients enrolled following a hospital weight restoration) showing somewhat greater short-term benefit from individual supportive therapy, while the second, purely outpatient study showed that both family therapy and psychodynamic psychotherapy were superior to individual supportive therapy. Therefore, the role that families may have in the treatment of adult patients remains largely unclear. Several other individual therapies have received considerable research attention for adult patients with AN (CBT, IPT and specialist supportive clinical management), and adults with BN (CBT, IPT). That said, involving the spouse or partner of the adult patient in treatment that leverages this relationship to support the patient's struggle with AN (Uniting Couples [in the treatment of] Anorexia Nervosa, or UCAN), has shown some considerable promise.

Conclusions

The effectiveness of family therapy for adolescents with AN is now quite well established. For most patients who are medically fit for outpatient treatment, involving the families in the care of the adolescent should be considered an effective initial treatment. Family therapy for adolescents with BN would appear to be a viable option, but unlike the clarity that has emerged in the case of AN, other treatments, such as CBT, seem equally effective. Family therapy for adults with an eating disorder seems much less effective compared to this mode of treatment for their adolescent counterparts, and research in this domain is mostly dormant. In contrast, research and clinical practice of family therapy for adolescent eating disorders have now been established at several centers across the world and further dissemination and adaptations are under way.

Suggested Reading

Agras, W. S., Lock, J., Brandt, H., Bryson, S. W., Dodge, E., Halmi, K. A., et al. (2014). Comparison of 2 family therapies for adolescent anorexia nervosa: A randomized parallel trial. *JAMA Psychiatry, 71*(11), 1279–1286.—The largest RCT for adolescents with AN, this study demonstrates that outcome in a specific eating disorder-focused family therapy is no different than that in a more generic systemic family therapy.

Eisler, I., Dare, C., Hodes, M., Russell, G., Dodge, E., & Le Grange, D. (2000). Family therapy for adolescent anorexia nervosa: The results of a controlled comparison of two family interventions. *Journal of Child Psychology and Psychiatry, 41*(6), 727–736.—This RCT shows that there are few differences in outcome between conjoint family therapy and separated family therapy, in which, in the latter, the adolescent and parents are not seen together in treatment.

Eisler, I., Dare, C., Russell, G. F., Szmukler, G., Le Grange, D., & Dodge, E. (1997). Family and individual therapy in anorexia nervosa: A 5-year follow-up. *Archives of General Psychiatry, 54*(11), 1025–1030.—This first long-term follow-up of a psychotherapy trial for eating disorders, to some extent, underscores the durable effect of family therapy for adolescents with AN.

Eisler, I., Simic, M., Blessitt, E., Dodge, L., et al. (2016). Maudsley service manual for child and adolescent eating disorders. Available at *www.national.slam.nhs.uk/wp-content/uploads/2011/11/Maudsley-Service-Manual-for-Child-and-Adolescent-Eating-Disorders-July-2016.pdf*.

Eisler, I., Wallis, A., & Dodge, E. (2015). What's new is old and what's old is new. In K. L. Loeb, D. Le Grange, & J. Lock (Eds.), *Family therapy for adolescent eating and weight disorders: New applications* (pp. 6–43). New York: Routledge.—In this chapter, the authors provide a historical perspective of the involvement of families in the treatment of eating disorders.

Le Grange, D., & Lock, J. (2007). *Treating bulimia in adolescents: A family-based approach.* New York: Guilford Press.—A treatment manual that outlines a family-based approach for adolescents with BN.

Le Grange, D., Hughes, E., Court, A., Yeo, M., Crosby, R., & Sawyer, S. (2016). Randomized clinical trial of parent-focused treatment and family-based treatment for adolescent anorexia nervosa. *Journal of the American Academy for Child and Adolescent Psychiatry, 55,* 683–692.—This third RCT highlights the utility of family therapy for AN and also demonstrates that CBT can be a helpful alternative treatment.

Le Grange, D., Lock, J., Agras, S., Bryson, S., & Jo, B. (2015). Randomized clinical trial of family-based treatment and cognitive-behavior therapy for adolescent bulimia nervosa. *Journal of the American Academy of Child and Adolescent Psychiatry, 54,* 886–894.—The third, and now the largest, RCT for adolescents with BN is a comparison of FBT-BN versus CBT for adolescents with BN. This RCT demonstrated a clear statistical and clinical benefit for FBT over CBT at the end-of-treatment as well as at the 6-month follow-up. However, there were no statistical differences between these two treatments at the 12-month follow-up mark.

Lock, J., & Le Grange, D. (2013). *Treatment manual for anorexia nervosa: A family-based approach* (2nd ed.). New York: Guilford Press.—A treatment manual of a family-based approach for adolescents with AN, highlighting treatment strategies across three phases of therapy.

Lock, J., Le Grange, D., Agras, W. S., Moye, A., Bryson, S. W., & Jo, B. (2010). Randomized clinical trial comparing family-based treatment with adolescent-focused individual therapy for adolescents with anorexia nervosa. *Archives of General Psychiatry, 67*(10), 1025–1032.—This RCT demonstrates the benefits of a family approach compared to an individual adolescent-focused approach at follow-up, but not at the end of treatment.

Madden, S., Miskovic-Wheatley, J., Wallis, A., Kohn, M., Lock, J., Le Grange, D., et al. (2015). A randomized controlled trial of inpatient treatment for anorexia nervosa in medically unstable adolescents. *Psychological Medicine, 45*(2), 415–427.—This is the only published RCT showing that long-term hospital refeeding in adolescent AN does not provide additional benefit over brief refeeding for medical stabilization, provided that the inpatient's stay is followed up by family therapy.

Schmidt, U., Lee, S., Beecham, J., Perkins, S., Treasure, J., Yi, I., et al. (2007). A randomized controlled trial of family therapy and cognitive behavior therapy guided self-care for adolescents with bulimia nervosa and related disorders. *American Journal of Psychiatry, 164*(4), 591–598.—The second of only three published RCTs for adolescents with BN, showing that there are few differences in outcome between family therapy and CBT guided self-care.

Psychopharmacological Treatment of Anorexia Nervosa and Bulimia Nervosa

LAUREL E. S. MAYER

While psychological and behavioral interventions are generally viewed as the first-choice treatments for patients with eating disorders, medications provide an additional therapeutic option. Advances in the pharmacological treatment of bulimia nervosa (BN) have been more rapid than those for anorexia nervosa (AN). The increased prevalence of BN relative to AN, and the fact that most patients with BN can be treated on an outpatient basis, have made the treatment studies of BN much simpler logistically and less costly than similar studies of AN. In addition, the significant weight loss and starvation characteristic of AN may confer a metabolic state that interferes with the expected therapeutic effect of psychotropic medications.

Pharmacotherapy for AN

Treatment of AN is possibly the most vexing among the treatments of eating disorders. Its salient features—a relentless pursuit of thinness accompanied by an intense fear of weight gain, despite being significantly underweight—become highly entrenched and curiously resistant to change. Evidenced-based treatment approaches for weight gain rely on behavioral strategies, in part, due to the surprising lack of efficacy of medications. Medications known for their propensity to lead to (unwanted) weight gain in other populations seem inert when used to enhance weight gain in patients with AN. Furthermore, the "intense fear of weight gain" inhibits many patients from even considering a trial of such medications. Therefore, behavioral and psychosocial treatments remain the standard, and the search for effective pharmacological interventions continues.

Antidepressants

Selective Serotonin Reuptake Inhibitors

This class of antidepressant medications is among the most commonly prescribed for treatment of AN. A rationale supporting their use is the shared symptoms and comorbidities with depressive, anxiety, and obsessive–compulsive disorders, for which the efficacy of selective serotonin reuptake inhibitors (SSRIs) is now well established. Although not devoid of side effects, SSRIs are less dangerous and better tolerated than the previous generation of antidepressants (e.g., tricyclic antidepressants [TCAs], monoamine oxidase inhibitors [MAOIs]). Thus, the utility of SSRIs in the treatment of AN is of substantial clinical and theoretical interest.

Of the SSRIs, fluoxetine is the most studied. Whether prescribed to aid acute weight gain or to prevent relapse, studies do not support fluoxetine's superiority over placebo. In a randomized, double-blind, placebo-controlled study of 31 inpatients, weight and mood improved, but without a significant difference between the fluoxetine and placebo groups. An early study examining fluoxetine's effect on relapse prevention suggested greater benefit from fluoxetine compared to placebo. However, later, in a larger relapse prevention trial, fluoxetine conferred no benefit over placebo in time to relapse in the year following hospitalization. All participants had normalized weight on an inpatient unit or a partial hospitalization program prior to randomization, and received outpatient cognitive-behavioral therapy following discharge. Participants were stratified for presence of comorbid depression and subtype (binge–purge vs. restricting), but the results were similar: Fluoxetine had no significant effect on outcome.

Tricyclic Antidepressants

Known for their potential side effect of weight gain and their impact on mood and appetite, TCAs were studied as potential treatments before the introduction of the SSRIs. Clomipramine compared to placebo increased self-reported hunger but did not result in additional weight gain. In two placebo-controlled trials, amitriptyline showed no benefit over placebo. However, an inpatient study of amitriptyline compared to cyproheptadine suggested a modest reduction in the number of days needed to reach target weight (32 ± 17 days for amitriptyline vs. 36 ± 20 days for cyproheptadine vs. 45 ± 18 days for placebo). Because underweight patients with AN are at increased risk of cardiac conduction abnormalities, caution must be exercised when using TCAs because of associated cardiac side effects (e.g., slowing of electrical conduction, potential risks of prolonged QT interval).

Serotonin–Norepinephrine Reuptake Inhibitors

Serotonin–norepinephrine reuptake inhibitors (SNRIs) have not been studied in a controlled fashion; a few open-label trials exist, but, consistent with studies of SSRIs, they do not appear to offer much promise.

Antipsychotics

First-Generation Antipsychotics

The introduction of chlorpromazine in the 1950s was accompanied by great excitement regarding improved treatment of serious psychiatric illnesses, including AN. In early studies that used historical controls rather than randomization to placebo, chlorpromazine appeared to promote weight gain, but it also seemed to trigger binge eating and purging behaviors, thus limiting its utility. Small trials of pimozide and sulpiride were conducted in the early 1980s, but results were disappointing.

Second-Generation Antipsychotics

The introduction of second-generation antipsychotics with their improved side effect profile renewed interest in the potential efficacy of this class of medications for AN. Olanzapine appears to be the most promising to date, for its potential effects on both weight and anxiety. In a study of day hospital patients, those receiving olanzapine compared to placebo demonstrated a greater rate of weight gain, earlier achievement of target weight, and significant reductions in obsessive symptoms. Another small pilot study demonstrated superiority of olanzapine over placebo for weight gain in outpatients. A large and, it is hoped, definitive olanzapine versus placebo outpatient trial is currently (as of the writing of this chapter) being conducted at five sites. Evidence for the utility of other second-generation antipsychotics (e.g., aripiprazole, quetiapine, and risperidone) is lacking.

Anxiolytics and Other Classes of Medications

Given the intense fear and anxiety associated with eating and weight gain among patients with AN, other pharmacotherapy trials have focused on the anxiolytic properties of medications. A small trial of oral tetrahydrocannabinol (THC) compared to the benzodiazepine diazepam (Valium®) revealed increased agitation in the oral THC group but no effect on weight. A preliminary, crossover design study of dronabinol, a synthetic cannabinoid agonist, was suggestive of greater weight gain compared to placebo, but full interpretation was limited by a substantial order effect and a significant increase in physical activity. A more recent study aimed to increase meal intake (and by extension promote weight gain) by attempting to decrease premeal anxiety using alprazolam (Xanax®) compared to placebo. Although alprazolam was associated with increased sleepiness, no differences were detected between the drug and placebo groups in either premeal anxiety or food intake.

A small trial of lithium suggested a positive effect on weight gain, but the numerous monitoring requirements reduce enthusiasm for its use. Trials of zinc supplementation have been reported with mild benefits, and prokinetic agents (e.g., cisapride, since withdrawn from the U.S. market) have also been studied, without dramatic effect.

Pharmacotherapy for BN

In stark contrast to the absence of a significant role for medications in the treatment of AN, the utility of pharmacotherapeutic interventions for the treatment of BN is well established. A large number of medication trials have been conducted, and many have reported clinically significant reductions in the frequencies of binge eating and purging.

Antidepressants

SSRIs

The antidepressants are the most commonly studied class of medications for the treatment of BN, and fluoxetine is the only antidepressant with a U.S. Food and Drug

Administration (FDA)-approved indication for BN. In a seminal study comparing fluoxetine 60 mg/day to 20 mg/day to placebo, only the higher dose was found to be superior to placebo. This finding is the basis for the recommendation that if an antidepressant, particularly an SSRI, is prescribed to treat BN, a target dose at the upper therapeutic range for that medication should be chosen. Other SSRIs studied as potential treatments for BN include sertraline, citalopram, escitalopram, and fluvoxamine, all with good result.

Bupropion is also effective in reducing symptoms, but it has been associated with increased seizure risk in women with BN and is therefore contraindicated. Trazodone also significantly reduces binge–purge frequency, but it is not commonly used.

TCAs and MAOIs

Earlier studies with TCAs (e.g., nortryptiline, imipramine, desipramine) and MAOIs (e.g., phenelzine) demonstrated benefit compared to placebo in reducing bulimic symptoms. Because of the dietary restrictions required with MAOI use, this class of medication is rarely used for patients with BN. In part, this is because easing dietary restriction is often a behavioral treatment goal, and the conflicting recommendations relating to diet are potentially confusing. Additionally, the impulse dyscontrol behaviors common in BN may manifest as eating tyramine-containing foods, thus increasing risk of a hypertensive crisis.

Strategic Antidepressant Use

While many trials have demonstrated that medications offer significant reductions in binge eating–purging frequency, complete resolution of symptoms is less common. However, the absence of abstinence is not evidence of complete pharmacotherapy failure. Rather, in the case of persistent or minimally improved symptoms, switching to a different antidepressant medication, either within or between classes of antidepressants, may improve outcome. For example, in a study of desipramine (DMI) compared to placebo, those who were not significantly improved after 8 weeks discontinued DMI and were switched to fluoxetine. After 8 weeks of treatment, additional patients had improved.

Also of note, while depressive symptoms are common in BN, the presence of depressive symptoms does not predict the degree of improvement in bulimic symptoms with antidepressant treatment. That is, with respect to the eating disorder symptoms, patients with BN and depression and BN without depression respond similarly to antidepressant medication. This intriguing finding suggests that the mechanism of action of antidepressant response in BN may differ from that in depression.

Mood Stabilizers

In addition to the many options within the antidepressant class of medications, mood stabilizers have been examined as potential treatment options. Early controlled studies of phenytoin and carbamazepine did not demonstrate a robust response, although there was a suggestion that a small number of patients might benefit. Lithium may be effective in reducing BN symptoms, but only in patients with comorbid depression.

Topiramate has been more successful in reducing the urge to binge and purge, often concomitant with a decrease in appetite. However, topiramate use may also be accompanied by significant weight loss, a complicated issue for patients with BN, who struggle with body image issues and often a desire to lose weight, despite usually being within a healthy range. For these reasons, topiramate should be used judiciously in patients with BN.

Other Classes of Medications

Opiate Antagonists

Given the striking similarities between BN and addictive disorders, there is recurrent interest in using opiate antagonists as a novel treatment approach for BN. High-dose naltrexone has been shown to have modest benefit in decreasing purging frequency, although effects of lower doses of this medication did not differ from placebo effects. The lack of robust response and the increased side effects accompanying higher doses of naltrexone significantly reduce enthusiasm for its use.

Other Medications

The 5-HT3 antagonist and antinausea medication, ondansetron, has been shown to be effective in decreasing binge eating and purging, and its mechanism of action may be related to modifying vagal afferent activity. Given the documented delayed gastric emptying in patients with BN, a preliminary trial of the prokinetic antibiotic, erythromycin, was conducted, but results were disappointing. While gastric emptying modestly increased, there was no clinically significant effect on symptoms.

Support for Combined Psychopharmacology and Psychotherapy

A salient issue is not which medication should be prescribed, but whether combination treatment (i.e., psychotherapy and psychopharmacology) is more effective than either treatment alone. One meta-analysis of four randomized trials ($N = 141$) found the higher remission rate with combined treatment remission did not reach statistical significance when compared to medication alone, but another meta-analysis of six trials suggested that combined treatment *is* more efficacious than psychotherapy alone. Combined treatments are frequently complicated by higher dropout rates compared to psychotherapy-alone interventions, likely related to medication side effects. Thus, while not definitive, study results suggest that combination approaches may be more effective, and, for those who are willing, an appropriate initial treatment choice.

Conclusion

The search for effective pharmacotherapeutic interventions for AN remains an important ongoing challenge; in contrast, the pharmacological options for treatment of BN are broader and likely to expand with the introduction of new antidepressants to the market. For AN, while behavioral interventions to promote weight gain remain the primary treatment approach, olanzapine may offer adjunctive benefit. In BN, multiple solo, sequential, or combination treatment approaches can be confidently recommended.

Suggested Reading

Aigner, M., Treasure, J., Kaye, W., & Kasper, S. (2011). World Federation of Societies of Biological Psychiatry (WFSBP) guidelines for the pharmacological treatment of eating disorders. *World Journal of Biological Psychiatry, 12*(6), 400–443.—Review and practice guidelines from the World Federation of Societies of Biological Psychiatry, based on data available through 2011.

Attia, E., Haiman, C., Walsh, B. T., & Flater, S. R. (1998). Does fluoxetine augment the inpatient treatment of anorexia nervosa? *American Journal of Psychiatry, 155*(4), 548–551.—Trial of fluoxetine in 31 hospitalized patients demonstrating no difference in rate of weight gain or clinical outcome between drug and placebo.

Bacaltchuk, J., Trefiglio, R. P., Oliveira, I. R., Hay, P., Lima, M. S., & Mari, J. J. (2000). Combination of antidepressants and psychological treatments for bulimia nervosa: A systematic review. *Acta Psychiatrica Scandinavica, 101*(4), 256–264.—Meta-analysis of the literature suggesting combination psychotherapy and psychopharmacology is more effective than pharmacology alone in the treatment of BN.

Bissada, H., Tasca, G. A., Barber, A. M., & Bradwejn, J. (2008). Olanzapine in the treatment of low body weight and obsessive thinking in women with anorexia nervosa: A randomized, double-blind, placebo-controlled trial. *American Journal of Psychiatry, 165*(10), 1281–1288.—Double-blind trial suggesting subjects' greater weight gain and decreased obsessionality on olanzapine compared to placebo.

Levine, L. R. (1992). Fluoxetine in the treatment of bulimia nervosa. *Archives of General Psychiatry, 49*, 139–147.—Definitive, multisite, randomized, double-blind, 8-week outpatient trial of two doses of fluoxetine compared to placebo, demonstrating superiority of 60 mg/day of fluoxetine compared to 20 mg/day and placebo in the treatment of BN.

Walsh, B. T. (2013). The enigmatic persistence of anorexia nervosa. *American Journal of Psychiatry, 170*(5), 477–484. Review.—Describes the history of AN, including the remarkable conservation of presentation throughout time, and relative resistance to treatment, culminating in the proposal of a new model of understanding the illness.

Walsh, B. T., Kaplan, A. S., Attia, E., Olmsted, M., Parides, M., Carter, J. C., et al. (2006). Fluoxetine after weight restoration in anorexia nervosa: A randomized controlled trial. *Journal of the American Medical Association, 295*(22), 2605–2612.—Large, multisite, relapse prevention trial demonstrating no benefit of fluoxetine over placebo in preventing relapse in the year following discharge from inpatient treatment for AN.

Walsh, B. T., Wilson, G. T., Loeb, K. L., Devlin, M. J., Pike, K. M., Roose, S. P., et al. (1997). Medication and psychotherapy in the treatment of bulimia nervosa. *American Journal of Psychiatry, 154*(4), 523–531.—Early study comparing different treatment modalities including psychotherapy alone, medication alone, and their combination for the outpatient treatment of BN, and demonstrating the benefit of initiating treatment with fluoxetine following unsuccessful treatment with desipramine.

Psychopharmacological Treatment of Binge Eating Disorder

JAMES I. HUDSON
HARRISON G. POPE, JR.

lthough binge eating disorder (BED) is the most common of the eating disorders, it was not widely recognized as a distinct diagnostic category until the last two decades. Thus, pharmacological trials in BED did not begin until approximately the mid-1990s. Since then, however, more than 25 randomized placebo-controlled trials have assessed medications from several chemical families as monotherapies in BED, and there have been many other trials that involved a non-placebo control group, used medications in combination with other treatments, or were performed on an open-label basis. Several recent reviews have summarized these trials and offered guidelines, formally or informally, for pharmacological treatment of BED (see Suggested Reading). In this chapter, we do not attempt to duplicate these reviews; instead we offer some general perspectives on the available evidence for drug efficacy and its implications for decision making among health care providers who treat patients with BED.

Goals of Treatment

There is a broad consensus about the goals of treatment for BED. The primary goal is, of course, to achieve cessation, or at least marked reduction, in binge eating. Important secondary goals are to reduce or eliminate associated psychopathological features, such as persistent thoughts about binge eating and urges to binge-eat; dissatisfaction with body weight and shape; and, among patients with concurrent obesity, to reduce body weight.

Summary of Evidence for Efficacy

In this section, we summarize evidence of the efficacy of various types of medications. We do not review medications that have been studied in BED but have now been withdrawn from the market (e.g., *d*-fenfluramine and sibutramine). Although we consider all available evidence, we focus primarily on the results of randomized placebo-controlled trials that have compared a medication given as monotherapy (i.e., not in conjunction with another form of treatment) versus placebo. We refer to these trials hereafter as simply "placebo-controlled trials," without reiterating the monotherapy requirement. In these trials, the primary outcome has almost invariably been the frequency of binge eating, expressed as the drug–placebo difference in frequency of binge eating episodes or frequency of binge days (days on which one or more binge eating episodes have occurred). Many trials have also used the criterion of cessation of binge eating for some period of time (e.g., 1 week or 1 month prior to end point) as a primary measure. Secondary measures of pathology associated with BED have included global severity; attitudes toward eating and body image; obsessive and compulsive features associated with BED; and concurrent symptoms of depression and anxiety. Change in body weight or body mass index has also represented an important outcome measure in all studies. In the discussion below, we focus primarily on the outcomes measures of frequency of binge eating and body weight, since measures of associated psychopathology generally respond in a manner that is highly correlated with frequency of binge eating.

Antidepressants and Related Compounds

Tricyclics

Tricyclic antidepressants have been evaluated in only two placebo-controlled studies in BED, both involving a small number of participants, using imipramine and desipramine, respectively. Both studies showed a modest effect on binge eating and associated psychopathology but no clear effect on body weight.

Selective Serotonin Reuptake Inhibitors

Selective serotonin reuptake inhibitors (SSRIs) have been evaluated in many placebo-controlled trials, including studies with escitalopram, citalopram, sertraline, fluvoxamine, and fluoxetine. However, most studies involved a small number of participants, with only two available trials evaluating more than 30 participants per treatment group, and none evaluating more than 60 participants per group. The most consistent evidence for efficacy comes from studies of escitalopram, citalopram, and sertraline—each of which was the subject of one published study. For fluoxetine and fluvoxamine, there is a larger number of studies, with some showing efficacy and others failing to show significant differences between drug and placebo. However, when considering these latter negative studies, it should be noted that none has shown that fluoxetine or fluvoxamine was "nonsuperior" to placebo—that is, the studies had insufficient power to exclude a clinically meaningful effect. Moreover, no study in BED has found that one medication was not superior to placebo, while simultaneously showing that another medication was superior to placebo, thereby providing evidence of "assay sensitivity" (i.e., evidence that the trial was capable of detecting a medication effect if a genuine effect existed). Thus, trials that have not demonstrated drug–placebo differences are less informative because it is not clear whether they represent truly "negative" studies (indicating nonsuperiority of medication to placebo), as opposed to simply "failed" studies (in that they were unable to distinguish a genuinely efficacious treatment from placebo). With these caveats in mind, and given the likelihood of a "class effect" for SSRIs (i.e., they probably have roughly similar efficacy because of similar chemical properties), it is our view that the available evidence favors similar efficacy across SSRIs. Specifically, these medications appear to have a moderately beneficial effect on reducing frequency of binge eating but little effect on reducing weight. Despite this modest profile of efficacy, the SSRIs currently appear to represent the class of medications most frequently prescribed for BED, perhaps because they are familiar to clinicians and relatively easy to use.

Serotonin–Norepinephrine Reuptake Inhibitors

Duloxetine was found effective in one controlled study of participants with BED plus major depression, and venlafaxine was found effective in a small, open-label investigation. Atomoxetine (also used in attention-deficit/hyperactivity disorder [ADHD]) proved effective for both frequency of binge eating and body weight in a single, small controlled trial. Reboxetine, widely marketed internationally as an antidepressant but not approved for use in the United States, was found modestly efficacious in one open-label study of nine patients.

Bupropion

Bupropion failed to reduce binge eating in a single placebo-controlled trial of individuals with BED and obesity, but it produced somewhat greater weight loss than placebo.

In summary, most antidepressants, with the exception of bupropion, have exhibited at least modest efficacy in binge eating but generally have not produced substantial weight loss.

Anti-Epileptics

Topiramate

Topiramate demonstrated impressive efficacy in treatment of BED in two placebo-controlled trials, as well as a third trial comparing topiramate plus cognitive-behavioral therapy versus placebo plus cognitive-behavioral therapy. In all three trials, substantial proportions of participants achieved a complete remission of binge eating and a marked reduction in body weight. However, adverse effects, most notably adverse neurocognitive effects, compromised the tolerability of topiramate in these studies and represent a well-known limitation of this compound.

Zonisamide

Zonisamide was found efficacious for treatment of BED in a single placebo-controlled trial, but it also was not well tolerated.

Lamotrigine

Lamotrigine, an anti-epileptic of known efficacy for mood disorders, failed to improve symptoms of BED or to reduce weight in one placebo-controlled trial.

Anti-Obesity Medications

The lipase inhibitor orlistat has been studied in controlled trials in which it has been given as monotherapy, compared with placebo plus a hypocaloric diet, or as an augmentation (vs. placebo) for cognitive-behavioral therapy or weight loss treatment. In these studies, orlistat showed little effect on frequency of binge eating and produced mixed results in terms of enhancing weight loss.

Opioid Antagonists

The novel opioid antagonist *ALKS-33* failed to outperform placebo in a single placebo-controlled trial in BED. However, some preliminary data suggest that the opioid antagonists naloxone and naltrexone might have some promise in reducing binge eating.

Psychostimulants

Lisdexamfetamine, an agent initially marketed for treatment of ADHD, has now become the most extensively studied medication for treatment of BED. Lisdexamfetamine showed marked evidence of efficacy both in reduction of binge frequency and in weight loss, in three placebo-controlled trials (including two large Phase 3 registration studies). In addition, a placebo-controlled relapse prevention study showed that lisdexamfetamine was associated with a markedly lower risk of relapse than placebo over 6 months. Lisdexamfetamine was approved by the U.S. Food and Drug Administration (FDA) for treatment of BED in January 2015. It represents the first and, at present, the only FDA-approved medication for BED.

Miscellaneous Medications

Several other medications from different chemical families, including baclofen, acamprosate, disulfiram, chromium picolinate, rimonabant, *N*-acetylcysteine, and sodium oxybate, have all shown some preliminary evidence of efficacy in BED, but data at present are too limited to permit confident conclusions.

Efficacy of Pharmacological versus Nonpharmacological Treatment

It is difficult to compare the efficacy of pharmacological versus nonpharmacological treatments for BED. First, there have been few direct comparisons of these modalities, and no study has compared psychological treatments with the two apparently most efficacious pharmacological treatments, namely, topiramate and lisdexamfetamine. Second, even if there were a rigorously designed comparison of this type, interpretation of the results would be compromised because drug treatment is typically administered under double-blind conditions, whereas psychological treatment is effectively "open-label."

One of the consequences of this disparity is that patients and investigators may be biased by expectational effects when receiving nonblind psychological treatment. Bias may also be introduced by what we have called the "responsibility effect." Specifically, if study participants fail to respond to a drug, they will likely conclude that the drug has failed. But if they respond poorly to a psychological therapy, they may feel that they themselves have failed—and may counter this disappointment by providing overly optimistic ratings of their response to psychological therapy.

Finally, when one moves from a consideration of comparative *efficacy*, as demonstrated in clinical trials, to comparative *effectiveness* in real-life treatment settings—where one encounters issues such as patient preference, availability of treatment modalities, adherence, cost and burden of treatment, and varying sequences and combinations of treatment modalities—it becomes even more difficult to provide empirical support for one given approach relative to another.

Approaches to Pharmacological Treatment

Given the previously discussed considerations, one must be hesitant to attempt any global recommendations for treatment approaches in patients with BED. Some patients may not desire, or may fail to adhere to, a given treatment modality, and particular treatments may or may not be available or affordable in a given setting. In addition, at present, there is a paucity of information about the long-term benefits and risks of pharmacological treatment for BED. While keeping these reservations in mind, it would seem that if pharmacotherapy is selected, lisdexamfetamine would likely represent the most attractive initial option given the present state of knowledge, provided that patients do not exhibit contraindications to the use of psychostimulants. Patients exhibiting prominent symptoms of depression in conjunction with BED, however, might be more suited to initial treatment with one of the various antidepressants shown to be effective in BED. Topiramate may often represent the next option in patients with an inadequate response to initial treatment, and this drug can generally be combined with lisdexamfetamine or antidepressants without serious interactions. Although large doses of topiramate (e.g., 400 mg/day) may produce unacceptable cognitive effects, smaller doses may often prove tolerable and may be sufficient to augment the effects of the primary agent. Psychological therapies, if not already in place, can easily be initiated simultaneously with pharmacological therapies, with the nature and duration of psychological therapy adapted to the needs of the patient.

There is little information at present to guide decisions on duration of pharmacological treatment of BED, and such judgments will likely be made on an individualized basis in actual practice. Fortunately, there exist substantial data on the long-term safety of the primary drugs used in BED because these drugs were all widely prescribed for other indications in the past (lisdexamfetamine for ADHD; topiramate for epilepsy and migraine; and antidepressants and related medications for mood and anxiety disorders, among other indications) before being applied for the treatment of BED. Finally, given the advances in pharmacotherapy for BED over the last two decades, along with the inclusion of BED as an official mental disorder diagnosis in the fifth edition of the *Diagnostic and Statistical Manual of Mental Disorders* (DSM-5) in 2013, together with increasing recognition of the public health burden of BED, it seems likely that we will see substantial further progress in this field in future years.

Suggested Reading

Aigner, M., Treasure, J., Kaye, W., & Kasper, S. (2011). World Federation of Societies of Biological Psychiatry (WFSBP) guidelines for the pharmacological treatment of eating disorders. *World Journal of Biological Psychiatry, 12*(6), 400–443.—Review and practice guidelines from the World Federation of Societies of Biological Psychiatry, based on data available through 2011.

American Psychiatric Association Work Group on Eating Disorders. (2006, July). Practice guideline for the treatment of patients with eating disorders, third edition. *American Journal of Psychiatry, 163*(Suppl.), 1–54.—The most recent practice guidelines for BED from the American Psychiatric Association. Although now dated, this article provides an excellent review of studies available through 2005.

Brownley, K. A., Peat, C. M., La Via, M., & Bulik, C. M. (2015). Pharmacological approaches to the management of binge eating disorder. *Drugs, 75*(1), 9–32.—Review of treatment studies available through 2014.

Hudson, J. I., Hiripi, E., Pope, H. G., Jr., & Kessler, R. C. (2007). The prevalence and correlates of eating disorders in the National Comorbidity Survey Replication. *Biological Psychiatry, 61*(3), 348–358.—Documents the prevalence and public health burden of BED in the United States, using data from the National Comorbidity Replication Survey.

Keck, P. E., Jr., Pope, H. G., Jr., & Hudson, J. I. (2004). Bulimia nervosa: Persistent disorder requires equally persistent treatment. *Current Psychiatry, 3*(1), 12–22.—Provides further discussion about the methodological difficulties encountered when attempting to compare psychological and pharmacological treatment for eating disorders, and introduces the term "responsibility effect."

McElroy, S. L., Guerdjikova, A. I., Mori, N., & Keck, P. E., Jr. (2015). Psychopharmacologic treatment of eating disorders: Emerging findings. *Current Psychiatry Reports, 17*(5), 35.—Reviews studies since 2011, intended as an update, using methodology patterned after that used in the World Federation of Societies of Biological Psychiatry guidelines (see Aigner et al., 2011), although it does not represent an official update by this body.

McElroy, S. L., Hudson, J., Ferreira-Cornwell, M. C., Radewonuk, J., Whitaker, T., & Gasior, M. (2016). Lisdexamfetamine dimesylate for adults with moderate to severe binge eating disorder: Results of two pivotal Phase 3 randomized controlled trials. *Neuropsychopharmacology, 41*(5), 1251–1260.—Reports results from two large registration studies of lisdexamfetamine, which formed the basis for FDA approval of lisdexamfetamine for treatment of moderate to severe BED.

Reas, D. L., & Grilo, C. M. (2015). Pharmacological treatment of binge eating disorder: Update review and synthesis. *Expert Opinion on Pharmacotherapy, 16*(10), 1463–1478.—Review of treatment studies available through early 2015.

Psychological Treatment of Binge Eating Disorder

CARLOS M. GRILO

Binge eating disorder (BED), a formal diagnosis in the fifth edition of the *Diagnostic and Statistical Manual of Mental Disorders* (DSM-5), is defined by recurrent binge eating, marked distress about the binge eating, and the absence of inappropriate weight compensatory behaviors. BED is associated strongly with obesity, and is associated with elevated rates of psychiatric/medical comorbidities and with heightened levels of eating disorder (e.g., overvaluation of shape/weight) and general psychological (e.g., depression, poor self-esteem, interpersonal difficulty) disturbances. Thus, ideally, effective treatments should be able to eliminate or substantially reduce binge eating, associated eating disorder and general psychopathology, and, if necessary, reduce excess weight and associated medical problems. Considerable progress has been achieved in developing and testing treatments for BED during the 20 years since the field trials and inclusion of BED as a "research diagnosis" earlier in DSM-IV. Early treatments for BED evolved and were adapted from the treatment literatures for bulimia nervosa (e.g., specialized psychological treatments such as cognitive-behavioral therapy [CBT] and interpersonal psychotherapy [IPT]) and for obesity (e.g., behavioral weight loss [BWL]).

This chapter provides an overview of the current status of psychological treatments for BED. Positive long-term empirical support exists for two specialist psychological treatments (CBT and IPT); positive short-term empirical support exists for an additional specialist psychological treatment (i.e., dialectical behavior therapy [DBT]), for guided-self-help versions of CBT, for BWL, and for certain specific combinations of pharmacotherapy with CBT or BWL. Despite the positive findings for some treatments, even the treatments with the best outcomes fail to help a substantial proportion of patients attain remission from binge eating, and most result in little to no weight loss. This chapter also provides an overview of the current status of research on predictors and moderators of treatment outcomes, which could lead to more effective treatment strategies, along with challenges around treatment scalability and dissemination.

Psychological (Specialist) Treatments

To date, two psychological treatments—CBT and IPT—have been intensively studied and have received strong empirical support. Both CBT and IPT approaches for BED are based largely on specific methods developed initially and empirically supported for bulimia nervosa.

CBT for BED, the most intensively studied approach, is based on cognitive-behavioral and restraint models of binge eating. CBT focuses on establishing normalized and more structured eating patterns (e.g., regular pattern of meals and snacks to decrease unhealthy dietary restriction), addressing maladaptive cognitions (e.g., to reduce overvaluation of shape/weight) via cognitive restructuring and behavioral experiments, goal-setting and problem-solving techniques to identify and overcome emotional and situational triggers to binge eating, and incorporating healthy eating with flexible restraint.

CBT, a focal short-term approach (e.g., generally 16 weeks, but studies range from 12 to 24 weeks), has received consistent empirical support in controlled trials testing both group and individual modes of delivery. CBT generally results in binge remission rates of roughly 50–60% at posttreatment, along with robust reductions in eating disorder psychopathology and associated depression, but it fails to produce weight loss. The short-term outcomes (binge eating and eating-related pathology) achieved with CBT have been found—in several studies—to be superior to various controls, including active treatment comparisons such as antidepressant medications and BWL, but have not differed from IPT. The outcomes achieved with CBT are generally durable, with studies indicating good maintenance through 48 months following treatment. Follow-up studies of CBT for BED have, for example, reported remission rates (no binge eating) of roughly 50% or greater at 12-, 24-, and 48-month follow-up; these maintenance outcomes for CBT are superior to those reported in comparisons to antidepressant medications and BWL, but not to IPT. Importantly, although CBT does not produce weight loss, follow-up studies through 48 months have reported stable weight over time, suggesting that CBT may protect against further weight gain over time in patients with BED.

IPT for BED follows adaptations of IPT for depression to IPT for bulimia nervosa, is based on interpersonal models of binge eating, and focuses on addressing difficulties in four primary areas (interpersonal deficits, role conflicts, role transitions, and loss/grief), with the goal of tolerating/expressing feeling and improving interpersonal and psychosocial functioning. This model follows findings that interpersonal stressors and psychosocial ineffectiveness lead some individuals to utilize binge eating as a means to cope and attempt to regulate/suppress negative affect; the binge eating, an ineffectual strategy, contributes to a worsening of interpersonal relations and social isolation. IPT for BED focuses exclusively on these interpersonal difficulties, without attention to eating disorder pathology, and without employing the techniques specific to CBT.

IPT for BED, a focal short-term (e.g., generally 24 weeks) manualized treatment delivered via both group and individual methods, has received strong empirical support in controlled trials, with acute and long-term outcomes comparable to CBT. IPT delivered in group and individual sessions has produced acute remission rates of roughly 65%. Follow-up studies of IPT for BED have reported excellent maintenance and durability of outcomes, with one study reporting roughly 65% remission (i.e., binge abstinence) at 24-month follow-up, and a second study reporting 54% binge abstinence at 12-month follow-up, increasing to 77% at 48-month follow-up; these maintenance outcomes for IPT did not differ from those reported for CBT but were superior to those reported for BWL in controlled studies. Importantly, although IPT—like CBT—does not produce weight loss, follow-up studies reported stable weight over time, suggesting that IPT may help to prevent further weight gain over time in patients with BED.

A third specialist treatment, DBT, has also demonstrated some promise for the treatment of BED. DBT for BED, a focal therapy developed and empirically supported for treating problems with emotion and behavioral regulation (e.g., borderline personality disorder, suicidality, substance abuse) and adapted for BED, has received initial support in two controlled trials. DBT is based on models of mood intolerance and emotion regulation difficulties that are thought to lead to maladaptive behaviors such as self-injurious behaviors, or in the case of BED, binge eating as an attempt to cope with distress. DBT focuses on teaching mood tolerance and healthy methods to regulate affect by focusing on four primary areas (mindfulness skills, distress tolerance, emotional regulation, and interpersonal difficulties).

DBT was been found to be superior to a waiting list in one study, and a second study found that group DBT had significantly greater acute efficacy through posttreatment than an active group comparison therapy (ACGT). At 12-month follow-up, however, DBT and ACGT did not differ significantly, with both group interventions having with good remission rates and good maintenance of benefits (e.g., binge abstinence rates of 64% for DBT and 56% for ACGT). DBT was associated with especially high retention rates; there are clinical suggestions that this treatment approach might be especially acceptable and useful for complex and multi-impulsive patient subgroups. Further research with DBT is needed to determine its effectiveness and treatment specificity.

Behavioral Weight Loss

BWL has also received considerable attention as a treatment approach for BED. The early literature produced mixed findings, and this fueled debate regarding whether BWL might be contraindicated given concerns that "dieting" might exacerbate binge eating. More recently, rigorous research has demonstrated that structured BWL methods do not worsen BED and may represent an alternative effective treatment for BED. Several trials have indicated that BWL can produce binge eating remission rates that approximate those achieved by CBT at posttreatment and through 12-month follow-up, with the advantage of producing greater weight loss. However, longer-term follow-ups suggest that weight regain occurs, and that by 24 months, weight loss with BWL is no longer significantly different from specialist CBT and IPT treatments, which maintain higher binge eating remission rates. Such findings, however, do support BWL as a viable alternative treatment for BED that may be especially attractive because it is more widely available and easier to disseminate (i.e., it can be delivered by a broader range of health care providers and is less costly) than specialist treatments such as CBT and IPT. With regard to dissemination, a recent study indicated that BWL produced good outcomes (roughly 50% binge eating remission rates through 6-month follow-up after completion of treatments) in low-socioeconomic-status and Spanish-speaking-only Latina/o patients with complex psychiatric problems at a community mental health center.

Self-Help and Guided Self-Help ("Scalable") Treatments

An important development in treatment research for BED has been findings that certain self-help formats of BED can be effective for a sizable portion of patients. Unguided self-help (i.e., patient self-directed use of a book containing the self-care version of a CBT program) and guided-self-help (i.e., a self-care CBT-based book augmented by guidance provided by a therapist in brief focused meetings) approaches have been tested in several studies. Research has generally supported guided-self-help (gsh) versions of CBT as effective for BED, with some research documenting good durability of outcomes through 24 months of follow-up. Some research suggests the advantage of CBTgsh over pure self-help in both specialist and generalist settings, and a recent study indicated that CBTgsh was superior to BWL over the long term.

Psychological and Behavioral Treatments Combined with Pharmacotherapy

To date, eight controlled comparative treatment trials have tested additive approaches with psychological or behavioral treatments delivered in combination with pharmacotherapy using various medications. Overall, within these comparative trials, CBT and the combination of medications with either CBT or BWL produce superior binge eating outcomes to pharmacotherapy-only over both short-term and longer-term follow-ups. Within these comparative trials, combining medications with CBT or BWL does not significantly enhance binge eating outcomes (except for one study with topiramate), but the addition of specific medications known to produce weight loss (e.g., topiramate and orlistat) enhances weight losses, albeit quite modestly.

Collectively, the combination approaches for BED tested to date have not shown much advantage over monotherapy with CBT, although there are hints of greater short-term weight loss with the addition of topiramate. Topiramate, unfortunately, has a complex adverse event profile, and future research should test combination methods using new, FDA-approved anti-obesity medications that might work in a more complementary fashion with CBT and BWL than medications tested thus far.

Predictors, Moderators, and Process of Change

Although several effective psychological, behavioral, and combination treatment approaches have been developed for BED, even the leading approaches leave a substantial proportion of patients with significant symptoms, and most with minimal to no weight loss. Recent years have witnessed increasing attempts to explore predictors and moderators of outcomes in the hope that findings might lead to evidence-based recommendations to specific treatments to improve outcomes. Unfortunately, reliable predictors–moderators have been difficult to identify. Recent converging research has suggested that greater eating disorder psychopathology, most notably overvaluation of shape/weight, signals the need for specialized treatments such as CBT and IPT rather than BWL and medication approaches.

Research has identified a treatment process variable (i.e., rapid response to treatment) that has reliably shown significant and specific prognostic significance. In contrast to CBT, in which rapid or nonrapid response does not predict substantially different long-term outcomes, research has shown that patients who fail to show a rapid response to either BWL or to medications are unlikely to derive further benefit, suggesting that clinicians should consider alternative treatments as soon as possible in such instances. Rapid response to BWL, in contrast, is associated with excellent outcomes in both binge eating and weight losses. Thus, one treatment strategy might be to begin with BWL and, in cases in which a rapid response is not observed, to switch to a specialist treatment (CBT or IPT) and/or add pharmacotherapy.

Future Directions

Larger studies with longer-term follow-up are needed to establish more definitively which treatment approaches are the most durable and for whom. Treatment research needs to identify optimal methods and combinations to assist patients with better weight control over the long term. Therapist training and maintaining fidelity in using evidence-based methods in clinical practice represent additional challenges. Developing and disseminating scalable interventions for BED represent another priority. There is a need to perform treatment studies with more diverse patient groups across diverse clinical settings in order to increase knowledge regarding generalizability of interventions. Larger studies with greater diversity in patient demographical and clinical characteristics are needed to allow for integration of adequately powered analyses testing predictors and moderators of outcome, and especially to initiate studies of potential mediators of change.

Acknowledgment

Preparation of this chapter was supported, in part, by National Institutes of Health Grant Nos. K24 DK070052 and R01 DK49587.

Suggested Reading

Grilo, C. M., Crosby, R. D., Wilson, G. T., & Masheb, R. M. (2012). 12-month follow-up of fluoxetine and cognitive behavioral therapy for binge eating disorder. *Journal of Consulting and Clinical Psychology, 80*(6), 1108–1113.—Twelve-month follow-up data after completion and discontinuation of 16-week treatments of CBT and fluoxetine alone and in combination for BED indicate the specificity of the effectiveness for CBT relative to fluoxetine at posttreatment and through 12 months of follow-up, and highlight the pressing need for pharmacotherapy research to investigate maintenance approaches.

Grilo, C. M., Masheb, R. M., & Crosby, R. D. (2012). Predictors and moderators of response to cognitive behavioral therapy and medication for the treatment of binge eating disorder. *Journal of Consulting and Clinical Psychology, 80*(5), 897–906.—This article summarizes empirical studies testing potential predictors and moderators of treatment outcomes for BED, and identified overvaluation of shape/weight as the most salient predictor and moderator of treatment outcomes; these findings persisted even after researchers controlled for negative affect.

Grilo, C. M., Masheb, R. M., Wilson, G. T., Gueorguieva, R., & White, M. A. (2011). Cognitive-behavioral therapy, behavioral weight loss, and sequential treatment for obese patients with binge eating disorder: A randomized controlled trial. *Journal of Consulting and Clinical*

Psychology, 79(5), 675–685.—This study found that CBT was superior to BWL for reducing binge eating through 12-month follow-up, whereas BWL had statistically greater weight losses during treatment.

Grilo, C. M., & White, M. A. (2013). Orlistat with behavioral weight loss for obesity with versus without binge eating disorder: Randomized placebo-controlled trial at a community mental health center serving educationally and economically disadvantaged Latino/as. *Behaviour Research and Therapy, 51,* 167–175.—This study, performed at a community-based mental health clinic serving SES-disadvantaged Latino/as, reported outcomes for BWL plus orlistat/placebo that are roughly comparable to the treatment literature with more restrictive BED and obese samples.

Grilo, C. M., White, M. A., Wilson, G. T., Gueorguieva, R., & Masheb, R. M. (2012). Rapid response predicts 12-month post-treatment outcomes in binge eating disorder: Theoretical and clinical implications. *Psychological Medicine, 42,* 807–817.—This study revealed that rapid response to treatment has prognostic significance through 12-month follow-up, with different time courses and outcomes for CBT and BWL; these findings have implications for stepped-care treatment approaches.

Hilbert, A., Bishop, M. E., Stein, R. I., Tanofsky-Kraff, M., Swenson, A. K., Welch, R. R., et al. (2012). Long-term efficacy of psychological treatments for binge eating disorder. *British Journal of Psychiatry, 200,* 232–237.—This study found that the robust acute outcomes achieved with CBT and IPT are durable over 48 months of follow-up.

Reas, D. L., & Grilo, C. M. (2014). Current and emerging drug treatments for binge eating disorder. *Expert Opinion on Emerging Drugs, 19,* 99–142.—This article, which reviews pharmacotherapy for BED, includes a thorough review of controlled trials testing treatment approaches involving the combination of medications with CBT and behavioral treatments.

Safer, D. L., Robinson, A. H., & Jo, B. (2010). Outcome from a randomized controlled trial of group therapy for binge eating disorder: Comparing dialectical behavior therapy adapted for binge eating to an active comparison group therapy. *Behavior Therapy, 41,* 106–120.—This study found that group DBT had significantly greater acute efficacy through posttreatment, but not at 12-month follow-up, than an AGCT.

Thompson-Brenner, H., Franko, D. L., Thompson, D. R., Grilo, C. M., Boisseau, C. L., Roehrig, J. P., et al. (2013). Race/ethnicity, education, and treatment parameters as moderators and predictors of outcome in binge eating disorder. *Journal of Consulting and Clinical Psychology, 81*(4), 710–721.—This study, which pooled data across several research sites testing psychological treatments for BED, revealed that black participants had lower treatment completion rates and that lower education levels were associated with poorer outcomes; however, race/ethnicity and education did not moderate treatment outcomes.

Wilson, G. T., Wilfley, D. E., Agras, W. S., & Bryson, S. W. (2010). Psychological treatments of binge eating disorder. *Archives of General Psychiatry, 67,* 94–101.—At posttreatment, CBTgsh, IPT, and BWL did not differ in binge remission and decreases in eating disorder psychopathology or depression, but BWL was associated with greater weight loss; at 2-year follow-up, CBTgsh and IPT were superior to BWL in terms of binge eating remission, and BWL was no longer associated with greater weight loss.

Wilson, G. T., & Zandberg, L. J. (2012). Cognitive-behavioral guided self-help for eating disorders: Effectiveness and scalability. *Clinical Psychology Review, 32,* 343–357.—This article provides a thorough review of CBT self-help and CBTgsh for eating disorders, including BED, and addresses issues regarding scalability and dissemination.

Intensive Treatment of Anorexia Nervosa and Bulimia Nervosa

JANET TREASURE

Inpatient care, particularly for anorexia nervosa, was central to the management of eating disorders in the 20th century. However, there has been a move to more community-centered care, with hospital care restricted to the patient group with severe medical risk and/or a failure to respond to outpatient care. The main goal of inpatient treatment is to reduce medical risk by improving nutrition. This usually involves meals supervised by nurses. Facilities with less than 24 hours per daycare, such as partial hospitalization or daycare, are used as an alternative to inpatient care, or as the second phase in a form of stepped care. As the effect of treatment is often transient, inpatient care is less often used for bulimia nervosa, unless comorbidity with problems such as diabetes increases the medical risk. This chapter describes the history and theoretical background of inpatient care. The available systematic reviews and randomized trials are noted. However, there is very little high-quality evidence.

The History of Inpatient Treatment

Hospital admission, so that nurses could support eating and restore weight to normal, was advocated as treatment for anorexia nervosa by Sir William Gull in the 19th century. A century later, care was mainly sited within specialized psychiatric units. Relapse post-discharge was common, but a seminal study of aftercare found that in young people in the early stage of illness (less than 3 years), family-based psychotherapy reduced relapse more effectively than individual therapy. However, neither form of therapy reduced relapse in those with a longer or later-onset form of illness.

Theoretical Background

The theoretical underpinning of the nursing approach to refeeding has changed over time. Gull described nurses using "moral authority." Later, behavioral principles were followed, with reward given or privileges reinstated, contingent on weight gain. However, evidence from a cohort study reported that a strict behavioral approach was less acceptable to nurses and patients, and produced an equivalent amount of weight gain to that in a more lenient approach. Meal support can be problematic, with mealtimes reported as taxing and confusing. In a recent survey of nurses in specialized U.K. units, some patients and nurses described meals as a battle. Such a conflictual mealtime environment may deepen negative memories associated with food and embed eating disorders behaviors more deeply. The importance of staff skills was emphasized by a study in which teaching nurses to use an intervention devised to train family members in the skills of mealtime support led to a more cost-effective inpatient stay. Moreover such a joint approach may bridge the transition period and allow changes to be sustained postdischarge.

Clinical Practice

Levels of anxiety are high before, during, and after meals. These times may be marked by intense emotional displays, but more often patients have a "poker face," with restricted facial expression of emotions. This blocks an empathetic reaction from staff members, who can become frustrated and hostile. On the other hand, if others recognize the terror associated with food, they may be drawn into accommodating to the illness, enabling patients to persist in eating disorder behaviors. Thus, careful planning and supervision is needed to achieve a balance between avoidance and coercion. Eating is non-negotiable. On the other hand, the form and content of food-related activities can be individualized to a degree. Advance planning and review, and a rule of no negotiations during meals themselves, are helpful strategies. Implementation interventions (i.e., "if . . . , then . . . " plans, can be helpful. For example, "If you are not able to eat all of your meal, then you will have liquid food replacement. If you are taking too long, then I will give you a reminder at half-time and every 10 minutes." The skills of motivational interviewing (warmth, open reflections, sidestepping resistance) are particularly helpful for managing the ambivalence and resistance that meals evoke.

   The principles of extinction learning have been applied. However, there is tension between the gradual individualized plan used in exposure therapy and (1) safely ameliorating medical risk by restoring nutrition in a timely manner, and (2) managing meal support with limited resources, often within a group setting. Exposure therapy uses a hierarchy of goals to tackle avoidance and accommodation behaviors used by patients and possibly also by those close to them. However, the new learning involved in extinction of fear memories is context-specific. This may explain why there is often a failure to sustain changes accomplished during inpatient stay after discharge.

Supplemental Treatments

Multidisciplinary interventions are regarded as a necessary part of a high-quality eating disorder inpatient program. In addition to nutrition, these interventions target the range of eating disorder features (e.g., cognitive and emotional style, body image work). A recent systematic review examined supplementary treatments to inpatient care. Four randomized controlled trials compared an antidepressant with placebo and found minimal effects. Four studies compared antipsychotic drugs with placebo, and, again, the overall effect was small; the largest effect was found in young people with anorexia nervosa. Minimal effects were also found in the four studies using randomized controlled designs to compare psychological treatments; possibly, the detrimental effects of starvation on brain plasticity and function may reduce the experiential benefits from psychotherapy. Case–control designs suggested that nasogastric feeding may be superior to oral feeding, particularly with the group with binge–purge symptoms.

It is challenging to develop a strong evidence base regarding interventions in inpatient settings because randomization to different forms of intervention within the inpatient setting can be problematic, and it is difficult to find effects over and above those resulting from standard care. On the other hand, an admission can provide time, space, and motivation for psychological change to begin.

Admission Criteria

There is no international agreement on the admission criteria for intensive care, and the thresholds specified in national guidelines vary. In part, the criteria depend on the facilities available and the amount of risk they are able to manage. Patients with extreme medical risk and multiple organ failure are usually admitted to general medical hospitals. In the United Kingdom, in 2014, the Royal College of Psychiatrists developed the "MARSIPAN: Management of Really Sick Patients with Anorexia Nervosa" (adult and junior) protocol to describe the care pathway for such cases and to optimize the liaison between physical and psychiatric care (*http://rcpsych.ac.uk/usefulresources/publications/collegereports/cr/cr189.aspx*).

Discharge Criteria

The traditional goal of inpatient care was to restore weight to normal. The underlying assumption was that normal physiology and eating habits would then resume. Indeed, low weight at discharge increases the likelihood of relapse and readmission. However, the outcome of inpatient care is confounded by many factors, such as the level of motivation, and randomized controlled trials (e.g., those described below) are essential to interpret findings. Shorter periods of inpatient stay and lower discharge body mass index (BMI) are part of current practice. For example, in the United States, over a 14-year period, the average length of inpatient admission decreased from 149.5 days to just 23.7 days, and discharge BMIs decreased over the years from 19 kg/m^2 (full restoration) to 17 kg/m^2 (medical stabilization). Results from two recent randomized trials validate this practice for young patients, as short admissions for medical stabilization, rather than normalization of weight, produced a similar improvement in symptoms. Moreover, the shorter (medical stabilization) admissions were associated with less service use in the year following discharge. It remains to be seen whether such an approach is useful for people in the enduring stage of illness.

Aftercare

The relapse rate following inpatient care ranges from 20 to 50%, and approximately one-third of patients are readmitted in the following year. Psychological interventions for patients and/or caregivers delivered face-to-face or through various form of technology have been found to reduce the rate of relapse. On the other hand, dietary advice or medication had no impact. A subgroup of patients has repeated or protracted involuntary admissions undertaken under the aegis of mental health legislation. In the United Kingdom, there have been a series of recent applications to the courts for best interest decisions regarding continuing treatment in these circumstances.

Key Issues

- There is now evidence from two randomized controlled trials suggesting that for adolescents with a short duration of illness, short admissions to stabilize medical risk followed by outpatient care involving the family may be the most cost-effective strategy.

- The question of the optimal length of stay for adults with an enduring illness and high medical risk remains unanswered.

- There is the suggestion, which requires further validation, that training nurses with skills in meal support may improve the inpatient experience and optimize outcomes. Postadmission care may be improved by providing caregivers with this form of training.

- Uncertainty remains in the management of treatment-resistant adult patients. Judgments of best interest decisions need to be made on an individual basis.

Future Directions

Inpatient treatment now has a much smaller place in the management of anorexia nervosa than was the case 20 years or more ago, particularly for young patients with a short history. The form and content of inpatient care may differ according to the stage of illness, but there is uncertainty about the management of patients with a severe, enduring form of illness. More attention to nursing and psychological interventions targeting the core symptoms both during and following admission may be needed to manage the profound psychosocial, cognitive, and emotional problems that influence the eating disorder features of patients in the later stage of illness, and to ensure that change is sustainable.

Suggested Reading

Couturier, J., & Mahmood, A. (2009). Meal support therapy reduces the use of nasogastric feeding for adolescents hospitalized with anorexia nervosa. *Eating Disorders, 17*(4), 327–332.— The use of nasogastric feeding was reduced following an intervention in which nurses were trained with a form of meal support therapy originally devised for parents as part of family-based therapy.

Herpertz-Dahlmann, B., Schwarte, R., Krei, M., Egberts, K., Warnke, A., Wewetzer, C., et al. (2014). Day-patient treatment after short inpatient care versus continued inpatient treatment in adolescents with anorexia nervosa (ANDI): A multicentre, randomised, open-label, non-inferiority trial. *Lancet, 383,* 1222–1229.—The outcomes of adolescent patients randomized to either a standard length inpatient admission or a shorter intervention followed by daycare were similar after 1 year.

Long, S., Wallis, D. J., Leung, N., Arcelus, J., & Meyer, C. (2012). Mealtimes on eating disorder wards: A two-study investigation. *International Journal of Eating Disorders, 45*(2), 241–246.—This study of mealtime practices within U.K. eating disorders units concluded that specialized mealtime implementation training was needed because most nurses did not have a clear rationale or plan for meal support management.

Madden, S., Hay, P., & Touyz, S. (2015). Systematic review of evidence for different treatment settings in anorexia nervosa. *World Journal of Psychiatry, 5*(1), 147–153.—A review of the literature up to July 2014, largely focusing on adolescents, concludes that a less restrictive form of management than inpatient care may have advantages.

Madden, S., Miskovic-Wheatley, J., Wallis, A., Kohn, M., Lock, J., Le Grange, D., et al. (2015). A randomized controlled trial of in-patient treatment for anorexia nervosa in medically unstable adolescents. *Psychological Medicine, 45*(02), 415–427.—Adolescent patients randomized to a short intervention for medical stabilization versus an admission for weight restoration had similar outcomes at 1 year, although the costs for those in the medical stabilization condition were slightly lower.

Steinglass, J. E., Albano, A. M., Simpson, H. B., Wang, Y., Zou, J., Attia, E., et al. (2014). Confronting fear using exposure and response prevention for anorexia nervosa: A randomized controlled pilot study. *International Journal of Eating Disorders, 47*(2), 174–180.—An intervention focusing on meal support using exposure and response prevention improved eating outcomes (calories consumed) compared with a cognitive remediation intervention.

Suárez-Pinilla, P., Peña-Pérez, C., Arbaizar-Barrenechea, B., Crespo-Facorro, B., Del Barrio, J. A. G., Treasure, J., et al. (2015). Inpatient treatment for anorexia nervosa: A systematic review of randomized controlled trials. *Journal of Psychiatric Practice, 21*(1), 49–59.—A summary of the literature up to September 2013 relating to treatments (pharmacological, psychological, nutritional) used to supplement inpatient care.

Touyz, S. W., Beumont, P. J., Glaun, D., Phillips, T., & Cowie, I. (1984). A comparison of lenient and strict operant conditioning programmes in refeeding patients with anorexia nervosa. *British Journal of Psychiatry, 144*(5), 517–520.—A more lenient approach in managing behavioral contingencies to manage feeding and weight gain was preferred by nurses and patients alike.

Treasure, J., Crane, A., McKnight, R., Buchanan, E., & Wolfe, M. (2011). First do no harm: Iatrogenic maintaining factors in anorexia nervosa. *European Eating Disorders Review, 19*(4), 296–302.—This article describes possible ways in which inpatient units might inadvertently support processes that maintain symptoms (e.g., by overprotection or by coercive forms of management).

Weight Restoration in Anorexia Nervosa

ANGELA S. GUARDA
GRAHAM W. REDGRAVE

The Importance of Weight Restoration in Anorexia Nervosa

Weight restoration and reversal of the starved state in anorexia nervosa (AN) are treatment imperatives. Starvation increases preoccupation with food and weight; exacerbates compulsive behaviors and mood and anxiety symptoms; and results in physiological consequences, including impaired hunger and satiety signaling and functional gastrointestinal complaints that further sustain restricted eating patterns. Individuals with AN demonstrate limited dietary variety, a preference for low calorie-dense foods, and rigid, stereotyped eating and exercise patterns. Weight restoration and normalization of eating behavior are associated with improvement in both cognitive and affective symptoms, although these lag behind behavior change and physiological improvement. Because patients with AN are inherently ambivalent, or outright resistant to gaining weight, weight restoration is a therapeutic challenge for clinicians.

Relapse risk remains around 50% following inpatient weight restoration; however, most patients who maintain a normal weight for 6–9 months achieve full remission and demonstrate improvement in cognitive, affective, and behavioral symptoms; overall function; and quality of life. Partial weight restoration, by contrast, has not been shown to significantly impact recovery rates for AN, and lower body mass index (BMI) at hospital discharge is associated with likelihood of future weight loss and repeat hospitalization. Prompt weight restoration is additionally needed for normalization of endocrine status and bone health. Osteoporosis is a frequent complication of AN, and resumption of menses in women with amenorrhea is an important indicator of recovery.

There remains a lack of consensus with regard to target weight, ideal rate of weight gain, and treatment setting for weight restoration. Additionally, controversy exists around the role of supplemental enteral or parenteral feeding approaches, and the circumstances and clinical settings in which these may be indicated. Finally, treatment approaches and considerations differ between adolescents and adults with AN, and between recent-onset and severe and enduring AN.

Establishing Target Weights

The definition of target weight in adults with AN varies, most commonly ranging from a BMI of 18.5–21 kg/m². The lower end of this range, 18.5 kg/m², is problematic because it is associated with low body fat, as well as significant rates of amenorrhea, and is commonly used as a diagnostic cutoff for recruitment into treatment studies of AN. Lower percent body fat following short-term, inpatient weight restoration has been associated with elevated relapse risk at 1-year follow-up, and athletes and those with low fat mass may need to reach a BMI > 21 kg/m² for return of menses and full physiological recovery. A higher target may also apply to individuals with a higher premorbid weight. A useful index of target weight is the weight at which menses cease, which is typically higher than the weight at menarche. Body fat following short-term weight restoration in AN has been shown to exhibit a central truncal distribution that normalizes within 1 year of weight maintenance (this is helpful information to transmit to patients, who are often anxious about this aspect of the refeeding process).

In adolescents who have not yet reached their adult height and are still growing, and whose body composition is changing, a variety of indices are used to assess target weight, including growth charts, median BMI percentiles, percent of expected body weight based on BMI percentiles, and BMI standard deviation scores. Reaching and maintaining a target weight between the 15th and 20th BMI percentile was recently found to predict return of menses within 12 months of weight restoration in a large cohort of adolescents with AN.

Refeeding Syndrome

Refeeding syndrome is a potentially life-threatening complication of weight restoration and includes a constellation of clinical findings, including electrolyte abnormalities, postprandial hypoglycemia, edema, and Wernicke–Korsakoff syndrome. Hypophosphatemia is traditionally viewed as its cardinal symptom and is more common in severely starved individuals with a BMI less than 14 kg/m². Refeeding syndrome can be avoided by slowly advancing calorie intake during refeeding. Traditional recommendations have been to "start low and go slow"; however, recent reports suggest that higher calorie approaches to inpatient refeeding are safe in the presence of close medical monitoring and prompt correction of hypophosphatemia and other electrolyte imbalances. Indeed, hypophosphatemia appears to be more strongly associated with very low BMI than with the rate of weight gain. Given the increased constraints on hospital lengths of stay, there is interest in optimizing rates of weight gain and refeeding strategies, and a need for long-term data comparing outcomes utilizing protocols that employ faster versus slower rates of refeeding.

Caloric, Macronutrient, and Micronutrient Dietary Requirements for Weight Restoration

Little is known regarding the optimal macronutrient content for refeeding in AN. Most programs follow currently recommended dietary guidelines of 25–35% calories from fat, 15–20% from protein, and 50–60% from carbohydrates. Maintenance calories for the average adult woman are around 1,800–2,400 cal/day. An extra 1,000 calories/day are needed above maintenance requirements to gain 2 pounds/week, so to achieve consistent weight gain, dietary intake must be 3,000–4,000 calories/day. Most programs initiate refeeding protocols at 1,200–2,000 calories/day and advance to 3,000–4,000 calories/day over 10–14 days. Some data suggest that patients with AN require higher than normal caloric intakes to gain weight, in part due to excessive activity and refeeding-associated increases in thermogenesis. Patients with the purging subtype of AN have been shown to require less calories than those with the restricting subtype, perhaps in part due to higher rates of edema and water retention following the sudden cessation of purging behavior during early inpatient refeeding.

Variety of food choice and fat intake at discharge from hospital-based weight restoration have been shown to predict relapse. This finding suggests that broadening food repertoire and incorporating fats in the diet should be an explicit treatment target. Several studies have identified micronutrient deficiencies in clinical samples of patients with AN, most commonly vitamins D and B_{12}, zinc, and calcium. Supplementation of calcium and vitamin D is recommended for all patients with AN given their risk for osteoporosis.

Outpatient Strategies for Weight Restoration

Outpatient weight restoration is always preferable in medically stable patients, though it is not always effective, especially for adult or chronically ill individuals. A minimal acceptable rate of weight gain for outpatients is 0.5–1.0 pounds/week. Failure to meet this target consistently over 6–8 weeks of outpatient treatment, or medical instability, indicates the need for a higher level of care.

In adolescents with AN, family-based treatment (FBT) is the most evidence-based outpatient approach. In 50–75% of adolescents who have been ill with AN for 3 years or less, FBT is effective in weight restoration to >95% of ideal body weight for age. FBT relies on training parents to refeed their child over 10–20 treatment sessions spread across 6–12 months and is relatively inexpensive compared to inpatient or residential treatment. When hospitalization is necessary in adolescents due to acute medical instability, a brief admission for medical stabilization followed by a course of outpatient FBT has been shown to be effective. The best predictor of weight restoration and remission with FBT is weight gain by week 6–8 of treatment. Early weight gain as an outcome predictor has also been linked to weight restoration for individual adolescent focused therapy, and may not be specific to FBT.

A caveat when comparing adolescent and adult treatment response rates in AN is the fact that adolescent AN encompasses a large proportion of mild or self-limited cases that remit spontaneously, or with relatively short nonspecific outpatient or inpatient interventions. For example, systemic family therapy and FBT yielded similar remission rates at the end of treatment in a recent study, although weight gain occurred earlier and treatment cost was lower for FBT. Another study found that an enhanced form of cognitive-behavioral therapy (CBT-E), in which most sessions are individual and do not involve parents, was able to restore weight in 65% of adolescents with AN but only 36% of adults. Chronic AN, lasting longer than 3 years, may therefore represent a subgroup with a more severe disorder, perhaps with a stronger genetic diathesis, or in whom social and/or biological consequences of restricting and purging behavior have made AN more resistant to treatment.

Indeed, no outpatient intervention has been found to reliably restore weight for a majority of adult patients with AN. Most controlled trials of adults with AN have low rates of weight restoration and high dropout rates. Some adult patients respond to outpatient behavioral interventions including supportive therapy, nutritional counseling or cognitive-behavioral approaches; however, many with severe and enduring AN who have been ill for years, or with serious medical complications, require more intensive behavioral specialty treatment.

Intensive Behavioral Treatment Settings: Inpatient, Residential, and Partial Hospitalization Programs

Inpatient behavioral specialty programs offer the highest level of care, including 24-hour nursing care and medical coverage, and are indicated for severely ill patients with a very low BMI less than 15 kg/m^2, or for medically or psychiatrically unstable patients. Most inpatient specialty programs employ lenient behavioral protocols that do not include bed rest but do have explicit behavioral guidelines and expectations, allowing for increasing levels of independence over food choice and exercise that are contingent on completing meals and achieving an adequate rate of weight gain. Lengths of stay average a few weeks or less, and patients are usually transitioned to either residential or partial hospitalization programs once stable and partially weight restored. Rates of weight gain are typically lower in these less intensive treatment settings than in inpatient specialty units, and programming often includes therapeutic meal-based activities including shopping and preparing meals; eating in social settings; and practicing normal eating behaviors—skills viewed as important to relapse prevention, although empirical data supporting their importance are needed.

The majority of patients reach their target weights in competent specialty inpatient programs with rates of weight gain of 3–4 pounds/week; however, there is a paucity of long- and short-term outcome data on weight restoration, especially for adults with AN in residential and partial hospitalization settings in which rates of weight gain are typically slower. In adolescents, a recent, large multicenter German study demonstrated comparable BMI outcomes at 1 year for inpatient weight restoration compared to transition from inpatient to partial hospitalization following 3 weeks of medical stabilization and initiation of refeeding. No equivalent data exist for an adult population. Given the current pressures to shorten hospital stays, there is a need for studies clarifying what elements of treatment are most helpful, as well as empirically driven refeeding guidelines and standards for target rates of weight gain and weight restoration across levels of care.

Access to specialty behavioral programs for AN is limited by both insurance and geographic constraints. Patients are therefore often admitted to general medical units for brief admissions aimed at medical stabilization and initiation of refeeding, or are treated on general psychiatric units. There are no data on the efficacy of these nonspecialty settings with respect to weight restoration outcomes for adults with AN.

Mode of Feeding: Oral, Enteral, and Parenteral Refeeding

The preferred and safest mode of refeeding is meal-based, oral refeeding aimed at broadening food repertoire, extinguishing fears of consuming calorie-dense foods, normalizing eating behavior, and restoring weight. Rates of weight gain of 2–3 pounds/week are typical of most behavioral inpatient specialist settings, with some hospital-based programs achieving average rates of weight gain of 4 pounds/week with oral refeeding alone.

Other programs employ supplemental nocturnal nasogastric feeds to boost lower rates of weight gain from 2 to up to 4 pounds/week. Additionally, short-term nasogastric feeding is utilized routinely on some adolescent units to initiate weight gain prior to transition to meal-based refeeding and transfer to a lower level of care. In adult AN populations, enteral feeding is prescribed only in cases with suboptimal rates of weight gain, if at all. Enteral feeding may also be employed on medical units when access to a specialty behavioral program is lacking, or when a patient is medically unstable and not compliant with meal-based refeeding. When enteral feeding is prolonged, gastrostomy tubes are sometimes used, although there is limited evidence to support chronic enteral feeding in AN. Treatment-resistant cases are as likely to sabotage enteral feeding as they are to refuse to eat adequate food to sustain weight gain. Complications from chronic nasogastric or gastrostomy feeding are also a risk, especially if patients are tampering with the equipment. Use of parenteral nutrition is not recommended in the presence of a functional gastrointestinal tract given the high risk of sepsis and hepatic complications in malnourished and severely underweight patients. Referral to a tertiary care, hospital-based specialty program with expertise in treatment-resistant AN is preferable when attempts at oral or enteral refeeding fail. In life-threatening AN, when competence to refuse treatment is in question, involuntary treatment can be effective. Comparisons of voluntary and involuntary admissions to behavioral specialty programs utilizing meal-based refeeding protocols have demonstrated equivalent short-term outcomes with respect to weight restoration.

Conclusions and Gaps in the Literature

To navigate their way out of AN, patients need to "eat first and understand second." Psychological insight alone does not equal treatment progress, whereas weight restoration is often accompanied by a decrease in ambivalence toward treatment. In general, behavioral treatment approaches are associated with the highest rates of weight restoration. These include FBT in adolescents and inpatient, meal-based behavioral refeeding in adults or adolescents in whom outpatient behavioral psychotherapeutic interventions fail. For adolescents, an emerging literature suggests that shorter inpatient stays followed by FBT or partial hospitalization may be effective alternatives to protracted hospitalization. Data on adults are lacking.

Increasing limitations on inpatient length of stay and stricter medical necessity criteria for hospital-based care have led to a drastic decrease in the length of hospital admissions for AN. This change has been accompanied by a drop in discharge BMI and an increase in readmission rates. Recently, residential treatment programs have developed to fill this gap. These programs provide a less expensive specialty setting for the 24-hour care and behavioral supervision needed to help patients in whom outpatient attempts at weight restoration have failed; however, there is a need for evidence demonstrating their effectiveness, especially in adults with chronic AN. Similarly, long-term outcome studies comparing fast versus slow approaches to refeeding, nasogastric versus meal-based refeeding, and the development and assessment of interventions aimed at relapse prevention following weight restoration are needed. Given the high cost of treatment of AN, future research should also routinely examine the economic implications of differing treatments, both in the short and in the long term, as well as ethical issues surrounding the role of involuntary treatment or other coercive measures aimed at weight restoration for individuals with life-threatening AN.

Suggested Reading

Bodell, L. P., & Mayer, L. E. (2011). Percent body fat is a risk factor for relapse in anorexia nervosa: A replication study. *International Journal of Eating Disorders, 44*(2), 118–123.—A replication study demonstrating that lower percent body fat following short-term weight restoration is associated with greater risk for relapse within a year of hospital discharge.

Calugi, S., Dalle Grave, R., Sartirana, M., & Fairburn, C. G. (2015). Time to restore body weight in adults and adolescents receiving cognitive behaviour therapy for anorexia nervosa. *Journal of Eating Disorders, 3,* 21.—A comparison of CBT-E for weight restoration in adolescents versus adults with AN.

Carter, J. C., Mercer-Lynn, K. B., Norwood, S. J., Bewell-Weiss, C. V., Crosby, R. D., Woodside, D. B., et al. (2012). A prospective study of predictors of relapse in anorexia nervosa: Implications for relapse prevention. *Psychiatry Research, 200*(2), 518–523.—A prospective study of relapse in the year following discharge for 100 weight-restored patients with AN treated in an inpatient partial-hospitalization program for eating disorders.

Dempfle, A., Herpertz-Dahlmann, B., Timmesfeld, N., Schwarte, R., Egberts, K. M., Pfeiffer, E., et al. (2013). Predictors of the resumption of menses in adolescent anorexia nervosa. *BMC Psychiatry, 13*(1), 308.—A prospective study of clinical parameters associated with resumption of menses in 172 female adolescents with AN.

Garber, A. K., Sawyer, S. M., Golden, N. H., Guarda, A. S., Katzman, D. K., Kohn, M. R., et al. (2016). A systematic review of approaches to refeeding in patients with AN. *International Journal of Eating Disorders, 49*(3), 293–310.—A systematic review of the literature on refeeding in adolescents and adults with AN.

Herpertz-Dahlmann, B., Schwarte, R., Krei, M., Egberts, K., Warnke, A., Wewetzer, C., et al. (2014). Day-patient treatment after short inpatient care versus continued inpatient treatment in adolescents with anorexia nervosa (ANDI): A multicentre, randomised, open-label, non-inferiority trial. *Lancet, 383,* 1222–1229.—A randomized comparison of inpatient weight restoration compared to 3 weeks of inpatient followed by day hospital weight restoration in 172 adolescents with AN.

Marzola, E., Nasser, J. A., Hashim, S. A., Pei-an, B. S., & Kaye, W. H. (2013). Nutritional rehabilitation in anorexia nervosa: Review of the literature and implications for treatment. *BMC Psychiatry, 13*(1), 290.—A recent review of nutritional rehabilitation literature in the treatment of AN.

Murray, S. B., & Le Grange, D. (2014). Family therapy for adolescent eating disorders: An update. *Current Psychiatry Reports, 16*(5), 1–7.—A review of studies of FBT for adolescent AN.

Redgrave, G. W., Coughlin, J. W., Schreyer, C. C., Martin, L. M., Leonpacher, A. K., Seide, M., et al. (2015). Refeeding and weight restoration outcomes in anorexia nervosa: Challenging current guidelines. *International Journal of Eating Disorders, 48*(7), 866–873.—A cohort study of 361 consecutive admissions to a meal-based behavioral refeeding specialty program employing a rapid refeeding protocol with medical monitoring.

Schebendach, J. E., Mayer, L. E., Devlin, M. J., Attia, E., Contento, I. R., Wolf, R. L., et al. (2011). Food choice and diet variety in weight-restored patients with AN. *Journal of the American Dietetic Association, 111*(5), 732–736.—A study linking variety of food choice at discharge from hospital-based weight restoration to relapse risk.

Self-Help Treatments for Eating Disorders

ROBYN SYSKO

Effective psychological treatments are available for bulimia nervosa (BN) and binge eating disorder (BED). However, despite the utility of these interventions, access to specialized therapies is often limited for several important reasons, including lack of experienced providers, effort needed to train and supervise new therapists, economic barriers to accessing care, and intensity of these therapies. Self-help treatments based on the standard outpatient version of cognitive-behavioral therapy for BN or BED have been developed as a way to make these specialized therapies more accessible to patients with eating disorders.

Self-Help Interventions

Self-help programs, delivered in book or electronic (e.g., CD-ROM, Internet-based) forms, typically include (1) didactic information intended to inform patients about eating disorders and (2) specific strategies to reduce symptoms. Programs are typically delivered as either *guided self-help (GSH),* a combination of the self-help program with a limited number of brief therapist visits to assist patients in implementing the treatment program, or *pure self-help,* which refers to following the program without additional assistance. How guided self-help is delivered (e.g., in person or remotely via telephone calls/Internet), the number of sessions, and the background of the therapist (e.g., mental health professional vs. primary care provider) varies, but a consistent feature is the lower intensity of the treatment in comparison to traditional psychotherapy. For example, standard cognitive-behavioral therapy for BN typically consists of twenty 50-minute individual sessions over 4–5 months, whereas self-help versions of this treatment can be administered in eight 20-minute sessions over 3–4 months.

Efficacy of Self-Help for BN, BED, and Their Variants

A number of studies have evaluated the efficacy of self-help treatments for BN, BED, and related variants of these disorders (e.g., recurrent binge eating). In general, despite limited therapist contact, self-help forms of cognitive-behavioral therapy are superior to control interventions and achieve comparable outcomes to specialized treatment (cognitive-behavioral therapy, interpersonal psychotherapy, family-based therapy) for adolescents and adults with BED or BN. It is notable that a substantial proportion of published trials compared self-help treatments to a waiting list control, and the superiority of self-help found in studies using this design only supports the use of self-help when no other treatment is available. Like standard cognitive-behavioral therapy, these treatments appear to work rapidly, producing significant reductions in binge eating and/or purging within the first month of treatment. Patients enrolled in these trials tend to rate self-help treatments as acceptable, but attrition and adherence have been identified as significant issues for delivering this type of intervention. Specifically, dropout appears to be influenced by the method with which self-help was delivered, diagnosis, and eating disorder symptoms (see "Suggested Reading"). Moreover, in comparison to other outpatient treatment options for eating disorders, self-help forms of cognitive-behavioral therapy have been shown to be more cost-effective even when utilizing specialized providers.

However, the aforementioned largely positive results noted across trials of self-help treatments employed in clinics specializing in the treatment of eating disorders contrast with two large controlled studies conducted in primary care settings, one for BN and one for BED (see "Suggested Reading"). Both trials failed to identify a significant benefit of self-help, which raises concerns about whether self-help methods are effective treatments for BN and BED outside of specialty settings. Factors influencing this observed variability in outcomes are not yet clear; however, there are several important differences between primary and tertiary care that may influence the provision of self-help interventions, including training of self-help providers, investment of providers in the expected efficacy of the self-help treatment in comparison to a medication treatment, and the lack of provider involvement in pure self-help.

Self-Help Treatments for AN

In contrast to BN and BED, little empirical evidence supports any particular form of psychological or pharmacological intervention for the acute treatment of anorexia nervosa (AN). Given the lack of available treatment options, as with many other treatment options, self-help approaches have been considered for patients with AN. One study (see "Suggested Reading") found that a self-help treatment administered prior to inpatient treatment was associated with a significant decrease in the number of days of hospitalization required. In addition, ongoing studies are exploring the use of self-help interventions for patients with AN to augment treatment or in collaboration with their families.

Future Research

Since the publication of the previous edition of this book, a substantial amount of research on self-help treatments has been published; however, several important questions about the use of these interventions remain unanswered. First, as described earlier, self-help treatment may be less effective in primary care settings, and studies are needed to understand better the conditions under which GSH can be delivered successfully, including the optimal training methods for delivering this treatment. Second, although predictors and mediators of outcome have been examined in several studies of BN, it is not yet possible to personalize the use of self-help treatments, or to determine for whom this type of intervention has the greatest likelihood of succeeding. Furthermore, while self-help treatments have documented efficacy, there is room for improvement. Existing well-studied manuals have already begun expanding skills included in the programs to address other areas, such as body image concerns, a fundamental symptom among patients with eating disorders. It may also be possible to incorporate other aspects of evidence-based treatments (e.g., emotion regulation strategies from dialectical behavior therapy) in future iterations of these manuals.

Finally, although GSH forms of cognitive-behavioral therapy for BN and BED are effective, few individuals utilize these treatments. There are a number of explanations for this observation, but an important concern relates to participant burden. The main skill employed throughout cognitive-behavioral forms of self-help is self-monitoring, a technique that is uniquely effective in reducing binge eating episodes; however, traditional pencil-and-paper versions of self-monitoring are time-intensive and cumbersome. In addition, other behavioral strategies utilized in cognitive-behavioral self-help (e.g., the development of a pattern of regular eating) require a high degree of participant engagement outside of session. Novel technologies, such as those available via smartphones, offer a potentially important means for reducing time spent by patients for these self-help treatments. Technology is likely to play a significant role in efforts to disseminate empirically supported treatments. Because the optimal format for making these treatments more widely available is not known, it is hoped that future studies will focus on identifying the best methods for utilizing smartphone technology for the use and dissemination of self-help treatments.

Suggested Reading

Beintner, I., Jacobi, C., & Schmidt, U. H. (2014). Participation and outcome in manualized self-help for bulimia nervosa and binge eating disorder: A systematic review and metaregression analysis. *Clinical Psychology Review, 34,* 158–176.—A review of factors influencing dropout and outcomes in studies and self-help, including duration, guidance, type of treatment, and diagnosis to help guide the use of this type of treatment for patients with BN and BED.

Fairburn, C. G. (1995). *Overcoming binge eating.* New York: Guilford Press.—The best studied cognitive-behavioral self-help manual for the treatment of BN and BED; a second edition was published in 2013, with additional elements focusing on body image disturbance.

Fichter, M., Cebulla, M., Quadflieg, N., & Naab, S. (2008). Guided self-help for binge eating/purging anorexia nervosa before inpatient treatment. *Psychotherapy Research, 18,* 594–603.—This controlled trial utilizing cognitive-behavioral self-help for AN prior to hospitalization found modest effects on duration of inpatient treatment (~5 days less) for patients receiving guided self-help.

Grilo, C. M., White, M. A., Gueorguieva, R., Barnes, R. D., & Masheb, R. M. (2013). Self-help for binge eating disorder in primary care: A randomized controlled trial with ethnically and racially diverse obese patients. *Behaviour Research and Therapy, 51,* 855–861.—Pure self-help, when used for patients with BED, was not effective in comparison to usual care, which raises concerns about the utility of self-help interventions in primary care.

Hilbert, A., Hildebrandt, T., Agras, W. S., Wilfley, D. E., & Wilson, G. T. (2015). Rapid response in psychological treatments for binge eating disorder. *Journal of Consulting and Clinical Psychology, 83*(3), 649–654.—Patients with BED who demonstrated a rapid response (i.e., within the first 4 weeks of treatment) to a GSH version of cognitive-behavioral therapy showed significantly greater rates of remission from binge eating than nonrapid responders, improvements that persisted over a 2-year follow-up.

Mitchell, J. E., Agras, S., Crow, S., Halmi, K., Fairburn, C. G., Bryson, S., et al. (2011). Stepped care and cognitive-behavioural therapy for bulimia nervosa: Randomised trial. *British Journal of Psychiatry, 198*, 391–397.—In the largest controlled study of patients with BN (*n* = 293), similar outcomes were noted for individuals receiving cognitive-behavioral GSH and cognitive-behavioral therapy (twenty 50-minute sessions); however, in comparison to other studies, the outcomes (abstinence rates) for cognitive-behavioral therapy were not as positive.

Schmidt, U., Lee, S., Beecham, J., Perkins, S., Treasure, J., Yi, I., et al. (2007). A randomized controlled trial of family therapy and cognitive behavior therapy guided self-care for adolescents with bulimia nervosa and related disorders. *American Journal of Psychiatry, 164*(4), 591–598.—One of a small number of trials for adolescents, in which a guided self-help form of cognitive-behavioral therapy was superior to a specialized treatment (family-based treatment) in reducing binge eating for full and subthreshold BN in the short-term, and comparable in long-term outcomes. The mean cost of self-help treatment was also significantly lower than that for family-based treatment.

Striegel-Moore, R. H., Wilson, G. T., DeBar, L., Perrin, N., Lynch, F., Rosselli, F., et al. (2010). Cognitive behavioral guided self-help for the treatment of recurrent binge eating. *Journal of Consulting and Clinical Psychology, 78*, 312–321.—A large portion of the sample (41%) did not meet criteria for BN or BED, but significant improvements were noted with cognitive-behavioral self-help, and there were no differences between full and subthreshold cases.

Walsh, B. T., Fairburn, C. G., Mickley, D., Sysko, R., & Parides, M. K. (2004). Treatment of bulimia nervosa in a primary care setting. *American Journal of Psychiatry, 161*, 556–561.—A comparison of cognitive-behavioral GSH and medication (fluoxetine/placebo) for patients with broadly defined BN in a primary care setting in which the self-help treatment conferred no measurable effect on bulimic symptoms.

Wilson, G. T., & Zandberg, L. J. (2012). Cognitive-behavioral guided self-help for eating disorders: Effectiveness and scalability. *Clinical Psychology Review, 32*, 343–357.—This comprehensive review includes summaries of studies evaluating the efficacy of self-help interventions for BN, BED, and eating disorder not otherwise specified; considers data on the acceptability, cost-effectiveness, and scalability of this type of treatment; and proposes future directions for research on GSH.

Dissemination of Evidence-Based Treatment

G. TERENCE WILSON

The primary focus of research on the treatment of eating disorders has been on the demonstration of efficacy using well-controlled randomized clinical trials (RCTs). As a result, it is now well established that there are evidence-based psychological treatments for both bulimia nervosa (BN) and binge eating disorder (BED). The consensus is that they are the first-line treatments of choice for these eating disorders. Moreover, accumulating evidence indicates that these findings from conventional RCTs can generalize to "real-world" clinical settings. The latter typically include more heterogeneous patient samples and therapists who are likely to have received limited training and less supervision than in standard RCTs. In contrast, evidence for the efficacy of treatments for anorexia nervosa (AN) is largely lacking. Currently, evidence-based treatment for AN is limited to family-based therapy for adolescents.

The major problem in the field, however—as with mental health disorders as a whole—is the lack of access to psychological treatment in general, and to evidence-based treatment in particular. Patients are not receiving effective treatments in routine clinical care, and even when they do receive these treatments, their implementation may not be optimal. Research on dissemination and implementation of evidence-based treatments is a priority in the mental health field.

Dissemination and Implementation: Obstacles and Solutions

Criteria for Evaluating Suitability of Different Treatments

In addition to outcome efficacy and effectiveness, selection criteria for implementing treatment for an eating disorder necessarily require consideration of the following features: clinical range (breadth of applicability), brevity, cost-effectiveness, acceptability to specific patient populations, and scalability. Treatments that rate positively on the aforementioned criteria are clearly better suited to dissemination across different settings and diverse patient populations. They can more easily implemented by therapists/counselors with limited training and less expertise than the more complex therapy packages that require greater professional qualifications. Critically, they are more scalable. Disadvantages of most current forms of psychological treatment are that they tend to be complex and multifaceted, and, hence, challenging to learn.

Availability of Therapists

The default model of treatment in clinical psychology and psychiatry in the United States remains individual, face-to-face psychotherapy with doctoral-level professionals. This method of treatment is inherently inadequate for providing the needed access to effective treatment even in resource-rich settings as the United States, let alone low-resource countries. A workable solution is known as task shifting (task sharing) in which less highly trained individuals, including practitioners who are more available and affordable members of the health service or community, implement specific treatment interventions in which they have been trained.

An obvious concern is that quality of care will suffer using this task-shifting model. However, impressive results have been achieved in major studies targeting depression and posttraumatic stress in global settings. Early findings suggest that this model is also applicable to the treatment of both BN and BED.

Training Therapists in the Implementation of Evidence-Based Treatments

To be successful, psychological treatments much be delivered in a competent manner. This requires that therapists/counselors be effectively trained in their implementation, but training has been a largely neglected subject. Training as usual is typically a workshop plus the provision of a therapy manual. Follow-up supervision is often impractical or unavailable, and evidence indicates that this model fails to increase necessary therapist skills. There is a need to develop effective and practical training methods (i.e., evidence-based training).

Two innovative training options are currently under consideration. One is the train-the-trainer model, in which an expert trains less qualified individuals to be future trainers. In addition, if the trainer is part of clinical service organization, he or she is able to provide continuing or follow-up consultation and supervision to the staff trainees. The early findings have been promising. However, this strategy would still produce a limited number of competent therapists/counselors. It would not provide a sufficiently large number of mental health care providers who could offer adequate access to evidence-based treatment especially in low-resource settings.

The second option that is currently under investigation in the use of enhanced cognitive-behavioral therapy (CBT-E) is Web-centered training. The training is based on a specifically designed website that provides detailed clinical instruction in the application of the treatment to specific eating disorder psychopathology. The website can be used on its own or in conjunction with guidance from a counselor, ideally, a nonspecialist in CBT for eating disorders, thereby increasing the scalability of this guided form of self-directed training. Were such Web-centered training shown to be effective in training therapists/counselors to administer treatment competently, it has the potential to greatly expand the number of available therapists in the field.

The impact of effective Web-centered training could be dramatic. It would provide for the first time a means of training that is widely available, cost-effective, and uniquely scalable. Web-based training might also address a well-documented problem, namely, how well the training of therapists is sustained over time. The term "therapist drift" denotes the reality that therapists increasingly become nonadherent to structured treatment protocols. A website might provide continuing "booster" opportunities for trainees to reengage in the treatment and possibly acquire new skills as treatment protocols are revised and improved.

Therapist Competence

Competence can be defined as the therapist's ability to implement treatment in the manner that it was implemented in the RCTs that provided the evidence justifying its adoption. Unfortunately, evaluations of this critically important aspect of treatment integrity have been infrequent in the psychological treatment of mental disorders generally. More commonly, studies have assessed simply whether the therapist adhered to the specific treatment protocol. However, as the saying goes, it is possible to do anything poorly. It is the *quality* of implementation that is decisive, and competence should be the primary aim of therapist training. Innovative ways of assessing therapist competence in CBT-E, including the development of an online measure, have been developed.

Failure to ensure competence can undermine dissemination. Although the findings of RCTs have been shown to generalize to routine clinical care in many instances, there are also reports that the benefits of evidence-based treatments drop off when the interventions are scaled up to new and different clinical settings—the so-called "implementation cliff." The problem might not be the treatment but the way it is implemented—a question of therapist competence.

Innovative Technology

In recent years, there has been an explosion of interest in the use of Internet-based and mobile-device applications (E-therapy) for the treatment of mental health problems, including eating disorders. One of many advantages is the potential for enhancing dissemination because of scalability.

In the treatment of eating disorders, the available evidence is mixed. Early reports were positive suggesting that E-therapy was a practical alternative to more traditional face-to-face therapies. A subsequent analysis, however, has provided a more sobering set of findings. Using the United Kingdom's NICE (National Institute for Health and Care Excellence) methodology, a recent meta-analysis of existing RCTs indicated that no firm conclusions can be drawn about Internet-based treatment. Few positive effects were observed, and no RCTs evaluating apps were identified.

Self-Help Interventions

Significant progress has been made in the dissemination of evidence-based treatment for eating disorders using a self-help approach. A prime example has been the development of cognitive-behavioral guided self-help (CBTgsh) which is an adaptation of full-scale CBT for use with BN and BED. The intervention typically comprises 8–10, 20- to 25-minute sessions in which the therapist provides focused guidance in the implementation of a manual-based CBT self-help program. Importantly for ease of dissemination, the guidance is mainly of a supportive and facilitative nature. It does not require specific expertise in CBT. The goal is to maintain a focus on the eating disorder, help patients monitor their progress, and address failure to engage in the program. CBTgsh is not simply an abbreviated session of full-scale CBT.

Current evidence shows that this brief CBTgsh treatment is an effective intervention. It has been shown to be as effective as full specialty therapy (e.g., interpersonal psychotherapy [IPT]) at posttreatment and 2-year follow-up for BED. Even if it were somewhat less effective than a longer specialty therapy, it would have the decided advantage of greater scalability, namely, being able to reach a much larger number of patients. CBTgsh is cost-effective. It requires fewer treatment sessions and can be more readily administered by less highly trained therapists, with more limited supervision than full-scale CBT or IPT. Research in a large health maintenance organization has shown that CBTgsh resulted in significantly lower total societal cost than treatment as usual.

CBTgsh lends itself to task shifting. With adequate training and some level of continuing supervision, CBTgsh can be implemented effectively by relatively inexperienced practitioners lacking formal professional credentials. It also fits well with the train-the-trainer model. In one study, after receiving expert-led instruction, a master's-level graduate student trained and supervised other clinically inexperienced beginning graduate students in CBTgsh for BN and BED. Results showed significant reductions in eating disorder psychopathology, general psychopathology, and functional impairment, as well as high ratings of acceptability by both referring clinicians and patients.

Future research on self-help interventions promises to enhance the value of this means of dissemination of evidence-based treatment for eating disorders. To date, the implementation of CBT self-help has relied on the use of a written treatment manual. It has been suggested that a still more effective and scalable delivery system would be via an interactive Web-based system. This would allow greater individualization of the self-help program. Intervention would be more easily tailored to the particular maintaining mechanisms of the individual's eating disorder. It is also likely that a longer and more clinically rich form of the program will be developed that has a greater clinical range while still providing a cost-effective and scalable alternative to specialty treatment.

Suggested Reading

Beintner, I., Jacobi, C., & Schmidt, U. H. (2014). Participation and outcome in manualized self-help for bulimia nervosa and binge eating disorder—a systematic review and metaregression analysis. *Clinical Psychology Review, 34*(2), 158–176.—Comprehensive review of applications of manual-based self-help.

Fairburn, C. G., Bailey-Straebler, S., Basden, S., Doll, H. A., Jones, R., Murphy, R., et al. (2015). A transdiagnostic comparison of enhanced cognitive behaviour therapy (CBT-E) and interpersonal psychotherapy in the treatment of eating disorders. *Behaviour Research and Therapy, 70*, 64–71.—A well-controlled RCT showing that CBT-E is broadly effective in the treatment of eating disorders and significantly superior to an alternative evidence-based psychological treatment.

Fairburn, C. G., & Patel, V. (2014). The global dissemination of psychological treatments: A road map for research and practice. *American Journal of Psychiatry, 171*(5), 495–498.—An analysis of the potential value and applicability of Web-based dissemination of evidence-based treatment.

Kazdin, A. E., & Blase, S. L. (2011). Rebooting psychotherapy research and practice to reduce the burden of mental illness. *Perspectives on Psychological Science, 6*, 21–37.—An influential analysis of how to improve dissemination based on innovations in the delivery of psychological treatments.

Loucas, C. E., Fairburn, C. G., Whittington, C., Pennant, M. E., Stockton, S., & Kendall, T. (2014). E-therapy in the treatment and prevention of eating disorders: A systematic review and meta-analysis. *Behaviour Research and Therapy, 63*, 122–131.—A critical appraisal of the methodological adequacy of existing E-therapy studies.

Lynch, F. L., Dickerson, J., Perrin, N., DeBar, L., Wilson, G. T., Kraemer, H., et al. (2010). Cost-effectiveness of treatment for recurrent binge eating. *Journal of Consulting and Clinical Psychology, 78*, 322–333.—A study demonstrating the cost-effectiveness of CBT guided self-help in terms of total societal cost estimated by using patient and health plan costs.

McHugh, R. K., & Barlow, D. H. (2012). *Dissemination and implementation of evidence-based psychological interventions.* New York: Oxford University Press.—A comprehensive review and analysis of the problems of dissemination and their possible solutions.

Shafran, R., Clark, D. M., Fairburn, C. G., Arntz, A., Barlow, D. H., Ehlers, A., et al. (2009). Mind the gap: Improving the dissemination of CBT. *Behaviour Research and Therapy, 47*(11), 902–909.—A review and analysis of the lack of access to CBT in routine clinical care and potential means of overcoming existing obstacles.

Wilson, G. T., & Zandberg, L. (2112). Cognitive-behavioral guided self-help for eating disorders: Effectiveness and scalability. *Clinical Psychology Review, 32*, 343–357.—A detailed review of the nature and outcome of guided self-help interventions.

Zandberg, L. J., & Wilson, G. T. (2013). Train-the-trainer: Implementation of cognitive behavioral guided self-help for recurrent binge eating in a naturalistic setting. *European Eating Disorders Review, 21*, 230–237.—A study showing the effectiveness of CBTgsh administered using the train-the-trainer model with BN and BED patients.

Prevention of Eating Disorders

TRACEY D. WADE

Prevention of eating disorders in youth represents an intuitively and objectively worthy endeavor, resulting in a proliferation of public health approaches, most of which have no evidence base. Indeed, some are associated with evidence showing ineffectiveness. Unfortunately, this lack of evidence base has not impeded dissemination of ineffective approaches. However, there is cause for optimism because evidence that has accumulated over the last 15 years supports a handful of promising directions in the prevention of eating disorders. This chapter provides an overview of these approaches.

Risk Factors Informing Prevention Targets

The 2008 Medical Research Council guidelines on developing and evaluating complex interventions emphasizes the use of theory for informing the development of effective interventions. This also requires evidence that supports the putative risk factors, processes, and outcomes. This is a particularly important focus in prevention work because there has been some concern about the direct targeting of eating-disordered behaviors, especially in prevention efforts targeting an entire population, due to the potential iatrogenic effects of such information. While empirical support for this concern is not strong, it does seem responsible to adhere to a "do no harm" approach; thus, most effective approaches have focused on risk factors for eating disorders, either distal or proximal, depending on which is most developmentally appropriate. One of the risk factors most commonly targeted includes *media internalization,* which refers to strong investment in societal ideals of size and appearance to the point that they become rigid guiding principles (sometimes called "thin ideal" internalization when related to females). Also commonly targeted are pressure (from media, peers, family) on the person to conform to a thin (girls) or muscular (boys) ideal, body dissatisfaction, and the undue influence of control over weight, shape, and eating on self-worth. Given that the conduct of these interventions is as important as the content, researchers also seek to change important risk factors in the way in which interventions are delivered, such as modeling flexible solutions in order to break down unhelpful perfectionism and the associated self-criticism, building up self-efficacy or effectiveness through acquisition of new skills, and modeling more helpful discussions and behaviors among peer groups in order to reduce pressures on appearance.

Types of Prevention

There are three types of prevention as defined by the 2009 National Research Council and Institute of Medicine: universal, selective, and indicated. Universal prevention targets the general public or a whole population group that has not been identified on the basis of individual risk, with an intervention that is desirable for everyone in that group. Selective interventions target individuals or a subgroup of the population whose risk of developing an eating disorder is significantly higher than average (e.g., girls). Indicated prevention targets high-risk individuals who are identified as having minimal but detectable signs or symptoms of an eating disorder (e.g., females with body image disturbance).

Overview of Efficacy

Studies were considered if they appeared in peer-reviewed journals and used designs that met the criteria previously outlined by Chambless and Hollon (1998) for empirically supported psychological therapies, which include (1) a comparison to another condition, including a placebo or control condition; (2) utilization of repeated measures; (3) sample size exceeding 25 in each cell; (4) follow-up assessment greater than 10 weeks after the cessation of the program; and (5) use of reliable and valid measures. *Prevention effects* can be defined as preventing an increase over time in these risk factors or eating disorder symptoms, such that there is significantly less elevation in the risk factor compared to the control condition. *Treatment effects* are defined as a decrease in risk factor or eating disorder symptom intensity over time compared to the control group.

Universal Prevention

In populations in which eating disorders and their symptoms are not yet manifested by the majority, prevention requires careful consideration of relevant outcomes. Inclusion of eating disorder symptoms will necessarily be attended by a floor effect, in which the low level of symptoms will preclude significant changes. It also requires an exceptionally lengthy follow-up time to observe a prevention effect in disordered eating in the typically younger age groups involved in these studies. Hence, most outcomes at this level focus on proximal risk factors for eating disorders, such as weight and shape concern, body dissatisfaction, and dieting.

Approaches to universal prevention are summarized in Table 56.1. The studies were conducted in classroom settings, included both boys and girls, and if an effect was present, showed positive significant change for both boys and girls, though typically stronger and/or for a greater range of variables for the latter. The greatest body of support is associated with media literacy approaches, which aim to empower participants to adopt a critical evaluation of media content so that they can identify, analyze, challenge, and propose alternatives to stereotypical and unhealthy messages presented in the mass media. It targets media internalization and also ineffectiveness by giving participants tools with

TABLE 56.1. Status of the Evidence for Universal Prevention

Broad approach	Degree to which evaluated[a]	Robustness of effect at follow-up[b] (longest follow-up period)
Dove Body Think: body image and self-esteem	Low	None (3-month)
Internalization of cultural appearance ideals, including appearance-related conversations, comparisons, teasing	Low	Promising (3-month)
Internalization of cultural appearance ideals, media literacy, and mindfulness	Low	Medium (12-month)
Media literacy	Substantial	Promising (30-month)
Self-esteem	Low	Medium (12-month)

[a]Number of studies: low < 5; medium ≥ 5 to ≤ 10; substantial > 10 studies.

[b]Judged on the proportion of studies supporting a significant difference at follow-up favoring the intervention across a number of eating disorder risk factors, ranging from none, medium, and promising.

which to stand up to unhealthy messages. A significant prevention effect for weight and shape concern compared to a control condition has been found in two different examinations of Media Smart (with 12-month and 30-month follow-up, respectively), a media literacy approach developed by Simon Wilksch and myself. Associated with few studies, but showing some promise, are interventions developed by Susan Paxton's group that target media internalization as they are expressed mainly in peer relationships. This approach is currently being investigated in randomized controlled trials in the classroom by Dove, who is seeking to adopt an evidence-based approach to replace Body Think. To date, no universal approaches have been evaluated with respect to prevention of eating disorder symptoms.

Selective Prevention and Indicated Prevention

As it is sometimes difficult to distinguish between these two types of prevention and there is some debate about this, both are considered together here. The most efficient way to approach this type of prevention is to examine which eating disorder risk factors moderate response to the intervention in universal prevention studies (i.e., a baseline characteristic that is not correlated with treatment, and that can be shown to have an interactive effect with the intervention on outcome). Previously examined moderators in eating disorders include weight and shape concern, depression, and sex (Table 56.2), and there are also studies that only investigate the efficacy of an intervention in girls. While many of the approaches show some degree of promise, there are few rigorous examinations to date.

This type of prevention often takes place in populations where there are minimal but detectable symptoms of eating disorders, so this research has the capacity to detect prevention effects with respect to the onset of eating disorders. Three programs have been shown to be associated with such prevention effects in females with elevated body image concerns, including the *Body Project* and the *Healthy Weight Intervention* devised by Eric Stice and colleagues, which have produced a 60% reduction in DSM-IV eating disorders over a 3-year follow-up period relative to a control condition, and *Student Bodies*,

TABLE 56.2. Status of the Evidence for Selective Prevention

Broad approach	Degree to which evaluated[a]	Robustness of effect at follow-up[b] (longest follow-up period) for which group
Cognitive-behavioral therapy (psychoeducation)	Medium	Medium (3-month) for females
Cognitive dissonance related to thin ideal	Low	Promising (8-month) for college-age females
Media literacy	Low	Promising (30-month) for participants with high levels of baseline depression
Mindfulness	Low	Promising (6-month) for females

[a]Number of studies: low < 5; medium ≥ 5 to ≤ 10; substantial > 10 studies.

[b]Judged on the proportion of studies supporting a significant difference at follow-up favoring the intervention across a number of eating disorder risk factors, ranging from none, medium, and promising.

an online cognitive-behavioral approach, devised by Barr Taylor and colleagues, that has been shown to prevent onset of eating disorders over a 2-year period in participants with a body mass index (BMI) ≥ 25, compared to 11.9% of the control group that developed an eating disorder.

The Body Project is distinguished from the other two by a large body of research characterized by rigorous testing and dissemination. It consists of four 1-hour sessions in a face-to-face group format, and uses a cognitive dissonance approach by examining the costs for women in pursuing the thin ideal. There is also inclusion of a self-affirmation exercise, body exposure, and developing the skills to stand up to the pressure of the thin ideal. There are further randomized controlled trials of this approach being funded by Dove for use with the World Association for Girl Guides and Girl Scouts, and emerging evidence suggests that an online application of the Body Project is as efficacious as the group intervention. The Healthy Weight Intervention was initially developed as a placebo comparison to the Body Project and includes various techniques to discourage unhealthy dieting behaviors while facilitating guidance for achieving a healthier lifestyle, including regular exercise and a healthy diet.

Student Bodies is an 8-week program that has the core goals to reduce weight and shape concerns, enhance body image, promote healthy weight regulations, reduce binge eating, and increase knowledge about risks associated with eating disorders. Included in the interactive software are video and audio presentations, a body image journal, online discussion groups, self-quizzes, goal-setting, personalized feedback, and accompanying weekly assignments. The program is currently being revised to include more content on managing negative affect and negative comments from others about eating, weight, or shape.

Factors That Influence Outcome Apart from Content

As noted previously, the conduct of these interventions can also influence outcome, with larger effect sizes achieved with the use of interactive rather than didactic approaches, multiple sessions (at least 4 hours of content) rather than just one or two sessions, and expert facilitators as opposed to task shifting to minimally trained presenters.

Key Issues

In a relatively short period of time, the outlook for prevention of eating disorders has changed from one of gloom to one of promise. However, there are important challenges that currently limit the successful dissemination of such approaches. First, decreased effect sizes when task shifting to less trained "in-house" providers requires an active and creative consideration of how to increase effectiveness in these settings. Second, competition in the market place, especially in classroom-based settings, means that we need to show transdiagnostic outcomes related to our interventions, especially in relation to negative affect and obesity. Third, pressure to reduce the hours of content below that which is likely to be effective should be resisted. The desire to do something positive and a positive outcome should not be conflated. Fourth, ongoing maintenance of these programs in real-world settings will provide a challenge that requires further attention.

Future Directions

There are a number of aspects of prevention that require investigation in future research:

- Online applications of prevention approaches.
- Evidence of larger and more persistent effects across a number of transdiagnostic targets in universal classroom settings, including growth of disordered eating behaviors and syndromes, obesity, and mental health issues related to negative affect.
- The efficacy and effectiveness of interventions that tackle some of the "road less traveled" risk factors, such as perfectionism and managing negative affect.
- Moderators that inform our understanding of what works for whom and under what circumstances.
- Mediators of interventions and outcomes that allow us to refine the connection between theory and intervention in order to improve our interventions by understanding how and why they work.

Suggested Reading

Atkinson, M., & Wade, T. (2015). Mindfulness-based prevention for eating disorders: A school-based cluster randomised controlled study. *International Journal of Eating Disorders, 48*(7), 1024–1037.—This research compared a classroom approach to mindfulness and cognitive dissonance to control and found 6-month follow-up effects favoring mindfulness over control across a number of outcomes, including eating disorder symptoms.

Austin, S. B. (2011). The blind spot in the drive for childhood obesity prevention: Bringing eating disorders prevention into focus as a public health priority. *American Journal of Public Health, 101*(6), e1–e4.—Recognizes the lack of connection between eating disorders and obesity prevention efforts, recommending an integration of these two in order to increase leverage in the generally unsuccessful efforts to prevent obesity.

Becker, C. B., Plasencia, M., Kilpela, L. S., Briggs, M., & Stewart, T. (2014). Changing the course of comorbid eating disorders and depression: What is the role of public health interventions in targeting shared risk factors? *Journal of Eating Disorders, 2,* 15.—If you read only one article on prevention, then this should be it because it provides an excellent and balanced overview of all the various prevention approaches in eating disorders.

Chambless, D. L., & Hollon, S. D. (1998). Defining empirically supported therapies. *Journal of Consulting and Clinical Psychology, 66,* 7–18.

Stice, E., Becker, C. B., & Yokum, S. (2013). Eating disorder prevention: Current evidence base and future directions. *International Journal of Eating Disorders, 46,* 478–485.—Provides an overview of two of the three indicated prevention approaches found to have prevention effects for eating disorder onset, as well as thoughts about future direction in the field.

Watson, H. J., Joyce, T., French, E., Willan, V., Kane, R. T., Tanner-Smith E. E., et al. (2016). Prevention of eating disorders: A systematic review of randomized, controlled trials. *International Journal of Eating Disorders, 49,* 833–862.—A new meta-analysis of the studies in this area that provides a very useful summary of what shows promise and what does not.

Wilksch, S. M., & Wade, T. D. (2015). Media literacy in the prevention of eating disorders. In L. Smolak & M. Levine (Eds.), *The Wiley-Blackwell handbook of eating disorders.* New York: Wiley-Blackwell.—A summary of the body of media literacy research in eating disorders prevention, with discussion of future directions in this field.

Yager, Z., Diedrichs, P. C., Ricciardelli, L. A., & Halliwell, E. (2013). What works in secondary schools?: A systematic review of classroom-based body image programs. *Body Image, 10,* 271–281.—An examination of the state of universal prevention in eating disorders.

Does Advocacy for Eating Disorders Really Work?

KITTY WESTIN
SCOTT CROW

Never doubt that a small group of thoughtful, committed citizens can change the world; indeed, it's the only thing that ever has.
—MARGARET MEAD

Have you ever asked yourself whether your voice matters, or wondered whether grassroots advocacy really makes a difference? We use the terms "grassroots advocate" and "citizen activist" interchangeably. Both phrases refer to someone who is activated, engaged, and ready to take action. A strong and important legacy of advocacy exists within the field of eating disorders, with a growing number of passionate and effective advocates. In this chapter, we review the benefits of grassroots advocacy and, more importantly, inspire you to use your voice and become an activist. We write this from an American perspective, as it is the one we know. However, we believe the principles we articulate are likely applicable across the free world.

The need for effective advocacy is great. In many areas, care systems and coverage for eating disorders lag behind those available for other illnesses. Moreover, research resources directed at eating disorders are woefully limited. For example, a search of the NIH RePORTER database in April 2015 shows 1,835 funded studies of schizophrenia, but only 60 studies of anorexia nervosa—despite the fact that this eating disorder is as common as schizophrenia, and carries a higher mortality risk.

One of the biggest challenges for those affected by eating disorders is getting the attention of the policymakers who have the power to enact laws and enforce existing policies that impact the eating disorders community. Until fairly recently, eating disorders were dismissed by the public (including elected officials) as simple behavioral problems or choices rather than serious, life-threatening mental illnesses. This mistaken belief has made it difficult to get policymakers to see the need to address eating disorders as serious health issues affecting millions of Americans. It has taken years of effort to dispel the many myths and misconceptions about eating disorders, but progress has been made through the efforts of advocacy organizations and the grassroots efforts of thousands of sufferers, families, friends, caregivers, and professionals.

Is Advocacy Important?

Advocacy is at the heart of change. Advocacy is the product of passion, commitment, and the desire to influence policy and practice. Grassroots advocacy is often driven by personal experience. There is impressive power in bringing together a group of people who share a common goal and are willing to work together to achieve that goal. Grassroots advocacy and community organization have been responsible for many (if not most) of the progressive social changes in the 21st century. Grassroots advocacy is a powerful tool in setting the policy agenda for individual provinces or states, or for an entire country. Efforts by citizen activists have the power to influence policymakers by demonstrating that a particular issue has widespread support and therefore voter support.

Minnesota's late Senator Paul Wellstone was well known for his ability to motivate and organize grassroots advocates. He believed that grassroots organizing was essential to building a "constituency for change" (Wellstone Action, 2005). Without citizen advocates who are passionate about their cause, we doubt that the groundbreaking Mental Health Parity Act would ever have passed, and mental health services may not have been included in the essential benefits in the Affordable Care Act. Advocacy is an essential component of change, and the most powerful advocates are often ordinary people who believe in something and are willing to speak out publicly to defend their views and fight for change. A study examining the effectiveness of grassroots lobbying suggests that the effect of e-mail campaigns on legislators is substantial, but that more personal contacts are far more effective than less personal contacts.

Why Is Advocacy Important?

A truth: Big companies, big money, and big business hire teams of highly paid lobbyists to "sell" their idea, product, or initiative to policymakers and the community. Lobbyists typically have ready access to members of Congress, and they are sometimes able to "buy" the support of a member. Grassroots advocates understand that in order to compete, we need to be in the game, we need to be at the table, and we need to speak out until we are heard.

Grassroots advocacy is a proven method of spreading the word about the multiple issues that the eating disorder community faces and, with widespread use of social media, messages can be seen by thousands of people, and calls to action can be sent in a matter of minutes. Advocacy efforts help us educate the community and equip patients, families, friends, and colleagues with information to help people understand the devastating impact of eating disorders. Community organizing brings much needed attention to a disease that can cause lifelong health issues or even death, and it can mobilize thousands of people to send a message, write a note, make a call, or in some other way demand that our policymakers give attention to eating disorders.

Who Can Be an Advocate?

Sadly, many grassroots advocacy organizations and efforts are the result of a tragedy. For example, Americans for Responsible Solutions, a nonprofit organization that supports gun control, was founded by U.S. House Member Gabrielle Giffords and her husband after she was shot while meeting with constituents. The Anna Westin Foundation was founded by the Westin family in 2000, after Anna died from an eating disorder. Her family was outraged when her insurance company denied coverage for the care that could have saved Anna's life.

However, researchers and clinicians are also often in a unique position to serve as effective advocates, providing a perspective to counter assertions made by others. Working with accurate facts and figures can be decisive. For instance, during the fight to pass the Paul Wellstone and Pete Domenici Mental Health and Addiction Equity Act, the business community and the insurance industry routinely reported that passing mental health parity would increase the cost of insurance by as much as 12%. The grassroots advocates who were working on this issue thought that a 12% increase seemed inflated, so they asked the Congressional Budget Office to make an assessment. The truth, as reported by the Congressional Budget Office, was a cost increase of only 0.9%. Once this more accurate number was reported, the Mental Health Parity Bill gained additional support, and it was finally passed into law on October 3, 2008.

Anyone can be an advocate, and many people step into an advocacy role almost daily, often without realizing it. Every time a therapist submits a preauthorization form for a client, he or she is serving as an advocate. Each time a psychiatrist helps a patient write an appeal or calls an insurance company on someone's behalf, he or she is acting as an advocate. Every time a researcher presents data to policymakers, advocacy occurs. Advocacy is part of our daily lives and the move from advocating for one individual or small group to advocating for a larger group is not as hard as some might think.

We believe that the qualities that help people be effective advocates include passion, commitment, integrity, honesty, and courage. Advocacy is about believing in something and being willing to speak openly, honestly, and often about that belief. The most effective advocacy occurs when ordinary people are brought together as a group and, after some training or coaching, are allowed to use their voices and speak for themselves. Most people find that becoming an advocate is easy because often they are advocating for something they know well and in which they believe. Grassroots activists are typically people who are driven by the belief that they have a story to tell, and that their story is important. This is distinctly different from a paid lobbyist who works for a company and seldom has a personal connection or interest in the "product" he or she is "selling."

Our experience on Capitol Hill has illustrated the power of citizen activists. Repeatedly, while speaking with a member of Congress or a staff person, we have been able to convince a member to support the eating disorder community by signing on to legislation, signing letters to colleagues, writing letters to government offices such as the Centers for Disease Control and Prevention (CDC), or hosting Congressional Briefings. We have been told that our presence and perseverance is what convinced them to support us, and that until we appeared in their office, they knew little or nothing about eating disorders.

Grassroots advocates are generally volunteers who travel to their capitols on their own time, without an expense account. Grassroots advocates do this because they have a story to tell, an experience to share, and in-depth knowledge about their cause. Because grassroots advocates are not working for a company or expected to recite the party line, they can be creative and use their voices in ways that are unencumbered by political or economic conflicts.

What Are Eating Disorder Advocates Working On?

The issues that are in need of advocacy efforts change over time. In the 1990s, getting anyone to pay attention to mental health disorders was a challenge, and many advocates were working to ensure that people who struggled with mental illness had their basic human rights upheld. In the early 2000s, the eating disorders community began to realize that there was a need for targeted advocacy efforts to ensure that eating disorders were getting much needed attention from policymakers. Today, there is a coordinated effort to address the many issues that face the eating disorder community. Currently, advocates are addressing eating disorders at the federal level with a bipartisan bill designed to offer training to help clinicians recognize signs and symptoms of eating disorders; to uphold the Mental Health Parity Act of 2008; and to demonstrate that digitally altered advertising images adversely impact young people. In addition, many states have enacted or are working on legislation to expand access to treatment for people with eating disorders. There are advocacy groups focusing their efforts on such things as combating the misuse of diet pills; ensuring that girls, boys, women, and men who choose modeling as a career are able to work in a safe environment; that there is accurate and timely information available to teachers, counselors, and families related to eating disorders; and that prevention is offered across the United States in schools and communities.

How Do You Advocate?

Advocacy is simple. It is about preparing, practicing, and telling a story. Grassroots advocates have the advantage of being interested in one issue and having a deep understanding of that issue. Clinicians and researchers must be prepared, with clear and compelling facts and figures. The steps necessary to be an effective advocate start with a passion or a mission. The first, and possibly the most important, step is to define what the passion or mission is. It is important to gather all the information before going into a meeting with a legislator. Do your homework. It is vitally important to be able to tell your story succinctly and to know what your most important points are. It is usually best to have only one or two key messages and an "ask." You typically only have few minutes with a legislator or staff person, and you must use the time wisely. Arrive at your meeting on time and be ready to present your case. Prior to the meeting, we suggest that you practice so that you feel confident and are able to communicate your key messages in your allotted time. The key messages lead to the ask, which is vital; it is what you want the legislator to do, such as cosign a bill, write a letter, host a briefing, or help you get a hearing.

After your meeting, be certain to follow-up with a thank-you letter or phone call. Ask if there are any additional questions or if you can help the legislator in any way.

Effective grassroots advocacy is about forming relationships and being persistent. It is about never giving up and being willing to return to your House member or Senator's office as often as necessary. It is about believing in your cause and working until you achieve your goal.

There is power in advocacy, and one must never underestimate the power of a single voice.

> It is from numberless diverse acts of courage and belief that human history is shaped.
> Each time a man stands up for an ideal, or acts to improve the lot of others, or strikes

out against injustice, he sends forth a tiny ripple of hope, and crossing each other from a million different centers of energy and daring those ripples build a current which can sweep down the mightiest walls of oppression and resistance.

—ROBERT KENNEDY (1966)

The future will belong to those who have passion and are willing to work hard to make our country better.

—PAUL WELLSTONE (1998)

Suggested Reading

Bolder Advocacy: An initiative of Alliance for Justice. Retrieved from *http://bolderadvocacy.org/ tools-for-effective-advocacy/evaluating-advocacy/international-advocacy-capacity-tool.*— A screening tool useful for assessment for capacity to engage in advocacy efforts.

Center for Nonprofits. *www.centerfornonprofitexcellence.org/resources/advocacy.*—A website that provides useful resources and information, as well as links to other advocacy sites.

Cogan, J. C., Franko, D. L., & Herzog, D. B. (2005). Federal advocacy for anorexia nervosa: An American model. *International Journal of Eating Disorders, 37*(Suppl. 1), S101–S102.— Article reviewing past eating disorder advocacy efforts in the United States.

Eating Disorders Coalition. *www.eatingdisorderscoalition.org.*—A U.S.-based group that is highly active in advocating for eating disorder issues.

Wellstone Action. (2005). *Politics the Wellstone way: How to elect progressive candidates and win on issues.* Minneapolis: University of Minnesota Press.—A book that provides overview of the legislative process with useful insights for advocates; the founder was a major advocate for eating disorder issues.

Part III

OBESITY

EPIDEMIOLOGY AND ETIOLOGY OF OBESITY

Obesity Is a Global Issue

TIM LOBSTEIN

Despite the remarkable gains in population health witnessed in the previous century, with greater prosperity, improved food supplies, better housing, and rising general living standards, the world now faces a new challenge to health caused by these very same advances in affluence. Obesity—a consequence of falling world food prices (especially for sugars, oils, and starches) and reduced physical exertion—is bringing a new wave of chronic disease and rising medical costs that challenge the budgets of many countries around the globe.

The number of adults who are obese (body mass index [BMI] $\geq$ 30 kg/m^2) worldwide now exceeds 500 million, or 10% of all adults, while a further 800 million adults are overweight but not obese (BMI 25–30 kg/m^2). The number of adults who are either overweight or obese now exceeds the number of underweight adults in every region of the world. Indeed, the World Health Organization (WHO) estimates that two-thirds of the world's people live in countries where overweight and obesity kill more people than does underweight. The costs of treating the diseases that follow obesity—cardiovascular disease, diabetes, liver disease, several cancers—and the costs of lost productivity due to excess bodyweight are estimated to exceed $2 trillion annually, equivalent to nearly 3% of global gross domestic product (GDP).

The rise in the spread of obesity has been very rapid: Global estimates suggest that in the 30 years following 1980, excess bodyweight (obesity and overweight combined) rose by some 27% among adults and a remarkable 47% among children. By the year 2020, the world will have passed a new, significant milestone: By that year, the number of undernourished children will be exceeded by those who are overnourished. Even the most vulnerable group of children—those under the age of 5 years—will show this "nutrition transition": some 142 million are likely to be affected by stunting, the commonest form of undernutrition, while more than 160 million will suffer excess bodyweight.

The trends among school-age children are equally alarming. While the rapid rise in obesity appears to be easing in some developed countries, albeit at a very high level, the prevalence of child obesity in developing economies is showing a faster increase than was experienced by developed economies (see Figure 58.1). For these newcomers to the obesity crisis, the number of children affected has doubled and even trebled within a generation.

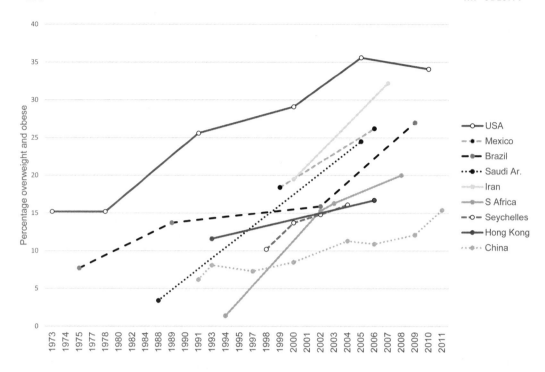

FIGURE 58.1. The rapid rise in the percentage of school-age children with excess body weight. Data from the World Obesity Foundation.

On the African continent, over 20% of children are overweight or obese in Nigeria, and over 30% in Libya. In South America, many countries report more than 25% of children are overweight or obese. In India and Malaysia, the figure is around 20%, and in China, 15%, up from just 5% barely 20 years earlier. Some of the worst figures come from the Middle East, with Bahrain and Qatar recently reporting that over 30% of adolescents are overweight or obese, and Kuwait reporting over 50%.

Many low- and middle-income countries now face the traditional health problems caused by nutritional deficiencies and food shortages, combined with the new problems of overweight and obesity, amounting to a "double burden" of problems caused by poor diets. It might be assumed that undernutrition and overweight will not affect the same population groups, but the reality is that the two problems may be closely allied: The WHO reports that it is not uncommon to find undernutrition and obesity existing side by side within the same community and even the same household. The WHO adds:

> Children in low- and middle-income countries are more vulnerable to inadequate pre-natal, infant and young child nutrition. At the same time, they are exposed to high-fat, high-sugar, high-salt, energy-dense, micronutrient-poor foods, which tend to be lower in cost but also lower in nutrient quality. These dietary patterns, in conjunction with lower levels of physical activity, result in sharp increases in childhood obesity while under-nutrition issues remain unsolved. (p. 1)

It is not just in lower income countries that this double burden can be seen: Data from the United Kingdom shows that population groups with the highest levels of child obesity also have the highest levels of mild and moderate stunting. In the United States, there is increasing evidence that the diets of obese children may be deficient in essential micronutrients—the vitamins and minerals needed for optimal growth and health.

Changing Dietary Patterns

Surveys in developing countries show how diets are changing. In Mexico, over the 11-year period 1988–1999, the percentage of dietary energy from fats and oils increased from 24 to 30%, while purchases of sugar increased 6%, and of sweetened sodas by 37%. By the early 2000s, Mexicans were the greatest per capita consumers of sugar-sweetened beverages worldwide. Similarly, in South Africa, the number of rural adults drinking sugar-sweetened beverages daily doubled in the 5-year period 2005–2010, and the proportion of adults exceeding recommended sugar intake levels rose from 24 to 43%.

Similar patterns are found in children's diets. In Mexico, in 2012, flavored milk beverages, sugar-sweetened soda, and high-fat milk were the top three major contributors to total daily energy intake in all children ages 1–19 years. In Saudi Arabia, 9% of children who ate their meals largely at home were obese, while 53% of children who ate outside the home more than five times per week were obese. In Jordan, among children ages 4–5 years, a survey in 2002 revealed that more than 50% consumed carbonated sugary beverages, 71% regularly consumed biscuits and cakes, and 76% consumed confectionery products.

Surveys of adolescents' consumption of sugar-sweetened beverages indicate high levels of daily intake (see Table 58.1), with as many as three-fourths of children ages 15–16 saying they have at least one such drink each day in a wide range of countries. These young people are moving into the peak reproductive age, when their nutritional intake

TABLE 58.1. Proportion of Youth Ages 13–15 Years Who Drink One or More Servings of Carbonated Beverages Daily

Country	Boys	Girls
Barbados	75%	72%
Bolivia	63%	63%
Egypt	60%	51%
Ghana	54%	58%
Jamaica	75%	71%
Kuwait	75%	74%
Maldives	36%	31%
Pakistan	28%	49%
Peru	55%	53%
Samoa	55%	53%
Tonga	55%	58%
United States	32%	31%
Canada	16%	11%
England	43%	39%
France	33%	27%
Greece	15%	9%

Note. Data from the World Health Organization.

should be at its optimum, but instead they risk being overweight or even obese in parent-hood, itself a risk factor for raising an overweight child, thus replicating the obesity crisis from generation to generation.

Infant Feeding

Even very young children are affected by the nutrition transition. A survey in South Africa of the quality of the labeling of commercially made complementary foods found several major shortfalls that would undermine continued breast-feeding and encourage overconsumption. Of 160 discrete infant feeding products, the labels on 68% of them were difficult to read, 88% failed to state the importance of continuing to breast-feed, 51% failed to state how much of their product should be given to an infant daily, and 17 out of 18 products for babies ages 6–9 months encouraged excessive consumption for a breast-fed baby, and the same was true for 11 out of 12 products for infants ages 9–12 months. Not only are commercial infant foods likely to be less nutritious than family foods, but the purchase of these widely advertised and prominently displayed products is a drain on the resources of low-income families, thus threatening their ability to buy healthy foods for other members of the family.

In theory, weaning foods help an infant to transfer from a milk-based diet to a diet based on family foods. In contrast, leading multinational companies offer products that rely on starches, oils, sugars, milk powder, and other ultraprocessed ingredients, supplemented with flavorings such as chocolate, strawberry, vanilla, and banana. The ingredients and flavorings match the range of foods the same companies produce for older children: breakfast cereals, snack foods, milk shakes, fruit-flavored soft drinks, and cookies. There is a danger that rather than being weaned onto a diet of traditional family foods, children are being weaned onto a diet of highly processed, branded foods.

Poor infant feeding practices are already common in developed economies. In the United States, the National Health and Nutritional Examination Surveys show that more than four out of 10 infants ages 12–23 months eat cookies, cakes, or pastries on any given day; almost one-third eat chips, popcorn, or pretzels; one-fifth eat candy; and one-third consume sugar-rich soda, fruit, or sports drinks daily. In the United Kingdom, the baby food market has been predicted to grow at 7% per year, with market analysts stating that familiar brands are "attaining the trust of parents," with nearly 80% of babies under age 12 months routinely consuming commercial baby products.

Global Nutrition Security

Although the United Nations Committee on World Food Security recognizes the importance of nutrition security, it has not yet turned its attention to the new threats that undermine nutrition security by influencing consumption patterns. Nutrition security includes "food security" (sustainable and adequate supplies, widespread availability, and affordable and accessible to all) and the *actual consumption* of healthful diets. Consumption depends on not only individual choice, of course, but also on the household distribution of foods; cultural and social norms and practices; education and skills; and information, product labeling, and persuasive marketing practices. These all determine what is actually eaten and, hence, the health outcome. Nutrition security depends on whether these latter factors are promoting or impeding healthy dietary behavior, and supporting or undermining optimum nutrition for each individual.

Threats to nutrition security are found in many areas, including ignorance, illiteracy, or mistaken beliefs, but one area that merits special attention is the conscious use of marketing activities to encourage the consumption of foods that do not fulfill national food-based recommendations, and that add to the burden of ill health. Used carefully, promotional marketing practices can support nutrition security but equally they can, as we have seen with baby formula milk products, undermine nutrition security.

Economic Development Plans

Global economic development is currently being revised through the Post-2015 Development Agenda, a process led by the United Nations to help define the future global development framework. The nutrition debate remains dominated by concern over food shortages, with a focus on undernutrition and nutrient deficiency. The discourse of undernutrition is one that helps to justify an expansion of the markets for processed food, especially food products with added fortification. However, there is an urgent need to reframe the discourse to take into account excess consumption of fats, salt, sugars, and overprocessed products. For these products, the message is now "eat less." Such a message fits with improved health, better environmental sustainability, less degrading agriculture, less atmospheric pollutants, and reduced global warming—but it does not fit with continued market freedom.

Companies are investing significantly into expanding their markets into lower-income countries and from urban into increasingly remote rural areas. For example, in Brazil, the world's largest global food company, Nestlé, is training door-to-door entrepreneurs to distribute their products in poorer city neighborhoods, and has built a "floating supermarket" to reach remote communities of the upper Amazon with snack foods, soft drinks, and infant formula. In Africa and Asia, Coca-Cola has developed a program for "women's empowerment," which includes loans and training schemes to help rural women set up distribution points and roadside stalls to sell the company's beverages.

Such economic development and inward investment is likely to be welcomed by government treasuries and ministries for finance. But the consequences of unhealthy food supplies are not considered in the equation: They are externalities born by the economy as whole, and by the individuals and their families who suffer the ill health that arises.

There is little space here to describe the similar changes that have led to reduced physical activity and the rise in high levels of sedentary behavior, primarily screen watching. The benefits of reduced car use, for the health of individuals and the planet, are obvious. Reduced screen watching also has significant health benefits. In both cases, however, there are commercial interests encouraging greater car use and more screen-watching behavior, including the automobile, fuel, and construction industries, and the entertainment, electronics, and advertising industries, and once again, the economic benefits accrue to the companies while the health costs are externalized to the community.

In September 2011, the United Nations held a special summit dedicated to a discussion of the issue of obesity and chronic disease, and agreed a target of "no increase in obesity on 2010 levels," indicating that any further rise should be reversed and eliminated by the year 2025. For many countries this will be an immense challenge, requiring nutrition and food supply policies that are at least as demanding as the policies needed to reduce stunting, and implying a need for market interventions to improve nutrition security, increase levels of physical activity, and reduce incentives for sedentary behavior. It is unlikely that a single country on its own can achieve the size of change needed, and civil society organizations are increasingly calling for internationally agreed conventions to protect and promote health, to hold companies to account for their actions, and to defend health as a basic human right.

Suggested Reading

Consumers International and World Obesity Federation. (2014). Recommendations towards a Global Convention to protect and promote healthy diets. Retrieved from *www.worldobesity.org/what-we-do/policy-prevention/advocacy/global-convention.*—This document is an example of the calls being made by civil society for stronger international agreements that, in turn, can support government actions to ensure that food supplies fully support health policies.

Dobbs, R., Sawers, C., Thompson, F., Manyika, J., Woetzel, J. R., Child, P., et al. (2014). Overcoming obesity: An initial economic analysis [Discussion paper]. Available at *www.mckinsey.com/industries/healthcare-systems-and-services/our-insights/how-the-world-could-better-fight-obesity.*—This report by an international consultancy highlights the costs of failing to tackle the obesity epidemic and the need for a wide range of actions by governments, individuals and the private sector.

Gomes, F. S., & Lobstein, T. (2011). Food and beverage transnational corporations and nutrition policy. *SCN News, 39,* 57–65.—This is one of a set of articles published by the United Nations Standing Committee on Nutrition concerning the opportunities and threats posed by the inclusion of commercial operators in the development of national and international nutrition policies.

Jenkins, B., Valikai, K., & Baptista, P. (2013). *The Coca-Cola company's 5by20 Initiative: Empowering women entrepreneurs across the value chain.* Cambridge, MA: CSR Initiative at the Harvard Kennedy School and Business Fights Poverty.—This document describes the Coca-Cola company's strategy to support women in lower-income communities as retailers and distributors for company products, offering loans, training, and start-up supplies. The initiative chimes with the Millennium Development Goal of improving women's economic status. (See also the company's statement "Women's Economic Empowerment" in the *Coca-Cola 2011/2012 Sustainability Report.*)

Lobstein, T. (2015). Post-2015 agenda: Sustainable and healthy food systems for preventing the crisis in child obesity. *SNC News, 41,* 19–26.—This is one of a set of articles published by the United Nations Standing Committee on Nutrition concerning the post-2015 development agenda. This one argues for market interventions to protect and promote healthful diets.

Lobstein, T., Jackson-Leach, R., Moodie, M. L., Hall, K. D., Gortmaker, S. L., Swinburn, B. A., et al. (2015). Child and adolescent obesity: Part of a bigger picture. *Lancet, 385,* 2510–2520.—This article is part of a *Lancet* series on obesity. It focuses on the rapid rise in child obesity worldwide and suggests that both overnutrition and undernutrition in childhood can be reduced through measures to limit the marketing of unhealthful food products and incentives for sedentary behavior.

Moodie, R., Stuckler, D., Monteiro, C., Sheron, N., Neal, B., Thamarangsi, T., et al. (2013). Profits and pandemics: Prevention of harmful effects of tobacco, alcohol, and ultra-processed food and drink industries. *Lancet, 381,* 670–679.—This article frames the rise in noncommunicable diseases as a societal problem and, especially, a commercial issue requiring policies that hold the suppliers to account.

Nestlé Brazil. (2010). Nestlé launches first floating supermarket in the Brazilian north region [Press release]. Retrieved from *www.nestle.com/asset-library/documents/media/*

press-release/2010-february/nestl%c3%a9%20brazil%20press%20release%20-%20 a%20bordo.pdf.—This is an example of the methods used by global food companies to extend their marketing to low-income populations in remote areas in the world, in this case by stocking a "floating supermarket" to reach communities in the upper Amazon.

Stuckler, D., & Nestle, M. (2012). Big food, food systems, and global health. *PLoS Medicine,* 9(6), e1001242.—This the first of several articles in the *PLoS Medicine* Series on Big Food, which look critically at the role of commercial food suppliers in shaping consumers' diets and health.

World Health Organization. (2014). *Global Nutrition Targets 2025: Childhood overweight policy brief.*—This briefing paper for governments describes the need for initiatives to meet the 2025 targets for "no increase in child obesity prevalence" and suggests measures ranging from individual education to national economic policies. It should be read alongside the subsequent Report of the WHO Commission on Ending Childhood Obesity (2016), available at *www. who.int/end-childhood-obesity/final-report/en.*

59

Connections between Undernutrition and Obesity

JUAN A. RIVERA
CLAUDIA IVONNE RAMIREZ-SILVA
LILIA S. PEDRAZA

Undernutrition and obesity in the past were considered two opposite conditions, with unrelated or even divergent determinants, occurring in different segments of the population: undernutrition among the poor and obesity amid the rich. The two conditions were often cited as examples of polarization in the health transition. However, evidence is now available about connections between the two conditions, including long-term associations between undernutrition during the early stages of human development and obesity and its comorbidities later in life, shared risk factors throughout the life course and coexistence of the two conditions within communities, and households and individuals at different points in time during their life.

We present in the next sections evidence of these connections, the potential or actual mechanisms explaining the apparent paradox of the links between conditions once considered contradictory, and we end with policy implications derived from these associations.

Effects of Famine and Undernutrition during Gestation on Obesity and Chronic Diseases Later in Life

Studies in animals have shown that poor nutrition during gestation is associated with increased disease susceptibility and mortality. Studies of cohorts born around the Dutch Hunger Winter in 1944–1945 (a.k.a. the Dutch famine) allowed the characterization of effects of maternal undernutrition during different stages of gestation on the future health of the offspring. Results show that exposure to famine during gestation is associated with obesity and cardiometabolic risk factors later in life, and that the effects on health depend on the time during gestation when the nutrition deprivation occurs.

For example, exposure to famine during any stage of gestation has been associated later in life with glucose intolerance and type 2 diabetes. Individuals' exposure during early gestation is associated with adiposity, atherogenic lipid profiles, hypertension, coronary heart disease, and altered blood clotting compared to individuals not exposed to famine or exposed during middle to late gestation.

In addition to the evidence linking famine with later obesity and comorbidities there are indications that less severe forms of undernutrition during the early stages of development are also associated with these health risks in adulthood.

Epidemiological studies from industrialized countries have shown evidence of an association between low birth weight and later occurrence of central obesity, insulin resistance, type 2 diabetes, and cardiovascular disease.

In the 1980s, Barker observed that differences in death rates from coronary heart disease in different areas of England and Wales paralleled differences in death rates among newborn babies in the early years of the century, when most causes of deaths in newborns were low birth weight. This observation suggested that low rates of growth before birth are linked to later development of coronary heart disease. Theses associations were later confirmed by additional studies.

Evidence from members of populations in low- and middle-income countries, exposed to different degrees of nutrition deprivation during gestation, and followed to adulthood, show somewhat different findings. Analysis of five prospective cohort studies from Brazil, Guatemala, India, the Philippines, and South Africa, which recruited newborns between 1969 and 1990 and followed them to adult age indicate that *a higher birth weight* was consistently associated with an adult body mass index (BMI) greater than 25 kg/m² (odds ratio 1.28, 95% confidence interval 1.21–1.35); and with decreased risk of dysglycemia (0.89, 0.81–0.98). Thus, growth during gestation was associated with higher risks of excess BMI but was protective against risk of type 2 diabetes. Further analyses of these studies suggest that the association between birth weight and BMI can be possibly explained through lean mass rather than fat mass. Additional studies in these populations support the association between birth weight and central obesity, as well as cardiometabolic alterations and cardiovascular disease. However, findings have been inconsistent.

It is worth noting that most individuals from these birth cohorts were followed from birth to adulthood during the 1970s–1980s, at a time when environments in these countries were not as obesity promoting ("obesogenic") as they are now. Therefore, nutrition deprivation during gestation was not followed by obesogenic environments during the postnatal period as opposed to cohort studies in high-income countries presented earlier.

Studies of Asian indigenous populations have documented a particular phenotypic adaptation to malnutrition that is associated with increased visceral adiposity and insulin resistance. Infants from India have been shown to have increased visceral fat at birth despite being underweight.

In summary, studies of humans exposed to acute undernutrition (famine studies) and to less severe nutrition deprivation during gestation have shown increased risk of obesity and risk factors for noncommunicable diseases during adult age. This has been particularly true for populations in which early undernutrition was followed by high availability of food and low physical activity during the life course of the participants in the cohorts studied.

Hypothesis to Explain Epidemiological Findings

Barker hypothesized that the mechanisms linking undernutrition during gestation and disease later in life might be structural changes in organs induced during early development or epigenetic modification during conception and the prenatal period that cause permanent modifications on patterns of gene expression. Both structural changes in organs and gene expression can affect organic functions that persist at several stages throughout life. Although the suggestion that events in childhood influence the pathogenesis of the disease was not new at the time when Barker presented his studies, this author postulated a clear hypothesis about the developmental origins of health and disease.

Other authors have suggested an independent effect of postnatal growth patterns on later adiposity and adult disease.

Epigenetic Changes

The studies of famine exposure during different stages in gestation, such as the Dutch famine studies and other epidemiological studies, including those conducted by Barker and his group, have suggested that adult disease risk is associated with adverse environmental conditions early in development. Although the mechanisms explaining these associations are not clear, an involvement of epigenetic dysregulation has been hypothesized.

Basically, the epigenetic changes on DNA are induced by nucleotide methylation of cytosine in the guanine–cytosine sequence. These sequences are generally identified in promotor regions, which regulate the transcription of genes. Specific nutrients are cofactors or regulators of genetic expression; thus, deficiencies of "methyl donor" nutrients and other micronutrients in early development can cause epigenetic changes. Findings from experimental studies in animal and humans have shown that periconceptional deficiencies of zinc, magnesium, manganese, and iron are associated with alterations on mechanisms of regulation of the appetite, higher fat mass, and less fat-free mass later in life, which could explain the link between undernutrition during early life and future obesity.

Postnatal Growth Patterns

Findings of studies from developed countries indicate that postnatal weight gain has an independent effect on obesity and cardiovascular disease.

The five prospective cohort studies analysis that recruited newborns between 1969 and 1990 and followed them to adult age, described earlier, found associations between postnatal growth patterns and several outcomes at adult age, including increased BMI.

The growth patterns studied were linear growth (length gain) and weight gain independent of linear growth (relative weight gain) in three age periods: 0–2 years, 2 years to midchildhood, and midchildhood to adulthood. The researchers found that faster weight gain independent of linear growth was associated with an increased risk of adult overweight (age 2 years, 51% increased risk; midchildhood, 76% increase) and elevated blood pressure (age 2 years, 7% increased risk; midchildhood, 22% increase) and was not associated with dysglycemia.

Micronutrient malnutrition during the postnatal period may indirectly impact the risk of overweight/obesity and chronic diseases through its contribution to childhood stunting and subsequent short adult stature in the nutrition transition context.

Double Burden: Coexistence of Undernutrition and Obesity

The coexistence of undernutrition (stunting, anemia, and micronutrient deficiencies) in children under 5 years of age and overweight/obesity at older ages, known as "double burden," has been described in low- and middle-income countries with important economic disparities and undergoing a nutrition transition (i.e., countries that have shifted from traditional diets to less healthy diets and from active to sedentary lifestyles). This double burden can be observed at the national level, within households, and even in the same individuals throughout life.

The coexistence of these conditions, as well as observations indicating that stunted children are more likely to accumulate central adipose tissue and to be in a prechronic disease state compared to normal height children, suggests that stunting might predispose individuals to future obesity.

A recent analysis of the double burden of malnutrition in low- and middle-income countries in Latin America assessed whether the coexistence of the two conditions was solely the result of the independent occurrence of each one of them by comparing the observed and the expected prevalence of the double burden, under the assumption that the two conditions were uncorrelated. The conclusions were that undernutrition and excess body weight risks seem to be largely unrelated at the individual and household levels. However, the fact remains that both types of conditions are very common at the national level in Latin America and other low- and middle-income countries: Overweight and obesity coexist with undernutrition (either stunting, anemia, or micronutrient deficiencies) at the national level. As a result of the high prevalences of the two conditions, the joint prevalence or co-occurrence of the double burden is common. It is therefore clear that the double burden does exist in Latin American countries, creating a double challenge for the health care systems. These findings indicate the need of policies and programs to tackle both conditions simultaneously in a coordinated fashion.

Shared Dietary Factors of Undernutrition and Obesity Throughout the Life Course

Undernutrition and obesity share some dietary risk factors. One example is inadequate food environments and eating behaviors, characterized by infant feeding practices that are inconsistent with international recommendations: lack of breast-feeding, exclusive breast-feeding less than 6 months, or short duration of any breast-feeding; early introduction of complementary foods; and/or low nutrient quality of foods provided to infants and toddlers. These practices lead to undernutrition at early stages of life and at the same time to overweight/obesity at later stages.

Also, food patterns throughout life characterized by high intake of sugar-sweetened beverages (SSBs) and energy-dense, nutrient-poor foods (ultraprocessed foods) and the concomitant high intake of added sugars displace nutrient-rich basic foods present in traditional diets. The combination of diets with high-energy density and liquid calories (both associated with obesity) and low density of nutrients per calorie (associated with undernutrition) is especially problematic. A stunted and anemic child may start to gain weight after 2 years of age but become an overweight and short-for-age school-age child (with a history of stunting) who also may be anemic and at high risk of becoming an overweight/obese adult.

Policy Implications

The fact that undernutrition and obesity share some risk factors means that policies for the prevention of the double burden may also share policy actions. The coexistence of the conditions indicates the need to reformulate policies and programs around the notion of "healthy eating" and "healthy lifestyles," including the promotion of physical activity during the different phases of the life course.

Some currently proposed actions include promotion of adequate infant feeding practices (breast-feeding and high-quality complementary foods), as well as regulations and legislation aimed at modifying the food and physical activity environments, so that healthy eating and an active life become the defaults, coupled with effective communication strategies to promote these healthy behaviors.

Suggested Reading

Adair, L. S., Fall, C. H., Osmond, C., Stein, A. D., Martorell, R., Ramirez-Zea, M., et al. (2013). Associations of linear growth and relative weight gain during early life with adult health and human capital in countries of low and middle income: Findings from five birth cohort studies. *Lancet, 382,* 525–534.—These authors present evidence from five cohorts from low- and middle-income countries, on the association of birth weight and growth (both linear growth and weight gain) during the first 2 years and during childhood, with several outcomes in adult age, including schooling and risk factors for chronic disease.

Arranz, C. T., Costa, M. Á., & Tomat, A. L. (2012). Orígenes fetales de las enfermedades cardiovasculares en la vida adulta por deficiencia de micronutrientes [Fetal origins of cardiovascular disease in adults due to micronutrient deficiencies]. *Clínica e Investigación en Arteriosclerosis, 24*(2), 71–81.—Authors of this review discuss the association between micronutrient deficiencies during fetal and postnatal life and the development of cardiovascular disease, as well as the benefits of micronutrient supplementation during pregnancy.

Corvalán, C., Kain, J., Weisstaub, G., & Uauy, R. (2009). Impact of growth patterns and early diet on obesity and cardiovascular risk factors in young children from developing countries. *Proceedings of the Nutrition Society, 68*(3), 327–337.—This article presents evidence indicating that actions to prevent obesity and nutrition-related chronic diseases in developing countries should start early in life considering the short- and long-term health consequences as well as the stage of the nutritional transition of the population.

Eckhardt, C. L. (2006). *Micronutrient malnutrition, obesity, and chronic disease in countries undergoing the nutrition transition: Potential links and program/policy implications.* Washington, DC: International Food Policy Research Institute.—A discussion of the potential long-term effects of micronutrient deficiency in early childhood on the later presence and severity of obesity and related diseases. Also stressed is the importance of programs and policies that jointly address undernutrition, in all its forms, and obesity.

Gluckman, P. D., Hanson, M. A., & Beedle, A. S. (2007). Early life events and their consequences for later disease: A life history and evolutionary perspective. *American Journal of Human Biology, 19,* 1–19.—This article details the "developmental origins of health and disease

(DOHaD) paradigm" and its application to understand human adaptation and development through adverse intrauterine environments.

Heijmans, B. T., Tobi, E. W., Stein, A. D., Putter, H., Blauw, G. J., Susser, E. S., et al. (2008). Persistent epigenetic differences associated with prenatal exposure to famine in humans. *Proceedings of the National Academy of Sciences USA, 105*(44), 17046–17049.—This article presents data supporting the hypothesis that early life environmental conditions can cause epigenetic changes in humans that persist throughout life.

Rivera, J. A., Pedraza, L. S., Martorell, R., & Gil, A. (2014). Introduction to the double burden of undernutrition and excess weight in Latin America. *American Journal of Clinical Nutrition, 100*(6), 1613S–1616S.—The authors present evidence indicating that overweight and obesity coexist with undernutrition (stunting and micronutrient deficiencies) in several Latin American countries and point out the critical need for policies and programs to tackle both conditions simultaneously.

Roseboom, T. J., Painter, R. C., van Abeelen, A. F., Veenendaal, M. V., & de Rooij, S. R. (2011). Hungry in the womb: What are the consequences? Lessons from the Dutch famine. *Maturitas, 70*(2), 141–145.—This review examines the effects on later health of prenatal undernutrition due to the Dutch famine. Increased risk of schizophrenia, depression, atherogenic plasma lipid profiles, worse cognitive performance, and type 2 diabetes were observed in people exposed to prenatal undernutrition. The effects seemed to be greatest during early gestation.

Tzioumis, E., & Adair, L. S. (2014). Childhood dual burden of under- and over-nutrition in low- and middle-income countries: A critical review. *Food and Nutrition Bulletin, 35*(2), 230–243.—This critical review describes patterns, trends, and predictors of the dual burden of undernutrition and obesity in low- and middle-income countries in the context of the nutrition transition.

Victora, C. G., Adair, L., Fall, C., Hallal, P. C., Martorell, R., Richter, L., et al. (2008). Maternal and child undernutrition: Consequences for adult health and human capital. *Lancet, 371*, 340–357.—This article reviews the association between maternal and child undernutrition in low- and middle-income countries with human capital and risk of disease in adulthood, concluding that the prevention of early life undernutrition is associated with later health, educational, and economic benefits.

Prevalence and Demographics of Obesity in the United States

HANNAH G. LAWMAN
CYNTHIA L. OGDEN

Over one-third of adults (34.9%) and approximately 17% of children in the United States have obesity. A high rate of obesity in the U.S. population has significant implications for the nation's medical, psychosocial, and economic health. Obesity is a function of energy balance, with multiple interacting influences at a variety of levels, including individual (e.g., genetics and behavioral factors), social (e.g., family and peers), community (e.g., built environment), and national and cultural (e.g., policy, societal, and heritage factors) influences. Other chapters in this book describe the etiology and treatment of obesity, as well as global obesity trends. This chapter summarizes published historical (since the 1970s) and recent (past decade) trends and current estimates and demographic differences in U.S. obesity prevalence.

U.S. Data Source and Definitions

U.S. surveillance of height and weight has been a part of the National Health and Nutrition Examination Survey (NHANES) since it began in the 1970s. Since 1999, NHANES has been continuously collecting data, which are released publicly in 2-year cycles. These data are used to routinely monitor trends in U.S. obesity prevalence, as well as many other health topics. NHANES uses a complex sampling design to provide a nationally representative sample of the noninstitutionalized civilian U.S. population. NHANES has oversampled various subgroups depending on the survey period, including some racial/ethnic minorities. Children and adolescents ages 2–19 years are included in all NHANES survey periods.

The survey includes an in-person home interview and a separate visit to a mobile examination center during which medical, physiological, anthropometric, and laboratory measures are collected. Height and weight are measured according to standardized protocols. During the exam, values are compared to age- and sex- specific ranges of previously collected NHANES height and weight data to reduce the potential for out-of-range values by prompting the examiner to verify any high values. Data are then electronically transmitted automatically to an NHANES database. These strategies have been used since the 1999–2000 cycle and help to maximize the quality of NHANES anthropometric data, which are considered to be more valid than other height and weight data based on self-report or collected by examiners with variable training and equipment.

Obesity is defined using body mass index (BMI), which is calculated as weight in kilograms divided by height in meters squared. For adults, *obesity* is defined as a BMI at or above 30, and can be further classified as grade 1 (BMI 30–34.9), grade 2 (BMI 35–39.9), and grade 3 (BMI ≥ 40, sometimes called *extreme obesity*). Due to the growth of children and natural increases in BMI as children age, *childhood obesity* among youth ages 2–19 years is defined by comparisons to age- and sex-specific distributions of BMI. Obesity in U.S. children is defined as a BMI that is at or above the age- and sex-specific 95th percentile of the 2000 Centers for Disease Control and Prevention (CDC) growth charts. This means, for example, that a boy with a BMI at the 97th percentile has a higher weight in relation to height than 96 of 100 boys of the same age in the CDC growth charts. *Extreme obesity in children* is often defined as a BMI at or above 120% of the 95th percentile.

U.S. Obesity Prevalence and Demographics

Obesity Trends from 1971–1974 to 2011–2012

Analyses and results presented in this chapter may be examined in greater detail (see "Suggested Reading"). Figure 60.1 shows the prevalence of obesity among U.S. children and adolescents ages 2–19 years beginning in 1971–1974 and ending with 2011–2012, the most recent NHANES data currently available. A dramatic increase in childhood obesity occurred predominantly during the 1980s and 1990s, and began to stabilize in the early to mid-2000s. Data from the last decade have shown no significant change in overall childhood obesity prevalence (ages 2–19 years) from 2003–2004 to 2011–2012. Specifically, the prevalence of obesity among preschool children ages 2–5 years rose from 5.0 to 13.9% between 1976–1980 and 2003–2004, then significantly decreased to a current 2011–2012 prevalence of 8.4%. The prevalence of obesity in 6- to 11-year-old children rose from 6.5% in 1976–1980 to 18.8% in 2003–2004 and has since stabilized with no significant differences since 2003–2004. In adolescents ages 12–19 years, the prevalence of obesity rose from 5.0 to 17.4% between 1976–1980 and 2003–2004, and showed no statistically significant differences since 2003–2004.

The prevalence of obesity in adults has shown similar trends, with an increase in obesity prevalence during the 1980s and 1990s, and stabilization over the last decade. Specifically, between 1976–1980 and 2003–2004, the prevalence more than doubled (14.5 to 32.9%), and was then followed by a period of recent stability from 2003–2004 to 2011–2012, in which there was no statistically significant change (32.9 to 35.3%).

The prevalence of obesity among U.S. adults and children is of great public interest. The issue of childhood obesity in particular has garnered much attention and some

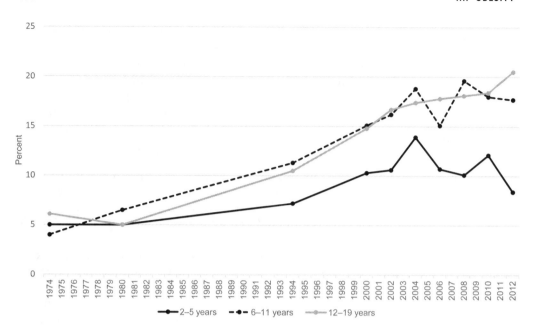

FIGURE 60.1. Prevalence of obesity among children and adolescents ages 2–19 years by sex: United States, selected years 1971–1974 through 2011–2012. Data from Fryar, Carroll, and Ogden (2014).

debate regarding trends in the last 10–15 years. The differences in the interpretation of trends in obesity prevalence reflect, in part, the initial time point chosen for examination. For example, as can be seen in Figure 60.1, time trends comparing 1976–1980 to 2011–2012 show an increase between the years, whereas time trends comparing 2003–2004 to 2011–2012 do not. Regardless of any differences in the interpretation of time trends, obesity remains a public health concern.

Current Obesity Prevalence

Figure 60.2 shows the variation in obesity prevalence by sex and race and Hispanic origin among U.S. youth ages 2–19 years in 2011–2012. Non-Hispanic white and non-Hispanic Asian youth had a significantly lower prevalence of obesity compared to non-Hispanic black and Hispanic youth. Non-Hispanic Asian youth also had a significantly lower prevalence compared to non-Hispanic white youth, but non-Hispanic black youth and Hispanic youth did not differ significantly from each other. The patterns of racial/ethnic differences are generally consistent across boys and girls. The disparities across sex and race and Hispanic origin groups are often large. For example, the obesity prevalence in Hispanic boys is approximately double the prevalence in non-Hispanic white boys (24.1 vs. 12.6%, respectively).

Differences in the prevalence of obesity by sex and race and Hispanic origin observed in childhood persist into adulthood and, in some cases, widen. During 2011–2012 (Figure 60.3), the overall prevalence of obesity ranged from a low of 10.0% in non-Hispanic Asian men to a high of 56.6% in non-Hispanic black women. Another way of thinking about obesity in the United States is in terms of the number of individuals with obesity

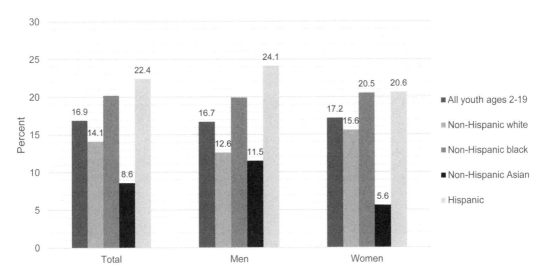

FIGURE 60.2. Prevalence of obesity by sex and race and Hispanic origin among youth ages 2–19 years: United States: 2011–2012. Data from Ogden, Carroll, Kit, and Flegal (2014).

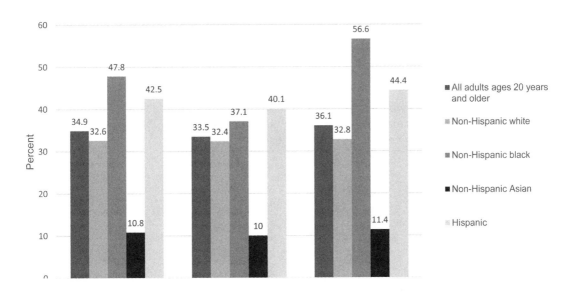

FIGURE 60.3. Age-adjusted prevalence of obesity by sex and race and Hispanic origin among adults ages 20 and over: United States, 2011–2012. Data from Ogden, Carroll, Kit, and Flegal (2014).

rather than percentage of the population. Overall, approximately 78.6 million U.S. adults ages 20 years and older were affected by obesity in 2011–2012. This includes 50.2 million non-Hispanic white adults, 13.4 million Hispanic adults, 12.2 million non-Hispanic black adults, and 1.2 million non-Hispanic Asian adults. Thus, while the population prevalence of obesity is highest among non-Hispanic black and Hispanic adults compared to non-Hispanic white adults (42.5–47.8 vs. 32.6%, respectively), the overall burden of obesity is highest among non-Hispanic white adults due to the greater number of affected individuals (50.2 vs. 25.6 million in non-Hispanic black and Hispanic adults combined).

Extreme obesity in adults has been associated with a substantially increased risk of mortality primarily due to increased risk of death from heart disease, cancer, and diabetes. Approximately 4.5% of men and 8.6% of women in the United States met criteria for extreme obesity in 2011–2012. These estimates can be compared to 0.6% of men and 2.0% of women who met criteria for extreme obesity in 1971–1974. Extreme obesity has also been documented in children and adolescents.

Summary

The current prevalence of obesity in U.S. children and adults is stable but more than one-third of adults and almost 2 in 10 children have obesity. The national obesity prevalence estimates from NHANES have been critical to informing a number of public health campaigns, policy decisions, and research agendas, and are an especially useful reference due to the high quality of the measurements. For example, First Lady Michelle Obama's Let's Move campaign relies on NHANES obesity prevalence data. While cross-sectional data collected on a national scale are unable to inform questions about why obesity prevalence rates may be increasing, decreasing, or stabilizing, the public availability and long-standing history of NHANES height and weight data have provided a benchmark for assessing progress.

There are often substantial differences in obesity prevalence by sex, age, and race and Hispanic origin, which makes it difficult to summarize a single overall trend. Moreover, subgroup differences in obesity prevalence do not necessarily correspond to similar patterns in cardiometabolic risk factors. For example, while Hispanics displayed a higher prevalence of obesity compared to non-Hispanic whites and Asians, Mexican Americans have been shown to have a lower level of some uncontrolled cardiometabolic risk factors, including uncontrolled hypertension and dyslipidemia, and smoking. While Asians showed the lowest prevalence of obesity, they have been shown to have higher excess body fat and higher diabetes risk at lower BMI levels compared to other race/ethnic groups. Subgroup differences are further complicated by sex, age, and racial/ethnic differences in the correlation of BMI to excess body fat.

Despite its wide use and convenience as a public health measure, BMI does not capture gradations in excess body fat distribution that are associated with cardiometabolic health outcomes. That is, BMI does not assess visceral adiposity or distinguish between fat and muscle, which are both associated with poorer health outcomes and vary by sex, age and race/ethnicity. Consequently, the prevalence of obesity using BMI may not completely reflect true population cardiovascular disease and diabetes risk associated with body fat.

Suggested Reading

Ahima, R., & Lazar, M. (2013). Physiology: The health risk of obesity—better metrics imperative. *Science, 341*, 856–858.—This article reviews the challenges associated with measuring obesity using BMI and controversies surrounding the "obesity–mortality paradox."

Blair, S. N., & Church, T. S. (2004). The fitness, obesity, and health equation: Is physical activity the common denominator? *Journal of the American Medical Association, 292*(10),

1232–1234.—The authors discuss the relative contributions of fitness and obesity to overall health and conclude that physical activity is an actionable treatment for both.

Centers for Disease Control and Prevention. (2012). National Health and Nutrition Examination Surveys: NHANES 2011–2012. Retrieved March 15, 2015, from *wwwn.cdc.gov/nchs/nhanes/search/nhanes11_12.aspx*.—This link contains the 2011–2012 NHANES data and documentation.

Flegal, K. M., Kit, B. K., Orpana, H., & Graubard, B. I. (2013). Association of all-cause mortality with overweight and obesity using standard body mass index categories: A systematic review and meta-analysis. *Journal of the American Medical Association, 309*(1), 71–82.—This systematic review found higher mortality among individuals with grade 2 and grade 3 obesity, but not grade 1 obesity, and lower mortality among overweight individuals compared to individuals in the normal weight category.

Flegal, K. M., Wei, R., Ogden, C. L., Freedman, D. S., Johnson, C. L., & Curtin, L. R. (2009). Characterizing extreme values of body mass index-for-age by using the 2000 Centers for Disease Control and Prevention growth charts. *American Journal of Clinical Nutrition, 90*(5), 1314–1320.—This study describes different approaches for characterizing extreme values of BMI in youth based on the CDC growth charts and suggests using a percentage of the 95th percentile.

Fryar, C. D., Carroll, M. D., & Ogden, C. L. (2014). Prevalence of overweight and obesity among children and adolescents: United States, 1963–1965 through 2011–2012. National Center for Health Statistics Health E-Stats. Available at *www.cdc.gov/nchs/data/hestat/obesity_child_11_12/obesity_child_11_12.htm*.—This Web publication contains a table with childhood obesity prevalence estimates using NHANES data from 1963–1965 through 2011–2012.

Fryar, C. D., Carroll, M. D., & Ogden, C. L. (2015). Prevalence of overweight, obesity, and extreme obesity among adults: United States, 1960–1962 through 2011–2012. National Center for Health Statistics Health E-Stats. Available at *www.cdc.gov/nchs/data/hestat/obesity_adult_11_12/obesity_adult_11_12.htm*.—This Web publication contains a table with adult obesity prevalence estimates using NHANES data from 1960–1962 through 2011–2012.

Fryar, C. D., Chen, T. C., & Li, X. (2012). *Prevalence of uncontrolled risk factors for cardiovascular disease: United States, 1999–2010*. Washington, DC: U.S. Department of Health and Human Services, Centers for Disease Control and Prevention, National Center for Health Statistics.—This study describes the prevalence, demographic differences, and recent trends in uncontrolled hypertension, dyslipidemia, and smoking.

Institute of Medicine (United States), Committee on Accelerating Progress in Obesity Prevention, & Glickman, D. (2012). *Accelerating progress in obesity prevention: Solving the weight of the nation*. Washington, DC: National Academies Press.—This report contains an evaluation of obesity prevention strategies and recommendations for new strategies to improve progress.

Ogden, C. L., Carroll, M. D., Kit, B. K., & Flegal, K. M. (2014). Prevalence of childhood and adult obesity in the United States, 2011–2012. *Journal of the American Medical Association, 311*(8), 806–814.—The study presents the most recent (as of September 2015) U.S. obesity prevalence information and analyzes by age the last 10 years' trends in obesity.

Early-Life Risk Factors for Childhood Obesity

ELSIE M. TAVERAS

In the past three decades, rates of overweight and obesity among children have substantially increased worldwide, with all but the poorest countries now struggling with a high prevalence of obesity and its related noncommunicable diseases. In the United States alone, the prevalence of overweight and obesity in children and adolescents is 32%. Although obesity prevalence among some U.S. subpopulations appear to have stabilized, overall rates remain at historically high rates and racial/ethnic differences appear to be widening, particularly among Latino children. The elevated prevalence of overweight and obesity even among children ages 2–5 years has led to a growing recognition that risk factors in early life may be crucial to the development—and therefore the prevention—of obesity and its consequences. Epidemiological studies suggest that adverse exposures in pregnancy, such as intrauterine exposure to maternal smoking, excessive weight gain, or elevated glucose levels, and, in early childhood, rapid infant weight gain, poor feeding practices, too much television viewing, and short sleep duration, may increase short- and long-term risks for obesity and its sequelae. For these reasons, national reports emphasize the important role of early-life risk factors in obesity development and the need for interventions in early life to prevent obesity.

Overview of Childhood Obesity

The obesity epidemic has spared no age group, including young children. Recent data indicate that even infants have experienced a rise in excess weight in the past 20 years, implying that the roots of the epidemic can be found as early as infancy, and before. In the United States, one-third of children ages 2–19 years are affected by overweight or obesity (sex-specific body mass index [BMI] ≥ 85th percentile for age). Approximately 8.1% of U.S. children under age 2 years have weight-for-length ≥ 95th percentile, predisposing them to obesity. Among preschool-age children ages 2–5 years, the 2007–2008 National Health and Nutrition Examination Survey reported an obesity prevalence of 10.4%. Obesity in children is associated with both short- and long-term adverse outcomes, including both physical and psychosocial consequences and even perhaps shortened lifespan. Children who are overweight tend to become overweight adults and, once present, obesity is notoriously hard to treat.

The Life-Course Approach to Understanding Obesity and the First 1,000 Days

The life-course approach to chronic disease prevention posits that factors may act in the prenatal period and extend into infancy, childhood, and beyond to determine risk of chronic disease. These factors can range from the social/built environment (macro) through behavior, physiology, and genetics (micro). Factors interact with each other over the life course, with different determinants being more or less important at different life stages. When risk factors have much more influence at a particular life stage than either before or after, it is called a "sensitive period." The first 1,000 days is one such sensitive period (i.e., the period from conception through age 2 years that is increasingly recognized as a critical period for development of childhood obesity and its adverse consequences). Here we review risk factors for obesity that emerge in the first 1,000 days and emerging solutions for prevention.

Early-Life Risk Factors

Prepregnancy and Pregnancy

Perhaps the strongest and most reliable early-life risk factor for offspring obesity is higher maternal prepregnancy BMI. Infants born to overweight mothers are more likely to be born large for gestational age, are less likely to be breast-fed, and are at higher risk for obesity and type 2 diabetes in later life.

Excess gestational weight gain also has consistently been found to increase risk for childhood overweight. Higher gestational weight gain is associated with higher infant birth weight for gestational age, which predicts offspring weight and risk of overweight in later life.

Children born to mothers with impaired glucose tolerance during pregnancy are more likely to be macrosomic and have higher body fat at birth, and subsequently may be at elevated risk for becoming overweight and developing related complications such as higher blood pressure and risk for type 2 diabetes. The link between a mother's glucose tolerance during pregnancy and her child's weight and glucose tolerance appears to result from not only shared genes and behaviors but also a direct influence of the adverse intrauterine environment on the fetus.

Maternal smoking during early pregnancy is associated with elevated risk for the offspring of having a BMI that exceeds the 85th percentile for age and sex, higher BMI z-score, and higher systolic blood pressure at age 3 years. A meta-analysis of 14 studies showed that smoking during pregnancy is associated with a 50% increased odds of obesity during childhood.

Other studies have found that maternal stressors, such as antenatal depression, are associated with offspring obesity. Other characteristics and behaviors during pregnancy, including diet and diet quality, may influence weight gain and obesity among offspring, but these factors remain understudied. Quite absent from the literature are *paternal* risk factors and behaviors that might increase their offspring's risk of overweight. The few studies that have examined paternal factors have shown associations between higher paternal BMI, and possibly also prenatal paternal BMI, and child overweight.

Infancy

In the first 2 years of life, the primary determinants of later obesity appear to be accelerated weight gain and type and duration of infant feeding. Higher birth weight, rapid early-infancy weight gain, and higher absolute weight-for-length during the first 2 years of life are associated with later BMI increases in childhood or adulthood.

Research on the early determinants of obesity has also focused on the role of infant feeding practices and mode. Findings illustrate that discordant feeding practices, or feeding infants when they are not hungry (e.g., feeding to soothe), are linked with increased frequency of feeding and accelerated infant weight gain. Conversely, responsive feeding practices (e.g., caregiver awareness of, and appropriate response to, infant cues of hunger) may protect against accelerated weight gain. The evidence is mixed for infant feeding mode. Some studies suggest that early introduction of solids (at age 4 months or earlier) may increase obesity risk, and breast-feeding initiation and prolonged duration may reduce short-term risk of obesity. Yet a large randomized controlled trial involving 13,000 children followed for more than 6 years provided no evidence of an effect of breast-feeding on child obesity.

In contrast to what is known about infant feeding practices and mode, less is known about the role of sleep, physical activity, and screen time on accelerated infant weight gain and childhood overweight. Several reviews and meta-analyses of longitudinal studies examining links between sleep and obesity overwhelmingly show that short sleep duration, even during infancy, is linked with higher subsequent risk of obesity in children.

An emerging risk factor for obesity in infancy is antibiotic exposure and its adverse effects on growth, likely mediated through alterations in the infant microbiome.

Beyond the First 1,000 Days

After the first 2 years of life, several risk factors can increase the risk of later obesity. Among school-age children, there is strong evidence from both observational and experimental research that television viewing is positively associated with risk of overweight. Short sleep duration persists as a potential risk factor for obesity in childhood. Over the last 30 years, consumption of fast food has paralleled the rise in childhood obesity prevalence. Sugar-sweetened beverage consumption is highly prevalent among young children and, among school-age children, intake of sugar-sweetened beverages has been associated with greater caloric intake and increased BMI. Additionally, greater consumption of fast food has been found to be associated with poorer diet quality and is usually accompanied by other unhealthy dietary exposures such as large portion sizes and high energy density, which are known to contribute to body weight.

Racial/Ethnic and Socioeconomic Differences

Research has demonstrated that children from racial/ethnic minority groups have a higher prevalence of several early-life risk factors for obesity than do their white counterparts.

These early-life risk factors are often modifiable and may contribute substantially to disparities in later childhood obesity. For example, among black and Latino children, differences in prevalence as compared to white children can be found in maternal depression during pregnancy, more rapid infant weight gain, lower rates of exclusive breast-feeding, short sleep duration, more infants receiving solid foods before 4 months of age, higher prevalence of a television set in the room where the child sleeps, and higher intake of sugar-sweetened beverages or fast food.

Previous studies among both children and adults have examined the extent to which racial/ethnic disparities in obesity are confounded or explained by socioeconomic status, a multidimensional construct that is known to exert a profound influence on health. The relationship between socioeconomic status, usually measured as parental income or education, and childhood obesity is complex. Although several U.S. studies of the relationship between socioeconomic status and childhood obesity have shown that low socioeconomic status and minority groups have a higher prevalence of obesity, more recent data have shown some conflicting results. A study of 8,984 children ages 12–17 years participating in the National Longitudinal Study of Youth, found that although parental income and maternal educational level partially explained observed black–white and Hispanic–white differences in BMI, a large portion of these differences remained unexplained. The exact role of socioeconomic status in the relationship between race/ethnicity and obesity is unclear, but the findings do suggest that social conditions and their effects on children's environments are important for understanding how disparities in childhood obesity originate.

Given that socioeconomic status may not fully explain racial/ethnic differences in obesity prevalence, increased attention has been given to culture, acculturation, and neighborhood environments as factors that may contribute to racial/ethnic disparities in obesity.

Emerging and Promising Solutions for Early-Life Obesity Prevention

Early childhood is a key period for not only understanding etiology but also delivering potentially effective preventive interventions. From a life-course perspective, the pregnancy and early childhood periods may provide a unique opportunity for preventing childhood obesity. Pregnancy and early childhood represent periods of maximal environmental dependence and parental care, and a developmentally plastic period during which behaviors are modifiable. Early childhood seems particularly promising and highly sensitive to interventions; there are multiple settings to access parents (primary care, child care, early education settings, etc.), and parents and caregivers are highly sensitized to children's needs.

In recognition of the growing evidence of the importance of assessing the beginnings of obesity and instituting preventive measures in the early years, the Institute of Medicine's Standing Committee on Childhood Obesity Prevention published a report examining strategies to prevent overweight and obesity from birth to 5 years, with a focus on nutrition, physical activity, and sedentary behavior.

Obesity prevention efforts in early childhood will need to engage parents and families in behavior change and, through creative communication, provide evidence to counter popular and cultural beliefs about healthy weight in young children. Seeking solutions from "positive deviants" (i.e., families who have succeeded where many others have not to change their health behaviors, maintain their child's BMI, and develop resilience in the context of sometimes adverse environments) could provide strategies for interventions that can be generalized and promoted to improve the outcomes of other children.

To date, few interventions have been conducted in the period between conception and age 2 years, and most of the existing studies have demonstrated an effect by focusing on individual- or family-level behavior changes through home visits, individual counseling, or group sessions in clinical settings, or using a combination of home and group visits; interventions with hydrolyzed protein formula curtailed infant growth, while protein-enriched formulas increased risk of childhood obesity. Across completed studies, the majority targeted individual-level behaviors of mothers and infants, and most were conducted in clinical settings. Overall, systems- and policy-level interventions are underrepresented.

Summary and Recommendations

Despite growing evidence for the role of early-life interventions in preventing childhood obesity, a 2010 review of interventions to prevent or treat overweight among children younger than 2 years yielded only 10 published studies of poor or fair quality. In addition, national funding initiatives continue to exclude children younger than 2 years, a missed opportunity for both obesity prevention and reduction of related racial/ethnic disparities.

There remain a number of gaps in the literature that should be filled to advance childhood obesity research in early life. First, future research during pregnancy should extend beyond the first months of life to examine the mechanisms through which intrauterine risk factors lead to offspring risk of overweight. Second, there is no single measure of adiposity that can be continuously used across fetal, infant, and early childhood lifecourse periods. A continuous measure of child growth during the first years of life would facilitate future research on high fetal and infant weight. Third, future research should include information on the role of fathers, partners, and other caretakers, in addition to the mothers, on child weight comes.

Effective interventions for addressing childhood obesity and eliminating related disparities will require multilevel, multisector strategies, especially those that invoke change at the social environment level and draw lessons from a life-course understanding of the etiology of obesity. In addition, to reduce obesity prevalence, there is an important need to identify effective levers of sustainable change and a move toward paradigm-shifting research and interventions that integrate translational, transformational, and transdisciplinary thinking and approaches.

Acknowledgments

Preparation of this chapter was supported, in part, by Grant No. 1K24DK105989-01 from the National Institutes of Health. We thank Ines Castro for her editorial assistance.

Suggested Reading

Dixon, B., Peña, M. M., & Taveras, E. M. (2012). Lifecourse approach to racial/ethnic disparities in childhood obesity. *Advances in Nutrition, 3*(1), 73–82.—By the preschool years, racial/

ethnic disparities in obesity prevalence are already present, suggesting that disparities in childhood obesity prevalence have their origins in the earliest stages of life. Understanding the risk factors during pregnancy, infancy, early childhood, and beyond, as well as racial/ethnic differences, may help to inform the design of clinical and public health interventions and policies to reduce the prevalence of childhood obesity.

Lumeng, J. C., Taveras, E. M., Birch, L., & Yanovski, S. Z. (2015). Prevention of obesity in infancy and early childhood: A National Institutes of Health Workshop. *JAMA Pediatrics, 169*(5), 484–490.—In fall 2013, the National Institute of Diabetes and Digestive and Kidney Diseases convened a multidisciplinary workshop to summarize the current state of knowledge regarding the prevention of infant and early childhood obesity and to identify research gaps and opportunities.

McGuire, S. (2012). Institute of Medicine (IOM) early childhood obesity prevention policies. *Advances in Nutrition, 3*(1), 56–57.—A published report examining strategies to prevent overweight and obesity from birth to 5 years, with a focus on nutrition, physical activity, and sedentary behavior.

Nader, P. R., Huang, T. T. K., Gahagan, S., Kumanyika, S., Hammond, R. A., & Christoffel, K. K. (2012). Next steps in obesity prevention: Altering early life systems to support healthy parents, infants, and toddlers. *Childhood Obesity* (formerly *Obesity and Weight Management*), *8*(3), 195–204.—Altering early life systems that promote intergenerational transmission of obesity holds promise for interrupting the continuing cycle of the obesity epidemic. A review of evidence from basic science, prevention, and systems research supports an approach that (1) begins at the earliest stages of development and (2) uses a systems framework to simultaneously implement health behavior and environmental changes in communities.

Ogden, C. L., Carroll, M. D., Kit, B. K., & Flegal, K. M. (2014). Prevalence of childhood and adult obesity in the United States, 2011–2012. *Journal of the American Medical Association, 311*(8), 806–814.—The authors provide a recent national estimate of childhood obesity, analyze trends in childhood obesity between 2003 and 2012, and provide detailed obesity trend analyses among adults. In conclusion, there were no significant changes in obesity prevalence in youth or adults between 2003–2004 and 2011–2012. Obesity prevalence remains high; therefore, it is important to continue surveillance.

Oken, E., & Gillman, M. W. (2003). Fetal origins of obesity. *Obesity Research, 11*(4), 496–506.—A new paradigm for prevention, which evolved from the notion that environmental factors *in utero* may influence lifelong health, has emerged in recent years. The combination of lower birth weight and higher attained BMI is most strongly associated with later disease risk. Prevention of obesity starting in childhood is critical and can have lifelong, perhaps multigenerational, impact.

Redsell, S. A., Edmonds, B., Swift, J. A., Siriwardena, A. N., Weng, S., Nathan, D., et al. (2016). Systematic review of randomised controlled trials of interventions that aim to reduce the risk, either directly or indirectly, of overweight and obesity in infancy and early childhood. *Maternal and Child Nutrition, 12*(1), 24–38.—This review identified interventions designed to reduce the risk of overweight/obesity that were delivered antenatally or during the first 2 years of life, with outcomes reported from birth to 7 years of age. Six electronic databases were searched for articles reporting randomized controlled trials of interventions published from January 1990 to September 2013. Despite the known risk factors, very few intervention studies for pregnant women continue during infancy, which should be a priority for future research.

Weng, S. F., Redsell, S. A., Swift, J. A., Yang, M., & Glazebrook, C. P. (2012). Systematic review and meta-analyses of risk factors for childhood overweight identifiable during infancy. *Archives of Disease in Childhood, 97*(12), 1019–1026.—Thirty prospective studies were identified to determine risk factors for childhood overweight during the first year of life to facilitate early identification and targeted intervention. Several risk factors for both overweight and obesity in childhood are identifiable during infancy.

Health Risks Associated with Obesity

ADELA HRUBY
FRANK B. HU

Obesity increases risk for or exists concomitantly with nearly every preventable chronic condition, from type 2 diabetes to dyslipidemia, to poor mental health. Its impacts on risk of stroke and heart disease, certain cancers, osteoarthritis, and, ultimately, quality of life are particularly significant. This chapter reviews the most common comorbidities and sequelae of obesity, including its role in premature mortality.

Diabetes

Excess weight and diabetes are so tightly linked that the American Diabetes Association recommends that physicians test for type 2 diabetes and assess risk of diabetes in *asymptomatic* individuals over 45 years old, simply if they are overweight or obese. In addition, the Association recommends testing for diabetes regardless of age if a patient is severely obese. Although not every overweight or obese individual has diabetes, some 80% of those with diabetes are overweight or obese. Being overweight raises risk of developing type 2 diabetes by a factor of three, and being obese raises risk of type 2 diabetes by a factor of seven, compared to being normal weight. Excess weight in childhood and in young adulthood, and weight gain through early to midadulthood are also strong risk factors for diabetes. Abdominal adiposity, beyond overall body mass, is also independently associated with incident diabetes. The presence of abdominal adiposity may further stratify risk of diabetes in overweight individuals: Having Class 2 obesity (body mass index [BMI] $\geq$ 35 kg/m^2) and a large waist circumference (> 102 cm in men, or > 88 cm in women) increases one's chances of developing diabetes by a dramatic 22- to 32-fold compared to those with normal weight and waist circumference.

Obesity itself raises diabetes risk even in the absence of other metabolic dysregulation (insulin resistance, hypertension, and dyslipidemia). While metabolically healthy obese individuals are estimated to have half the risk of their metabolically unhealthy counterparts, they still have four times the risk of those who are normal weight and metabolically healthy. In addition, the metabolically healthy obese phenotype tends to be transitory, especially for those who gain weight over time.

Although some studies have suggested that obesity in individuals with diabetes may be protective against mortality (as per the obesity paradox, discussed further below), a recent analysis of U.S. health professionals with diabetes followed for up to 16 years, found that excess body weight in those who had never smoked was linearly related to risk of all-cause, cardiovascular, and cancer mortality. In those who had ever smoked, linear trends were not as evident, but obesity nevertheless tended to be associated with higher risk of all-cause mortality. In addition, in those who were diagnosed with diabetes before age 65, linear trends between increasing BMI and higher risk of death were evident regardless of smoking status. The effect of quitting smoking on body weight—which is typically associated with weight gain—may explain why overweight does not *always* associate with higher mortality risk.

Heart and Vascular Diseases

Excess body weight is a well-known risk factor for heart disease and ischemic stroke, including their typical antecedents—dyslipidemia and hypertension. Recent studies have consistently shown that when it comes to the heart, benign obesity is a myth; overweight and obesity add to risk of heart disease and stroke beyond their implications for hypertension, dyslipidemia, and hyperglycemia.

Given childhood obesity rates, research has also increasingly focused on the role of obesity in early life and subsequent adulthood disease. Obesity in childhood or adolescence has been associated with twofold or higher risk of adult hypertension, heart disease, and stroke. A recent study pooling data from four child cohorts with follow-up into midadulthood, observed that compared with individuals who were normal weight in childhood and nonobese as adults, those who were normal weight or overweight in childhood but became obese as adults, or who were obese as children and stayed obese into adulthood, were considerably more prone to develop high-risk dyslipidemia, hypertension, and worse carotid intima-media thickness. Notably, those individuals who were overweight or obese as children, but nonobese as adults, had similar risk profiles to those individuals who were never obese, indicating that the potential health effects of childhood obesity can be offset by weight loss and maintenance prior to or while entering into adulthood.

Cancer

Beyond being a major risk factor for diabetes, which itself is a risk factor for several cancers, obesity is associated with increased risk of developing esophageal, colon, pancreatic, postmenopausal breast, endometrial, and renal cancers. More recently, evidence has accumulated that overweight and/or obesity raises risk for cancers of the gallbladder, liver, ovaries (epithelial), and prostate, as well as leukemia.

While excess body weight contributes to risk of developing certain cancers, the effects of excess body weight on cancer survival, cancer recurrence, and cancer mortality are less clear. However, therapy- and diagnosis-induced weight and lifestyle changes, as well the timing of BMI assessment (i.e., during induction or latency periods, or during or after diagnosis) and its relevancy to cancer outcomes, add complexity to the present understanding of these relationships. Nonetheless, evidence suggests that prediagnosis obesity is associated with decreased survival among breast cancer patients.

Trauma and Infection

Although specific medical complications of adult obesity are discussed in this volume (Chapter 73), several epidemiological observations are worth mentioning here. A nearly decade-long retrospective study of Pennsylvania trauma centers indicated that in-hospital mortality and risk of major complications of surgery were increased in obese patients as compared to nonobese patients. Severely obese patients had upwards of 30% increased risk of trauma mortality than nonobese patients, double the risk of major complications, and over 2.5 times the risk of developing acute renal failure. Severely obese females also had greater than 2.5-fold risk of developing wound complications, and greater than four-fold risk of developing decubitus ulcers. This and other analyses of obesity in trauma care conclude that obesity is associated with 45% increased odds of mortality, longer stays in the intensive care unit, and higher rates of complications, and tend to be associated with longer durations of mechanical ventilation and longer stays in the hospital overall, compared to nonobese patients, despite equivalent injury severity. However, these poorer outcomes may not be purely a result of physiological differences in how obese patients need to be treated; they may also signal bias, or lack of knowledge or training, on the part of health care practitioners in treating these patients.

While higher risk of preventable chronic disease seems to be an obvious consequence of obesity, recent research has also focused on obesity's relationship to risk of infection and infectious disease, including surgical-site, hospital-acquired catheter, bloodstream, nosocomial, urinary tract, cellulitis, and other skin infections; community-acquired infections, such as flu; and less optimal recovery outcomes owing to higher risk of flu, pneumonia, bacteremia, and sepsis. A purported underlying mechanism of obesity's role in infectious disease may be the impaired immunological response associated with excess body weight. Recent research has demonstrated lower vaccine efficacy and serological response to vaccination in obese individuals. For example, a recent study estimated an eightfold increase in the odds of nonresponsiveness to hepatitis B vaccination in obese versus normal-weight women. The consequences of a global obesity epidemic may therefore also forebode a greater global burden of infectious disease.

Mental Health

Dissecting the role of weight in mental health is more complex than that in other comorbidities and sequelae primarily owing to the challenge of determining the causal order of disease, as well as the corelationship of obesity itself with eating disorders and other weight-related disorders, potentially predisposing individuals to or following on other mental health disorders. Nevertheless, obesity and excess adiposity have documented associations with both anatomical and functional changes in the human brain. In older adults, higher BMI is associated with smaller brain volume. Furthermore, compared to their normal-weight counterparts, those who are obese show more atrophy in the frontal lobes, anterior cingulate gyrus, hippocampus, and thalamus, whereas those who are overweight exhibit basal ganglia atrophy and corona radiata of white matter. Notably, anatomical changes have been shown to occur in childhood obesity as well, including smaller orbitofrontal cortex gray-matter volume coupled with poorer performance in certain domains of executive function (e.g., inhibitory control).

Overweight and obesity in midlife are related to increased risk of depression, Alzheimer's disease, dementia, and some aspects of reduced executive function, such as poor decision making, planning, and problem solving. The depression–obesity link, one that is particularly susceptible to reverse causation, has recently been evaluated in a meta-analysis of 15 longitudinal studies, revealing that the relationship is indeed bidirectional. The authors observed that with obesity as the exposure, there was a 57% higher risk of depression in baseline obese versus normal-weight individuals. With baseline depression as the exposure in initially normal-weight individuals, depression was associated with 40% higher risk of obesity, and a nonsignificant 20% increase in risk of overweight. However, in the studies that had follow-up periods of 10 years or more, depression was associated with an 81% increased risk of overweight, suggesting that exposure to depression could have more pronounced effects on weight in the long term.

Physical activity may help mitigate the cognitive decline observed in overweight/obese individuals. Several researchers have observed that middle-aged adults who are overweight and at least modestly active are not at increased risk of poor mental function or dementia compared to those who are normal weight and active. However, being inactive and overweight considerably increases risk of poor mental function and dementia. Thus, being physical active and maintaining a healthy weight are both important for preventing cognitive decline.

Other Conditions

Obesity affects conditions well beyond those we described earlier. Adding to the immense cumulative burden of obesity are elevated risk of osteoarthritis, gallstones and gallbladder disease, nonalcoholic fatty liver disease, pain, impaired mobility, and other physical disability. Social and professional sequelae—among them weight bias and stigma, absenteeism, loss of productivity, and overall poor health-related quality of life, irrespective of comorbidities—further compound the burden.

Overall Mortality

Obesity confers a significantly elevated risk for premature death. Fifteen percent of deaths in the United States in 2000 were attributable to excess weight caused by poor diet and physical inactivity. Overweight and obesity in middle age shortens life expectancy by an estimated 4–7 years. Many long-term studies, as well as major syntheses of pooled data from established cohorts, unequivocally show that obesity over the life course is associated with excess risk of total mortality, and death from cardiovascular disease, diabetes, cancer, or accidental death. These studies have typically been able to account for the confounding impact of smoking history, chronic disease status, and/or intentionality of weight loss—factors that tend to skew the relationship between BMI and mortality.

However, the role of obesity in premature death continues to be the subject of considerable debate, with some suggesting that excess body weight may be protective against mortality from certain chronic conditions—the so-called "obesity paradox." However, most studies that have shown an obesity paradox, or no association between obesity and mortality, have been conducted in groups of older individuals (ages 65 years and older) or in those with chronic conditions, or have inadequately accounted for smoking—important confounding factors noted earlier. Indeed, the role of excess adiposity in old age is unclear. While the protective effects of overweight in specific instances of diseased older populations may be real, the observations belie the limitations of generalizing excess adiposity's supposed benefits to younger populations over the life course, not least because excess body weight leads to higher chronic disease incidence to begin with. Other limitations include the limited utility of BMI in assessing adiposity in older age groups, particularly in the presence of sarcopenic obesity; the confounding generated by disease-free or well-managed disease survival into old age; that weight loss in old age is frequently unintentional, a sign of underlying disease; frailty; history of smoking; and poor nutrition in old age. Finally, additional complexity arises when cardiovascular fitness, abdominal adiposity, and fat mass versus lean mass (as in sarcopenia) are considered when evaluating the obesity–mortality relationship. Because of these complexities, the data on the relationship between BMI and mortality, especially in older individuals and those with chronic diseases, should be interpreted cautiously.

Summary

The consequences of obesity are numerous and potentially devastating, compounded by the fact that obesity is a preventable condition for the vast majority of people. The deteriorations of physical and mental health associated with obesity described here are often magnified by the disease's socioeconomic burdens.

Suggested Reading

Glance, L. G., Li, Y., Osler, T. M., Mukamel, D. B., & Dick, A. W. (2014). Impact of obesity on mortality and complications in trauma patients. *Annals of Surgery, 259*(3), 576–581.—A decadelong study of 147,680 patients admitted to Pennsylvania trauma centers found that severely obese patients were more than 30% more likely to die than nonobese patients, and twice as likely to experience major complications.

Hu, F. B. (2008). *Obesity epidemiology*. New York: Oxford University Press.—A textbook on the epidemiology of obesity, its risk factors, comorbidities, and consequences.

InterAct Consortium. (2012). Long-term risk of incident type 2 diabetes and measures of overall and regional obesity: The EPIC-InterAct Case–Cohort Study. *PLoS Medicine, 9*, e1001230.— In a total cohort of 340,234 participants that comprised 12,403 incident type 2 diabetes cases and a stratified subcohort of 16,154, BMI and waist circumference were each independently associated with type 2 diabetes, with waist circumference being a stronger risk factor in women than in men. Among overweight individuals, high waist circumference identified a subgroup of overweight people whose 10-year cumulative incidence was comparable to that of obese people.

Juonala, M., Magnussen, C. G., Berenson, G. S., Venn, A., Burns, T. L., Sabin, M. A., et al. (2011). Childhood adiposity, adult adiposity, and cardiovascular risk factors. *New England Journal of Medicine, 365*(20), 1876–1885.—This study followed 6,328 children for a mean 23 years into midadulthood; children who were obese in childhood and adulthood had 1.8- to 5.4-fold increased risk for type 2 diabetes, hypertension, high low-density lipoprotein cholesterol, low high-density lipoprotein cholesterol, high triglycerides, and carotid artery atherosclerosis, compared to children who were normal weight in childhood and not obese in adulthood.

Kramer, C. K., Zinman, B., & Retnakaran, R. (2013). Are metabolically healthy overweight and obesity benign conditions?: A systematic review and meta-analysis. *Annals of Internal Medicine, 159*(11), 758–769.—A meta-analysis of "metabolically healthy" obesity in relation to all-cause mortality and cardiovascular events in eight studies of 61,386 participants estimated that obesity, even in the presence of metabolic health, raised risk by 24% in obese compared with normal-weight individuals.

Lu, Y., Hajifathalian, K., Ezzati, M., Woodward, M., Rimm, E. B., & Danaei, G. (2014). Metabolic mediators of the effects of body-mass index, overweight, and obesity on coronary heart disease and stroke: A pooled analysis of 97 prospective cohorts with 1.8 million participants. *Lancet, 383*, 970–983.—Authors of this massive analysis of the relationship between obesity and cardiovascular disease in the latter half of the 20th century reported that the risk of heart disease increased 27%, and risk of stroke 18%, for every 5 kg/m^2 above 20 kg/m^2.

Luppino, F. S., de Wit, L. M., Bouvy, P. F., Stijnen, T., Cuijpers, P., Penninx, B. W., et al. (2010). Overweight, obesity, and depression: A systematic review and meta-analysis of longitudinal studies. *Archives of General Psychiatry, 67*(3), 220–229.—This meta-analysis considered the bidirectional relationship between obesity and depression, in which baseline obesity increased odds of incident depression by 55%, while baseline depression increased odds of incident obesity by 58%.

Raji, C. A., Ho, A. J., Parikshak, N. N., Becker, J. T., Lopez, O. L., Kuller, L. H., et al. (2010). Brain structure and obesity. *Human Brain Mapping, 31*(3), 353–364.—Cognitively normal older adult overweight/obese individuals exhibited differential atrophy in frontal, temporal, and subcortical brain regions compared to normal-weight counterparts, and in overweight/obese individuals, higher BMI was associated with lower brain volume.

The Global BMI Mortality Collaboration. (2016). Body-mass index and all-cause mortality: Individual-participant-data meta-analysis of 239 prospective studies in four continents. *Lancet, 388*, 776–786.—In nearly 4 million never smoking adults initially free of chronic disease, above a BMI of 25 kg/m^2, every 5 kg/m^2 increment was shown to increase risk of all cause-mortality by 29–39%.

Tobias, D. K., Pan, A., Jackson, C. L., O'Reilly, E. J., Ding, E. L., Willett, W. C., et al. (2014). Body-mass index and mortality among adults with incident type 2 diabetes. *New England Journal of Medicine, 370*(3), 233–244.—In health professionals followed for 15.8 years after diabetes diagnosis, a J-shaped association with all-cause mortality was observed across BMI categories; with 22.5–24.9 kg/m^2 as the reference, those with a BMI greater than 35 kg/m^2 had 33% higher risk of death, while those with a BMI less than 22.5 kg/m^2 had 29% higher risk, with stronger associations with increasing BMI among those who had never smoked.

Obesity in U.S. Racial/Ethnic Minority Populations

SHIRIKI K. KUMANYIKA

Effective obesity treatment and prevention in minority populations is of high priority from both clinical and population health perspectives. The minority segment of the U.S. population continues to increase in size. The need for special attention to obesity prevention and treatment in minority populations relates to the higher than average prevalence of obesity in these populations and associated health implications.

Minority Population Diversity

Minority populations in the United States include black/African Americans (13.2%), Hispanic or Latino Americans (17.4%), American Indians or Alaska Natives (1.2%), Asian or Pacific Islander Americans (5.4%), and Native Hawaiians and other Pacific Islanders (0.2%). These populations combined now comprise more than one-third of the U.S. population and more than half of the populations of several states and many counties. The broad categories are internally very diverse as well, ethnically, and in other ways, such as fertility rates; family structures; living arrangements; poverty; wealth; educational attainment; occupation; residence distribution across U.S. regions and urban, suburban, and rural areas; and the percentage that is foreign born, their ages at immigration, and duration of U.S. residence. Social-structural factors related to discrimination and opportunity result in more poverty and unemployment, lower education attainment, poorer housing, and other types of social disadvantage in minority populations, not all of which are related to resource limitations. Social disadvantage is less common among Asian Americans compared to other minority populations.

Prevalence, Trends, and Health Implications

Obesity prevalence data for several racial/ethnic minority populations are included in Table 63.1. Prevalence is higher than that among whites for all minority populations except Asian Americans. However, data on the relationship of body mass index (BMI) to body fatness indicate that BMI-based definitions of obesity using standard cutoffs underestimate obesity-related health risks in people of Asian descent. Asian Americans on average have a higher percent body fat at a given BMI level in comparison to other populations. They may also have relatively more fat in the abdominal region. Therefore, use of lower BMI cutoff points to identify target populations for obesity interventions is recommended for Asian populations (e.g., BMI $\geq$ 25 rather than $\geq$ 30. This lower cutoff was used in the analysis of National Health Interview Survey data for Asian/Pacific Islander subgroups shown in Table 63.1. A substantial gender difference (higher prevalence in women) is observed in blacks and some Hispanic subgroups when obesity is defined using BMI $\geq$ 30. Grade 3, or severe, obesity (BMI $\geq$ 40) is more common among women in all groups but is notably more prevalent in blacks compared to whites, Hispanics, and Asian Americans.

Trends in obesity prevalence in minority populations show increases that are consistent with trends in the U.S. population as a whole. In some cases, the rate of increase in obesity prevalence is higher in minority populations and still increasing, while prevalence in whites appears to be stabilizing. Severe obesity is increasing in all population groups.

Obesity prevalence and trends also vary by income and education, and these associations differ by race/ethnicity and gender. Higher education or income does not appear to be protective, or as protective, in minority populations as one would expect based on data from non-Hispanic white populations. This may reflect a "nutrition transition" effect; in economically upwardly mobile populations and societies, increased obesity prevalence is initially observed in the more advantaged segments of the populations.

Cardiovascular diseases, cancer, and type 2 diabetes—all obesity-related—are among the major causes of premature death in the U.S. population overall. Where studied, an association between obesity and higher total mortality in minority populations is not observed consistently. These analyses are complicated by aspects of health profiles other than obesity (e.g., different patterns with respect to other risk factors and also differential access to early treatment). In addition, the *relative* risks associated with obesity are smaller when obesity prevalence is very high within a population. Data linking obesity, either generalized or in the abdominal region, to health risks or adverse health outcomes have been reported for one or more minority populations in relation to numerous conditions, including diabetes, hypertension, dyslipidemia, subclinical atherosclerosis, coronary heart disease, left ventricular hypertrophy, sleep apnea, and musculoskeletal problems. Asian Americans have a higher than average prevalence of type 2 diabetes, the health outcome most closely associated with obesity, in spite of less obesity by standard BMI definitions. This may reflect a greater tendency to develop diabetes at a lower BMI level due to the previously noted differences in body composition and fat patterning, or due to other reasons.

Modifiable Pathways for Eliminating Disparities

As with obesity in all populations, causal pathways involve interactions among biological, behavioral, and environmental factors that influence energy intake, output, and metabolism. The search for causes of obesity *disparities*, however, focuses specifically on modifiable pathways that vary on the basis of race- or ethnicity-related aspects of social structures (i.e., apart from intra- and interpersonal differences within a given population)

TABLE 63.1. Obesity Prevalence in U.S. Racial/Ethnic Subgroups

Data source and subgroup	Time period, ages, obesity definition	Percent obese	
		Men	Women
National Health Interview Survey (NHIS)[a]			
Non-Hispanic white	Years: 2008–2010	27.0	24.5
Non-Hispanic black		31.0	42.1
Mexican American	Ages ≥ 18 years*	33.1	35.6
Native American/Alaska Native	BMI ≥ 30 kg/m²	39.3	41.9
Asian American		10.8	9.5
Native Hawaiian or other Pacific Islander		48.0	44.5
National Health and Nutrition Examination Survey (NHANES)[b]			
Non-Hispanic white	Years: 2011–2012	32.4	32.8
Non-Hispanic black		37.1	56.6
Non-Hispanic Asian	Ages ≥ 20 years*	10.0	11.4
Hispanic	BMI ≥ 30 kg/m²	40.1	44.4
Non-Hispanic white		*3.8*	*7.4*
Non-Hispanic black	BMI ≥ 40 kg/m²*	*6.9*	*16.4*
Non-Hispanic Asian		*0.2*	*1.4*
Hispanic		*3.7*	*7.6*
Hispanic Community Health Study (HCHS)[c]			
All	Years: 2008–2011	36.5	42.6
Cuban		33.6	38.9
Dominican	Ages 18–74 years*	38.6	42.5
Mexican	BMI ≥ 30 kg/m²	36.8	41.5
Puerto Rican		40.9	51.4
Central American		32.7	41.6
South American		26.8	30.8

Data source and subgroup	Time period, ages, obesity definition	Men and Women
National Health Interview Survey (NHIS)[d]		
Non-Hispanic white		60.8
All Asian/Pacific Islander	Years: 2006–2011	41.4
Chinese		27.9
Asian Indian	Ages ≥ 18 years	44.4
Filipino		53.2
Korean	BMI ≥ 25 kg/m²	30.1[#]
Vietnamese		24.4[#]
Japanese		34.6[#]
Hawaiian and Pacific Islander		73.8

[a]Based on self-reported height and weight; U.S. national probability sample, age-adjusted (Schoenborn et al., *Vital and Health Statistics, 10*(257), 2013).

[b]Based on measured height and weight; U.S. national probability sample; age adjusted to the Census 2000 projected population. Italics indicate estimates with a large standard error (Ogden et al., *Journal of the American Medical Association, 311*(8), 806–814, 2014).

[c]Based on measured height and weight; cohort recruited from a random sample (in the Bronx, NY; Chicago, IL; Miami, FL; San Diego, CA); age adjusted to Census 2010 population (Daviglus et al., *Journal of the American Medical Association, 308*(17), 1775–1784, 2012).

[d]Based on self-reported height and weight; U.S. national probability sample, age adjusted; # data for these populations are for 2004–2006; these groups were not reported separately in the latter period. Note that the cutoff point is lower in these data and includes both overweight and obesity where standard definitions are used (Singh & Lin, *ISRN Preventive Medicine*, Article ID 898691, 12 pp., 2013).

that may predispose individuals to excess weight gain or have implications for how interventions are approached.

Evidence suggests that higher than average obesity prevalence in minority populations can be explained on the basis of known or suspected obesity risk factors. Available data support environmental pathways that promote obesity more strongly than pathways related to genes. This is partly because racial/ethnic minority categories define groups that are genetically highly heterogeneous. These classifications define population groups with common geographic and cultural origins in a very broad sense as people who may share risks in terms of their social or economic positions or political status. The once popular hypothesis that genes predisposing to greater efficiency in energy utilization conferred a survival advantage during exposure to food shortages is no longer considered viable. Such genes have not been identified, and these explanations are no longer plausible in the context of the obesity epidemic. Moreover, studies of the African diaspora and of Asian and Hispanic migrants have demonstrated gradients of increased obesity, with increased exposure to obesity-promoting environments. Increases in obesity with successive generations of U.S. immigrants are also evidence of environmental rather than genetic influences. On the other hand, biological pathways that reflect exposure *in utero* could contribute to excess obesity risks in minority populations intergenerationally, for example, in association with high maternal weight preconception or excess pregnancy weight gain. Environmental factors that predispose to and perpetuate excess weight gain in minority populations are readily identifiable—starting with factors for populations as a whole, then focusing on those for which minority populations have higher exposure or may be more strongly impacted. In this sense, environments are understood as neighborhoods, work and school environments, exposure to recreational facilities, and considering interactions among environments and between people and environments.

Blacks, Hispanic Americans, and American Indians are more likely than whites to live in communities with other ethnic/minority residents. Many of these communities are in socially disadvantaged settings. Social and economic disadvantages concentrate obesity-promoting forces in living environments and limit individual capacity for effectively navigating these environments, both overall and in response to preventive or therapeutic interventions. The mix of foods available in low-resource neighborhoods is skewed toward overconsumption of calories and fat and insufficient consumption of dietary fiber; physical activity options are skewed toward relatively low levels. Deterrents to healthy eating and physical activity patterns may include lack of neighborhood access to retail outlets that sell appealing, healthy foods at affordable prices, combined with an excess of fast-food outlets, lack of neighborhood fitness and recreational facilities, and crime or other conditions that discourage being outdoors. Both discretionary income and discretionary time may be limited for individuals who have low incomes, high housing costs, more than one job, and child care or family responsibilities—further limiting lifestyle options.

Attitudes and preferences in minority populations are influenced by sometimes longstanding sociocultural norms that may increase the vulnerability to obesity-promoting forces. The ubiquity of inexpensive, highly palatable, high-calorie foods and beverages may be especially problematic in sociocultural contexts where, although once unavailable or unaffordable, they can now be readily obtained and consumed routinely. In addition, preferences and norms that favor consumption of fried or other high-calorie foods or sugar-sweetened beverages are amplified by food marketing in minority communities. The relatively greater availability of these products, coupled with advertisements and promotions that directly target ethnic minorities in both intensity and content are synergistic stimuli for higher consumption. The excess exposure to such targeted marketing is well documented with respect to black and Hispanic populations, especially youth.

On the output side of the energy balance equation, there is convincing evidence that leisure-time physical activity levels are lower and sedentary behavior is higher in many minority populations. This may reflect a lack of environmental support for active living in concert with attitudes and norms that favor the use of cars or engaging in sedentary entertainment.

Prevention and Treatment

Many individuals in minority populations express a strong desire to lose weight, yet several factors detract from motivations and social support for weight control, over and above the previously described environmental and sociocultural challenges. The higher the level of obesity in a population, the more likely that obesity may be viewed as normative (i.e., because so many peers are also overweight). In addition, cultural attitudes toward obesity and large body size are generally less negative in minority populations compared to those observed in white populations and more likely to include some positive aspects. The positive aspects relate to associating larger body sizes with robustness, whereas thinness is associated with terminal illness or severe poverty. Accordingly, the belief that excess weight impairs health may also be less common.

The continuing trends of increase in obesity prevalence in some minority populations suggest a need for more targeted strategies designed to have above-average effectiveness. Engaging high-risk communities directly in the planning and implementation of interventions and using whole-community approaches are recommended increasingly to address this need. Approaches that are equally effective in minority and nonminority populations will maintain the status quo, and disparities could widen if strategies are less effective.

Evidence from studies of high-quality obesity treatment interventions indicates that weight losses sufficient to improve health status can be achieved under ideal conditions for minority as well as white populations. However, reports of smaller weight losses in minority populations compared to whites in the same study suggest a need to improve the environmental relevance, specificity, and long-term sustainability of these interventions.

Minority Children and Youth

The picture of obesity prevalence in children and youth in racial/ethnic minority populations is very similar to the one described here for adults (i.e., above-average prevalence except for Asian Americans, and still increasing trends in some race/ethnicity–age–gender groups). The health burden of obesity with childhood onset begins sooner and, if not addressed, will be of longer duration. The occurrence of type 2 diabetes in 10- to 19-year-olds, although fortunately still infrequent, is two or more times higher than that in whites in all racial/ethnic minority groups. Intervention considerations for obesity prevention and treatment in minority children both include and mirror those described for adults. The neighborhood influences are as relevant or more relevant to children, both directly and through effects on parental or caregiver behaviors—especially for young children. Black and Hispanic youth are major focal points for targeted marketing of unhealthy foods and beverages, both as potential consumers and as trend setters who influence norms and behaviors of other youth. In this context, the reach and apparent effectiveness of school- and child care-based interventions in several racial/ethnic groups are promising for addressing disparities in these settings.

Conclusion

Prevention and treatment of obesity in minority populations are among the most significant yet challenging domains for future obesity research. Identifying modifiable factors in pathways that predispose racial/ethnic minority populations to higher than average obesity prevalence is still a work in progress. Developing programs that can have an enduring impact in minority communities will require a higher priority for the inclusion of these populations in etiological and intervention research, a commitment to designing interventions that will align with their needs and preferences, and a willingness to empower community members within the research enterprise.

Suggested Reading

Caprio, S., Daniels, S. R., Drewnowski, A., Kaufman, F. R., Palinkas, L. A., Rosenbloom, A. L., et al. (2008). Influence of race, ethnicity, and culture on childhood obesity: Implications for prevention and treatment. *Obesity (Silver Spring), 16*(12), 2566–2577.—Obesity expert consensus statement that provides a detailed examination of racial/ethnic disparities in childhood obesity, potential causes, prevention, and treatment implications.

Grier, S. A., & Kumanyika, S. K. (2008). The context for choice: Health implications of targeted food and beverage marketing to African Americans. *American Journal of Public Health, 98*(9), 1616–1629.—Systematic review of evidence related to the disproportionate exposure of black Americans to targeted marketing of unhealthy foods and beverages.

Institute of Medicine. (2013). *Creating equal opportunities for a healthy weight: Workshop summary*. Washington, DC: National Academies Press.—Summaries of presentations that explored health equity issues in population-based obesity prevention undertaken in various settings.

Isasi, C. R., Ayala, G. X., Sotres-Alvarez, D., Madanat, H., Penedo, F., Loria, C. M., et al. (2015). Is acculturation related to obesity in Hispanic/Latino adults?: Results from the Hispanic Community Health Study/Study of Latinos. *Journal of Obesity, 2015,* Article 186276.—Analyzes variation in obesity levels among Hispanic population subgroups by demographic variables and shows that length of U.S. residence is a major factor in the pathway to obesity.

Kumanyika, S., Taylor, W. C., Grier, S. A., Lassiter, V., Lancaster, K. J., Morssink, C. B., et al. (2012). Community energy balance: A framework for contextualizing cultural influences on high risk of obesity in ethnic minority populations. *Preventive Medicine, 55*(5), 371–381.—Proposes a comprehensive framework to aid in understanding determinants of obesity and related intervention pathways in racial/ethnic minority populations in the United States and other high-income countries.

Lovasi, G. S., Hutson, M. A., Guerra, M., & Neckerman, K. M. (2009). Built environments and obesity in disadvantaged populations. *Epidemiologic Reviews, 31,* 7–20.—Reviews evidence of built environment influences on obesity in disadvantaged populations and supports the importance of access to healthy food and places to exercise, and safety.

May, A. L., Freedman, D., Sherry, B., & Blanck, H. M. (2013). Obesity: United States, 1999–2010. *Morbidity and Mortality Weekly Report, 62*(3), 120–128.—Reports obesity prevalence and recent trends for U.S. adults and children by race–ethnicity–gender groups and by socioeconomic status within these groups.

Whitt-Glover, M. C., Kumanyika, S. K., & Haire-Joshu, D. (2014). Introduction to the special issue on achieving healthy weight in black American communities. *Obesity Reviews, 15*(Suppl. 4), 1–4.—This special issue includes 10 systematic reviews of obesity interventions in black adults and children in various settings.

Williams, J. D., Crockett, D., Harrison, R. L., & Thomas, K. D. (2012). The role of food culture and marketing activity in health disparities. *Preventive Medicine, 55*(5), 382–386.—Explores the complex relationship between food culture and marketing activities that potentially contribute to obesity-related health disparities.

World Health Organization Expert Consultation. (2004). Appropriate body-mass index for Asian populations and its implications for policy and intervention strategies. *Lancet, 363,* 157–163.—Recommends that BMI cutoffs lower than the standard WHO international definitions should be used as appropriate to identify overweight- and obesity-related risk in populations of Asian descent.

Epidemiology and Causes of Obesity in Children and Young Adults

TIMOTHY GILL

The World Health Organization (WHO) has labeled childhood obesity as one of the most serious global public health challenges of the 21st century. Its assessment was based on the level of childhood overweight and obesity throughout the world, the rapid rate at which this level has risen, and the potential health consequences of the condition. Childhood obesity often progresses to adult weight problems, but there are also immediate health consequences in children and especially adolescents. These range from increased levels of cardiovascular disease risk factors and type 2 diabetes to orthopedic complications, sleep apnea, and fatty liver, in addition to psychosocial problems, including low self-esteem and depression. More recent assessments indicate that many of these conditions are beginning to emerge in children and adolescents and to become established in early adulthood, leading to lifelong chronic conditions.

Definitions of Childhood Overweight and Obesity

Obesity is commonly defined as abnormal or excessive fat accumulation that presents a risk to health. Body mass index (BMI) has been shown to be a reasonable proxy for fatness, and cut points have been set to define overweight and various grades of obesity in adults. However these cut points cannot be applied to children and adolescents given that BMI changes continuously during this stage of rapid growth and development in which height increases and body composition changes with age. It is therefore necessary to compare a child's weight status against standard growth curves that are based on the usual changes in height and weight that occur across childhood and adolescence. A number of countries have developed their own growth curves based on historical data, and international growth curves have been generated by combining data from a range of countries. However, a number of different systems to define overweight and obesity in childhood and adolescence remain, making international comparisons challenging (see Table 64.1). This lack of consistency of definitions not only causes disparities in estimates of the prevalence in weight problems among children but also has the potential to influence research into identifying factors promoting obesity in children.

Prevalence and Trends in Overweight and Obesity in Children, Adolescents, and Young Adults

Defining the true level of overweight and obesity in children and young adults throughout the world is extremely difficult because of not only the problems of varying definitions but also the scarcity of quality data on height and weight in many countries or regions. Most developed countries such as the United States, the United Kingdom, and Australia have regular health surveys, but many poorer countries often do not have well established data collection systems. However, a number of recent studies have brought together multiple data sets and analyzed these using a common standard to provide a realistic estimate of the weight status of children at a global level.

Preschool Children

In 2010, the WHO gathered together data on the weight status of children under 5 years of age from 144 countries to identify prevalence and trends in overweight and obesity using WHO standards. It estimated that the global prevalence of overweight and obesity was about 6.8%, or about 42.8 million children worldwide. The prevalence in developed countries was almost twice that in developing counties (11.7 vs. 6.1%), but the absolute number of children with a weight problem in developing countries was around 35 million, or almost four times as great as that in developed countries, reflecting the huge number of young children living in developing regions of the world. There were great variations in the rates of overweight throughout the various regions of the world, with countries within South Asia reporting levels of overweight of around 3.5%, whereas North Africa and the Middle East had levels of 17% or more. Very poor countries such as Nepal and North Korea had the lowest rates of overweight with less than 1%, whereas Balkan countries such as Albania and Bosnia and Herzegovina had levels greater than 25%.

TABLE 64.1. Competing Definitions of Childhood Obesity

Organization	Age range (years)	Growth standard	Overweight	Obesity
World Health Organization (WHO)	0–5	WHO child growth standards	2 SD above median	3 SD above median
	6–19	National Center for Health Statistics/WHO growth reference	1SD above median	2 SD above median
U.S. Centers for Disease Control and Prevention	2–20	CDC growth charts	≥ 85th– < 95th percentile	≥ 95th percentile
International Obesity Task Force (IOTF)	2–18	IOTF international reference standards	Correspond to adult BMI of 25	Correspond to adult BMI of 30

The global prevalence of overweight and obesity increased 60% between 1990 and 2010 and was projected to reach 9.1% (or 60 million preschool children) by 2020. Once again, there are variations: The rate of change is higher in developing countries (an increase of 65%) than in developed countries (an increase of 48% between 1990 and 2010).

School-Age Children and Adolescents

Data on the weight status of children older than age 5 years is less consistently available than data on preschoolers because they are beyond the monitoring reach of maternal and child health services. As a consequence, estimates of rates of overweight across the world often rely on extrapolation and projection from available data sets. In 2004, The International Obesity Task Force (IOTF) conducted an assessment of childhood weight status applying the IOTF standards to data from national surveys across the world. They estimated that 10% of the world's children (or 155 million) were overweight, with around 2–3% (or 30–45 million) of these being obese. North America, Europe, and parts of the Western Pacific had the highest prevalence of overweight among children (20–30%), whereas countries within Southeast Asia and much of sub-Saharan Africa had the lowest prevalence. The 2013 Global Burden of Disease Study used data from a wide range of sources to estimate the levels of overweight and obesity in children ages 2–19 years in 188 countries at various time points between 1980 and 2013, based on IOTF standards. These estimates indicate that around 24% of boys and 23% of girls in developed countries were overweight, having risen rapidly from levels of around 16% for boys and girls in 1980. The rate of increase was as marked in developing countries, with overweight and obesity increasing from around 8 to 13% for both girls and boys between 1980 and 2013. Regions with the highest levels of child and adolescent obesity included the Middle East and North Africa (especially for girls) and the Pacific Island and Caribbean nations. Age-standardized prevalence of obesity in children and adolescents ranged from more than 30% for girls in Kiribati and the Federated States of Micronesia to less than 2% in Bangladesh, Nepal, Laos, and a number of African countries.

Young Adults

The years between ages 18 and 25 are a time of transition from adolescence to adulthood, with rapidly changing circumstances and competing priorities. These years are now viewed as a significant stage in the development of health behaviors and long-term weight status. Although overall prevalence of obesity in young adults is lower than that in older age groups, recent studies have identified the alarming rates of weight gain that occur at this stage of life. This weight gain in early adulthood is associated with a greater risk of chronic diseases, such as diabetes and heart disease, than similar weight gain later in life. Longitudinal studies in both developed and emerging countries have found that weight increases at around 0.5–1.0 kg each year in young adults, which is faster than that for any other stage of adulthood. The weight changes of American college students has been extensively studied, and although the fabled "freshman 15" (which purported that college students gain 15 pounds in their first year) has been found to be an exaggeration, the stress and adjustments associated with study do result in substantial weight gain in many students over the course of their degree.

A Plateau in the Level of Overweight and Obesity in Children

Although there has been an alarming rise in rates of childhood overweight and obesity across the world since the 1980s, data from the United States, Australia, Japan, the United Kingdom, and some European countries indicate that these rates may now be plateauing, albeit at unacceptably high levels. The reasons behind this plateau in rates are hotly debated, and questions remain as to whether this leveling is real or just a statistical quirk, or is possibly the product of declining participation rates in surveys. Some studies have noted concomitant improvements in diet and physical activity behaviors, and it is feasible that these improvements in children's weight status can be attributed to the impact of health promotion actions to address childhood obesity. Closer assessment of national survey data in the United States and Australia have revealed significant disparity in obesity rates between advantaged and disadvantaged groups. Children from higher socioeconomic status (SES) groups have shown marked improvements in their weight status, while rates of overweight and obesity for those from lower SES groups continue to rise.

Causes of Childhood Obesity

The drivers of the obesity epidemic have been addressed in detail elsewhere in this book, but there are issues that are of specific concern in the development of obesity in childhood and adolescence. The basic foundation of weight gain and obesity is an energy imbalance in which energy intake in the form of food and beverages exceeds energy expenditure from body metabolism and activity. However, in reality, the causes are far more complex because a wide range of interrelated and interacting genetic, physiological, environmental, social, psychological, and cognitive factors influence diet and activity behaviors, and the regulation of body weight. In children, many of these factors are beyond their direct control.

In Utero *and Early-Life Factors*

Recent research has demonstrated that *in utero* exposure to a variety of factors sets the potential for the development of excessive fatness and obesity in childhood. The diet, smoking, and physical activity behaviors and weight status of the mother, together with the resulting physiological environment of high insulin and glucose or circulating lipids, creates changes in the developing fetus that influence body composition and functioning. These lead to adaptive responses that predispose the child to later obesity, particularly when the postnatal environment differs greatly from that experienced *in utero*. Very rapid early growth of infants in the first year of life, which greatly exceeds the normal growth curves, has also been associated with increased risk of childhood and early adulthood obesity. In addition, excessive weight gain in the first 3 months of life has been associated with greater risk of diabetes and cardiovascular disease in adulthood.

Infant feeding patterns have also been linked to childhood obesity and later disease. Studies suggest infants fed breast milk substitutes have a higher postnatal growth and higher levels of fatness, whereas exclusive breastfeeding has been shown to promote slower growth and leaner infants who have a modest reduction in the risk of later overweight and obesity. There is no indication that early introduction of appropriate complementary feeding exacerbates weight gain.

Early Childhood Diet and Activity Behaviors

The recent period of rapid increase in child obesity rates has been accompanied, and perhaps driven, by significant shifts in dietary and physical activity behaviors. The diet of children today is characterized by large intakes of highly processed, hyperpalatable, ready-to-consume food snacks and sweetened beverages, all of which have been associated with consumption of excess calories and weight gain. In highly developed countries, these products can contribute 40–50% of total dietary energy intake, and in developing countries their consumption is increasing rapidly. Physical activity patterns have also altered markedly, with fewer children walking or cycling to school or other destinations, and passive recreational pursuits such as video games replacing more active play. There is particular concern around these changes because activity and food preferences and behaviors established in childhood usually track into adulthood. There is some indication of an association between short sleep duration in infants and higher levels of overweight in later childhood, which is thought to be mediated, in part, by exacerbating diet and activity behaviors that contribute to weight gain.

Environmental Factors

Children's' diet and activity behaviors are also influenced by a number of changes that have occurred in their living environment and the broader society that encourage behaviors associated with excessive weight gain and obesity. High levels of car traffic, loss of neighborhood play areas, and increasing crime rates in some areas have discouraged parents from allowing children to play freely outside. Marketing of snack foods and sweetened beverages, and sedentary leisure pursuits have increased dramatically in recent decades and now targets young children directly with persuasive messaging that encourages children to demand the purchase of these products through "pester power." Growing personal income and the wide availability of snack foods and beverages around schools, sporting stadiums, and other places where children and adolescents congregate also encourage and enable children and adolescents to overconsume food products most associated with excess energy intake.

Summary and Conclusions

Childhood and adolescent obesity rates have increased dramatically over the last three decades, to the point that 20–30% of school-age children in developed countries now have a weight problem. The prevalence of childhood overweight and obesity continues to increase at alarming rates in developing countries, but it appears to be leveling out in many developed countries. However there remain great disparities in the rates of obesity, with much of the improvement in prevalence being driven by improvements in high income groups, while children of low SES continue to gain weight. Of particular concern is the high level of inappropriate weight gain in young adults that puts them at risk of early development of a number of chronic conditions and threatens a lifetime of ill health. We are developing a better understanding of how overweight and obesity develops so early in life and the impact of intrauterine and early-life influences. However, eating and activity behaviors that drive energy imbalance and weight problems in children continue to deteriorate, driven by changes in marketing and access of food, as well as social structures and family behaviors. Urgent and sustained action is required to address these issues.

Suggested Reading

Centers for Disease Control and Prevention. (2015). Childhood obesity causes and consequences. Retrieved May 26, 2015, from *www.cdc.gov/obesity/childhood/causes.html*.—Overview of key environmental factors driving childhood obesity and the major health consequences. Updated regularly.

Cole, T. J., Bellizzi, M. C., Flegal, K. M., & Dietz, W. H. (2000). Establishing a standard definition for child overweight and obesity worldwide: International survey. *British Medical Journal, 320,* 1240–1243.—Original article from the IOTF clarifying the need for a universal definition of childhood obesity and setting out a methodology for childhood obesity standards that are linked to those for adults.

De Onis, M., Blössner, M., & Borghi, E. (2010). Global prevalence and trends of overweight and obesity among preschool children. *American Journal of Clinical Nutrition, 92*(5), 1257–1264.—First major study of the weight status of preschool children from across the world. Data are presented from an analysis of 450 nationally representative cross-sectional surveys from 144 countries.

Gupta, N., Goel, K., Shah, P., & Misra, A. (2012). Childhood obesity in developing countries: Epidemiology, determinants, and prevention. *Endocrine Reviews, 33*(1), 48–70.—A different perspective on the problem via a comprehensive overview of prevalence, causes, and management of obesity within developing countries.

Lobstein, T., Baur, L., & Uauy, R. (2004). Obesity in children and young people: A crisis in public health. *Obesity Reviews, 5*(Suppl. 1), 4–85.—A major advocacy report from the IOTF detailing the size of the childhood obesity problem and its likely growth together with a call for action at all levels.

Lobstein, T., Jackson-Leach, R., Moodie, M. L., Hall, K. D., Gortmaker, S. L., Swinburn, B. A., et al. (2015). Child and adolescent obesity: Part of a bigger picture. *Lancet, 385,* 2510–2520.—An excellent summary of the latest understanding around the development, trends, and required action to address childhood obesity.

Ng, M., Fleming, T., Robinson, M., Thomson, B., Graetz, N., Margono, C., et al. (2014). Global, regional, and national prevalence of overweight and obesity in children and adults during 1980–2013: A systematic analysis for the Global Burden of Disease Study 2013. *Lancet, 384,* 766–781.—A rich collection of data brought together for the Global Burden of Disease and reanalyzed to provide comparable information on the trends in child and adolescent obesity in 188 countries.

Oddy, W. H. (2012). Infant feeding and obesity risk in the child. *Breastfeeding Review, 20*(2), 7–12.—A good overview of the range of factors and potential mechanisms for influencing child weight status and later obesity.

Paes, V. M., Ong, K. K., & Lakshman, R. (2015). Factors influencing obesogenic dietary intake in young children (0–6 years): Systematic review of qualitative evidence. *BMJ Open, 5*(9), e007396.—An overview of the behavioral and environmental factors that influence the dietary behaviors most associated with obesity in young children.

Rokholm, B., Baker, J. L., & Sørensen, T. I. A. (2010). The levelling off of the obesity epidemic since the year 1999—a review of evidence and perspectives. *Obesity Reviews, 11*(12), 835–846.—One of the first assessments to analyse the plateauing of data in child obesity prevalence in developed countries and to assess the likely causation and implications.

Economic Causes and Consequences of Obesity

JOHN CAWLEY

This chapter explains what is known about the economic causes of obesity (e.g., food prices, income, education, macroeconomic conditions, and peers) and economic consequences of obesity (e.g., higher medical care costs and worse labor market outcomes). In many cases, it would be infeasible or unethical to use randomized controlled trials to investigate the causes and consequences of obesity; as a result, many studies have exploited natural experiments to identify causal effects.

Collectively, the research suggests that there is no single dominant economic cause of obesity; many factors may contribute a modest amount to the risk of obesity, and these factors may be different for different subgroups. There are much stronger and more consistent results regarding the economic consequences of obesity; morbid obesity significantly raises medical care costs, and additional weight (even below the threshold of obesity) lowers wages for women.

Economic Causes of Obesity

Food Prices

Since 1980, when the prevalence of obesity began rising in the United States, the real (i.e., inflation-adjusted) price of energy-dense foods has decreased, while the real price of fresh fruits and vegetables has increased. Several studies have exploited natural experiments in order to test whether this correlation between food prices and obesity is causal. One study examined the effect of variation in minimum wage laws, which in turn creates variation in fast-food prices, and found that fast-food prices have no detectable effect on obesity. Another study exploited the natural experiment of Wal-Mart expansion and found evidence that the entry of a Wal-Mart into an area is associated with a higher prevalence of obesity; that study interprets this as evidence that a new Wal-Mart (which is the largest grocery chain in the United States) drives down the prices of groceries, leading nearby residents to consume more calories.

Income

Among women, there is a strong negative correlation between income and weight (i.e., higher-income women are less likely to be obese). There is not a consistent correlation between income and obesity in men. In order to test whether these correlations are causal, one study utilized the natural experiment of variation in payments in the Earned Income Tax Credit program and estimated that additional income leads to small increases in weight for the low-income women in the program, but no change in weight for the low-income men in the program. Another study examined payments in the Social Security program that were due to legislative accident (i.e., the Social Security Benefits "notch") and found no detectable effect of income on weight for either women or men. Consistent with this, studies have estimated that the impact of income on food expenditures in developed countries is very small.

Education

In general, college-educated individuals are less likely to be obese; this correlation is stronger for women than for men. A series of articles has exploited changes in compulsory schooling laws as natural experiments in order to estimate the causal effect of education on weight. One of the strongest such studies, based on data from the United Kingdom, found no evidence that additional education affects the probability of overweight or obesity. A series of studies that used data from several European countries found inconsistent results. There is some evidence from the United States that early childhood interventions and the preschool program Head Start decrease the probability of obesity in the years after the intervention, but these effects disappear at older ages.

Macroeconomic Conditions

Studies have also investigated whether weight and obesity are sensitive to the macroeconomy. A high unemployment rate could affect diet and physical activity through the mechanisms of employment, income, or stress. The results of these studies are inconsistent; some find that a high unemployment rate is associated with a lower probability of obesity, while others find that it is associated with a higher probability of obesity. These widely varying results may be due to studies using different methods and data, and examining different time periods and subgroups.

Peer and Neighborhood Effects

People's decisions and behavior regarding diet, physical activity, and weight may be influenced by peers. One study tested for peer effects using randomized roommate assignment among college freshmen and found that girls who are randomized to have a heavier roommate tend to gain more weight during their freshman year; there was no such peer effect on weight among boys. However, there is evidence of peer effects in boys' physical activity. A study at the U.S. Air Force Academy took advantage of the random assignment of cadets to squadrons and found that cadets score higher on physical fitness tests after they have been assigned to a squadron with a higher starting physical fitness score. Studies have also found evidence of neighborhood effects on weight. A randomized experiment that gave low-income families rent vouchers if they moved to higher-income neighborhoods found that the offer led to a lower probability of obesity 5 years later, and a lower probability of morbid obesity 12 years later. It is unclear what aspects of the neighborhoods are responsible for these effects; it could be beneficial peer effects from the new neighbors, closer proximity to full-service grocery stores, more walkable neighborhoods, and/or spending more time outdoors in response to the greater safety.

In summary, there is no single dominant economic cause of obesity. There is convincing evidence of peer and neighborhood effects on weight, and there is evidence of small effects of food prices on weight and, for low-income individuals, small effects of income on weight. Estimates of the effect of macroeconomic conditions and education on weight are inconsistent.

Economic Consequences of Obesity

In contrast, the economic consequences of obesity are quite clear: higher medical care costs among the morbidly obese and lower wages among women.

Wages and Earnings

A large literature has estimated the effect of excess weight on wages or earnings. In order to estimate the causal effect, studies have exploited as a natural experiment the heritable component of weight. Studies of U.S. data tend to find that additional weight lowers the wages of women but has no detectable impact on the wages of men. Studies analyzing data from European countries tend to find that weight lowers wages for both women and men. Within the United States, there appear to be differences by race and ethnicity; for example, the obesity wage penalty is greater for white females than for African-American or Hispanic females.

To some extent, the lower wages may be due to obesity-related illness lowering productivity and increasing job absenteeism. Obese and morbidly obese individuals do tend to miss work for health-related reasons more often than do lighter individuals. However, women's wages begin declining with weight at levels far below the threshold for obesity. This suggests that the lower wages are not entirely due to worse health or impaired productivity, but are also due in part to discrimination on the basis of appearance.

Employment

In general, heavier individuals are less likely to be employed. However, a study that exploited the heritability of weight as a natural experiment was unable to reject the null hypothesis of no effect of obesity on employment in Great Britain.

An audit study paired equivalent resumes with photos that were manipulated by photo editing software to alter the perceived weight of the job applicant, and submitted them to actual job openings in Sweden (where photos commonly accompany job applications). The study found that applicants with a heavier appearance were significantly less likely to be contacted for an initial job interview than the applicants who appeared lighter but had equivalent qualifications. For more on the evidence of discrimination against obese individuals in various settings, see Chapter 21.

Higher Medical Care Costs

Because obesity raises the risk of heart attack, stroke, cancer, and type 2 diabetes, it should not be surprising that it is also associated with higher medical care costs.

To estimate the causal effect of weight on medical care costs, researchers have exploited the natural experiment of the heritability of weight. The results suggest that the causal effects are even larger than the correlation. These studies estimated that in 2010, obesity raised medical care costs by $3,508 per obese individual. However, this is somewhat misleading because medical care costs were relatively constant with body mass index (BMI) around the threshold for obesity (BMI of 30); it was only in the morbidly obese range that medical care costs rose dramatically. In other words, it is only morbid obesity, not obesity generally, that raises medical care costs. These studies estimated that in 2010, the direct medical care costs of adult obesity in the United States totaled $315.8 billion, which equals 27.5% of health expenditures for noninstitutionalized U.S. adults.

Implications for Public Policy

The bulk of spending on obesity-related illness can be classified as external costs (i.e., costs of obesity that are paid by people other than the obese individuals). This is because 88.2% of the medical care costs of obesity are paid for by either health insurance companies (primarily funded by group insurance premiums that are not based on weight), Medicare (funded by payroll taxes), or Medicaid (funded by general government revenues). These negative externalities impose deadweight loss (inefficiency) on society in three ways: (1) the higher cost of private health insurance results in lower take-up of health insurance and therefore higher rates of uninsurance; (2) the higher costs in public health insurance programs (e.g., Medicare and Medicaid) are passed on to taxpayers in the form of higher taxes, which leads to decreased labor supply; and (3) because individuals do not pay anywhere near the full medical care costs of obesity or an unhealthy diet, there may be moral hazard—underinvestment in healthy diet, active lifestyle, and prevention of weight gain. The evidence is relatively strong that there is deadweight loss to society from the first two sources; there is less evidence of deadweight loss from the third source (moral hazard).

The substantial external medical care costs of obesity, and the deadweight loss that they impose, represent an important economic rationale for government intervention. Public policies can address this market failure by "internalizing" the external costs. This could be done several ways; the most commonly advocated way is to tax energy-dense foods. Increasingly, employers are seeking to reduce the externalities of obesity that operate through job absenteeism and health insurance by implementing workplace wellness programs that incentivize physical activity and healthy weight.

In summary, there is strong and consistent evidence on the economic consequences of obesity. Weight lowers wages, and this negative correlation begins at weights far below the threshold for obesity, so it is likely due in part to both discrimination and (at high levels of weight) worse health and/or lower productivity. Other evidence of discrimination is that an obese appearance lowers the probability of an initial job interview. Morbid obesity significantly raises medical care costs, and the resulting external costs that operate through health insurance represent an economic rationale for government intervention.

These consequences can be addressed through policies to internalize external costs and legal protections against discrimination.

Acknowledgments

Preparation of this chapter was supported by an Investigator Award in Health Policy Research from the Robert Wood Johnson Foundation.

Suggested Reading

Cawley, J. (2004). The impact of obesity on wages. *Journal of Human Resources, 39*(2), 451–474.—The author estimates the causal effect of weight and obesity on wages, and documents important differences by gender and race/ethnicity.

Cawley, J. (2010). The economics of childhood obesity. *Health Affairs, 29*(3), 364–371.—An accessible overview to the economics of childhood obesity.

Cawley, J. (2011). The economics of obesity. In J. Cawley (Ed.), *The Oxford handbook of the social science of obesity* (pp. 120–137). New York: Oxford University Press.—An accessible overview that explains the "economic way of thinking" (i.e., the intuition behind economic models) about obesity.

Cawley, J. (2014). The Affordable Care Act permits greater financial rewards for weight loss: A good idea in principle, but many practical concerns remain. *Journal of Policy Analysis and Management, 33*(3), 810–820.—Part of a point–counterpoint on the usefulness and appropriateness of health insurance companies and employers offering financial rewards for weight loss.

Cawley, J. (2015). An economy of scales: A selective review of obesity's economic causes, consequences, and solutions. *Journal of Health Economics, 43,* 244–268.—An exhaustive overview of the research on the economic causes and consequences of obesity, as well as economic approaches to treatment and prevention.

Cawley, J., & Meyerhoefer, C. (2012). The medical care costs of obesity: An instrumental variables approach. *Journal of Health Economics, 31*(1), 219–230.—The authors estimate the causal effect of obesity on medical care costs.

Cawley, J., Meyerhoefer, C., Biener, A., Hammer, M., & Wintfeld, N. (2015). Savings in medical expenditures associated with reductions in body mass index among US adults with obesity, by diabetes status. *Pharmacoeconomics, 33*(7), 707–722.—This article estimates the causal effect of obesity on medical care costs with a larger and more recent sample than the 2012 study listed above, and explores the nonlinearities in the cost curve, documenting that costs rise exponentially among those with extreme obesity.

Cawley, J., & Ruhm, C. J. (2012). The economics of risky health behaviors. In T. G. McGuire, M. V. Pauly, & P. P. Barros (Eds.), *Handbook of health economics* (Vol. 2, pp. 95–199), New York: Elsevier.—An exhaustive review of the economic research on risky health behaviors, such as alcohol abuse, smoking, illicit drug use, and the actions that contribute to obesity. Useful for seeing the similarities in the causes and consequences of risky health behaviors, as well as possible policies to reduce them.

66

Dietary Drivers of Obesity

ADELA HRUBY
FRANK B. HU

Prolonged periods of energy intake in excess of energy requirements are the primary drivers of weight gain leading to obesity. Energy needs have many determinants (growth and aging, body mass, genetics, physical activity, hormones, diseases, microbiota, etc.), which are discussed in the chapters throughout Part I of this volume. However, there are dietary qualities beyond energy needs and quantity of intake that play an important role in healthy weight maintenance, weight gain and loss, and weight loss maintenance. This chapter focuses on the dietary drivers of weight gain and obesity; the role of diet in weight loss and weight loss maintenance is discussed in chapters in this volume on the treatment of obesity.

Dietary Patterns

Evidence from clinical trials has almost universally shown that caloric restriction, regardless of dietary pattern (e.g., low-fat, low-carbohydrate, or Mediterranean diets, or those based on dietary guidelines emanating from various government and nongovernment entities), is associated with better weight outcomes. Although the metabolic nuances and relative merits of differing dietary patterns for various health conditions (comorbid with obesity) are still being investigated, the evidence seems to suggest that merely *adhering* to a diet—nearly irrespective of what type of healthy diet it is—has an impact on weight loss/control in the short term. However, beyond overall caloric intake to regulate body weight, a tremendous amount of research has attempted to resolve the roles of diet quality and dietary patterns in the primary prevention of obesity.

Evidence from long-term cohort studies indicates that diets that are considered "healthier" lead to better long-term weight maintenance, or at least mitigate weight gain typically associated with aging through middle age. Such "healthier" diet patterns include those that are rich in vegetables and fruits, whole grains, and fish, as compared to unhealthy diet patterns generally consisting of high amounts of red and processed meats, sweets and added sugars, and other refined and processed foods. Long-term research in U.S. health professionals indicates that average 4-year weight gain throughout middle age is strongly associated with increasing intake of potato chips and potatoes, sugar-sweetened beverages, and processed and unprocessed red meats, but inversely associated with increasing intake of vegetables, fruits, whole grains, nuts, and yogurt. Relatedly, a population-based study of adult men and women in Europe observed similar patterns with respect to increases in waist circumference over a 5-year period. Waist circumference is a proxy measure of abdominal adiposity, characterized by higher amounts of visceral fat, which is considered an important predictor of cardiometabolic disease. Smaller increases in waist circumference were evident in those who ate relatively higher amounts of vegetables, fruits, high-fat dairy products, and red meat, while higher intakes of potatoes, processed meats, poultry, and snack foods were positively associated with larger waist increases over time.

Additional research has found that diet patterns can and do change in the majority of adults, and not always for the better. Long-term trajectories from healthier toward unhealthy patterns—for example, moving from high intake of vegetables, fish, and legumes to high intake of meat and soda—are associated with increases in body mass index (BMI) and were found to raise risk of overweight and obesity twofold or more. However, given that changes in patterns are relatively frequent over the long term in adult populations, there are opportunities to change future patterns for the better, even if those changes are relatively small.

Adherence to specific traditional dietary patterns has also been associated with less weight gain and lower waist circumference over time. The Mediterranean diet is one example of such a pattern. Rich in vegetables, fish, nuts, and olive oil, and low in red meat and added sugar, it has been associated with lower odds of excessive weight gain in adulthood and smaller increases in waist circumference. While the Mediterranean diet has regional variations, studies of adults in Spain and France, for example, show that adhering to this traditional but regionally varying pattern is consistently associated with better weight outcomes.

In addition, adhering to guidelines from recognized medical organizations, such as the American Heart Association (AHA), has also been related to better weight outcomes. The AHA's 2020 ideal healthy weight dietary recommendations include five components identified as particularly important to cardiometabolic health: several daily servings of fruits, vegetables, and whole grains, at least two servings of fish per week, keeping sodium under 2,300 mg per day, and drinking fewer than 36 ounces per week of sugar-sweetened beverages. Young adults who scored low on the AHA's Healthy Diet Score had higher year-over-year increases in BMI, such that by the fourth year of follow-up in their mid- to late 20s, they were at least 0.5 kg/m^2 larger than their counterparts who had a higher diet score. Thus, higher adherence to a diet rich in vegetables, fruits, whole grains, and fish, and low in sugar-sweetened beverages, led to lower risk of experiencing the weight gain frequently observed to occur in early adulthood, potentially mitigating later adult weight gain, as well as premature incidence of related medical conditions.

Beverages

Evidence from trials and cohort studies lead us to conclude almost unequivocally that in both children and adults, sugar-sweetened beverages play an important role in weight;

their "empty" calories notably lead to weight gain and increasing abdominal obesity in adults when included in the diet, and healthy weight loss in children when removed from the diet. Behavioral studies on sugar-sweetened beverage consumption suggest that people tend to not be cognizant of "liquid" energy and therefore do not compensate by appropriately decreasing energy intake from foods, contributing to chronic energy consumption in excess of needs.

The role of "diet" or non-nutritive beverages—drinks sweetened with noncaloric or low-calorie sweeteners—in weight gain is unclear. In early observational studies, which were mostly cross-sectional, diet beverages tended to be associated with higher body mass. Prospective studies, however, have not yielded consistent results, suggesting that diet beverages do not play a major role in incident obesity but may be a viable substitute for sugar-sweetened beverages in weight loss attempts.

Although a long-recommended weight loss strategy, the role of water intake in weight loss has only recently been the subject of clinical research. Findings support the claim that higher water intake, for example, when consumed immediately prior to a meal, leads to greater weight loss in overweight/obese individuals. Long-term observational studies on the impact of water intake in weight gain through adulthood are few, although the limited evidence also points to higher water intake in place of sugar-sweetened beverages leading to less weight gain over time. Water may impact weight by affecting gastric distension, thus inducing feelings of fullness; it may be a replacement beverage for higher-calorie beverages; or it may act via novel physiological pathways currently under study.

Higher consumption of other beverages, such as tea and coffee, are also associated with slightly less weight gain in adulthood, as well as lower risk of cardiometabolic disease, and the findings are more consistent for coffee than for tea. Apart from containing few or no calories, other constituents of these beverages, such as caffeine and unique polyphenolic compounds, may have properties that contribute to maintaining energy balance.

Select Foods and Food Groups

Carbohydrate sources beyond added sugars are important as well. In terms of mitigating weight gain, whole grains (when replacing refined grains) and fiber (predominantly from grains, but other sources, such as nuts and pulses, are also important) are thought to add bulk to the diet, delay gastric emptying, and slow metabolic responses to ingestion, thus increasing fullness and satiety, potentially leading to better weight outcomes in the short and long term. Several studies have shown that individuals consuming higher amounts of fiber and/or whole grains experience less weight gain and smaller increases in waist circumference. Concomitantly, those with high or increasing intakes of refined grains, such as white bread, tend to gain more weight than those who consume low amounts or decrease their intake over time.

Consistent with the Mediterranean pattern described earlier, nut consumption (e.g., two or more servings per week of either tree nuts or peanuts) is associated with lower body mass, less weight gain over time, and lower risk of obesity in the long term. These observations run counter to previously long-held beliefs regarding the potentially weight-gain-inducing fat and energy content of nuts, and instead support nuts as an important source of protein, fiber, vitamins, minerals, and other phenolic compounds.

Another major food group that has been widely studied is dairy, although the evidence is equivocal. In short-term trials, dairy in the context of caloric restriction appears to facilitate body weight and body fat reduction better than caloric restriction without dairy. This may be due to the protein content of dairy, and in higher-fat formulas, to the satiating effects of both protein and fat. In contrast, longer-term observational studies on dairy and weight gain or obesity have generally shown no association with body weight across adulthood. Yogurt intake, a common food in healthier dietary patterns, is an exception: Higher intake frequently accompanies lower long-term weight gain.

Macronutrients

Protein is considered a weight-favorable macronutrient owing to its effects on increased thermogenesis and satiety. Higher relative levels of intake are frequently recommended in weight loss regimens, and weight loss trials have shown benefits of higher relative protein intake in the context of energy restriction. Over the long term, however, observational research has failed to support a clear relationship with total protein intake and weight gain and/or obesity prevention. As is true of all energy components, dietary sources and moderating intake relative to needs are warranted. For example, a pan-European study of adults showed that higher intake of total protein, as well as protein from animal sources (specifically, meat and poultry, rather than fish or dairy) was associated with weight gain in men and women over a 6-year period. However, there was no overall association between plant protein and weight change. Other studies have noted similar trends in which total protein intake does not appear to impact weight change over time, but animal protein associates directly and vegetable protein inversely with weight gain.

As noted earlier, whole grains and sugar-sweetened beverages, both important carbohydrate-based energy sources, have opposite effects on weight gain. Without distinctions between carbohydrate sources, carbohydrates as a broad class alone have a divergent relationship with weight. Other ways of classifying carbohydrate quality or the quality of diets high in carbohydrates, such as using the Glycemic Index, have shed little light on prospective excess weight gain in adults.

Although fat intake has intuitively been linked to obesity in the minds of many, the epidemiological evidence does not bear out a straightforward relationship. For weight loss, meta-analyses of weight loss trials with low-fat arms as compared to control/placebo diet arms have generally shown favorable shifts in weight in overweight/obese participants. However, low-fat interventions frequently have been accompanied by caloric restriction, have been short term, and have obviously not investigated normal-weight individuals. In addition, low-fat regimens have not necessarily been better than alternative diet approaches, such as Mediterranean or low-carbohydrate approaches to weight loss. Observational cohorts have yielded inconclusive results, but most studies show no long-term relationship between total fat intake and weight gain or loss. As with protein and carbohydrates, fatty acid types and sources may be more important than total quantity; higher intakes of polyunsaturated fatty acids and monounsaturated fatty acids, such as those found in olive oil, may be beneficial in terms of helping individuals limit weight gain and perhaps even contribute to moderate weight loss in adulthood. There is no strong evidence for an effect of saturated fat intake per se on incident obesity, although a

Western dietary pattern, which is typically high in saturated fat, has been associated with increased risk of weight gain and obesity.

Selected Eating Behaviors: Eating Out, Breakfasting, Snacking

Studies in the United States and Europe indicate that regularly eating meals prepared outside the home and frequently dining out in restaurants are associated with higher incremental weight and waist gain, greater risk of gaining substantial weight (e.g., 2 kg or more) per year, and higher risk of becoming overweight/obese (in those initially normal weight). In developing countries, merely increasing the availability of Western-style fast food at the community level is also associated with increasing adiposity. Research conducted on restaurants in the United States shows consistently high (1,000 kcal) or extremely high (>2,000 kcal) energy content of a single meal, energy that often exceeds an adult's energy requirements for an entire day.

Although the roles of eating breakfast and snacking have been the subject of debate in weight loss treatments and maintenance, the limited observational evidence presents an equivocal role for these behaviors in preventing incident obesity or long-term weight gain in the first place.

Summary

While the role of macronutrients in weight gain and incident obesity remains equivocal, both dietary patterns research and research on specific foods and beverages indicate that diets characterized by high intake of added sugars and refined grains, and low intake of whole grains and fiber, are associated with greater adult weight gain over time, increasing the likelihood of developing obesity-related conditions. Certain food groups, such as dairy, poultry, and fruits and vegetables, have less definitive relationships with adult weight gain but tend to be a part of healthier dietary patterns associated with favorable weight trajectories, suggesting that they may have a role in weight in the context of overall dietary behavior. There is little evidence to indicate that behavioral factors related to diet, such as snacking and having breakfast, have a role in preventing or promoting obesity, although the extreme calories associated with eating out appear to increase risk of obesity considerably in the long term.

Suggested Reading

Hu, F. B. (2013). Resolved: There is sufficient scientific evidence that decreasing sugar-sweetened beverage consumption will reduce the prevalence of obesity and obesity-related diseases. *Obesity Reviews, 14*(8), 606–619.—A review of scientific evidence supporting low or no sugar-sweetened beverage consumption as a vehicle for reducing and preventing obesity.

Lloyd-Jones, D. M., Hong, Y., Labarthe, D., Mozaffarian, D., Appel, L. J., Van Horn, L., et al. (2010). Defining and setting national goals for cardiovascular health promotion and disease reduction the American Heart Association's Strategic Impact Goal through 2020 and beyond. *Circulation, 121*(4), 586–613.—The authors identify seven health behaviors and metrics for the promotion of optimal cardiovascular health; among them is maintaining a healthy body mass.

Malik, V. S., Pan, A., Willett, W. C., & Hu, F. B. (2013). Sugar-sweetened beverages and weight gain in children and adults: A systematic review and meta-analysis. *American Journal of Clinical Nutrition, 98*(4), 1084–1102.—A comprehensive review and quantitative summary of the literature on sugar-sweetened beverages and weight gain.

Miller, P. E., & Perez, V. (2014). Low-calorie sweeteners and body weight and composition: A meta-analysis of randomized controlled trials and prospective cohort studies. *American Journal of Clinical Nutrition, 100*(3), 765–777.—A comprehensive review and quantitative summary of the literature on non-nutritive sweeteners on body weight.

Mozaffarian, D., Hao, T., Rimm, E. B., Willett, W. C., & Hu, F. B. (2011). Changes in diet and lifestyle and long-term weight gain in women and men. *New England Journal of Medicine, 364*(25), 2392–2404.—Authors investigated relationships between changes in diet and 4-year weight changes in 120,877 American men and women, observing an average 3.36-pound gain in each period through mid- to late life.

Pan, A., Malik, V. S., Hao, T., Willett, W. C., Mozaffarian, D., & Hu, F. B. (2013). Changes in water and beverage intake and long-term weight changes: Results from three prospective cohort studies. *International Journal of Obesity, 37*(10), 1378–1385.—A multicohort, long-term, prospective analysis of beverage intake, including water, and changes in weight across adulthood.

Summerbell, C. D., Douthwaite, W., Whittaker, V., Ells, L. J., Hillier, F., Smith, S., et al. (2009). The association between diet and physical activity and subsequent excess weight gain and obesity assessed at 5 years of age or older: A systematic review of the epidemiological evidence. *International Journal of Obesity, 33*(Suppl. 3), S1–S92.—A detailed review of the prospective literature on dietary factors and activity in relation to incident obesity and weight gain in children and adults.

Ye, E. Q., Chacko, S. A., Chou, E. L., Kugizaki, M., & Liu, S. (2012). Greater whole-grain intake is associated with lower risk of type 2 diabetes, cardiovascular disease, and weight gain. *Journal of Nutrition, 142*(7), 1304–1313.—A systematic examination of longitudinal studies and randomized trials investigating whole-grain and fiber intake in relation to weight gain estimates that consumers, compared to nonconsumers, experienced consistently less weight gain over up to 13 years of follow-up.

Physical Activity and Prevention of Obesity

RUSSELL R. PATE
JENNIFER I. FLYNN

Obesity is a condition that results from a gradual and excessive increase in fat mass, with the transition from normal weight to obese typically occurring over several years. On average, adult Americans gain approximately 1 kg/year of weight, and many gain 2–3 kg/year; the result is the current high prevalence of obesity. Treatment of established obesity is very difficult, and few obese adults succeed in losing a substantial amount of weight and maintaining that weight loss in the long term. For that reason, while treatment of obesity remains an important medical concern, the challenge for public health is to help people avoid becoming obese.

Physical activity is an important contributor to overall energy expenditure, and it exerts a powerful influence on regulation of body weight and composition. Accordingly, scientists, professionals, and the public have long viewed physical activity as playing a role in both prevention and treatment of obesity. However, because these groups typically have focused on treatment of obesity (i.e., weight loss in those who are already overweight), the potential role that physical activity can play in reversing the obesity epidemic is not well understood. While scientists know that a modest increase in physical activity, as a singular behavior change, will not produce a large weight loss in people who are obese, the same modest increase is likely to help those who are normal weight maintain their weight and avoid excessive weight gain.

This chapter addresses the contribution of physical activity to *prevention* of obesity. We summarize research studies that examine the role of physical activity in adiposity and weight status in persons who were initially at normal weight. Our purposes in this chapter are (1) to note the growing body of evidence pointing to the powerful influence of physical activity on development of adiposity during childhood and adulthood, and (2) to propose that clinicians and public health practitioners promote physical activity as a primary strategy for preventing excessive weight gain in individuals and populations.

Background

The scientific literature suggests at least three reasons that higher levels of habitual physical activity should be associated with reduced risk for developing obesity.

Closing the Energy Gap

Excessive weight gain occurs when energy intake chronically exceeds energy expenditure. In theory, an existing "energy gap" could be closed by reducing energy intake, increasing energy expenditure, or a combination of the two. In most people who are in a state of positive energy balance, the daily gap is small, typically less than 20 calories/day when averaged over weeks and months. Clearly, since 20 calories corresponds to about one-fourth mile of walking, it is entirely feasible for a modest increase in physical activity to close that gap.

Bucking the Secular Trend

The prevalence of obesity in the United States and other developed countries has increased dramatically since the 1970s. While we cannot be certain of the causes of this trend, it is clear that marked societal changes in physical activity behavior have occurred during that same period. These include reductions in physical activity energy expenditure in the occupational setting, resulting from dramatic decreases in physically demanding work, and substantial decreases in physical activity in and around the home setting, the result of decreased energy expenditure required to complete household chores. In addition, participation in sedentary activities, such as watching television and playing video games, has increased significantly. Reversing these trends will require that people build physical activity into their lifestyles through work or leisure activity.

Engaging the Body's Regulatory System

The body uses a complex and elegant system for regulating body weight and composition. That system evolved to support physically active people who were living the so-called "hunter–gatherer" lifestyle. Through most of human history, that system effectively maintained normal weight status in most people. However, as habitual physical activity decreases, the efficiency of the system that regulates weight and body composition decreases, and the risk of obesity increases. Maintaining a physically active lifestyle puts the body's powerful weight regulation system to work in ways that promote healthy weight and body composition.

Exemplary Research Studies

A number of studies have examined the relationship between physical activity and change in weight over time. The following section summarizes important observational and experimental studies, and includes studies conducted in both adults and children.

Observational Studies in Adults

The National Health and Nutrition Examination Survey Epidemiological Follow-Up Study examined the relationship between physical activity and changes in body weight in 9,325 men and women ages 25–74 years. Body weight was measured and physical activity was reported by participants at baseline and after 10 years of follow-up. The study found that men who reported low physical activity levels gained approximately 1.6 kg more across the 10 years than men who reported high physical activity. Women who reported low physical activity levels gained approximately 1.9 kg more than women who reported high activity levels. Men who decreased their physical activity across the 10 years were three times more likely to gain 8 kg or more compared to men who maintained a high level of physical activity. Women who decreased their physical activity were nearly six times more likely to gain at least 13 kg compared to women who maintained a high level of physical activity.

The Women's Health Study examined how changes in physical activity were related to changes in weight gain across 13 years of follow-up in 34,079 women who were 45 years of age or older at baseline. Participants reported their height, weight, and weekly time spent performing selected physical activities. Women who reported the lowest levels of physical activity were 11% more likely to gain at least 2.3 kg at follow-up, compared to women who reported the highest levels of physical activity. Additionally, women with a normal body mass index (BMI) who were physically active for at least 60 minutes per day were the least likely to gain 2.3 kg. No relationships between physical activity and weight gain for overweight or obese women were observed.

Experimental Trials in Adults

The Exercise Intervention to Prevent Excessive Gestational Weight Gain study, a randomized controlled trial to determine the effect of physical activity on excessive weight gain during pregnancy, was delivered 3 days per week for 50–55 minutes in a supervised setting. Each session included a warm up and a cool down, and 25–30 minutes of either resistance training or moderate intensity aerobic activity. The control group was asked to continue standard care with a physician or midwife. Gestational weight gain was categorized using the 2009 Institute of Medicine (IOM) weight gain recommendations for pregnancy. This intervention resulted in favorable outcomes related to weight gain and the prevention of excessive weight gain. The women in the intervention group gained less weight than the women in the control group. Additionally, women exposed to the intervention had a nearly 40% reduction in risk of gaining weight above the IOM recommendations. When the effect of the intervention was examined by BMI, women in the intervention who were categorized as normal weight were 50% less likely to gain weight above the IOM guidelines during their pregnancy compared to the control group. However, women who were overweight or obese had a similar risk of gaining weight in both groups.

The Health, Risk Factors, Exercise Training, and Genetics (HERITAGE) study examined a standardized exercise program conducted in 828 sedentary men and women ages 17–65 years. The exercise sessions were delivered 3 days per week in a supervised setting. Participants' exercise duration and intensity were gradually increased from 30 to 50 minutes and 55 to 75% of baseline fitness level, respectively. Aside from the sessions, participants were asked to maintain their usual lifestyle habits. At the beginning and end of the program, body weight, percent fat, and total fat mass were measured. Following the 20-week program, men significantly decreased their body weight by approximately 0.5 kg. Women maintained their body weight throughout the program. Men and women had similar decreases in percent body fat (0.7–0.9 %) and total fat mass (0.6–1.0 kg).

Observational Studies in Children

The Iowa Bone Development Study followed a cohort of more than 300 children ages 5–11 years to examine how physical activity influences adiposity in children. Fat mass was measured using dual-energy X-ray absorptiometry, and physical activity was measured using an accelerometer worn for 7 consecutive days over several years. The study examined how physical activity influenced changes in body fat mass over 3 years. The results indicated that children who had the highest levels of physical activity at age 5 years had the lowest body fat mass at age 8 years. Additionally, children with the highest levels of physical activity were less likely to gain fat mass across the 3-year span. In a follow-up study, the investigators assessed how physical activity influenced changes in body fat mass across 6 years. Similar to the previous findings, children who were the most active at age 5 had significantly lower body fat at age 8 and age 11 compared to the least active children.

The Avon Longitudinal Study of Parents and Children examined how physical activity influenced changes in fat mass in a cohort of 4,150 children (ages 12–14 years). Fat mass was measured using dual-energy X-ray absorptiometry, and physical activity was measured for 7 consecutive days via accelerometry. The results of the 2-year observation showed that girls and boys who accumulated the highest levels of moderate to vigorous physical activity (MVPA) at age 12 years had a 10–12% lower fat mass at age 14 years compared to children who participated in less MVPA. Additionally, the study provided important information about how physical activity can influence the trajectory of fat mass gains. Children whose MVPA increased 15 minutes/day from ages 12–14 years had an approximately 2.4% lower fat mass compared to children whose MVPA did not increase.

Experimental Trials in Children

The Intervention Centered on Adolescents' Physical Activity and Sedentary Behavior study, a randomized controlled trial, tested a physical activity intervention among 12- to 16-year-old children in schools in France. Schools were randomized into intervention and control groups. During the 4-year trial, students in the intervention group were exposed to new physical activity opportunities during lunchtime, class breaks, and after school. In addition, the intervention schools organized afterschool sporting events and active commuting days. Intervention schools also provided students with education about physical activity and sedentary behaviors, and engaged educators and parents in efforts to promote the new physical activity opportunities. Schools in the control group were asked to adhere to their regular school curriculum. BMI and fat mass, measured using bioelectrical impedance analysis, were measured annually. At 4-year follow-up, normal-weight students in the intervention group had 0.33 kg/m^2 lower increases in BMI and 0.20 kg/m^2 lower increases in fat mass index compared to students in the control group. Additionally, the incidence of becoming overweight was reduced in the intervention schools. Over the course of the intervention, only 4.2% of normal-weight children became overweight in the intervention schools compared to 9.8% in the control schools.

The Superkids/Superfit Exercise Program was evaluated in a randomized controlled trial conducted to determine the effects of a 30-week physical activity intervention to prevent obesity in kindergarten children (ages 4–5 years). Children in the intervention school participated in a 15-minute walk before class and a 20-minute dance session in the afternoon, 3 days/week. The control school adhered to its normal class schedule. At the beginning and end of the intervention, BMI, triceps skinfold thickness, and waist circumference were measured. Following the Superkids/Superfit Exercise Program, girls were 68% less likely to have increases in BMI compared to the control school. However, there was no intervention effect on BMI in boys and no changes in triceps skinfold thickness or waist circumference following the physical activity program.

Implications for Public Health and Medical Practice

There will be no quick, easy solution to the obesity epidemic that currently afflicts the developed societies of the world. But the best opportunity for reducing the prevalence of obesity lies in actions aimed at primary prevention of excessive weight gain. This chapter provides a rationale for emphasizing promotion of physical activity as a central strategy for prevention of overweight and obesity. Efforts to promote higher levels of physical activity in the day-to-day lives of Americans and residents of other developed nations will require actions in multiple societal sectors, including education, transportation, community planning, business/industry, recreation/parks, public health, and health care. If the health care sector is to make a meaningful contribution, greater attention will need to be given to early detection of excessive weight gain and referral of patients to community-based programs that are able to deliver effective interventions for modification of physical activity behavior. The public health sector should lead the effort to promote higher levels of physical activity at the population level, but its ability to do so will require establishing this goal as a much higher priority than has been the case so far.

Suggested Reading

Janssen, I., Katzmarzyk, P. T., Ross, R., Leon, A. S., Skinner, J. S., Rao, D. C., et al. (2004). Fitness alters the associations of BMI and waist circumference with total and abdominal fat. *Obesity Research, 12*(3), 525–537.—The results of the 20-week intervention showed that men significantly decreased their body weight by 0.5 kg and women maintained their body weight.

Janz, K. F., Kwon, S., Letuchy, E. M., Gilmore, J. M. E., Burns, T. L., Torner, J. C., et al. (2009). Sustained effect of early physical activity on body fat mass in older children. *American Journal of Preventive Medicine, 37*(1), 35–40.—The most active children at age 5 years had lower body fat at ages 8 and 11 years compared to the least active children.

Lee, I., Djoussé, L., Sesso, H. D., Wang, L., & Buring, J. E. (2010). Physical activity and weight gain prevention. *Journal of the American Medical Association, 303*(12), 1173–1179.—Women who maintained a normal-weight BMI reported a mean of 21.5 MET-hour/week (metabolic equivalent) of physical activity.

Lewis, C. E., Jacobs, D. R., McCreath, H., Kiefe, C. I., Schreiner, P. J., Smith, D. E., et al. (2000). Weight gain continues in the 1990s: 10-year trends in weight and overweight from the CARDIA study. *American Journal of Epidemiology, 151*, 1172–1181.—Weight gain of greater than 20 kg was more common in men and women of both race groups who were overweight.

Mo-suwan, L., Pongprapai, S., Junjana, C., & Puetpaiboon, A. (1998). Effects of a controlled trial of a school-based exercise program on the obesity indexes of preschool children. *American*

Journal of Clinical Nutrition, 68, 1006–1011.—This randomized controlled trial showed that an obesity prevention program implemented over 1 year resulted in 68% fewer girls in the overweight category.

Riddoch, C. J., Leary, S. D., Ness, A. R., Blair, S. N., Deere, K., Mattocks, C., et al. (2009). Prospective associations between objective measures of physical activity and fat mass in 12–14 year old children: The Avon Longitudinal Study of Parents and Children (ALSPAC). *British Medical Journal, 339,* b4544.—An extra 15 minutes per day of MVPA at age 12 years was associated with lower fat mass at age 14 years for boys and girls.

Ruiz, J. R., Perales, M., Pelaez, M., Lopez, C., Lucia, A., & Barakat, R. (2013). Supervised exercise-based intervention to prevent excessive gestational weight gain: A randomized controlled trial. *Mayo Clinic Proceedings, 88*(12), 1388–1397.—This randomized controlled trial showed that the intervention successfully reduced the risk of gaining weight above the IOM recommendations by 40%.

Simon, C., Schweitzer, B., Oujaa, M., Wagner, A., Arveiler, D., Triby, E., et al. (2008). Successful overweight prevention in adolescents by increasing physical activity: A 4-year randomized controlled intervention. *International Journal of Obesity, 32*(10), 1489–1498.—This randomized controlled trial showed that a 4-year intervention to prevent obesity resulted in lower incidence of overweight in the intervention school (4.2%) compared to the control school (9.8%).

Williamson, D. F., Madans, J., Anda, R. F., Kleinman, J. C., Kahn, H. S., & Byers, T. (1993). Recreational physical activity and ten-year weight change in a US national cohort. *International Journal of Obesity, 17,* 279–286.—Men and women who reported low physical activity gain nearly 1.6 kg and 1.9 kg, respectively, than men and women who reported high activity.

The Gut Microbiome and Obesity

PHILIP CHUANG
ILSEUNG CHO

The *human gut microbiome* refers to the community of 10^{14} bacteria, 100 times the number of cells in the body, residing on or within the human body. The symbiotic relationship that we have with our gut microbiome is irrefutable, and its role in the digestion of complex carbohydrates and the development of the immune system has long been clear. However, many of the bacteria that exist within the human gastrointestinal tract cannot be grown in standard culture media. These were termed the "unculturable microbial majority" by Rappe and encompass environments beyond that of just the gut microbiome. Despite this drawback, within the last decade, scientists have been able to study the microbiome by using high-throughput sequencing. By collecting a stool sample and sequencing the short ribosomal sequences that may be used to identify bacteria, scientists have become able to characterize an individual's microbiome. Using these techniques, researchers are now linking the gut microbiome to immune defense, inflammatory conditions, liver diseases, diabetes, and obesity.

Although there has always been circumstantial evidence linking the microbiome to metabolism, it was the advent of germ-free mice that began to demonstrate plausible physiological mechanisms of action. Early studies demonstrated that germ-free mice were statistically leaner than their conventional age-matched counterparts. Even when subjected to high-fat and high-sugar diets, these mice resisted gaining significant amounts of weight. Furthermore, transplanting the microbiome of *ob/ob* mice that were genetically obese due to leptin deficiency to germ-free mice resulted in mice that had statistically more adipose tissue and weight compared to the germ-free mice that received microbiota transplantation from wild-type mice. When the microbiome of both the donors and the recipients was sequenced, the microbiomes of both the donors and their respective recipients were taxonomically similar. Additionally, it was also found that the obese microbiome had not only a lower diversity of microbes, but also a lower *Bacteroidetes* to *Firmicutes* ratio. The Blaser lab subsequently replicated this change in microbial diversity in mice with the administration of low-dose antibiotics and further demonstrated an increased propensity toward obesity, likely through modulation of the gut microbiota. These groundbreaking studies demonstrated that obesity traits were a transmissible and externally susceptible characteristic of the gut microbiota and not only suggested some mechanistic possibilities, but also invited further studies.

There have been many hypotheses on the mechanisms by which the gut microbiome affects metabolism. These can be summarized into three theories. The first, and perhaps most widely accepted, is the "energy harvest" hypothesis. It is known that the body is unable to extract certain indigestible residues through inherent digestive processes. These indigestible residues include resistant starches and dietary fibers that require gut bacteria to be broken into short-chain fatty acids (SCFAs) that can be absorbed by the colonic mucosa. It is thought that this additional source of energy is equivalent to 10% of our daily caloric intake, and in a study comparing the amounts of fecal SCFAs between obese individuals and lean individuals, it was found that obese individuals had a 20% increase in energy extraction compared to their lean counterparts. This theory is further supported in a landmark study by Suez and colleagues (2014), showing that artificial sweeteners induce glucose intolerance in mice and humans through modulation of the gut microbiome partly through a mechanism involving increased SCFA production. In mice fed artificial sweeteners they found elevated SCFA levels in stool, and metaganomic analysis demonstrated increased starch, sucrose, fructulose, and mannose metabolism, as well as glycolipid and fatty acid production in the microbiome. In this same study they were able to end the deleterious effects of artificial sweeteners by administering antibiotics. Despite this increased energy extraction however, it is unclear whether the additional energy extracted from dietary fibers is enough to offset the innately low-energy density of dietary fibers. This suggested that SCFAs are not the only component of the "energy harvest" hypothesis.

Beyond being the primary energy source of colonic cells, many scientists hypothesize that SCFAs play a role in regulating metabolism. Those SCFAs that are not metabolized by colonocytes are absorbed into the portal venous circulation and subsequently filtered into the systemic circulation. There they exert downstream signaling effects on various cell types, including hepatocytes, muscle cells, and both brown and white adipose tissues. In both liver cells and muscle tissues they act via the adenosine monophosphate (AMP)-activated protein kinase (AMPK), which in turn activates peroxisome proliferator-activated receptor gamma coactivator (PGC)-1 alpha expression that controls transcriptional activity of several peroxisome proliferator-activated receptors (PPARs). These receptors are important regulators of cholesterol, lipid, and glucose metabolism. Ultimately, this leads to increased fatty acid oxidation in both liver and muscle, in addition to decreased fatty acid synthesis in the liver. Additionally, SCFA binding to free-fatty acid G-protein coupled receptors (Ffar) on colonocytes themselves stimulate upregulation of peptide YY (PYY). Based on both mouse models and human studies, this molecule has been shown to induce satiety by 33% when administered postprandially. It is thought that PYY acts through the arcuate nucleus of the brain in a gut–hypothalamic pathway.

The effects of SCFAs in adipocytes are also diverse. SCFAs increase not only expression of PGC-1 in brown adipocytes but also expression of uncoupling protein (UCP-1), leading to an added effect of thermogenesis. In white adipocytes, SCFAs influence fatty acid regulation via multiple pathways through the free fatty acid G-protein coupled receptor (Ffar2 or GPR43). The binding of SCFAs to Ffar2 has been shown to increase leptin and potentially decrease insulin signaling. Leptin is an adipokine that regulates energy expenditure and food intake, leading to increased satiety and increased fatty acid oxidation in both the liver and muscle. Although similar to PYY, its efficacy is limited in obese individuals; studies have shown that they tend to be resistant to its actions. Decreased insulin signaling inhibits fat storage and up-regulates the metabolism of lipids and glucose in the body. Finally, Ffar2 binding also leads to a multistep pathway that ultimately is thought to deactivate hormone-sensitive lipase (HSL) in adipose tissue, thereby leading to a decrease in lipolysis of fat tissues and decreasing overall free fatty acids in circulation.

The interplay between the gut microbiome, inflammation, and obesity has also been theorized as a potential mechanism. It is widely accepted that obesity is a proinflammatory state, associated with elevations in systemic inflammatory markers such as C-reactive protein and erythrocyte sedimentation rate. Despite this observation, studies have yet to demonstrate definitive evidence that would support the inflammation–microbiome–obesity connection. One proposed mechanism implicates metabolic endotoxemia. Cani and colleagues (2007) reported that increasing the circulation of lipopolysaccharides (LPSs) to two or three times the amounts in a normal mouse diet via subcutaneous infusion could induce a significant weight gain that was similar to that in mice fed a high-fat diet. This held true even though the LPS-infused experimental mice consumed fewer calories than the high-fat-diet experimental mice.

The amount of proinflammatory LPS that is translocated into systemic circulation is thought to be partly dependent on passive diffusion and intestinal permeability. *In vitro* studies have demonstrated that exposure of intestinal epithelial cells to bacteria, such as some *Bifidobacterium* and *Lactobacillus* strains, resulted in better preservation of tight-junction structures, thus decreasing intestinal permeability. Interestingly, these are the same bacteria that have reduced representation in obese mice. Decreased intestinal permeability is also seen with administration of SCFAs, the carbohydrate degradation products generated by the microbiota. As the main energy source of colonic epithelial cells, SCFAs are thought to enhance fluid and electrolyte uptake and increase mucin release, all of which maintain the integrity of intestinal mucosa. This was shown in rodent models, in which butyrate was perfused through a cecum, leading to a 50% reduction in a radio-labeled marker in mesenteric blood circulation. Despite all of these theories and the compelling evidence seen in mouse models described earlier, there have not been consistent data showing the same in humans.

Similar to previous mice studies, studies of the human microbiome by Turnbaugh and colleagues (2006, 2009) showed that obese individuals had statistically less diversity in their microbiome compared to lean individuals. Again this was associated with a larger proportion of *Firmicutes* compared to *Bacteroides*. When these obese individuals were placed on either low-carbohydrate or low-fat diets, they observed statistically significant increases in *Bacteroides* and decrease in *Firmicutes* in their gut microbiome. However, attempts at replicating these same results have met with variable success. Although some studies were able to show a similar pattern in microbial changes, many more showed either no changes or an isolated association of *Bacteroides* with obesity instead. This, however, does not preclude the role of the microbiome in obesity. There are myriad confounders in each study, such as ethnicities, diets, length of follow-up, or small sample size, making it difficult to extrapolate globally true observations. Additionally, there may be more effective metrics to help elucidate the effect of the microbiome.

In their study on the microbiome of monozygotic and dizygotic twins and their mothers, the Gordon lab was unable to show a shared core gut microbiome. Even comparisons between the microbiome of monozygotic and dizygotic twins did not show a significant difference in microbial similarity. It was clear from this that no microbial distribution was universal between individuals. They were, however, able to find shared microbial genes. By analyzing the gene sequences against gene databases, they were able to construct a metabolic "core" microbiome based on bacterial functional categories. They termed these "genetic modules." By analyzing these genetic modules between obese and lean twin pairs, they were able to find 383 significantly different genes between the two groups; 273 genes were enriched in obese individuals and were involved in carbohydrate, lipid, and amino acid metabolism. Of those obesity enriched genes, 75% were from *Actinobacteria* and 25% were from the *Firmicutes*. Of the 110 genes that were depleted in obese individuals, 42% of these genes were from the *Bacteroides*.

Ongoing research is beginning to demonstrate that the microbiome plays important roles in a variety of diseases, as well as obesity. While taxonomic studies have not provided a mechanistic link between the microbiome and obesity, metagenomic analyses of the gut microbiome hint at promising physiological links to metabolism and obesity. Already this method has already produced high-impact results, such as the link between artificial sweeteners and a microbiome that generates more SCFAs. However, their discovery of a reset switch using antibiotics should be interpreted with caution; perturbation of the microbiome with antibiotics can itself lead to obesity. Instead, therapeutics should focus on identifying bacteria expressing genetic modules associated with leanness. With this knowledge, a spectrum of dietary, prebiotic, and probiotic interventions could be developed that enhance specific bacterial phenotypes and favor a shift toward a lean microbiome.

Acknowledgements

Preparation of this chapter was supported, in part, by Grant No. 2014109 from the Doris Duke Charitable Foundation.

Suggested Readings

Bäckhed, F., Ding, H., Wang, T., Hooper, L. V, Koh, G. Y., Nagy, A., et al. (2004). The gut microbiota as an environmental factor that regulates fat storage. *Proceedings of the National Academy of Sciences USA, 101*(44), 15718–15723.—This study illustrates an increase in body fat in germ-free mice after conventionalization, but also further illustrates how angiopoietin-like protein 4 (also known as Fiaf), which is repressed in conventionalization, promotes leanness in mice.

Cani, P. D., Amar, J., Iglesias, M. A., Poggi, M., Knauf, C., Bastelica, D., et al. (2007). Metabolic endotoxemia initiates obesity and insulin resistance. *Diabetes, 56*, 1761–1772.—This article establishes that a high-fat diet in mice can induce weight gain and diabetes through low-grade endotoxemia. They further establish that low-grade endotoxemia can induce weight gain despite similar caloric intake to control mice.

Cho, I., & Blaser, M. J. (2012). The human microbiome: At the interface of health and disease. *Nature Reviews Genetics, 13*(4), 260–270.—This article provides an introduction to the characterization and analysis of the microbiome and its many effects on human health and a variety of disease states.

Cho, I., Yamanishi, S., Cox, L., Methé, B. A., Zavadil, J., Li, K., et al. (2012). Antibiotics in early life alter the murine colonic microbiome and adiposity. *Nature, 488*, 621–626.—This article illustrates the microbiome changes associated with low-dose antibiotics and its associated propensity toward obesity in mice.

Cox, A. J., West, N. P., & Cripps, A. W. (2015). Obesity, inflammation, and the gut microbiota. *Lancet Diabetes and Endocrinology, 3*(3), 207–215.—This article reviews the evidence and theories regarding perturbations of inflammation and gut permeability in the microbiome as a factor in obesity.

Den Besten, G., van Eunen, K., Groen, A. K., Venema, K., Reijngoud, D.-J., & Bakker, B. M. (2013). The role of short-chain fatty acids in the interplay between diet, gut microbiota, and host energy metabolism. *Journal of Lipid Research, 54*(9), 2325–2340.—This comprehensive review details the role of SCFAs in metabolism, ranging from their production by the gut microbiota to their contributions in regulating fatty acid metabolism.

Harley, I. T. W., & Karp, C. L. (2012). Obesity and the gut microbiome: Striving for causality. *Molecular Metabolism, 1*(1–2), 21–31.—This review analyzes various studies that link the gut microbiome to obesity and further compares their associated microbial shifts. It additionally reviews several mechanisms that may explain how the microbiota can contribute to obesity.

Holmes, E., Li, J. V., Athanasiou, T., Ashrafian, H., & Nicholson, J. K. (2011). Understanding the role of gut microbiome–host metabolic signal disruption in health and disease. *Trends in Microbiology, 19*(7), 349–359.—This review details the association between the microbiome and various disease states, including diabetes and obesity.

Suez, J., Korem, T., Zeevi, D., Zilberman-Schapira, G., Thaiss, C. A., Maza, O., et al. (2014). Artificial sweeteners induce glucose intolerance by altering the gut microbiota. *Nature, 514,* 181–186.—This article showed that artificial sweeteners could induce glucose intolerance through a change in microbiota. Additionally they showed that this phenotype is transmissible from human subjects to germ-free mice.

Tagliabue, A., & Elli, M. (2013). The role of gut microbiota in human obesity: Recent findings and future perspectives. *Nutrition, Metabolism and Cardiovascular Diseases, 23*(3), 160–168.—This article reviews the effect of the microbiome on obesity with regard to its effects via SCFAs in metabolism and lipopolysaccharides in inflammation. Additionally it compares various studies of obese versus normal-weight individuals and their microbiota before and after weight loss.

Tilg, H., & Kaser, A. (2011). Gut microbiome, obesity, and metabolic dysfunction. *Journal of Clinical Investigation, 121*(6), 2126–2132.—This article reviews how the microbiome's effect on energy harvest, epithelial integrity, and gene regulation can affect metabolism and contribute to obesity and metabolic dysfunction.

Turnbaugh, P. J., Hamady, M., Yatsunenko, T., Cantarel, B. L., Duncan, A., Ley, R. E., et al. (2009). A core gut microbiome in obese and lean twins. *Nature, 457,* 480–484.—A study demonstrating a "core" functional gut microbiome characterized by conserved consistencies in genetic potential.

Turnbaugh, P. J., Ley, R. E., Mahowald, M. A., Magrini, V., Mardis, E. R., & Gordon, J. I. (2006). An obesity-associated gut microbiome with increased capacity for energy harvest. *Nature, 444,* 1027–1031.—This article illustrates the transmissibility of the gut microbiome from obese mice to germ-free mice and its associated phenotype of increased efficiency of energy harvest leading to statistically significant adiposity.

Stress and Obesity

ASHLEY E. MASON
ELISSA S. EPEL

Several types of psychological stress influence eating behavior; however, these associations vary widely across a number of psychological and physiological individual differences. Some individuals tend to eat more when stressed, whereas others tend to eat less. Furthermore, eating can itself influence stress arousal. Eating and the experience of stress are critical survival functions that share neurobiological pathways that are regulated by overlapping neuroendocrine systems. Here we review classic and recent literature on mechanisms linking stress and obesity; the intersection of stress, reward, and eating; laboratory and longitudinal associations among stress, eating, and weight gain; and societal implications of this body of findings.

Mechanisms Linking Stress and Obesity

Acute, isolated stressors, as well as chronic, ongoing stressors, impact eating behavior in both animals and humans. Most animal studies demonstrate that eating decreases under stress, unless highly palatable food is available, in which case selective eating of highly palatable food increases. This aligns with human studies documenting increased eating of widely available, highly palatable, calorie-dense "comfort foods" in response to the experience of stress.

Stress responses involve a neural network that comprises neurons in the hypothalamus, brainstem, and afferent nerves, as well as several areas within the limbic system and frontal cortex. Stress responses operate along two interacting pathways. One pathway is the limbic–hypothalamic–pituitary–adrenocortical (LHPA) axis, which produces a cascade of hormone secretions that represent an endocrinological stress response. These hormones include corticotropin-releasing hormone (CRH), adrenocorticotropic hormone (ACTH), and glucocorticoids (GCs).

A second pathway, the sympathetic–adrenal–medullary (SAM) axis, is a part of the autonomic nervous system (ANS) that involves the catecholamines adrenaline and noradrenaline. Acute stress-induced catecholamine release leads to increased lipolysis (breaking down of triglycerides in the cell) and weight loss by stimulating beta-adrenergic receptors. Chronic stress, combined with a highly palatable diet, can lead to changes in the SAM and LHPA axes. In the SAM axis, this combination leads to impaired beta-adrenergic activation, release of neuropeptide Y (NPY), and subsequent growth of adipocytes. Chronic arousal of the LHPA axis leads to both larger adipocytes and dysregulated physiological satiety mechanisms. Hence, regulation of LHPA axis activity has a well-known, critical role in the neural regulation of eating and peripheral energy balance. Below, we focus on the intersection of dysregulation of the LHPA axis, stress, and obesity.

The LHPA Axis: An Intersection of Stress, Eating, and Obesity

The adrenal glands release GCs in response to real or perceived stress, and increases in GCs are associated with greater caloric intake, especially from highly palatable foods, in both humans and animals. Accordingly, experimental laboratory studies assessing eating behavior in response to acute stressors, naturalistic case–control studies examining longer-term changes in GCs and weight gain, and medical studies of hypercortisolism (as in Cushing syndrome), provide clear evidence linking chronically elevated GCs to greater adiposity, especially visceral adiposity.

One prominent mechanism by which activation of the LHPA axis alters glucose metabolism and hunger is via action on feedback loops involving appetite-regulating hormones. Specifically, increases in GCs are associated with elevations in insulin and leptin, which, paradoxically, are hormones that signal satiety. GCs can, however, reduce tissue sensitivities to both insulin and leptin. During chronic stress, sustained high levels of GCs can result in hyperinsulinemia, reduced insulin sensitivity, and resultant accumulation of visceral abdominal fat. That is, insulin resistance can blunt signaling in the satiety and reward areas of the brain, leading to reduced control of the physiological hunger system, overeating, and an increased drive to eat. Recent studies have suggested a similar pattern of increased leptin, leptin resistance, and reduced resting energy expenditure.

Chronic stimulation of the LHPA axis also inhibits the reproductive, growth, and thyroid hormonal axes. The effects of LHPA axis activation on these major endocrine axes serve to selectively redirect nutrients and all vital substrates to the brain and stressed areas of the body. Though adaptive in the short-term, prolonged, chronic stress can lead to long-term disruptions in metabolic homeostasis via these axes. These disruptions can contribute to weight gain, insulin resistance, and metabolic syndrome. For example, stress-induced activation of the LHPA axis decreases production of thyroid-stimulating hormone (TSH), which, in turn, can reduce basal metabolic rate and increase energy conservation.

Stress, Eating, and the Reward System

In addition to disruptions in the regulation of energy homeostasis, stress-induced LHPA axis activity can alter the mesolimbic reward area, which is replete with dopaminergic neurons. This can cause highly palatable, calorie-dense foods to be perceived as especially rewarding. Such foods have been termed "comfort foods" to signify their stress-dampening and rewarding properties. In animal models, stress-induced eating dampens the stress response by increasing dopamine secretion in the mesolimbic pathway, including the ventral tegmental area (VTA) and nucleus accumbens (NAc). LHPA axis activation amplifies this rewarding experience by stimulating the release of endogenous opioids, which increase palatable food intake and additional opioid release. This sustained opioid release decreases LHPA axis activity and attenuates the stress response in a negative feedback fashion.

Habitual behavior can become embedded in the stress–reward pathway. Repeated and strong opioid responses in the reward neural circuitry promote the encoding of habits in the basal ganglia, which regulate habit-based behavior. Memories involving strong emotions, and the solutions that people use to cope effectively with them, are especially likely to be encoded. Hence, stress-induced eating of comfort foods is easily learned, remembered, and repeated. Functional magnetic resonance imaging (fMRI) data indicate that upon viewing images of highly palatable food, individuals endorsing greater chronic stress show exaggerated activity in regions of the brain involving reward, motivation, and habitual decision making, and reduced activity in areas linked to strategic planning and emotional control. It is therefore not surprising that many people increase their eating of highly palatable comfort foods when stressed.

Longitudinal Associations between Stress and Obesity

Large studies have examined cross-sectional and longitudinal associations between weight change and chronic psychological stress, such as that following from work-related issues (e.g., low job control), psychosocial factors (e.g., interpersonal relationships, bullying, social rejection), and cumulative stressful life events (e.g., traumatic early life experiences). Most associations have been weak to moderate, possibly due to the heterogeneity in eating behavior in response to stress. Some individuals tend to eat more, whereas others tend to eat less, and averaging responses obfuscates these individual differences. Thus, this potential bimodal distribution may account for small effects reported in the literature. Furthermore, prospective studies have found that stress-induced weight gain is contingent on baseline weight status and biological sex. For example, the Midlife in the United States (MIDUS) study, which examined 1,354 adults over a 9-year period, found that psychosocial stress was associated with weight gain among those with a higher body mass index (BMI) at baseline. Additionally, the types of stress associated with weight change differed across men (e.g., work-related stress) and women (e.g., family relationship stress). The Whitehall II Study, which investigated 7,965 British civil servants over a 5-year period, found that work-related stress was associated with weight gain for the most obese men. In contrast, work-related stress was associated with weight loss for the leanest men. In summary, obese status is a risk factor for further stress-induced weight gain, and different types of stressors differentially impact men's and women's weight gain over time.

Stress Reactivity, Eating, and Obesity

Laboratory studies have documented associations between stress responses and weight, especially abdominal adiposity. Laboratory paradigms designed to induce acute psychological stress have allowed researchers to investigate associations among acute stress responses and adiposity. A number of findings show associations among these acute stress responses (e.g., GC and autonomic reactivity) and measures of adiposity (e.g., abdominal obesity, generalized obesity, elevated BMI). A growing body of evidence suggests that abdominal obesity, relative to general obesity, may be more strongly correlated with LHPA axis dysregulation (both hypo- and hyperreactivity) and slower cardiovascular and endocrine recovery following acute stressors.

Though earlier research documented positive associations between GC reactivity and eating of palatable food in the laboratory, recent studies have demonstrated mixed results that may be due to important individual differences in dietary restraint, disinhibition, food insecurity, adiposity, and chronic stress levels, which we examine next. It remains important for researchers to develop research designs that will maximally clarify the extent to which acute stress reactivity in the laboratory can predict real-world eating of highly palatable food.

The Special Case of Chronic Stress

Recent research suggests that chronic stress is one important determinant of the association between GC reactivity and obesity. While several studies indicate that greater GC reactivity in the laboratory is associated with increased eating of palatable foods and abdominal adiposity, new studies indicate that lower GC reactivity (hyporeactivity) is also a risk factor for stress-induced eating. These discrepant associations may be due to varying levels of chronic stress, as explained by the *chronic stress response network model* (Mary Dallman and colleagues), which posits that chronic stress increases eating of palatable food, which, in turn, increases abdominal fat and inhibits acute stress-induced LHPA axis responses. Thus, chronically stressed individuals who habitually overeat highly palatable food may evidence blunted GC reactivity in response to acute stressors. This model has been demonstrated in animal studies (e.g., rats, rhesus monkeys) and, more recently, has been observed cross-sectionally in humans. The phenotype of blunted GC reactivity is in fact a common profile in stress-related disorders, and it is possible that chronic eating of palatable food may partially underpin this profile. To test this idea, we recently examined the extent to which a high-sugar diet suppressed stress responses. Results showed that 2 weeks of increased sugar consumption dampened GC reactivity to acute stress, thus demonstrating a metabolism-to-brain negative feedback loop. In summary, data from animals, and a small but growing body of data from humans, suggest that chronic stress is associated with greater eating of palatable food, and that stress-induced eating of palatable food alters LHPA axis activity.

Conclusion and Future Directions

The eating of highly palatable, calorie-dense comfort foods to reduce stress can foster problematic weight gain. The neural networks that regulate eating and psychological stress are tightly intertwined. In the past three decades, the modern food environment has swelled with increasing cues and opportunities to eat highly palatable food, and researchers have documented small but significant population-level increases in psychological stress. Mechanistic and longitudinal studies in animals and humans have demonstrated that the experience of stress can promote eating of highly palatable foods which, in turn, can reduce stress responses. Coupled with increased chronic stress, widespread chronic eating of highly palatable foods promotes habitual stress-induced eating as an extremely accessible coping strategy.

Associations between stress and obesity depend on multiple risk factors and moderators. Chronic stress increases risk for weight gain among individuals who are already overweight or obese; however, there are important differences between men and women in terms of which types of stressors confer this risk. Furthermore, it is important to understand risk factors for stress-induced eating at multiple levels, which include prenatal stress exposure, trauma and poor nutrition in childhood, family and relationship issues, employment and work-related factors, food insecurity and neighborhood food accessibility, and individual differences in the experience of a drive to eat for reward and sensitivity to food cues.

In summary, mechanistic research has shed light on pathways linking stress and weight change in animals and humans, as well as some of the complexities of these associations. Although more basic research, especially with humans, is needed, we should use what we know about associations between chronic stress and eating behavior to inform prevention efforts that target individuals who are at increased risk for weight gain. We believe this will require societal efforts focused on reducing population-wide increases in psychosocial stress, cultivating stress resiliency across the lifespan, and fostering the growth of and access to healthy food environments.

Acknowledgments

Ashley E. Mason and Elissa S. Epel were supported by the National Institutes of Health (Grant Nos. NCCIH T32AT003997 and NHLBI 1U01HL097973, respectively). They are grateful to Mary Dallman for her review and feedback on this chapter.

Suggested Reading

Adam, T. C., & Epel, E. S. (2007). Stress, eating, and the reward system. *Physiology and Behavior, 91*(4), 449–458.—The authors propose a theoretical model of reward-based stress eating and uses animal and human literatures to explain how different types of psychological stress impact eating.

Block, J. P., He, Y., Zaslavsky, A. M., Ding, L., & Ayanian, J. Z. (2009). Psychosocial stress and change in weight among US adults. *American Journal of Epidemiology, 170*(2), 181–192.—This article reports on associations between weight gain and several domains of psychological stress among adults enrolled in the MIDUS study.

Dallman, M. (2010). Stress-induced obesity and the emotional nervous system. *Trends in Endocrinology and Metabolism, 21*(3), 159–165.—This article reviews emotional and regulatory brain networks, and outlines processes by which stress and GC secretion can impact behavior that increases risk for obesity.

Kyrou, I., Chrousos, G. P., & Tsigos, C. (2006). Stress, visceral obesity, and metabolic complications. *Annals of the New York Academy of Sciences, 1083*(1), 77–110.—The authors discuss stress physiology with an emphasis on metabolism, and highlight data suggesting that multiple neuroendocrine and inflammatory mechanisms impact the paths through which chronic stress can contribute to central obesity and metabolic syndrome.

Maniam, J., & Morris, M. J. (2012). The link between stress and feeding behaviour. *Neuropharmacology, 63*(1), 97–110.—This article reviews the neuropeptides that regulate eating behavior and how their function can be altered by cross talk with neuropeptides and hormones that also regulate the HPA axis.

Mietus-Snyder, M. L., & Lustig, R. H. (2008). Childhood obesity: Adrift in the "limbic triangle." *Annual Review of Medicine, 59,* 147–162.—This article reviewed three interacting neural systems that regulate eating and food choices—the ventromedial hypothalamus (hunger), the VTA, and the NAc (reward seeking), and the amygdala (emotional responding)—and how factors such as stress and leptin resistance can dysregulate these systems.

Nyberg, S. T., Heikkilä, K., Fransson, E. I., Alfredsson, L., De Bacquer, D., Bjorner, J. B., et al. (2012). Job strain in relation to body mass index: Pooled analysis of 160,000 adults from 13 cohort studies. *Journal of Internal Medicine, 272*(1), 65–73.—The authors performed a pooled analysis to examine cross-sectional and longitudinal associations between job strain and BMI in adults enrolled in 13 European studies.

Rosmond, R. (2005). Role of stress in the pathogenesis of the metabolic syndrome. *Psychoneuroendocrinology, 30*(1), 1–10.—This article reviews the pathways by which GC secretion plays a pathogenic role in the development of obesity and is associated with factors comprising metabolic syndrome.

Sinha, R., & Jastreboff, A. M. (2013). Stress as a common risk factor for obesity and addiction. *Biological Psychiatry, 73*, 827–835.—This article reviews the role of stress as a risk factor for obesity and addiction, and proposes an integrative heuristic model that outlines the hypothesis that chronically high stress levels alter stress biology and both appetitive and energy regulatory systems in ways that promote stress-induced overeating of highly palatable food, thereby increasing risk for weight gain.

Ulrich-Lai, Y. M., Christiansen, A. M., Ostrander, M. M., Jones, A. A., Jones, K. R., Choi, D. C., et al. (2010). Pleasurable behaviors reduce stress via brain reward pathways. *Proceedings of the National Academy of Sciences USA, 107*(47), 20529–20534.—This article presents experimental data showing that the hedonic properties of highly palatable foods have stress-reducing effects that can therefore increase motivation to eat in times of stress.

Food, Addiction, and Obesity

ERICA M. SCHULTE
MICHELLE A. JOYNER
ASHLEY N. GEARHARDT

Over the past several decades, significant changes have occurred in the food environment that may contribute to increasing rates of obesity. Highly palatable, highly processed foods are widely accessible, affordable, and available in large portion sizes. While some individuals maintain a healthy weight despite the current obesogenic climate, others may be more vulnerable to the rewarding properties of these high-fat, high-sugar foods and be triggered by cues in the environment to consume these foods. This potential pathway for problematic eating behavior and obesity has led to the hypothesis that some individuals may experience an addictive-like response to certain foods, which may be exacerbated by the abundance of highly processed foods and food cues in our environment. We describe in this chapter potential parallels between highly processed foods and drugs of abuse; examine overlapping mechanisms in obesity, eating disorders, and addiction; review existing evidence for "food addiction"; and discuss treatment implications.

The Role of Food

An addiction perspective posits that an individual's vulnerabilities (e.g., impulsivity, emotion dysregulation) interact with an addictive substance/behavior (e.g., cocaine, gambling). Applying this framework to eating behavior would suggest that, like drugs of abuse, certain foods may be capable of triggering an addictive process in at-risk individuals. Highly processed foods, with added amounts of fat and/or refined carbohydrates (e.g., white flour or sugar), may share features with drugs of abuse that increase their addictive potential. Specifically, addictive substances are made to be particularly rewarding due to a large, concentrated dose of an addictive agent that is absorbed rapidly by the system. For example, naturally occurring coca leaves have little addictive potential when chewed but can be processed into a highly addictive substance, cocaine, by increasing the concentration and the rate at which the addictive agent hits the system. In a similar manner, highly processed foods do not occur in nature but may be designed to be artificially rewarding by adding fat and/or refined carbohydrates with rapid delivery to the system (e.g., high blood sugar spike). Thus, it is likely that highly processed foods have a greater "addictive" potential than natural, minimally processed foods (e.g., fruits, vegetables).

Consistent with this idea, humans report that highly processed foods are more likely to be consumed in an addictive-like way (e.g., loss of control, continued use despite negative consequences), whereas minimally processed foods are not. Furthermore, highly processed foods with a high blood sugar spike seem to be more problematic for persons reporting addictive-like eating behavior, consistent with the idea that vulnerable individuals may be particularly sensitive to the highly rewarding nature of these foods.

Evidence for Food Addiction in Animal Models

Animal model studies provide evidence that highly processed foods may be associated with core biological and behavioral features of addiction. Rats given intermittent access to sugar begin to display behaviors similar to those seen in addiction, such as binge consumption and withdrawal symptoms. Additionally, when fed a diet of highly processed foods, such as cheesecake, rats begin to show dysfunction in reward-related neural systems, similar to that seen in rats given extended access to heroin or cocaine. Rats also endure aversive stimuli (e.g., foot shock, bright lights) to obtain access to the highly processed food despite having their chow available. Furthermore, rats appear to exhibit behavioral indicators of an addictive process in response to high-sugar, high-fat foods such as Oreo cookies and cheesecake but not to their typical chow. Binge-prone rats consume larger amounts of highly processed foods, but not normal chow, in response to stress, and rats fed a high-fat diet display a preference for this high-fat food over their standard chow. Surprisingly, there is also some evidence that ingredients in highly processed foods may be even more reinforcing than drugs of abuse, as rats offered a forced choice between sugar and an addictive drug (e.g., heroin, stimulants) exhibit a preference for sugar over the drug rewards. Thus, evidence in animal models suggests there may be similarities between highly processed foods and drugs of abuse.

Shared Mechanisms in Obesity, Binge Eating Disorder, and Addiction

Further evidence for the role of an addictive process in eating-related problems is that mechanisms implicated in addiction also appear to be involved in obesity and binge eating disorder (BED). In particular, addiction, obesity, and eating disorder perspectives all identify reward dysfunction, emotion dysregulation, and impulsivity as key contributors to excess food consumption.

Drugs and highly processed foods both activate reward-related neural systems, such as the mesolimbic dopaminergic pathway, to a greater degree than do naturally occurring rewards. Individuals with obesity and those who binge-eat demonstrate patterns of neural functioning that are implicated in addiction. For example, individuals with obesity or BED exhibit elevated activation in reward-related regions while viewing cues or anticipating receipt of highly processed foods compared to healthy controls. This pattern of reward responsivity is also observed in individuals with substance use disorders, relative to controls. Similar to individuals with addiction, persons with obesity or binge eating behavior also demonstrate an attentional bias for cues related to highly processed food and increased motivation to respond to them. Thus, disruption in reward processes may similarly contribute to problematic eating behaviors and addiction.

Emotion dysregulation is another mechanism that is relevant to both addiction and problematic eating behaviors. Akin to drug use among individuals with addictive disorders, persons with obesity or BED may consume highly processed foods in an attempt to regulate strong emotions. The experience of negative affect (e.g., sadness, anxiety) is associated with increased cravings for highly processed foods and is a predictor of overeating or binge eating episodes. Similarly, negative affect is also a trigger for excessive substance use. During negative affect, individuals with substance use disorders and eating-related problems exhibit increased activation in reward-related brain regions towards drug and food cues, respectively. Thus, intense emotional states may increase the likelihood of excess consumption of both drugs of abuse and food.

Impulsivity also seems to be implicated in addictive disorders and problematic eating behavior. Individuals with obesity and/or BED and persons with substance use disorders demonstrate greater behavioral impulsivity than do controls and have decreased activation in executive control regions (e.g., prefrontal cortex) during decision-making tasks. This behavioral and neurobiological pattern may explain why individuals with addictive disorders or eating-related problems may choose short-term rewards, such as drug or highly processed food consumption, over long-term goals of improving health outcomes.

In summary, overlapping mechanisms implicated in addictive disorders, obesity, and BED suggest that an addictive process may contribute to eating-related problems. Furthermore, animal model studies indicate that rats exhibit behavioral and biological markers of addictive-like behavior in response to highly processed foods. Thus, to examine whether some humans may be addicted to highly processed foods, the Yale Food Addiction Scale (YFAS) was developed.

The Yale Food Addiction Scale

The YFAS was developed using the DSM-IV criteria for substance dependence to examine whether some individuals may experience symptoms of an addictive disorder with respect to certain foods. The YFAS measures behavioral indicators of addictive-like eating, such as loss of control over consumption, continued use despite negative consequences, and inability to cut down on consumption despite a desire to do so. Higher scores on the YFAS have been associated with greater impulsivity, elevated craving, and dysfunction in emotion regulation. Neural correlates associated with addictive disorders also appear to be reflected in addictive-like eating. Individuals who report three or more symptoms of "food addiction" on the YFAS appear to have increased activation of reward-related regions in response to cues related to highly processed food and diminished activity in executive control regions upon food consumption, which is observed with relevance to drugs of abuse for persons with substance use disorders. Notably, addictive-like eating is indicative of these patterns of reward responsiveness even when accounting for body mass index (BMI).

Yet one question about the validity of the YFAS is its overlap with other eating-related problems. Higher YFAS scores are positively associated with obesity and even more strongly with BED, which may be expected because of shared contributing mechanisms.

However, there is also evidence of discrimination from these eating-related problems. For example, some individuals with elevated YFAS symptomatology do not meet criteria for BED or other eating disorders but exhibit clinical levels of impairment. Additionally, normal-weight individuals who report "food addiction" symptoms exhibit dysfunction and significant distress. Thus, "food addiction," as measured by the YFAS, may provide clinically meaningful information about problematic eating behavior, though more research is needed to evaluate its utility.

Future Research Directions

Although the literature on addictive-like eating has grown rapidly over the last decade, there are still a number of important future directions. An immediate next step in the evaluation of the "food addiction" construct is to examine whether highly processed foods, or ingredients in these foods (e.g., sugar) may be capable of triggering neuroplastic changes in the brain that drive compulsive consumption. For example, one potential avenue may be to examine whether individuals can develop tolerance to the hedonic properties of highly processed foods, as evidenced by diminished reward responsiveness during consumption over time. Preliminary evidence suggests that self-reported frequent consumption of a highly processed food (ice cream) is associated with blunted reward responsiveness when eating that food, but no previous studies have systematically examined whether prolonged exposure to highly processed foods alters the system enough to result in a diminished reward response. If tolerance to the hedonic properties of these foods can develop, this may be a potential explanation for the increase in portion sizes of highly processed foods in our modern food environment.

Another direction for future study may be to investigate whether withdrawal symptoms can develop when highly processed foods are removed from the diet. Previous research in animal models suggests that rats exhibit markers of withdrawal, such as teeth chattering and anxiety when sugar is taken out of their diet. However, no studies have examined the role that withdrawal may have for addictive-like eating in humans. Though it is unlikely that severe, physical withdrawal symptoms (e.g., vomiting) would be acutely present if highly processed foods were removed from an individual's diet, psychological withdrawal (e.g., preoccupation, irritability, anhedonia) may be related to continued, compulsive consumption. Psychological preoccupation may be triggered or exacerbated by cues, which may contribute to problematic eating behavior in an obesogenic food environment for addictive-like eaters. This underscores the necessity for future research on this topic, which may be clinically useful and informative for food policy initiatives.

Treatment Implications

If some individuals experience an addictive-like response to certain foods, efficacious treatments for substance use disorders may be adapted for clinical use among persons with "food addiction." Currently, cognitive-behavioral therapy (CBT) for substance use and eating disorders share many components, such as craving management, emotion regulation, and trigger identification. Thus, treatment for food addiction may also include these features. One controversial aspect regarding intervention for addictive-like eating behavior is whether abstinence from potentially addictive foods (e.g., highly processed foods) should be considered a treatment goal. While abstinence-based programs are used for the treatment of substance use disorders, there has been limited empirical investigation of existing abstinence-based, 12-step interventions for "food addiction." However, not all evidence-based interventions for substance use disorders emphasize abstinence, which may provide a useful model for the integration of addiction perspectives into the treatment of eating-related problems. For example, harm reduction approaches focus on reducing negative outcomes associated with drugs of abuse or addictive behaviors by encouraging moderate consumption and limiting use in triggering situations. Consistent with CBT, harm reduction approaches help the individual identify high-risk environments, develop skills to tolerate cravings, and regulate emotions. Though future research is needed, harm reduction techniques may also be effective for decreasing negative consequences associated with addictive-like eating behavior, without requiring abstinence from highly processed foods.

Concluding Remarks

Obesity and eating disorders continue to be major public health issues. There is growing evidence that mechanisms contributing to addictive disorders may also be relevant for eating-related problems (e.g., reward dysfunction, impulsivity). A burgeoning literature suggests that highly processed foods may be capable of triggering addictive-like responses in at-risk individuals. Future research is warranted to evaluate further the validity of addiction perspectives applied to eating behaviors, such as examining which foods or ingredients are implicated and whether core features of addiction (e.g., withdrawal, tolerance) contribute to problematic eating. If some individuals experience an addictive-like response to certain foods, an addiction framework may provide clinically useful information for treating and preventing eating-related concerns.

Suggested Reading

Avena, N. M., Rada, P., & Hoebel, B. G. (2008). Evidence for sugar addiction: Behavioral and neurochemical effects of intermittent, excessive sugar intake. *Neuroscience and Biobehavioral Reviews, 32*(1), 20–39.—This article reviews evidence of sugar dependence in animal models, such as bingeing, withdrawal, craving, and cross-sensitization.

Berridge, K. C., Ho, C. Y., Richard, J. M., & DiFeliceantonio, A. G. (2010). The tempted brain eats: Pleasure and desire circuits in obesity and eating disorders. *Brain Research, 1350,* 43–64.—The authors describe how neural systems of reward processes may contribute to obesity and eating-related problems.

Burger, K. S., & Stice, E. (2012). Frequent ice cream consumption is associated with reduced striatal response to receipt of an ice cream–based milkshake. *American Journal of Clinical Nutrition, 95*(4), 810–817.—This study provides evidence that frequent consumption of a highly processed food, ice cream, is associated with diminished reward responsivity in humans.

Gearhardt, A. N., Corbin, W. R., & Brownell, K. D. (2009). Preliminary validation of the Yale Food Addiction Scale. *Appetite, 52*(2), 430–436.—This article provides psychometric data on the YFAS, a self-report measure of behavioral indicators of addictive-like eating, based on DSM-IV criteria for substance dependence.

Gearhardt, A. N., White, M. A., & Potenza, M. N. (2011). Binge eating disorder and food addiction. *Current Drug Abuse Reviews, 4*(3), 201–207.—The authors discuss the shared and unique features of BED and food addiction.

Gearhardt, A. N., Yokum, S., Orr, P. T., Stice, E., Corbin, W. R., & Brownell, K. D. (2011). Neural correlates of food addiction. *Archives of General Psychiatry, 68*(8), 808–816.—This study measured patterns of reward-related neural circuitry in persons reporting addictive-like eating behavior. These individuals exhibited elevated activation in response to food cues, yet reduced activation to food receipt. This pattern is also observed in persons with substance use disorders with respect to drug cues and receipt.

Meule, A., & Gearhardt, A. N. (2014). Five years of the Yale Food Addiction Scale: Taking stock and moving forward. *Current Addiction Reports, 1*(3), 193–205.—This review summarizes prevalence rates of food addiction symptoms and diagnoses in various populations. Additionally, psychometric properties, adaptations, and proposed future directions of the YFAS are discussed.

Mole, T. B., Irvine, M. A., Worbe, Y., Collins, P., Mitchell, S. P., Bolton, S., et al. (2015). Impulsivity in disorders of food and drug misuse. *Psychological Medicine, 45*(4), 771–782.—The authors found that individuals with eating-related problems exhibit impulsive decision making, marked by a preference for short-term versus long-term rewards. This pattern is also observed in persons with substance use disorders.

Schulte, E. M., Avena, N. M., & Gearhardt, A. N. (2015). Which foods may be addictive?: The roles of processing, fat content, and glycemic load. *PLoS ONE, 10*(2), e0117959.—This study provides evidence that highly processed foods, with added fat and refined carbohydrates, are most associated with addictive-like eating behavior. The authors discuss similarities between highly processed foods and drugs of abuse, such as a high dose and rapid rate of absorption of rewarding ingredients.

Tang, D. W., Fellows, L. K., Small, D. M., & Dagher, A. (2012). Food and drug cues activate similar brain regions: A meta-analysis of functional MRI studies. *Physiology and Behavior, 106*(3), 317–324.—This meta-analysis examines similarities between neural systems implicated in cue reactivity to food and smoking stimuli, suggesting overlapping neural circuitry for food and drug rewards.

Food and Addiction

Reasons to Be Cautious

HISHAM ZIAUDDEEN
PAUL C. FLETCHER

Many of us at some point have experienced powerful cravings for certain foods (often ones we regard as indulgent or unhealthy), and struggled to resist and failed (leading to disappointment or guilt). These experiences seem akin to the cravings described by people with drug addiction. Even though it is unlikely that these cravings are as intense as those for drugs (at least for most of us), they nevertheless do make the idea of food addiction (FA) credible, both to scientists and the public. For scientists, it casts a problematic behavior, that is, overeating (and obesity), in terms of sophisticated and well-researched models of drug addiction. For individuals struggling to control their eating and weight, it provides an important explanatory narrative for their difficulties, one that may seem mercifully free of moral judgment.

However, being appealing or even useful does not necessarily make a concept valid or ultimately helpful. The idea must be examined on its scientific merits so far, whether FA exists and, if so, in whom, remains an open question. There is little direct or consistent evidence to support the idea of FA in humans, and we suggest that its widespread acceptance stems more from its conceptual and descriptive attractiveness than from its empirical support. Of course, in the face of incomplete evidence, one might wish to embrace this idea while gathering the relevant data, and some have chosen to do precisely this—a respectable position but a risky one. We caution against the ready acceptance of the FA concept, at least as it is understood now, for three main reasons. First, we need to be reasonably convinced that we have defined and identified a distinct and valid scientific and clinical entity. Second, we need to consider the treatment implications for those thought to be affected by FA. Third, we must be mindful of the implications for public health policy and food legislation. While, ultimately, the data must determine whether FA exists, we counsel against any firm position until those data do exist.

The Scientific and Clinical Evidence

There are two key ideas about the nature of FA. The first is that certain foods, specifically, highly palatable foods that are rich in fat and sugar, activate brain reward systems and induce patterns of overeating that resemble drug addiction (i.e., some foods are addictive). The second is that certain individuals (with obesity) show a pattern of food-related behavior characterized by loss of control over intake and compulsive consumption despite adverse consequences, which strongly resembles drug addiction (i.e., some people become addicted to food). These ideas are not mutually exclusive and are in fact strongly linked in the literature. The relationship to obesity is rather complex. Obesity could, of course, be a consequence of FA but not a necessary one, and since both would be associated with distinct and overlapping brain changes, any empirical work aimed at identifying underlying mechanisms becomes complex.

The animal literature presents compelling proof of concept for the FA model. This is very important, but unfortunately it does not help us identify a putative agent, and this becomes relevant when we consider the human FA syndrome. This is modeled on DSM-IV criteria for substance dependence, which have been adapted for food and operationalized in the now widely used Yale Food Addiction Scale (YFAS). The translation is not without problems (see Table 71.1). A key issue is that DSM-IV substance dependence criteria are defined with respect to an addictive agent and are difficult to apply without such an agent. Perhaps hyperpalatable and/or highly processed foods are key, though this has yet to be determined. Drug addiction results from the combination of an addictive agent, an individual with vulnerabilities to addiction, and time. Only 15% of individuals who use drugs develop dependence. This is especially critical when the substance (food) is universally consumed (though not necessarily in the aforementioned hyperpalatable forms), but some individuals may go on to develop a FA. Without some evidence for a putative addictive substance or underlying physiological process, there is a danger of circularity in defining FA purely in terms of clinical overlap and a dedicated questionnaire. Crudely put, FA exists because certain people are defined as food addicts on the YFAS; the YFAS is valid because it can identify FA. This is something of a caricature, but given the widespread acceptance of the YFAS as a diagnostic tool for FA it, we should bear this in mind. The recently published YFAS 2.0 has updated the original scale to be in line with the DSM-5 criteria for substance use disorder, but the above concerns remain.

FA is not generally considered to provide a general mechanism that explains overeating and obesity, but it does provide one that may be relevant to specific subgroups with obesity (though, theoretically, an individual with FA may not, or not yet, be obese). The strongest candidate here is binge eating disorder (BED). Here we have a behavioral syndrome, more convincingly like that of drug addiction, with loss of control of eating, escalating consumption, and possibly consumption to ameliorate dysphoric and negative effects. The face validity of the FA construct is strongest when it is applied to BED. An important caveat is that although BED is associated with obesity, a substantial number of people who show binge eating behavior are not obese, and most obese people do not have BED. High levels of comorbidity (41.5–72.0%) have been found between BED and FA (as per YFAS), and there is also significant overlap with other eating disorders such as anorexia and bulimia nervosa. This raises an important question: Is FA a unique nosological entity?

This is a critical question that in our view can only be answered by defining the natural history of the syndrome and exploring its underlying mechanisms. While the DSM

TABLE 71.1. Comparison of the DSM-IV Substance Use Criteria and the Yale Food Addiction Scale

Salient features of DSM-IV criteria for substance dependence	YFAS equivalent	Comment
Persistent desire for and unsuccessful attempts to reduce drug use.	Persistent desire for food and unsuccessful attempts to cut down the amount of food eaten.	Without a clear agent or substance, the YFAS applies severity and impairment thresholds to make this criterion meaningful. It asks about "certain foods" and gives examples of energy-dense and fast foods.
Larger amounts of drug are taken than intended.	Larger amounts of food eaten than intended.	As above.
Substance use is continued despite persistent harmful physical/psychological consequences.	Overeating is maintained despite persistent harmful physical/psychological consequences.	As above.
A great deal of time is spent on getting/using/recovering from use of the substance.	Great deal of time is spent eating.	As above. Less useful for foods given their easy availability in most developed societies.
Substance use leads to reduction or abandonment of important social, work, or recreational activities.	Activities are given up because of overeating or recovery from overeating.	
Tolerance: Increasing amounts of drug are required to achieve desired impact.	Increased amounts of food are required to get the same pleasure or relief from negative emotions.	Tolerance and withdrawal relate to physiological adaptations to sustained substance use. They are not seen with all substances and may not be relevant to foods; therefore, thus far they are not known for any foods. The YFAS equivalents are not convincing but, of concern, they are strongly endorsed by participants in studies using this measure.
Withdrawal symptoms upon drug discontinuation.	Withdrawal symptoms such as anxiety, agitation or other physical symptoms.	

criteria for drug addiction are behavioral, they have been validated by a large body of neuroscientific research that has examined their neural underpinnings, so much so that both the syndrome and the term "addiction" have come to imply a specific set of underlying neural mechanisms. Behaviors that look like addiction suggest but, on their own, do not confirm an addiction syndrome. In keeping with this, the researchers who have sought to characterize the neurobiology of FA have hypothesized that if this set of food-related behaviors is indeed reflective of addiction, then the neurobiological correlates of the two conditions should overlap. Three key features of drug addiction have been examined in this regard. The first is the finding of lower striatal dopamine (D_2) receptors in drug addiction. The second is an enhanced neural anticipatory response to an imminent drug reward, with a blunted consummatory response on receipt of the reward. The third is an enhanced neural response to drug-related cues.

The first and most influential finding in this area was that obese individuals had lower levels of striatal D_2 receptors than controls, a pattern very similar to that seen in drug-dependent individuals. This positron emission tomography (PET) study, however, compared severely obese individuals (body mass index [BMI] > 40) with controls (BMI < 30). The finding has been replicated twice, although at least three studies have failed to replicate it. The one study that specifically looked at obese individuals with BED did not find any difference in D_2 receptor levels compared to non-BED obese individuals. It may be that a more regionally specific examination is required. A recent study has shown that increasing BMI is related to increased D_2 receptor binding in the dorsal striatum and decreased binding in the ventromedial striatum.

Studies that have examined the relationship of key dopaminergic genes to FA have shown that these individuals may have some degree of upregulation in the dopamine system. However, whether obesity is associated with lower striatal D_2 receptors remains an open question. With respect to the other two neurobiological features of addiction, while there have been several functional magnetic resonance imaging (fMRI) studies in obesity, given the lack of consistency in their findings, no single mechanism has been consistently implicated in obesity, let alone an addictive one. One study has specifically examined people phenotyped using the YFAS, but only two of the 48 subjects in the study had a diagnosis of FA, as per the YFAS. The authors found that individuals with higher FA scores showed greater responses to anticipation of food (a chocolate taste) in the anterior cingulate cortex, orbitofrontal cortex, and amygdala. However, these findings were not entirely as predicted, and some of these effects were driven by a decreased response to the control taste rather than an increased response to the food. More importantly, since only two people in the study had FA, any interpretation of the findings depends on how valid the YFAS scale scores are, and any conclusions must necessarily be tentative.

In summary, the validity of the human FA concept has not yet been convincingly established, and there are important conceptual and methodological limitations to be considered in interpreting the extant literature.

Food Addiction in the Clinic

Despite its widespread informal adoption, FA is not recognized as a clinical disorder at present. It was considered by the DSM-5 committee but was not included because it was deemed to have insufficient evidence to merit inclusion even as a research diagnosis. The burden of proof is higher in the clinical context given the need and responsibility to make valid diagnoses and advise appropriate treatments. If FA can be validated as a distinct clinical disorder, it could suggest different treatment approaches. It has been suggested that treatment approaches from drug addiction could be adapted to FA. These may include controlled consumption of or abstinence from specific foods, psychological treatments such as individual cognitive-behavioral therapy (CBT), or 12-step programs to help individuals gain control over their eating. It is worth contemplating whether and how such approaches to food would differ from other kinds of weight loss treatment and support. Certainly there is a major difference between CBT approaches for binge eating and addiction treatments given that they do not advocate avoidance or abstinence but instead focus on decreasing dietary restraint and enhancing the individual's sense of control over food. While there is enthusiasm about the potential additional treatment approaches that may come from the addiction field, this should be tempered by the limited effectiveness of these approaches in drug addiction.

Food and Public Policy

Much has been written in the scientific literature about the public health and policy implications of FA. The main focus has been on foods that may be addictive rather than individuals with FA. The argument is that such addictive foods are widely available and represent a risk at the population level, and parallels are drawn with nicotine and smoking. Certainly, if we could establish that certain foods are addictive, this could reasonably demand a policy response that would look at the important issues of availability of and access to such foods, particularly in vulnerable groups such as children. The issue is not that we lack evidence from other lines of health research to justify such policies, but that there are multiple challenges including political will, industry agreement, issues of individual choice, and restricting access to particular groups and individuals. However, a true confirmation that a particular food is addictive could change the picture because it invokes a very specific model of state responsibility, such as that for substances known to be addictive. Such a confirmation would also provide more powerful means to address the role of the food industry. This brings us once again to difficult questions: What is the addictive agent? How much evidence do we need to support such a policy intervention? Given that there is, at present, insufficient evidence to support the notion of FA, it is of some concern that a part of the scientific community has been suggesting that FA mandates the modification of public health policy in much the same way that nicotine addiction did for smoking. This is surely premature and would scarcely withstand the scrutiny to which a defensive food industry would be likely to subject it.

It is worth giving some consideration to the ideas that are being suggested for policy change, such as restrictions on high-fat and high-sugar foods. These have proven difficult to implement, and attempts such as the ban on large drinks in New York and the fat tax in Denmark have been unsuccessful. We should be mindful of the valuable lessons from the world of substance addiction. The classifications of drugs of abuse (and therefore the attendant legal ramifications) are periodically reviewed, not necessarily based on scientific evidence alone (societal value judgments play a significant role). It is salutary to remember that, in such case, the addictive agents are already clear, in contrast to the case with food. Enforcing the relevant legislation is not always straightforward with drugs that are clearly identified, and this is likely to be far more problematic with foods. While the idea of an illegal cheesecake dealer is difficult to imagine, it is not too difficult to consider the problems that may arise in restricting some foods and not others from some people/groups. We conclude on this cautious note, which highlights that even if FA were to be validated as a disorder, we have much further to go to make it clinically useful, and the eagerly proposed formulation of public health policy around such a model would be quite complicated.

Suggested Reading

Avena, N. M., Gearhardt, A. N., Gold, M. S., Wang, G. J., & Potenza, M. N. (2012). Tossing the baby out with the bathwater after a brief rinse?: The potential downside of dismissing food addiction based on limited data. *Nature Reviews Neuroscience, 13*(7), 514–514.—This brief response to the Ziauddeen and colleagues' (2012b) review suggests tempering any conclusions that the FA model is not supported and instead argues that the evidence is not yet sufficient to draw conclusions one way or another.

Benton, D. (2010). The plausibility of sugar addiction and its role in obesity and eating disorders. *Clinical Nutrition, 29*(3), 288–303.—A comprehensive and critical review of the evidence for sugar as a putative addictive substance.

Wilson, G. T. (2010). Eating disorders, obesity and addiction. *European Eating Disorders Review,* *18*(5), 341–351.—A thorough and thoughtful review of how ideas of FA relate to what is currently known about overeating and binge eating, including familial and clinical patterns, as well as treatment regimens.

Ziauddeen, H., Farooqi, I. S., & Fletcher, P. C. (2012a). Food addiction: Is there a baby in the bathwater? *Nature Reviews Neuroscience, 13*(7), 514.—This article was written in response to Avena and colleagues (2012) and essentially agrees with them.

Ziauddeen, H., Farooqi, I. S., & Fletcher, P. C. (2012b). Obesity and the brain: How convincing is the addiction model? *Nature Reviews Neuroscience, 13*(4), 279–286.—This review focused on the emerging neuroimaging findings and questioned whether they were interpretable in terms of the FA model.

Ziauddeen, H., & Fletcher, P. C. (2013). Is food addiction a valid and useful concept? *Obesity Reviews, 14*(1), 19–28.—A comprehensive review of ideas about FA. In addition to considering the neurobiological evidence, it explores clinical and policy implications in light of the current lack of evidential support for or against the FA model.

CLINICAL CHARACTERISTICS OF OBESITY

Definition and Classification of Obesity

JUNE STEVENS

Obesity has been defined by the World Health Organization (WHO) as an excessive fat accumulation that presents a risk to health. This simple definition provides only a starting place for determining who is obese. For that purpose, body measurements assessed in the continuous form must be categorized using cutoff points that capture relations with health. This categorization needs relevance to a range of purposes in multiple settings and for individuals who differ in gender, age, ethnicity, and other characteristics.

The ability to identify and classify obesity is useful in comparing adiposity status across groups, identifying individuals and segments of populations in need of prevention or treatment regimens, forming a diagnosis, facilitating understanding of the role of adiposity in disease, and providing a basis for the evaluation of interventions. Measurements and cutoff points are needed by public health workers, medical care providers, insurance agencies, and the military, as well as many other parties, in order to fashion practical decision-making rules for actions. The types of body measurements that are feasible to collect vary by context. In addition, the determination of the amount of fat accumulation that presents a risk to health is enormously complex and, of course, is dependent on the specific diseases or functions used to define health. This chapter addresses the definition and classification of obesity using measurements of fatness or body mass in adults and youth (ages 2–20 years) separately. It also briefly addresses alternative anthropometric measurements and issues related to obesity classification across gender and ethnic groups.

Definition and Classification of Obesity in Adults

Percent Body Fat in Adults

There are numerous methodologies for accurate assessment of percent body fat in humans. Dual X-ray absorptiometry (DXA) is currently the most widely used method. However, the study of associations of percent body fat with disease outcomes generally requires large samples, and the expense of collecting precise percent body fat measures is usually prohibitive. Therefore, in studies of disease risk, body mass index (BMI; weight in kg/ height in meters squared) is often used as an indicator of adiposity because it is easily and inexpensively measured. An approximation of the levels of adiposity associated with different levels of health risk can be estimated by relating adiposity levels to BMI. According to research conducted by Heo and colleagues (2012) using U.S. nationally representative data from the National Health and Nutrition Examination Survey (NHANES), the percentage of body fat that corresponds to a BMI of 18.5, 25, 30, 35, and 40 kg/m^2 across race/ethnic and age groups ranged from 12.2 to 19.0%, 22.6 to 28.0%, 27.5 to 32.3%, 31.0 to 35.3%, and 33.6 to 37.6%, respectively, in men. The corresponding ranges in women were from 24.6 to 32.3%, 35.0 to 40.2%, 39.9 to 44.1%, 43.4 to 47.1%, and 46.1 to 49.4%, respectively.

To make assessment of percent body fat feasible in large studies and nonclinical settings, mathematical formulas have been created that use combinations of multiple demographic, anthropometric, and bioelectric impedance analysis (BIA) variables to provide estimates of percent body fat. Most of these equations were developed in small or moderately sized samples that were recruited by convenience sampling and often limited to a specific and narrowly defined group. Associations between anthropometric measurements and percent body fat can differ importantly by gender, age, and race/ethnicity; therefore, it is necessary to match these characteristics between the sample in which an equation was developed and the individuals to which it is applied. In order to produce more broadly applicable equations, NHANES data have also been used to produce percent body fat estimates for adults and children 8 years of age and older that are generalizable to the U.S. population (*http://abcc.sph.unc.edu*).

BMI Cutoffs in Adults

Although classic definitions of obesity emphasize adiposity, in practice, a BMI of ≥ 30 kg/ m^2 is currently the measure most often used to diagnose obesity. BMI provides a feasible, albeit imperfect, assessment of body mass that is independent of height, and has been shown in some studies to be more predictive of cardiometabolic risk factors than DXA-measured percent body fat. Nevertheless, since BMI cannot distinguish fat from lean tissue, some misclassification of obesity (defined as "excess adiposity") is inevitable. Across ethnic groups in the 1999–2006 NHANES, the coefficient of determination (R^2) of BMI as a predictor of percent body fat was .521 in men and .606 in women.

The WHO and the National Heart, Lung, and Blood Institute (NHLBI) have endorsed BMI cutoff points for obesity (30 kg/m^2) and other classifications of BMI with slight differences in terminology (Table 72.1). In 2013, a systematic evidence review sponsored by NHLBI and released under the auspices of the American Heart Association, the American College of Cardiology, and the Obesity Society indicated increased rates of cardiovascular disease in adults with a BMI of 25 kg/m^2 or more, and increased rates of all-cause mortality in adults with a BMI of 30 kg/m^2 or more.

Definition and Classification of Obesity in Youth

Percent Body Fat in Youth

Determination of operational cutoff points to define excessive fat accumulation that presents a risk to health in youth is more problematic than that in adults due to normal (and large) changes in body composition that occur with age and growth. To illustrate, a 30%

TABLE 72.1. BMI Cutoff Points and Labels as Defined by the NHLBI and the WHO

NHLBI			WHO					
			Standard cutoff points			Narrow cutoff points		
Label	Lower limit	Upper limit	Label	Lower limit	Upper limit	Label[a]	Lower limit	Upper limit
Underweight	—	<18.5	Underweight	—	<18.5	Severe underweight	—	<16.0
Normal	18.5	<25.0	Normal	18.5	<25.0	Moderate underweight	16.0	<17.0
Overweight	25.0	<30.0	Overweight	25.0	—	Mild underweight	17.0	<18.5
Obese	30.0	—	Pre-obese	25.0	<30	—	18.5	<23.0
Obese Class I	30.0	<35.0	Obese	30.0	—	—	23.0	<25.0
Obese Class II	35.0	<40.0	Obese Class I	30.0	<35.0	—	25.0	<27.5
Obese Class III	40.0	—	Obese Class II	35.0	<40.0	—	27.5	<30.0
			Obese Class III	40.0	—	—	30.0	<32.5
						—	32.5	<35.0
						—	35.0	<37.5
						—	37.5	<40.0

[a]Labels were not designated for BMI categories of 18.5 kg/m² and greater.

body fat level in girls in the Pediatric Rosetta study was at the 95th percentile in girls at age 7 years, but near the 50th percentile in girls at age 15 years.

Determination of associations between adiposity and health risk is also more problematic in youth than in adults due to the need for studies to span many decades in order to observe chronic disease outcomes. In addition, since the relation of childhood adiposity to disease is likely to be influenced by adult levels of adiposity, it is necessary to monitor body fatness using multiple measurements throughout life, then make decisions about how to integrate and interpret that information in a meaningful way. Gender- and age-specific body fat percentiles at the 85th or 95th percentiles have been used by some investigators to indicate excess body fatness; nevertheless, currently, there is no clear consensus of a definition of childhood obesity using measures of body fat.

BMI Cutoffs in Youth

Across ethnic groups in the 1999–2006 NHANES, the R^2 of BMI as a predictor of percent body fat was .285 in boys and .637 in girls 8–20 years of age. The low R^2 value in boys likely reflects the changes that occur with development, such as disproportionate increases in muscle compared to fat mass around the age of puberty. Because the association of BMI with body fatness varies with both age and gender in children, gender-specific BMI-for-age indices such as percentiles or z-scores are often used to diagnose excess adiposity. Two widely used classification systems in youth are the Centers for Disease Control and Prevention (CDC) growth charts and the International Obesity Task Force

(IOTF) cutoff points. Both systems are based on the distribution of BMI levels in nationally representative samples. The CDC growth charts issued in 2000 included smoothed, normalized percentiles of BMI for ages 2–20 based on American data from the 1960s and 1970s, with additional data from 1988–1994 for children under 6 years of age (boys: *www.cdc.gov/growthcharts/data/set2clinical/cj41c073.pdf*; girls: *www.cdc.gov/growthcharts/data/set2clinical/cj41c074.pdf*). The IOTF standards are based on data from six (largely high-income) countries. IOTF BMI-for-age *z*-scores of 18-year-old adolescents with BMIs of 25 and 30 kg/m² were used to determine BMI cutoff points at younger ages (*www.worldobesity.org/resources/child-obesity/newchildcutoffs*).

In 2007, an American Medical Association (AMA) expert committee report suggested that the 85th and 95th percentiles of the BMI-for-age from the CDC 2000 charts be called "overweight" and "obesity," respectively. This terminology has been adapted for use in publications from the U.S. National Center for Health Statistics (NCHS) and other CDC agencies, although a 2015 federal report confirmed that obesity conceptually refers to excess body fat rather than a high BMI-for-age. The IOTF-25 cutoff points for BMI are similar to the CDC 85th percentiles, and generally, the IOTF-30 cutoff points are higher than the CDC 95th percentiles.

An analysis from the Pediatric Rosetta Project, summarized by Freedman and Sherry, showed that in youth ages 5–18 years, only 75% of boys and 63% of girls at or over the 95th CDC percentile (obese) had excess body fat defined as being at or above the internal age- and gender-specific 85th percentile of DXA-assessed percent body fat. Nevertheless, BMI percentiles and their recommended cutoff points, used with caution, are considered to provide useful information for screening and public health surveillance of overweight and obesity in children.

Assessments of Obesity Using Other Measurements

Skinfolds are commonly used to provide assessments of subcutaneous fat. Although a single skinfold or the sum of multiple skinfolds assessed at different body sites have been used as an indicator of overall adiposity, greater correlation with percent body fat is gained by using skinfold measurements in prediction equations that include other types of anthropometric measures and coefficients.

Waist circumference has been used to provide an assessment of overall and abdominal fatness. Waist is also used in a ratio with hip circumference (waist/hip) and in a ratio with height (waist/height). Compared to total body fat or subcutaneous fat, visceral fat has been shown to be an as strong or stronger correlate with multiple cardiometabolic risk factors. Research to uncover mechanisms behind these correlations continues to unfold. Cutoff points for determining a high waist circumference in adults have been suggested by the WHO (94 cm in men, and 80 cm in women) and by NHLBI (102 cm in men, and 88 cm in women). The NHLBI cutoffs have also been endorsed by the WHO as indicators of *substantially* increased, as opposed to increased, risk of metabolic complications.

An absence of cardiometabolic risk factors has been used to distinguish adults with a BMI of 30 kg/m² or above as metabolically healthy obese versus metabolically unhealthy obese. Several studies have shown differences in development of cardiovascular disease and all-cause mortality in these two groups. Currently, the operational definition and usefulness of this designation to determine disease risk and recommendations for weight reduction treatment are under debate.

Impact of Age, Gender, Ethnicity, and Physical Activity on Obesity Classification

There are large differences between youth and adults in percent body fat, and different schemes are used to define obesity as a result of those differences. There are also systematic discrepancies between younger and older adults, with older adults tending to have a higher percent body fat at the same BMI. However, this trend is generally ignored in definitions of obesity. The large gender difference in percent body fat following puberty is well recognized but not incorporated into the BMI cutoff point used to define obesity, probably because the relative risk of mortality in obese men and women compared to those in the normal BMI range is similar, despite the wide dissimilarity in percent body fat. Smaller differences by ethnicity have also been noted, with percent body fat tending to be larger in Asians and smaller in blacks compared to whites. These differences, along with higher rates of some cardiometabolic conditions, have been used to advocate for race-specific BMI cutoff points for overweight and obesity (e.g., 23 kg/m^2 and 27 kg/m^2, respectively, in Asians). The promotion of higher BMI cutoffs in blacks has received little support, in part because rates of diabetes and hypertension are higher in blacks than in whites with the same BMI, despite the trend toward lower percent body fat in blacks. Finally, it is well known that physical activity increases muscle mass; hence, obesity can be misdiagnosed by BMI in athletes. This misdiagnosis tends to make BMI–assessed obesity rates appear somewhat higher than would be found with a percent body fat cutoff point, particularly in males. Despite this bias, and other biases related to age, gender, and ethnicity, BMI remains a widely used metric to diagnose obesity in adults, probably because of its low expense, low participant burden, and high reproducibility.

Acknowledgments

Preparation of this chapter was supported, in part, by Grant No. DK097046 from the National Institutes of Health. My thanks to Lauren Paynter for her editorial assistance.

Suggested Reading

Barlow, S. E., & the Expert Committee. (2007). Expert committee recommendations regarding the prevention, assessment, and treatment of child and adolescent overweight and obesity: Summary report. *Pediatrics, 120,* S164–S192.—An expert committee suggests that the 85th and 95th percentiles of the BMI-for-age from the CDC 2000 charts be called "overweight" and "obesity," respectively.

Fabbrini, E., Magkos, F., Mohammed, B. S., Pietka, T., Abumrad, N. A., Patterson, B. W., et al. (2009). Intrahepatic fat, not visceral fat, is linked with metabolic complications of obesity. *Proceedings of the National Academy of Sciences USA, 106*(36), 15430–15435.—The observed relationship between visceral adipose tissue and cardiometabolic risk may be due to correlations with intrahepatic fat.

Flegal, K. M., & Ogden, C. L. (2011). Childhood obesity: Are we all speaking the same language? *Advances in Nutrition, 2,* 159S–166S.—This review explores terminology and measures used in studies of weight and adiposity in children.

Freedman, D. S., & Sherry, B. (2009). The validity of BMI as an indicator of body fatness and risk among children. *Pediatrics, 124,* S23–S34.—This review examines the relationships between body fatness, BMI, and health risk in children, as well as whether these associations are impacted by race/ethnicity, skinfold thickness, and body circumferences.

Freedman, D. S., Wang, J., Maynard, L. M., Thornton, J. C., Mei, Z., Pierson, R. N., et al. (2005). Relation of BMI to fat and fat-free mass among children and adolescents. *International Journal of Obesity, 29*(1), 1–8.—A study of 5- to 18-year-olds indicates that a high BMI-for-age is a good indicator of excess fat mass, but performance is not strong among thinner children.

Heo, M., Faith, M. S., Pietrobelli, A., & Heymsfield, S. B. (2012). Percentage of body fat cutoffs by sex, age, and race–ethnicity in the U.S. adult population from NHANES 1999–2004. *American Journal of Clinical Nutrition, 95,* 594–602.—Corresponding ranges of percent body fat in adults are given for selected BMI levels.

Jensen, M. D., Ryan, D. H., Hu, F. B., Stevens, F. J., Hubbard, V. S., Stevens, V. J., et al. (2013). 2013 AHA/ACC/TOS guideline for the management of overweight and obesity in adults. *Circulation, 129,* S102–S138.—A systematic evidential review of associations between BMI and cardiovascular risk is presented.

Kramer, C. K., Zinman, B., & Retnakaran, R. (2013). Are metabolically healthy overweight and obesity benign conditions?: A systematic review and meta-analysis. *Annals of Internal Medicine, 159,* 758–769.—This article presents a systematic review of studies to examine the effect of metabolic status on risk for mortality and incident cardiovascular events in normal-weight, overweight, and obese adults.

Stevens, J. S., Ou, F.-S., Cai, J., Heymsfield, S. B., & Truesdale, K. P. (2016). Prediction of percent body fat measurements in Americans 8 years and older. *International Journal of Obesity (London), 40*(4), 587–594.—Equations to predict percent body fat from demographic and anthropometric measurements were developed and validated.

WHO Expert Consultation. (2004). Appropriate body-mass index for Asian populations and its implications for policy and intervention strategies. *Lancet, 363,* 157–164.—A WHO expert consultation identified public health action points along the continuum of BMI.

Medical Complications of Obesity in Adults

Tirissa J. Reid
Judith Korner

The Surgeon General's Call to Action to Prevent and Decrease Overweight and Obesity in 2001 was deemed necessary, based on the fact that as obesity prevalence increases, so do associated comorbidities, causing significant morbidity, mortality, and financial strain estimated to cost over $140 billion a year. This chapter reviews the myriad complications resulting from excess adiposity stemming from the fact that obesity adversely affects nearly every organ system in the body.

Cardiovascular Complications

Peripheral edema and varicose veins can result from mechanical pressure placed on the vasculature by increased body mass and increased circulatory volume needed to perfuse a greater body mass. This pressure can lead to valvular insufficiency in the lower extremities, with subsequent venous pooling or venostasis. Phlebitis may result from venostasis, since stagnant blood can result in inflammation and deep venous thrombosis, with the possibility of clot embolization to the lungs.

Other cardiovascular complications include dyslipidemia, which usually involves low levels of cardioprotective high-density lipoprotein (HDL) cholesterol and elevated levels of triglycerides and low-density lipoprotein (LDL) cholesterol, which can contribute to atherosclerotic plaque formation in the setting of inflammation, resulting in coronary and carotid atherosclerosis. An additional contributor to the atherosclerotic process is hypertension (HTN), which is twice as common in obese adults compared with normal-weight adults. Myocardial infarction, congestive heart failure, cerebrovascular infarction, and death are acute complications. Congestive heart failure can also develop chronically as a result of long-standing HTN, since the heart will remodel and increase its muscle mass to pump against elevated pressures in the periphery, but ultimately becomes weakened over time. Even in obese patients without HTN, there is an increase in blood volume and cardiac output to supply the increased body mass, which can ultimately result in ventricular dilation and hypertrophy, with subsequent atrial enlargement and an increased risk for atrial fibrillation.

Increased waist circumference, a surrogate measure of visceral adiposity, in conjunction with hypertriglyceridemia, low HDL-cholesterol, HTN, and elevated fasting blood glucose are all known to increase the risk for cardiovascular disease. The presence of three or more of these features in a single individual is termed "metabolic syndrome" and increases the risk for heart disease, stroke, and diabetes more than the sum of risk from the individual components. Obesity is a modifiable risk factor for this syndrome.

Endocrine Complications

The risk of developing type 2 diabetes mellitus (T2DM) increases as body mass index (BMI) increases. A man with a BMI of 30 kg/m^2 has a fivefold increased risk of developing T2DM compared to a person with a normal BMI of 21 kg/m^2; in women this risk would be at least 25 times greater. Over 80% of people with T2DM are overweight or obese. The diagnosis of T2DM is usually preceded by a period of insulin resistance, which can occur as a result of obesity in which cells do not respond appropriately to a normal amount of insulin. In this scenario, increased levels of insulin are required, placing additional strain on the pancreatic beta-cells to achieve glucose homeostasis. After years of hyperinsulinism, the beta-cells are unable to meet the increased demand required to achieve euglycemia and hyperglycemia results.

The effects of diabetes are far-ranging and when uncontrolled over a long period of time can lead to complications in multiple organ systems, including coronary artery disease, gastroparesis, retinopathy, neuropathy, and nephropathy. The vascular damage inflicted by diabetes is so severe that a diagnosis of diabetes is considered a coronary artery disease equivalent. Small vessel damage by diabetes is one of the leading causes of end-stage renal failure requiring dialysis and is responsible for at least half of all limb amputations.

Obese women of child-bearing age are frequently faced with fertility challenges. Women who are obese have an increased risk of polycystic ovarian syndrome (PCOS), which can include symptoms of hirsutism, acne, insulin resistance, menstrual irregularities such as amenorrhea, oligomenorrhea, and menometrorrhagia, along with infertility. Due to increased rates of infertility, achieving pregnancy in women with PCOS or obesity is more likely to require medication and/or assistive technology, and success rates are lower than those of their normal-weight counterparts. If pregnancy is achieved, having had prepregnancy maternal obesity is associated with an increased risk for preeclampsia, preterm birth, gestational diabetes, and macrosomia, with an increased risk of cesarean deliveries and postpartum hemorrhage.

Musculoskeletal Complications

Osteoarthritis occurs more commonly in patients with obesity as a result of repetitive trauma from carrying excess body weight on weight-bearing joints. Over time, this can result in severe joint destruction and pain, limiting mobility and necessitating the use of assistive devices to walk and carry out activities of daily living. Unfortunately, the destruction of a joint space that occurs when a joint is chronically placed under an excessive weight load is irreversible at some point. Even with joint replacement, without removing the precipitating factor, excess weight, the artificial joint will likewise deteriorate. Inflammatory cytokines secreted from adipose tissue are believed to play a role in osteoarthritis as well. The increased levels of tumor necrosis factor (TNF)-alpha and interleukin (IL)-6 that occur in obesity are associated with a loss of knee cartilage. Increased levels of leptin, also secreted from adipocytes, are found in osteoarthritic cartilage and are thought to cause apoptosis and activate matrix metalloproteinases, resulting in cartilage destruction. Visfatin, another adipokine, is able to activate matrix metalloproteinases to cause cartilage destruction. IL-10 and adiponectin are thought to have protective effects on chondrocytes, but are decreased in obesity, allowing increased destruction from other cytokines. While progressive weight gain increases the risk of developing osteoarthritis, the reverse is also true, the risk of developing osteoarthritis decreases with weight loss.

Rheumatoid arthritis occurs at a higher frequency in obese patients. Although the exact mechanism underlying this relationship is unknown, it is most likely related to an increased number of adipocytes secreting inflammatory factors, such as C-reactive protein, IL-6, and TNF-alpha, which are usually detected at higher levels in patients with rheumatoid arthritis.

Gout occurs at increased rates in obese patients. This is likely due to increased rates of insulin resistance in obese patients, resulting in elevated serum uric acid levels and decreased renal clearance of uric acid, so urate crystals are more likely to form in the joint spaces, causing gouty arthritic pain.

Renal Complications

Obese patients have an increased prevalence of focal segmental glomerulosclerosis and glomerulopathy with proteinuria, even without diagnoses of HTN, diabetes, or other disorders known to result in these abnormalities, with an unknown mechanism for their development. They also have higher rates of hyperfiltration, but the clinical significance of this abnormality is currently unclear.

There is nearly double the risk of nephrolithiasis in obese patients, partly due to the increased prevalence of insulin resistance, which can result in decreased urinary pH and elevated levels of urinary calcium through an unknown mechanism, and to diets that often have a high content of animal protein, resulting in elevated levels of urinary calcium, oxalate, and uric acid, all of which increase the risk of renal stone formation.

Gastrointestinal Complications

The gastrointestinal system of obese patients is more susceptible to complications compared with those who are normal weight. Increased mechanical pressure from excess weight in the abdominal region of obese patients can promote the movement of gastric acid in a retrograde fashion through the lower esophageal sphincter into the esophagus, causing gastroesophageal reflux disease (GERD), as well as increased rates of hiatal hernias, another risk factor for GERD. Over years, GERD can result in cellular changes along the esophagus, with the potential for malignant transformation.

Increased body fat results in increased cholesterol production, to be excreted through the biliary system, which can precipitate and form gallstones. The risk for gallstones is increased further in obese females and even more so with rapid weight loss, with greater levels of bile supersaturation and decreased gallbladder contractility. Gallstones can increase the risk of pancreatitis while moving throughout the biliary tree, with the possibility of causing inflammation and/or obstruction. Obese patients are more likely to have lipid deposition in the liver, nonalcoholic fatty liver disease (NAFLD), which may progress to more serious stages, such as nonalcoholic steatohepatitis, fibrosis, cirrhosis, and end-stage liver disease. It is predicted that given the severity of the current obesity epidemic, NAFLD will be the most common indication for liver transplantation within a decade.

Respiratory Complications

Excess external and internal soft tissues in the neck of obese patients can obstruct the flow of oxygen through the oropharynx, particularly when patients are supine. This can result in apneic episodes, and an absence of oxygen flow to the brain. If these episodes are frequent and of sufficient duration, patients are diagnosed with obstructive sleep apnea (OSA). If OSA is untreated, it increases the risk of HTN, heart failure, stroke, depression, obesity, and all-cause mortality.

Asthma is more prevalent in obese populations as well, likely due to the increased inflammatory environment created from excessive cytokine release from adipocytes, resulting in increased airway hyperreactivity and bronchoconstriction, although the exact mechanism is unknown.

Neurological and Neurocognitive Complications

Pseudotumor cerebri, a condition with increased intracranial pressure, which can progress to include papilledema and blindness if untreated, occurs most commonly in obese patients, particularly obese women of childbearing age. The risk for carpal tunnel syndrome, a neurological disorder with pain and paresthesias in the hands due to compression of the median nerve, is increased by at least 75% in obese patients compared with normal-weight patients, although the exact reason for this is unclear.

Obese adults of all ages have been noted to have cognitive deficits in the areas of attention, processing, and fine motor speed. In older adults who are obese, there is also an increased risk for deficits in executive functioning, and the risk for dementia is doubled. While the exact cause of these cognitive deficits has not been discovered, they are currently thought to be the result of the increased inflammatory environment that accompanies the obese state, and in the case of dementia in older adults, the increased rates of insulin resistance, hyperlipidemia, and vascular infarcts that occur in obese patients may be primarily responsible.

Oncological Complications

Obesity is associated with an increased risk for certain types of cancer, including endometrial, colon, gallbladder, prostate, renal, and postmenopausal breast cancer. The increased risk may relate to increased levels of inflammatory factors in obese patients for a majority of these cancers, and in breast and endometrial cancers specifically, an increased fat mass results in higher levels of estrogen in the circulation, due to the conversion of androgens to estrogen within fat tissue, which can stimulate the growth of breast and endometrial tissue. As a result, women who are overweight have a significantly increased risk of breast cancer after menopause and endometrial cancer compared to women who are normal weight. Obese women are less likely to have smaller breast masses detected by palpation, and while breast cancers are not more likely to be missed on mammography in obese women, they do have a higher rate of false positives, necessitating additional testing and stress. Mortality after diagnosis is increased in obese patients with breast and prostate cancers. Since patients with obesity are less likely to undergo routine health screenings, cancers are frequently detected in later stages and therefore have a worse prognosis.

Dermatological Complications

Intertrigo, a fungal infection, and hidradenitis suppurativa, a painful skin disorder involving the occlusion of sweat glands that can lead to the formation of nodules or abscesses, both occur with increased frequency in obese patients. Increased areas of skin friction and sweat retention in intertriginous areas, along with higher levels of inflammatory cytokines in the circulation of obese patients, present a prime environment for these disorders.

Hyperinsulinism can cause melanocyte hyperplasia, which manifests dermatologically as acanthosis nigricans, a darkening and thickening of the skin, most commonly found on the neck, axillae, and other skin folds, and patients may also have skin tags.

Conclusion

As evidenced by this review of complications resulting from obesity, the effects of obesity are far-reaching, and few body systems remain unaffected. The complications are mediated via hormonal changes, an inflammatory environment, and biomechanics. The morbidity and mortality related to these complications are numerous, severe, and costly, and remind us that the treatment of obese patients involves prevention and treatment of multiple disorders. In addition to efforts to combat the obesity epidemic, health care providers must have a multipronged approach that concurrently addresses obesity and its medical complications.

Suggested Reading

Byers, T., & Sedjo, R. L. (2015). Body fatness as a cause of cancer: Epidemiologic clues to biologic mechanisms. *Endocrine-Related Cancer, 22*(3), R125–R134.—Discussion of the known mechanisms relating obesity to cancer, such as excess estrogen stimulating breast and endometrial tissues, as well as possible mechanisms for the associations between obesity and other (e.g., renal and pancreatic) cancers.

Cohen, J. I., Yates, K. F., Duong, M., & Convit, A. (2011). Obesity, orbitofrontal structure and function are associated with food choice: A cross-sectional study. *BMJ Open, 1*(2), e000175.—Examines differences in cognitive testing between obese and lean adults to help explain how obesity may affect cognitive processing and food choices.

Conway, G., Dewailly, D., Diamanti-Kandarakis, E., Escobar-Morreale, H. F., Franks, S., Gambineri, A., et al. (2014). The polycystic ovary syndrome: A position statement from the European Society of Endocrinology. *European Journal of Endocrinology, 171*(4), P1–P29.—Reviews the different historical definitions of PCOS, including the increased rates of insulin resistance and obesity, along with a phenotypic division of patients, which is also useful for guiding therapeutic decisions.

Eknoyan, G. (2011). Obesity and chronic kidney disease. *Nefrologia, 31*(4), 397–403.—Reviews the effects of obesity on the kidneys along with descriptions of the pathogenic mechanisms involved.

Kahn, S. E., Hull, R. L., & Utzschneider, K. M. (2006). Mechanisms linking obesity to insulin resistance and type 2 diabetes. *Nature, 444*, 840–846. Describes the mechanisms linking obesity to the development of insulin resistance and ultimately type 2 diabetes.

Kenchaiah, S., Gaziano, J. M., & Vasan, R. S. (2004). Impact of obesity on the risk of heart failure and survival after the onset of heart failure. *Medical Clinics of North America, 88*(5), 1273–1294.—Discusses how excess weight can lead to structural changes in the heart and result in heart failure.

Lee, R., & Kean, W. F. (2012). Obesity and knee osteoarthritis. *Inflammopharmacology, 20*(2), 53–58.—Discusses the biomechanical and metabolic mechanisms linking these two conditions, including adipokines and how they have a role in osteoarthritis.

Poirier, P., Giles, T. D., Bray, G. A., Hong, Y., Stern, J. S., Pi-Sunyer, F. X., et al. (2006). Obesity and cardiovascular disease: Pathophysiology, evaluation, and effect of weight loss an update of the 1997 American Heart Association Scientific statement on obesity and heart disease from the Obesity Committee of the Council on Nutrition, Physical Activity, and Metabolism. *Circulation, 113*(6), 898–918.—Reviews the pathophysiology linking obesity to cardiovascular disease and how these changes are altered with weight loss.

Rinella, M. E. (2015). Nonalcoholic fatty liver disease: A systematic review. *Journal of the American Medical Association, 313*(22), 2263–2273.—Reviews the pathogenesis, diagnosis and treatment of NAFLD, including its association with obesity and other features of the metabolic syndrome, along with results of studies showing that diet and exercise interventions are effective treatments.

Romero-Corral, A., Caples, S. M., Lopez-Jimenez, F., & Somers, V. K. (2010). Interactions between obesity and obstructive sleep apnea: Implications for treatment. *CHEST Journal, 137*(3), 711–719.—Discusses the mechanisms linking the increased risk of OSA with obesity, including excess adiposity in the upper airways and thorax, along with other common disease states.

Medical Consequences of Obesity in Childhood and Adolescence

WILLIAM H. DIETZ

$\mathbf{W}$hen the first review of the medical consequences of childhood obesity was published in 1998, most of the frequent consequences of childhood obesity were already recognized. Since then, the literature has increased dramatically, such that much of the data in this chapter are derived from systematic reviews and meta-analyses. An important gap is that the mechanisms that account for many of the consequences remain unclear. Based largely on studies of adults, inflammation is likely to play a key role. Inflammation, a common consequence of obesity, may account for adverse consequences of childhood and adolescent obesity, such as fetal mortality, asthma, and nonalcoholic steatohepatitis. Markers of inflammation increase with the severity of obesity, and elevations as high as 75% have been found in preoperative adolescents with severe obesity. Other consequences, such as the psychosocial consequences, reflect the pervasive bias and stigmatization associated with obesity, despite how prevalent obesity has become. The frequency of the consequences of obesity is shown in Table 74.1, and the most common of these are reviewed here.

Pregnancy and the Perinatal Period

The risks of obesity to children begin at conception. A large meta-analysis has demonstrated that fetal death, stillbirth, and perinatal, neonatal, and infant mortality are all increased among women with obesity. Furthermore, risk increases with the severity of obesity. The mechanisms that explain these associations remain uncertain. Increases in fetal mortality and stillbirth persist after controlling for preeclampsia, elevated blood pressure, and gestational and type 2 diabetes. A second systematic review and meta-analysis has described a variety of congenital anomalies among infants born to mothers with obesity. These include neural tube defects, including spina bifida, hydrocephalus, cleft lip or palate, cardiovascular defects, anal atresia, and limb anomalies. Maternal

TABLE 74.1. Frequency of Comorbidities and Risk Factors Associated with Obesity in Childhood and Adolescence

Comorbidity or risk factor	Frequency
Frequent	
Asthma	6–9%
Nonalcoholic fatty liver disease	> 50%
Nonalcoholic steatohepatitis	8%
Hyperinsulinemia/abnormal GTT	20–25%
Low HDL-cholesterol	17%
Elevated blood pressure	25%
Knee joint malalignment	20%
Knee pain	21%
Impaired health-related QOL score	49%
Bullying victim	15–18%
Bullying perpetrator	9–13%
Persistence into adulthood	60–80%
Intermediate	
Polycystic ovarian syndrome	3%
Obstructive sleep apnea	5–7%
Tibia vara	1–2%
Slipped capital femoral epiphysis	1–2%
Type 2 diabetes mellitus	2–4%
Infrequent	≤ 1%
Congenital malformations	
Fetal and infant mortality	
Pseudotumor cerebri	

Note. The data in this table are derived from both population-based and clinical studies, so not all estimates are representative of the general population of children and adolescents with obesity. GTT, glucose tolerance test; QOL, quality of life.

diabetes and folic acid deficiency, both of which are increased in women with obesity, may contribute to these findings.

Maternal obesity, and particularly gestational diabetes, also affect neonatal outcomes. Macrosomia may lead to complications at delivery, which in turn may lead to the need for a caesarian section. Both increased fetal size, as well as other complications associated with obesity during pregnancy, may help explain why the frequency of caesarian section increases with the severity of obesity. Among women with severe obesity, the risk of caesarian section is almost threefold higher than its frequency among women at a healthy weight. Gestational diabetes increases the risk of neonatal hypoglycemia, because of the delay in compensation when the rich intrauterine supply of glucose ends with delivery.

Prevalent Consequences of Obesity

Asthma, nonalcoholic fatty liver disease (NAFLD), and cardiovascular disease risk factors are among the most prevalent consequences of obesity in children and adolescents. The prevalence of asthma among children and adolescents with obesity ranges from 6 to 9%. A large cohort study has demonstrated an increased incidence of asthma among children with obesity, and a dose–response relationship of asthma with the degree of obesity. The incidence of asthma was increased among white and black children compared to Hispanic children, and was greater in boys and in younger children. The severity of asthma, assessed by medical visits and medication use, also increased with the severity of obesity.

NAFLD, the most frequent liver disease in children, may progress to nonalcoholic steatohepatitis (NASH), an abnormality that can progress to cirrhosis and liver failure. The liver enzyme alanine aminotransferase (ALT) has been used as a marker of NAFLD. Elevated ALT has been found in approximately 17% of overweight 12- to 19-year-olds, and 38–52% of 12- to 19-year-olds with obesity. An autopsy study of children dying of a variety of nonmedical causes disclosed that the prevalence of NASH was 8.7% among children with obesity and fatty liver.

Abnormal glucose tolerance, which is the precursor of type 2 diabetes mellitus, occurs in 21% of children and 25% of adolescents with obesity studied clinically. In large population studies, the prevalence of type 2 diabetes mellitus in children and adolescents has been estimated at .24/1000, or .02%. However, clinical studies have found a prevalence of 2–4% of silent diabetes among children with obesity. The prevalence of type 2 diabetes accounts for only 5% of all diabetes in whites, but almost 38% in blacks, 35% in Hispanics, and 80% among Native American youth. Onset generally occurs after 10 years of age. Although type 2 diabetes is rare in adolescents, associated microvascular disease occurs earlier in those affected by type 2 diabetes, thereby increasing the risk of nephropathy and myocardial infarcts in early adulthood.

The prevalence of a number of cardiovascular disease risk factors is also increased in childhood obesity. A comprehensive systematic review demonstrated statistically significant increases in fasting glucose, insulin, triglycerides, systolic and diastolic blood pressures and left ventricular mass, and lower levels of high-density lipoprotein (HDL)-cholesterol. The prevalence of these abnormalities ranges from approximately 10–25%. Among children and adolescents with obesity, 30% have at least one cardiovascular disease risk factor, such as elevated blood pressure, abnormal lipids, or fasting insulin, and 60% have two or more. The magnitude of these increases is even greater among adolescents with severe obesity presenting for bariatric surgery, although selection bias could account for some of these differences.

Childhood and adolescent obesity increase the risk of orthopedic complications. Although tibia vara and slipped capital femoral epiphysis are uncommon, increased weight bearing increases the likelihood of fractures and musculoskeletal injuries. Although relatively few children develop tibia vara, misalignment of the femur and tibia probably contributes to the increased frequency of knee pain.

A comprehensive study that combined four prospective data sets provides insights into the long-term consequences of obesity. Four groups of children studied at a mean age of 11 years were followed up approximately 23 years later. Based on their childhood and subsequent adult weight, four groups were established: Group 1 included individuals who had a healthy weight in childhood and as adults; Group 2 developed obesity in childhood but returned to a healthy weight by adulthood; Group 3 had a healthy weight in childhood but developed obesity in adulthood; and Group 4 developed obesity in childhood that persisted into adulthood. The risk of type 2 diabetes, hypertension, reduced HDL cholesterol, and elevated low-density lipoprotein (LDL) cholesterol, triglycerides, and intima media thickness were all increased in adults with persistent obesity from childhood, as well as adults who developed obesity in adulthood. Those individuals who developed obesity in childhood but achieved a healthy weight by adulthood had levels of these risk factors that were comparable to those in individuals who never developed obesity.

The risk of adult obesity varied directly with child weight status. Fifteen percent of normal-weight children, 60% of overweight children, and 82% of children with obesity were affected by obesity in adulthood. Overweight children and adolescents with obesity accounted for 44% of adult obesity.

These observations raise several concerns. Childhood-onset obesity may be associated with more severe obesity in adulthood. In addition, the likelihood that an adult with obesity will achieve a healthy body weight is less than 1%, with even lower rates for adults with more severe obesity. These observations emphasize that the effective control of a substantial proportion of adult obesity must begin by preventing childhood obesity.

Psychosocial Consequences of Obesity

Although overweight and obesity affect over 30% of children and adolescents, bias and stigmatization remain common. The reaction to bias likely accounts for the lower health-related quality-of-life scores observed in children and adolescents with obesity compared to healthy children and adolescents. Both physical health and psychosocial health scores are significantly reduced. Psychosocial health scores are significantly lower for emotional functioning, social functioning, and school functioning domains. Impaired physical functioning is not unexpected because of the impact of obesity on the ease and energy costs of movement, both of which increase with increasing severity of obesity.

A second consequence of obesity, and at times a potential cause of stigmatization, is bullying. In school-age children, the frequency of becoming a victim of bullying ranges from 15% (boys)–18% (girls), and the frequency of perpetrating bullying ranges from 9% (girls)–13% (boys). These may be early signs of exposure to adverse childhood experiences, which predict severe obesity in adulthood.

Suggested Reading

Aune, D., Saugstad, O. D., Henriksen, T., & Tonstad, S. (2014). Maternal body mass index and the risk of fetal death, stillbirth, and infant death: A systematic review and meta-analysis. *Journal of the American Medical Association, 311*(15), 1536–1546.—This article presents a comprehensive view of obesity and the associated risk of fetal and perinatal mortality.

Black, M. H., Zhou, H., Takayanagi, M., Jacobsen, S. J., & Koebnick, C. (2013). Increased asthma risk and asthma-related health care complications associated with childhood obesity. *American Journal of Epidemiology, 178*(7), 1120–1128.—Large cohort study from Kaiser Permanente that demonstrates the significant disease burden asociated with asthma in children with obesity.

Fildes, A., Charlton, J., Rudisill, C., Littlejohns, P., Prevost, A. T., & Gulliford, M. C. (2015). Probability of an obese person attaining normal body weight: Cohort study using electronic health records. *American Journal of Public Health, 105*(9), e54–e59.—This recent study has shown the low odds of an adult with obesity achieving a healthy weight over a 9-year period of follow-up.

Janssen, I., Craig, W. M., Boyce, W. F., & Pickett, W. (2004). Associations between overweight and obesity with bullying behaviors in school-aged children. *Pediatrics, 113*(5), 1187–1194.—Population-based study of the association of obesity with victimization and perpetration of bullying.

Juonala, M., Magnussen, C. G., Berenson, G. S., Venn, A., Burns, T. L., Sabin, M. A., et al. (2011). Childhood adiposity, adult adiposity, and cardiovascular risk factors. *New England Journal of Medicine, 365*(20), 1876–1885.—This study combines four prospective cohort studies to describe the relationship of childhood obesity to subsequent adult obesity, diabetes, and cardiovascular risk factors.

Schwimmer, J. B., Burwinkle, T. M., & Varni, J. W. (2003). Health-related quality of life of severely obese children and adolescents. *Journal of the American Medical Association, 289*(14), 1813–1819.—Clincal study that compares health-related quality-of-life measures in children and adolescents with obesity to healthy controls and to children with cancer.

Schwimmer, J. B., Deutsch, R., Kahen, T., Lavine, J. E., Stanley, C., & Behling, C. (2006). Prevalence of fatty liver in children and adolescents. *Pediatrics, 118*(4), 1388–1393.—Autopsy study that demonstrates the prevalence of NAFLD and NASH.

Stothard, K. J., Tennant, P. W., Bell, R., & Rankin, J. (2009). Maternal overweight and obesity and the risk of congenital anomalies: A systematic review and meta-analysis. *Journal of the American Medical Association, 301*(6), 636–650.—This study presents a comprehensive analysis of the likelihood of a variety of congenital anomalies.

Taylor, E. D., Theim, K. R., Mirch, M. C., Ghorbani, S., Tanofsky-Kraff, M., Adler-Wailes, D. C., et al. (2006). Orthopedic complications of overweight in children and adolescents. *Pediatrics, 117*(6), 2167–2174.—Clinical study documenting the frequency of musculoskeletal complications of childhood obesity.

Effects of Weight Loss on Health Outcomes

RENA R. WING

A large number of epidemiological studies have examined the association between changes in weight and health outcomes. However, these observational studies have important methodological problems, including the inability to distinguish between intentional and unintentional weight loss (perhaps due to illness). Randomized controlled trials, in which some participants are randomly assigned to lose weight and others to serve as controls, provide far stronger conclusions about the benefits (or risks) of weight loss. To date, most randomized trials of weight loss have focused on the short-term effects of weight loss. Although these studies have consistently documented benefits of weight loss on health parameters, such as cardiovascular risk factors, their short duration precludes the ability to examine effects on more critical health outcomes related to morbidity and mortality. Recently there have been several randomized controlled trials examining the long-term health benefits of weight loss. This chapter focuses on these long-term randomized trials and the health benefits of weight loss in (1) prevention of diabetes and (2) individuals who already have type 2 diabetes. The chapter also addresses issues related to the magnitude of weight loss needed to produce health benefits and possible adverse effects of weight loss and weight cycling.

Weight Loss in the Prevention of Type 2 Diabetes

Type 2 diabetes is a major health problem because it occurs so frequently and has serious adverse effects on health. It provides a good model for prevention efforts for several reasons. First, prior to the development of type 2 diabetes, there is a period in which there are elevations in glucose levels, but these levels are not yet high enough to be diagnostic of diabetes. This provides an ideal window for prevention efforts. In addition, many of the risk factors for diabetes (including overweight and sedentary lifestyle) can be modified by lifestyle intervention.

There have been a number of trials examining the effect of lifestyle intervention on prevention of type 2 diabetes, including the Diabetes Prevention Program (DPP), which showed conclusively that the incidence of type 2 diabetes may be dramatically reduced by lifestyle intervention in those at high risk of developing this disease. This multicenter randomized trial involved 3,234 overweight or obese individuals, recruited at 27 centers throughout the United States, who had elevated glucose levels fasting (95–125 mg/dl) and 2 hours after a 75-gram oral glucose load (140–199 mg/dl). These participants were randomly assigned to one of three groups: lifestyle intervention, metformin, or placebo. The lifestyle intervention was delivered on a one-to-one basis, with 16 core sessions over the first 24 weeks, then frequent (typically monthly) individual follow-up meetings and group sessions. The goals of the lifestyle intervention were to lose 7% of initial body weight through a healthy low-calorie, low-fat eating plan, and to engage in at least 150 minutes per week of physical activity. Weight losses over the 16-week core curriculum averaged 6.5 ± 4.7 kg (or 6.9 ± 4.5% of initial weight) and 4.5 ± 6 kg (or 4.9 ± 7.4%) after 3 years of intervention. Participants reported 224 ± 141 minutes/week of activity at the end of the core curriculum, and 227 ± 212 at the end of the intervention.

The primary outcome of DPP, reported after an average follow-up of 2.8 years, was that the lifestyle intervention reduced the risk of developing diabetes by 58% compared to placebo, and metformin reduced the risk of developing diabetes by 31% compared to placebo. The lifestyle intervention was significantly more effective than metformin. Although the DPP lifestyle program included strategies to decrease dietary fat intake, increase physical activity, and lose weight, subsequent analyses showed that weight loss was the primary determinant of the reduced risk of diabetes. Increased physical activity and lowered fat intake predicted weight loss and maintenance, but it was the weight loss that predicted reduction in diabetes incidence. For every kilogram of weight loss, there was a 16% reduction in diabetes risk, adjusted for changes in diet and physical activity. These findings confirm the results of several other randomized trials, including the Finnish Diabetes Prevention Study and the Da Qing Study, showing that weight loss reduces risk of diabetes.

Equally striking are the longer-term outcomes of the DPP. Based on the positive initial effects of lifestyle intervention in preventing diabetes, DPP participants who had been randomly assigned to metformin or placebo were offered group-implemented lifestyle intervention, and all participants were invited to participate in continued follow-up over time. During the 10 years of follow-up from randomization, the lifestyle group gradually regained weight, although it still weighed 2 kg less at 10 years than it did at randomization. However, despite the regain, the beneficial effects of the lifestyle intervention were maintained. Across the entire 10 years, the incidence of diabetes was reduced by 34% in the lifestyle intervention and 18% in the metformin group compared with placebo. Thus, the effects of lifestyle intervention, focused primarily on weight loss, persisted for at least 10 years.

Weight Loss in Individuals Who Already Have Type 2 Diabetes

Although the DPP showed that weight loss could help prevent development of diabetes, it raised questions about those who already have this disease. Would lifestyle intervention in those who have diabetes help to reduce their risk of cardiovascular disease? Look AHEAD. a randomized trial of lifestyle intervention for individuals with type 2 diabetes, was designed to answer this question. In this trial, over 5,000 overweight or obese individuals with type 2 diabetes were recruited and randomly assigned to intensive lifestyle intervention (ILI) or diabetes support and education (DSE), the control group for this trial. The study population included 59% women, 37% ethnic minorities, and 14% individuals with a prior history of cardiovascular disease; the average body mass index (BMI) was 36 kg/m², and the average duration of diabetes was 6.8 years.

Participants assigned to ILI received a combination of group and individual sessions designed to help them lose 10% of their body weight. Weight loss was accomplished through a low-calorie, low-fat eating plan (with meal replacement products used to improve adherence to the plan) and 175 minutes/week of moderate-intensity physical activity. On average, participants in ILI lost 8.6% of their initial weight at 1 year, compared to 0.7% in DSE. At 4 years, weight losses were 4.7 and 1.1% in ILI and DSE, respectively, and at 8 years, weight losses were 4.7 and 2.1%, respectively. The ILI also produced significant improvements in cardiovascular fitness and changes in most risk factors (with the exception of low-density lipoprotein [LDL] cholesterol), and led to decreased use of insulin, hypertension medications, and lipid-lowering medications.

The primary outcome of Look AHEAD was a composite cardiovascular outcome, including fatal or nonfatal myocardial infarction or stroke, and hospitalization for angina. Despite the differences in weight loss, risk factors, and fitness changes, Look AHEAD found no differences between ILI and DSE on cardiovascular events. There were 403 patients in ILI who had a primary outcome, compared to 418 in the control group, which was not a statistically significant difference. There has been a great deal of speculation about these outcomes. It may be that larger weight losses are needed to observe beneficial effects. Alternatively, the fact that there was no difference in LDL cholesterol between ILI and DSE, and that lipid-lowering agents were used more frequently in DSE than in ILI, may have obscured difference between the two arms. Another possibility is that earlier intervention is needed to reduce the risk of heart disease.

Although Look AHEAD did not see beneficial effects of weight loss on cardiovascular morbidity and mortality, the study showed other important benefits of weight loss in this patient group. Of particular note are the following positive effects of ILI on important health outcomes. Participants in ILI, relative to those in DSE, were more likely to experience a complete or partial remission of their diabetes. At 1 year, 11.5% of ILI participants, compared with 2% of DSE participants, experienced remission; at 4 years, remission was seen in 7.3% of ILI participants and 1.5% of DSE participants. The lifestyle intervention also reduced incidence of very-high-risk kidney disease by 31%, improved urinary incontinence in both women and men, and improved quality of life. The declines in mobility that are typically seen with aging were reduced in ILI relative to DSE, as was knee pain. Finally, the ILI reduced the number of days in the hospital by 15% and resulted in cost savings for both hospitalizations and medication use. Thus, there were clearly a wide variety of beneficial effects of the ILI on the health of individuals with diabetes.

Weight Loss and Mortality

Observational studies have produced conflicting findings relative to the effects of weight loss on mortality, with some studies suggesting that weight loss is associated with lower risk of mortality, but others suggesting that it is associated with increased risk. The inability to distinguish between intentional and unintentional weight loss may be responsible for these conflicting findings. Few clinical trials have extended long enough to examine the effects of lifestyle intervention on all-cause mortality. In Look AHEAD, there was a nonsignificant reduction in total mortality in ILI relative to DSE, and follow-up is continuing to address this. In a meta-analysis of weight loss trials, lifestyle interventions led to a 15% reduction in all-cause mortality. Thus, this is an area in need of further study.

How Much Weight Loss Is Needed for Health Benefits?

An important, frequently asked question is "How much weight loss is needed for health benefits?" The answer appears to be that beneficial effects of weight loss are often seen with only modest weight reductions; thus, overweight and obese persons are frequently encouraged to lose 5–10% of their weight. However, it is also important to recognize that larger weight losses typically yield better results. Data from Look AHEAD suggest that such modest weight losses improve many health parameters, but often a clear dose–response relationship is seen between magnitude of weight loss and health outcomes. In addition, it is unclear whether the short- and long-term effects of a specific weight loss are equivalent, or whether sustained weight loss, without further weight reduction, loses its beneficial effect.

In Look AHEAD, the magnitude of weight loss was strongly associated with improvements in glycemia, blood pressure, triglycerides, and high-density lipoprotein (HDL)-cholesterol at 1 year, but not with changes in LDL-cholesterol. Compared with weight-stable individuals, those who lost 5–10% of their body weight at 1 year were more likely to achieve clinically significant improvements in hemaglobin A1c (HbA1c), diastolic and systolic blood pressure, triglycerides, and HLD cholesterol. However, those who lost 10% of their weight or more had even greater improvements on each of these parameters.

Modest weight losses improved not only risk factors but also disease outcomes, including hepatic steatosis and sleep apnea in persons with type 2 diabetes. Using proton magnetic resonance to assess fatty infiltration of the liver, participants who lost > 10% of their body weight at 1 year had significantly greater median percent reductions in steatosis compared to weight-stable individuals (79.5 vs. 13.7%). Likewise, when sleep apnea was assessed with home polysomnography, there were significant reductions in the Apnea–Hypopnea Index (AHI) with weight loss. Those individuals who lost ≥ 10 kg at 1 year experienced a reduction in AHI of 11.3 events/hour, which was significantly greater than that in all other weight loss categories. Weight losses at year 4 were also strongly associated with improvements in sleep apnea, suggesting long-term benefits of weight loss of at least 10 kg on this health outcome.

Potential Adverse Effects of Weight Loss

Although most of the effects of weight loss on health outcomes are positive, there are a few important potential adverse outcomes. Gallstones and cholecystitis have been reported, especially with rapid weight loss. In addition, weight loss leads to reductions in lean body mass, which can affect muscle strength and bone density. Concerns about loss of lean body mass have raised questions about the risk–benefit ratio of weight loss in individuals over the age of 70. For the most part, however, the advantages of weight loss far exceed these concerns.

Concerns about Weight Cycling

Frequently, individuals who lose weight are unable to maintain it and may gradually regain back to baseline. This has raised concerns about possible negative effects of such weight cycles or "yo-yo dieting." Although, clearly, it is best to lose weight and maintain it, there is little evidence to support the statement that intentional weight loss followed by regain is detrimental to health, especially in overweight or obese persons. In a prospective study of weight changes and their association with changes in cardiovascular risk factors, those who lost weight and regained it had risk factors comparable to those who remained weight-stable throughout. In epidemiological studies, many of which are derived from the Nurses' Health Study, those women who lost weight intentionally and regained it several times did not appear to be at increased risk of health problems and mortality, after adjusting for BMI at age 18 and current BMI. Finally in the DPP, discussed earlier, there were long-term beneficial effects of weight loss despite the fact that much of the weight had been regained.

Conclusions

Lifestyle interventions for overweight and obese individuals produce important health benefits. Losing just 5–10% of body weight yields positive outcomes, although larger weight losses produce greater improvements. Efforts to achieve and maintain these weight losses should therefore be strongly encouraged.

Suggested Reading

Diabetes Prevention Program Research Group. (2002). Reduction in the incidence of type 2 diabetes with lifestyle intervention or metformin. *New England Journal of Medicine, 346*(6), 393–402.—Presents the primary findings of the DPP, showing that weight loss reduces risk of developing diabetes.

Diabetes Prevention Program Research Group. (2009). 10-year follow-up of diabetes incidence and weight loss in the Diabetes Prevention Program Outcomes Study. *Lancet, 374,* 1677–1686.—This report documents the long-term effects of lifestyle intervention on the risk of developing diabetes.

Jensen, M. D., Ryan, D. H., Donato, K. A., Apovian, C. M., Ard, J. D., Comuzzie, A. G., et al. (2014). Guidelines (2013) for managing overweight and obesity in adults. *Obesity, 22*(Suppl. 2), S1–S410.—This document provides a detailed discussion and considers the strength of the evidence for the effects of reduction in body weight on cardiovascular disease events and risk factors, morbidity, and mortality.

Kritchevsky, S. B., Beavers, K. M., Miller, M. E., Shea, M. K., Houston, D. K., Kitzman, D. W., et al. (2015). Intentional weight loss and all-cause mortality: A meta-analysis of randomized clinical trials. *PLoS ONE, 10*(3), e0121993.—This recent meta-analysis suggests that lifestyle interventions may have positive effects on mortality.

Pi-Sunyer, F. X. (1993). Short-term medical benefits and adverse effects of weight loss. *Annals of Internal Medicine, 119*(7, Pt. 2), 722–726.—This author does an excellent job of reviewing not only the positive but also the adverse effects of weight loss.

Wing, R. R., Bolin, P., Brancati, F. L., Bray, G. A., Clark, J. M., Coday, M., et al. (2013). Cardiovascular effects of intensive lifestyle intervention in type 2 diabetes. *New England Journal of Medicine, 369,* 145–154.—This article presents the primary results of the Look

AHEAD trial, showing that lifetyle intervention did not reduce the risk of cardiovascular events.

Wing, R. R., Jeffery, R. W., & Hellerstedt, W. L. (1995). A prospective study of effects of weight cycling on cardiovascular risk factors. *Archives of Internal Medicine, 155*(13), 1416–1422.— This article documents the effects of losing weight and regaining it, relative to never having lost weight at all, on cardiovascular risk factors.

Wing, R. R., Lang, W., Wadden, T. A., Safford, M., Knowler, W. C., Bertoni, A. G., et al. (2011). Benefits of modest weight loss in improving cardiovascular risk factors in overweight and obese individuals with type 2 diabetes. *Diabetes Care, 34*(7), 1481–1486.—Using data from Look AHEAD, this article shows the dose–response relationships between weight loss and cardiovascular risk factors.

Social and Psychological Effects of Weight Loss

LUCY F. FAULCONBRIDGE

Obesity is often experienced alongside an array of other negative health consequences, some physical and some psychological. Many obese individuals wish to lose weight, in part because they seek relief from the significant physical comorbidities that come with obesity, and in part because they covet freedom from the heavy psychological burden of obesity, which includes stigma and discrimination, poor body image and self-esteem, low mood, and poor quality of life. This chapter summarizes the research findings on the effects of intentional weight loss on mood, body image, and quality of life in overweight/obese individuals. Theoretical mechanisms for how weight loss could lead to either improvement or deterioration in mood are presented, and known predictors for negative psychological outcomes of weight loss are summarized. Each section addresses areas for further research.

Effects of Weight Loss on Mood

The debate about whether weight loss improves or worsens mood has been ongoing for more than half a century. A seminal study published in 1950 by Ancel Keys raised concerns about the effects of dieting and weight loss on psychological stability. In an experiment designed to develop optimal refeeding practices for military personnel who were returning from prisoner of war camps in an emaciated state, Keys and his colleagues recruited normal-weight men and induced dramatic weight loss (25% of initial weight). Prior to the refeeding phase, Keys noticed a deterioration in the psychological health of many of his participants, and some developed full-blown mental health disorders, including depression, anxiety, kleptomania, and food hoarding, exhibiting many of the same symptoms observed today in those with anorexia nervosa. The results of this study became a warning to researchers about the negative mental health implications of severe weight loss.

A second study, published in 1957, by Albert Stunkard fueled concerns about weight loss as it reported adverse psychological symptoms in a group of obese adults losing weight on a psychiatric inpatient ward. Indeed, this study coined the phrase "dieting depression" to characterize the nervousness and mental instability observed in these patients. Unfortunately, the conclusions from these studies, in which the samples were either normal-weight individuals losing dramatic amounts of weight or psychiatric inpatients with many comorbid mental health conditions, have been mistakenly applied to the majority of overweight/obese individuals undertaking moderate weight losses (5–10% of initial weight).

In fact, the majority of weight loss trials undertaken in nondepressed individuals reveal improvements rather than worsening of mood, as well as protection against the incidence of depression and suicidal ideation. For example, a large meta-analysis conducted by Fabricatore and his colleagues in 2011 found that across 31 studies analyzed, intentional weight loss was associated with modest improvements in mood, but the magnitude of weight loss was not correlated with the reduction in symptoms of depression. Furthermore, Faulconbridge and colleagues (2012) investigated changes in symptoms of depression over 1 year as individuals lost weight in the Look AHEAD (Action for Health in Diabetes) trial, a very large, nationally representative randomized controlled trial in which overweight/obese individuals with type 2 diabetes were assigned to an intensive lifestyle intervention (ILI) designed to induce a 7% weight loss, or to a usual care control group. Weight loss was not associated with precipitation of symptoms of depression; instead, it appeared to protect against development of depression.

The majority of studies finding overall positive effects of weight loss on mood were carried out in adult samples of a wide age range (18–70 years). In older individuals, there is mixed evidence about whether moderate weight loss results in improvements in mood. A recent population-based study in the United Kingdom, which analyzed the relationship between weight loss and mood over 2 years in overweight/obese adults over age 50, showed a greater incidence of depressed mood in individuals who lost at least 5% of their weight, compared to those who remained weight-stable or who gained weight. This difference remained significant, even when researchers controlled for baseline weight and mood, weight loss intention, and major life events. These results echo findings from two other studies, the Health and Retirement Study and the Health ABC study, which revealed no psychological benefit to weight loss, and found some evidence that weight loss was associated with deterioration in mood. Clearly, more research is needed to determine whether specific factors (e.g., age) determine the psychological response to weight loss.

Of particular note is the issue of the clinical significance of changes in symptoms of depression assessed in research trials. Depending on the sample size, small improvements in mood may be statistically significant but may not translate into any noticeable improvement for the patient. A fascinating area of future research might address how much change in mood is necessary to be clinically significant, and how much weight loss is typically required to achieve such improvements.

Theoretical Mechanisms for Improvements in Mood with Weight Loss

Most individuals experience a sense of accomplishment and pride as they lose weight and improve their body image and self-esteem. They are able to buy smaller clothes, and they report increased confidence at social occasions. Many of the significant psychological burdens associated with obesity, such as prejudice and social stigma, may be lifted as individuals lose weight. In addition, the positive reinforcement they receive from others as their weight loss is noticed can be very rewarding. The improvements in physical functioning that are seen with weight loss enable individuals to be more active and have fewer physical ailments, leading to an overall improved quality of life. Finally, there may be biological mechanisms associated with weight loss, such as reductions in inflammatory cytokines and leptin, which may result in improvements in mood, although this research is still in its infancy.

There is not yet good evidence to explain how losing moderate amounts of weight would cause psychological harm. Several theories have been proposed, however. Maintaining weight loss over the long term is notoriously difficult, and the personal demands required to be successful with weight loss may impair mood. Western environments offer so much opportunity to consume highly palatable foods at low cost that the levels of self-control that must be sustained over long periods may simply represent a high psychological tax. Such an environment predisposes many individuals to be unsuccessful at losing dramatic amounts of weight, leading individuals to be unhappy with more moderate (5–10% of initial weight) weight losses. As individuals lose weight, biological mechanisms may be initiated to restore lost fat, causing increases in hunger and making weight loss progressively harder.

Another potential pathway for weight loss to result in worsening mood symptoms concerns expectations about how weight loss will affect life overall. For example, some individuals mistakenly believe that weight loss will radically change their lives, making them more likable, solving their interpersonal problems, and bringing them more friends. As individuals find that weight loss does not necessarily lead to the fruition of these wishes, they may become extremely disappointed given all the work they invested to lose weight. Finally, some individuals may not like the increased attention that weight loss brings. Attention and compliments may not be well received by shy individuals who feel upset that they are now being treated differently simply because they are leaner. These changes can serve to highlight the poor treatment they received when they were heavier, paradoxically, causing them more pain.

Predictors of Worsening Mood in Weight Loss Trials

Clearly, there is mixed evidence about the relationship between weight loss and changes in mood. While the majority of overweight/obese individuals who lose moderate amount of weight can expect to enjoy improvements in their mood, some individuals do not. Identifying predictors for worsening mood in individuals losing weight is critically important, such that weight loss interventions can be tailored appropriately to assess and target worsening symptoms of depression. In 2009, Faulconbridge and colleagues examined changes in symptoms of depression in participants undergoing different weight loss treatments: behavior modification, pharmacotherapy (i.e., sibutramine), or their combination. Over the course of a year, they observed that 8.5% of individuals in the behavior modification alone group experienced significant worsening in symptoms of depression (defined as an increase of 5 or more points on the Beck Depression Inventory). Predictors of worsening symptoms of depression across treatments included a prior psychiatric history and suboptimal weight losses. Similarly, 6.3% of patients in the ILI in the Look AHEAD trial who were not depressed at baseline did report clinically significant symptoms of depression at 1 year, and this change was negatively associated with weight change. Busch and colleagues (2013) analyzed changes in mood in depressed participants in the Be Active Trial. In the lifestyle intervention condition, participants with a comorbid psychiatric diagnosis and attention-deficit/hyperactivity disorder (ADHD) symptoms at baseline were associated with nonresponse (i.e., no improvement in symptoms of depression), while higher baseline depression scores, lower hedonic capacity, and the absence of ADHD symptoms were associated with greater likelihood of experiencing an improvement in symptoms of depression. Taken together, these results suggest that a prior psychiatric history, moderate levels of depression at baseline, current symptoms of ADHD, and suboptimal weight loss during a lifestyle modification intervention may be predictors of worsening symptoms of depression. As such, we tentatively suggest that clinicians maintain a watchful eye for these symptoms and be ready to offer more support to those participants. Clearly, however, robust research into the identification of the potential predictors of worsening symptoms of depression while undertaking weight loss is lacking and represents an important area of further inquiry.

Effects of Weight Loss on Body Image

Research shows significant improvements in body image as participants lose weight. In a meta-analysis published in 2015, Chao found that improvements in body shape concerns, body size dissatisfaction, and body satisfaction all favored the intervention groups over control groups. Despite the improvements in body image observed with weight loss, the magnitude of change in body image does not always correlate with the amount of weight loss, such that the same improvements in body image are reported with moderate and significant weight losses. This finding suggests a potential threshold effect, such that moderate weight loss induces positive changes in body image that are not augmented by further weight losses.

Despite the improvements in body image associated with weight loss, some studies show that formerly overweight individuals experience more negative body image than people of the same weight who were never overweight. Even individuals who have experienced significant weight loss may retain negative feelings about their bodies, including shame, self-disgust, and distorted thoughts about their bodies. Further research needs to identify which individuals are apt to retain negative body image, and the mechanisms that improve or hinder body image during weight loss.

Effects of Weight Loss on Quality of Life

The majority of studies examining changes in quality of life with weight loss reveal improvements in both physical and psychological components of quality of life. This relationship has been observed across studies using different assessment instruments and appears to be independent of the means by which weight loss is achieved (lifestyle modification, pharmacotherapy, or bariatric surgery). Moreover, some studies suggest a correlation between the magnitude of weight loss and the degree to which quality of life improves. Despite the positive effect observed in individual studies, however, a 2005 meta-analysis of 34 randomized controlled trials conducted by Maciejewski and colleagues found very little consistent relationship between weight loss and changes in quality of life. One explanation for these discrepant findings may be due to the use of obesity-specific, as compared to generic, measurements of quality of life. Future research may need to focus on larger sample sizes and discriminate between participants losing moderate (5–10% of initial weight) and those losing significant amounts of weight (30–40% of initial weight).

Summary

Obesity is associated with many physical and psychological challenges. Research suggests that the overwhelming majority of overweight/obese individuals losing moderate amounts of weight will experience improvements in their mood, body image, and quality of life. For a significant minority, however, such improvements do not materialize, and for some, weight loss comes with either no improvement or deteriorations in functioning within these areas. We encourage more research in this area, so that individuals at risk for worsening mood, body image, and quality of life can be identified and given adjunctive treatment. As clinicians help patients make decisions about whether to undertake weight loss, the potential risks of weight loss for that individual must be tempered against the risks, both psychological and physical, of remaining obese.

Suggested Reading

Busch, A. M., Whited, M. C., Appelhans, B. M., Schneider, K. L., Waring, M. E., DeBiasse, M. A., et al. (2013). Reliable change in depression during behavioral weight loss treatment among women with major depression. *Obesity, 21*(3), E211–E218.—This study evaluated predictors of changes in mood in the Be Active Trial as participants lost weight.

Chao, H. L. (2015) Body image change in obese and overweight persons enrolled in weight loss intervention programs: A systematic review and meta-analysis. *PLoS ONE, 10*(5), e0124036.—This systematic review and meta-analysis showed that weight loss interventions significantly improved body shape concern, body image, and body satisfaction in obese/overweight persons compared to control groups.

Fabricatore, A. N., Wadden, T. A., Higginbotham, A. J., Faulconbridge, L. F., Nguyen, A. M., Heymsfield, S. B., et al. (2011). Intentional weight loss and changes in symptoms of depression: A systematic review and meta-analysis. *International Journal of Obesity, 35*(11), 1363–1376.—This meta-analysis examined changes in symptoms of depression with different weight loss interventions.

Faulconbridge, L. F., Wadden, T. A., Berkowitz, R. I., Sarwer, D. B., Womble, L. G., Hesson, L. A., et al. (2009). Changes in symptoms of depression with weight loss: Results of a randomized trial. *Obesity, 17*(5), 1009–1016.—This study examined changes in symptoms of depression in 194 obese participants in a 1-year randomized trial of lifestyle modification and medication. While mean symptoms of depression declined across all participants at 1 year, 13.9% of participants reported discernible increases in symptoms of depression.

Faulconbridge, L. F., Wadden, T. A., Rubin, R. R., Wing, R. R., Walkup, M. P., Fabricatore, A. N., et al. (2012). One-year changes in symptoms of depression and weight in overweight/obese individuals with type 2 diabetes in the Look AHEAD study. *Obesity, 20*(4), 783–793.—This study examined whether moderate weight loss in overweight/obese individuals with type 2 diabetes would be associated with incident symptoms of depression and suicidal ideation in the Look AHEAD (Action for Health in Diabetes) study.

Jackson, S. E., Steptoe, A., Beeken, R. J., Kivimaki, M., & Wardle, J. (2014). Psychological changes following weight loss in overweight and obese adults: A prospective cohort study. *PLoS ONE, 9*(8), e104552.—This prospective study examined cardiometabolic and psychological changes following weight loss in a cohort of almost 2,000 overweight/obese adults, and called into question the notion that weight loss is associated with improvement in psychological well-being.

Keys, A., Brožek, J., Henschel, A., Mickelsen, O., & Taylor, H. L. (1950). *The biology of human starvation.* Minneapolis: University of Minnesota Press.—This seminal work examined the psychological changes elicited by calorie restriction and dramatic weight loss.

Maciejewski, M. L., Patrick, D. L., & Williamson, D. F. (2005). A structured review of randomized controlled trials of weight loss showed little improvement in health-related quality of life. *Journal of Clinical Epidemiology, 58*(6), 568–578.—These reviewers examined the effect of weight loss interventions on health-related quality of life and symptoms of depression in randomized controlled trials and found mixed results.

Stunkard, A. J. (1957). The "dieting depression": Incidence and clinical characteristics of untoward responses to weight reduction regimens. *American Journal of Medicine, 23*(1), 77–86.—This author coined the term "dieting depression" to describe an array of unexpected adverse psychological consequences of calorie restriction and weight reduction in a minority of patients in a weight reduction clinic.

TREATMENT OF OBESITY

Clinical Assessment of Patients with Obesity

ROBERT F. KUSHNER

The clinical assessment of patients presenting with obesity is important for understanding the etiology of the disorder in the individual patient and for establishing a tailored treatment plan. Not all clinical assessments have to be conducted by a physician, although one has to be knowledgeable about the multiple determinants of obesity, assessment for the presence and extent of comorbidities, recommendations for further medical and laboratory evaluation, as needed, and recognition of individuals at high risk for complications of obesity. The clinical assessment includes a focused medical history, a careful physical examination, and, as appropriate, laboratory studies. In addition, evaluation of readiness, motivation for weight loss, and potential barriers to change need to be appraised.

Assessment

Screening Recommendations

Based on the burden of obesity and the benefits of treatment, the U.S. Preventive Services Task Force (USPSTF) recommends screening all adults for obesity and, that patients with a body mass index (BMI) ≥ 30 kg/m^2 receive intensive, multicomponent behavioral intervention, either in-office or by referral to another practitioner, registered dietitian, or commercial program. Monitoring BMI can help clinicians in primary care settings identify adult patients at risk for obesity complications. Accordingly, the 2013 Guidelines for Managing Overweight and Obesity in Adults recommends measuring height and weight and calculating BMI at annual visits or more frequently, depending on the patient's risk factors. The Centers for Medicare and Medicaid Services (CMS) has also mandated that electronic medical records (EMR) calculate BMI as part of Core Measures on Vital Signs. The EMR is also capable of tracking weight trajectory, so that intervention can occur at an earlier time point to prevent further weight gain.

Taking an Obesity-Focused History

Once a diagnosis of obesity is established and the patient has health reasons to lose weight, issues that will effect treatment decisions should be incorporated into the history. This "obesity-focused" history allows the physician to develop tailored treatment recommendations that are more consistent with the needs and goals of the individual patient. For many patients, weight gain initially occurs or is accelerated coincident to smoking cessation, initiation of a medication, or change in life events, such as a change in marital status, occupation, or illness. At-risk times for women also include pregnancy and menopause. Stressful life events often result in a change in eating and physical activity habits. Additional clinical information obtained from the interview is listed in Table 77.1.

For all patients, a dietary and physical activity history should be assessed prior to initiating counseling. Diet can be ascertained by taking a 24-hour recall, food frequency, or asking the patient to complete a food diary. Longitudinal studies have shown that cardiorespiratory fitness (as measured by a maximal treadmill exercise test) is an important predictor of all-cause mortality independent of BMI and body composition. Fit men and women who are obese have a lower risk of all-cause mortality than unfit, lean men and women. Consequently, fitness assessment is an important component of the clinical evaluation of patients with obesity. Assessment includes evaluation of cardiovascular risk and current engagement in physical activity. Detailed guidance on obtaining a physical activity history and providing fitness-related treatment recommendations can be found at Exercise is Medicine® and the 2008 Physical Activity Guidelines for Americans.

Assessment of psychological health and psychiatric history should be routinely obtained. Asking about mood disorders is important, since they are relatively common in the general population and occur in high rates among persons with obesity. Drug-induced weight gain should always be considered when there is a change in the trajectory of body weight coincident with starting a new medication. Common offenders include antidiabetics (insulin and sulfonylureas), antidepressants (amitriptyline, mirtazapine, and paroxetine), antipsychotics (olanzapine and clozapine), mood stabilizers (lithium and valproate), and corticosteroids. Substitution with a weight-neutral or weight-losing medication should be considered if possible.

Determining a patient's readiness to make lifestyle changes is an important part of the initial evaluation. The 2013 Guidelines recommend that physicians assess whether the patient is prepared and ready to undertake the measures necessary to succeed at weight loss before undertaking comprehensive counseling efforts. Many patients are ambivalent about changing long-standing lifestyle behaviors, fearing that it will be difficult, uncomfortable, or depriving. Motivational interviewing is a useful technique to elicit the patient's own motivation to change and to explore ambivalence, and has been shown to result in a modest amount of weight loss in patients with obesity.

Physical Examination of the Patient with Obesity

Accurate measurement of height and weight, which are used to calculate the BMI, is the initial step in the clinical assessment of the patient for obesity. Using BMI cutoff points to define healthy (18.5–24.9 kg/m²), overweight (25.0–29.9 kg/m²), and obese (≥ 30 kg/m²) states is useful for screening and treatment decisions. In addition to BMI, the 2013

TABLE 77.1. Obesity-Focused Clinical Information Obtained from Interview

1. What factors contribute to the patient's obesity?
   - Familial predisposition
   - Psychosocial life events (stress, emotional eating, time restraints)
   - Physical inactivity/excess caloric intake
   - Endocrine disorders (polycystic ovarian syndrome, hypothyroidism)
   - Iatrogenic drug-related weight gain
   - Psychiatric disorders (binge eating disorder, night eating syndrome)

2. How is the obesity affecting the patient's health?
   - Weight-related medical conditions and diseases (see Table 77.3)
   - Impaired quality of life
   - Self-esteem and body dissatisfaction

3. What is the patient's level of risk regarding obesity?
   - BMI classification
   - Waist circumference
   - Insulin resistance/metabolic syndrome
   - Severity and number of obesity-related conditions and diseases

4. What are the patient's goals and expectations?
   - Desired weight goal
   - Reduction in medication usage
   - Reduced morbidity and risk factors

5. What does the patient find hard about managing weight?
   - Life events, stress, and other responsibilities
   - Food preferences, cost and availability
   - Access to and time for increased physical activity
   - Boredom and monotony of diets

6. Is the patient motivated and engaged to enter a weight management program?
   - Contemplation, preparation, or action stage of change
   - Identifies short-term and long-term goals
   - Has social support
   - Identifies barriers and possible solutions

7. What kind of help does the patient need?
   - Dietary, physical activity, and behavioral guidance
   - Accountability
   - Psychological and emotional counseling
   - Pharmacotherapy
   - Bariatric surgery

Note. Bullet points provide examples of categories, topics, or patient responses.

Guidelines recommend measuring waist circumference for obesity-related comorbid conditions and risk factors. Complications of overweight and obesity are independently associated with excess abdominal fat and fitness level. Waist circumference, measured horizontally at the level of the iliac crest of the pelvis should be obtained on an annual basis and used to identify patients who may be at increased risk for cardiovascular disease. In the 2013 Guidelines, an elevated waist circumference is treated as a risk factor;

with a BMI greater than 25 but less than 35 kg/m², an elevated waist circumference is considered to be risk justifying medical intervention for weight loss. As shown in population studies, people with large waist circumferences have elevated obesity-related health risk compared to those with normal waist circumferences, despite having similar BMIs. The threshold for what is considered excessive abdominal fat varies between racial and ethnic groups, but cutoff points for waist circumference of more than 88 cm (> 35 inches) for women and more than 102 cm (> 40 inches) for men are generally recommended for North American populations. The classification of weight status (by BMI and waist circumference) and risk of disease is shown in Table 77.2.

Unique aspects of the physical examination for patients with obesity include attention to using appropriate size gowns, scales, and blood pressure cuffs. The following features are particularly important when identifying coexistent medical disorders and endocrinological abnormalities.

• *Blood pressure*: Should be taken using a cuff size appropriate for arm circumference. A bladder cuff that is not the appropriate width for the patient's arm circumference will cause a systematic error in blood pressure measurement. The error in blood pressure measurement is larger when the cuff is too small relative to the patient's arm circumference than when it is too large—a situation commonly encountered among the obese. The cuff should have a bladder length that is 80% and a width that is at least 40% of arm circumference (a length-to-width ratio of 2:1). Therefore, a large adult cuff (16 × 36 cm) should be chosen for patients with mild to moderate obesity (or arm circumference 14–17 inches) while an adult thigh cuff (16 × 42 cm) will need to be used for patients whose arm circumference is greater than 17 inches.

• *Skin*: Acanthosis nigricans suggests insulin resistance; red to purple depressed striae, hirsuitism, acne, and moon facies with plethora suggest Cushing syndrome; mild hirsuitism is also seen in polycystic ovarian syndrome; dry, coarse, cool, and pale skin suggests hypothyroidism.

• *Throat and neck*: Crowded oropharynx and large neck circumference (when accompanied by history of loud snoring, gasping, or choking episodes during sleep; excessive daytime sleepiness; and awakening headaches) suggest obstructive sleep apnea.

TABLE 77.2. Classification of Overweight and Obesity as Recommended by the NHLBI Guidelines

| | | | Disease risk[a] relative to normal weight and waist circumference[b] | |
	BMI (kg/m²)	Obesity class	Men: <102 cm Women: <88 cm	Men: >102 cm Women: >88 cm
Underweight	<18.5		—	—
Normal[b]	18.5–24.9		—	—
Overweight	25.0–29.9		Increased	High
Obesity	30.0–34.9	I	High	Very high
	35.0–39.9	II	Very high	Very high
Extreme obesity	≥ 40.0	III	Extremely high	Extremely high

[a]Disease risk for type 2 diabetes, hypertension, and CVD.

[b]Increased waist circumference can also be a marker for increased risk in normal-weight individuals. Measure waist circumference horizontally at the level of the iliac crest.

- *Fat distribution*: Truncal distribution with fat accumulation around the supraclavicular areas and dorsocervical spine (buffalo hump) suggest Cushing syndrome.
- *Edema*: Edema localized to lower extremities is common in moderate to severe obesity.

No single laboratory test or diagnostic evaluation is indicated for all patients with obesity, although a fasting glucose and lipid profile are consistent with current guidelines. The specific evaluation performed should be based on presentation of symptoms, risk factors, index of suspicion, and screening guidelines appropriate to the patient. It is important to focus attention on the laboratory tests that are most relevant to decision making about the overweight patient. Because diabetes, nonalcoholic fatty liver disease, gall bladder disease, heart disease, obstructive sleep apnea, and cancer have a relationship to obesity, these are important conditions to evaluate with laboratory and diagnostic tests when indicated.

Identifying the High-Risk Obese Patient

With the high prevalence of obesity and the imprecision of BMI and waist circumference measurement alone to estimate individual risk, identifying which patient to treat is an important clinical decision. The 2013 Guidelines recommend weight loss treatment for obese individuals with or without comorbidity(ies) and overweight individuals with one or more indicators of increased cardiovascular disease (CVD) risk (e.g., diabetes, prediabetes, hypertension, dyslipidemia, elevated waist circumference) or obesity-related comorbidities. A list of obesity-related medical conditions is seen in Table 77.3. The incidence and prevalence of these conditions varies by BMI class, gender, and age.

Although BMI and waist circumference are useful anthropometric markers to identify potential risk, they do not accurately reflect the presence or severity of the health risk. Analogous to other staging systems commonly used for congestive heart failure and chronic kidney disease, new functional staging systems for obesity have been proposed. These risk-stratification constructs, called the Edmonton Obesity Staging System (EOSS) and the complications-based clinical staging system, are intended to provide prognostic information independent of BMI and waist circumference. Future studies will need to determine whether new staging models improve risk stratification over other tools, such as the Framingham Risk Score.

Suggested Reading

Armstrong, M. J., Mottershead, T. A., Ronksley, P. E., Sigal, R. J., Campbell, T. S., & Hemmelgarn, B. R. (2011). Motivational interviewing to improve weight loss in overweight and/or obese patients: A systematic review and meta-analysis of randomized controlled trials. *Obesity Reviews, 12*(9), 709–723.—In this review, 11 studies were included for meta-analysis. Motivational interviewing was associated with a greater reduction in body mass in the intervention group compared to controls, and there was a significant reduction in body weight for those in the intervention group compared with controls.

Daniel, S., Soleymani, T., & Garvey, W. T. (2013). A complications-based clinical staging of obesity to guide treatment modality and intensity. *Current Opinion in Endocrinology, Diabetes,*

TABLE 77.3. Obesity-Related Comorbid Conditions by Organ Systems

Cardiovascular	Respiratory
Hypertension	Dyspnea
Congestive heart failure	Obstructive sleep apnea
Cor pulmonale	Hypoventilation syndrome
Varicose veins	Pickwickian syndrome
Pulmonary embolism	Asthma
Coronary artery disease	
Endocrine	Gastrointestinal
Metabolic syndrome	Gastroesophageal reflux disease (GERD)
Type 2 diabetes	Nonalcoholic fatty liver disease (NAFLD)
Dyslipidemia	Cholelithiasis
Polycystic ovarian syndrome (PCOS)/	Hernias
androgenicity	Colon cancer
Amenorrhea/infertility/menstrual disorders	
Musculoskeletal	Genitourinary
Hyperuricemia and gout	Urinary stress incontinence
Immobility	Obesity-related glomerulopathy
Osteoarthritis (knees and hips)	End-stage renal disease (ESRD)
Low back pain	Hypogonadism (male)
Carpal tunnel syndrome	Breast and uterine cancer
	Pregnancy complications
Psychological	Neurological
Depression/low self-esteem	Stroke
Body image disturbance	Idiopathic intracranial hypertension
Social stigmatization	Meralgia paresthetica
	Dementia
Integument	
Striae distensae (stretch marks)	
Stasis pigmentation of legs	
Lymphedema	
Cellulitis	
Intertrigo, carbuncles	
Acanthosis nigricans	
Acrochordon (skin tags)	
Hidradenitis suppurativa	

and Obesity, 20(5), 377–388.—A novel classification system designed to estimate cardiovascular risk among patients who are overweight or obese.

Emerging Risk Factors Collaboration. (2011). Separate and combined associations of body-mass index and abdominal adiposity with cardiovascular disease: Collaborative analysis of 58 prospective studies. *Lancet, 377,* 1085–1095.—In this analysis of 58 prospective studies, addition of information on BMI, waist circumference, or waist-to-hip ratio to a CVD risk prediction model containing conventional risk factors did not improve risk discrimination.

Jensen, M. D., Ryan, D. H., Apovian, C. M., Ard, J. D., Comuzzie, A. G., Donato, K. A., et al. (2014). 2013 AHA/ACC/TOS guideline for the management of overweight and obesity in adults: A report of the American College of Cardiology/American Heart Association Task Force on Practice Guidelines and The Obesity Society. *Circulation, 129*(25, Suppl. 2), S102–S138.—These guidelines review the assessment and risks of obesity, as well as the efficacy (as determined by randomized controlled trials) of dietary interventions, intensive lifestyle modification, and behavior therapy.

Jones, S., & Phillips, E. M. (Eds.). (2009). *ACSM's Exercise is Medicine: A clinician's guide to exercise prescription*. Philadelphia: Lippincott, Williams & Wilkins.—Exercise is Medicine™ is an American College of Sports Medicine initiative to "make physical activity and exercise a standard part of a disease prevention and treatment medical paradigm." This book teaches practitioners how to motivate and instruct patients on the importance of exercise, and how to design practical exercise programs for patients.

Kushner, R. F., & Bray, G. A. (2014). Classification and evaluation of the overweight patient. In G. A. Bray & C. Bouchard (Eds.), *Handbook of obesity: Vol. 2. Clinical applications* (4th ed.). Boca Raton, FL: CRC Press/Taylor & Francis Group.—This comprehensive chapter that addresses the assessment and evaluation of patients with obesity includes multiple tables and figures.

Moyer, V. A. (2012). Screening for and management of obesity in adults: U.S. Preventive Services Task Force recommendation statement. *Annals of Internal Medicine, 157*(5), 373–378.— Updated recommendations from the USPSTF that recommends screening all adults for obesity and offering or referring patients with a BMI ≥ 30 kg/m² to intensive, multicomponent behavioral interventions.

Seger, J. C., Horn, D. B., Westman, E. C., Lindquist, R., Scinta, W., Richardson, L. A., et al. (2013). American Society of Bariatric Physicians Obesity Algorithm: Adult Adiposity: Evaluation and Treatment, 2013. Available at *www.obesityalgorithm.org*.—The Obesity Algorithm, presented by ASBP, helps clinicians navigate the various steps involved in treating patients affected by overweight or obesity. This educational tool offers health care providers an overview of necessary principles to consider when evaluating patients and implementing personalized treatment plans.

Sharma, A. M., & Kushner, R. F. (2009). A proposed clinical staging system for obesity. *International Journal of Obesity, 33*(3), 289–295.—A novel staging systems that suggests classifying patients into four stages based on simple clinical assessments that include medical history, clinical and functional assessments, as well as simple routine diagnostic investigations.

Silk, A. W., & McTigue, K. M. (2011). Reexamining the physical examination for obese patients. *Journal of the American Medical Association, 305*(2), 193–194.—Brief guide on practice suggestions for performing the physical examination in patients with obesity.

Macronutrient Composition and Obesity Treatment

ARNE ASTRUP
JENNIE BRAND-MILLER

Principles for Diet-Induced Weight Loss

For overweight and obese patients the dietary goal is to decrease energy intake while maintaining the satiating effect of the diet and nutritional adequacy. Obese patients have, due to their enlarged body size, higher energy requirements for a given level of physical activity than their normal-weight counterparts. Reducing the obese patient's total energy intake to that of a normal-weight individual will inevitably cause weight loss, consisting of about 75% fat and 25% lean tissue, until weight normalization occurs at a new energy equilibrium.

The main aim of weight reduction diets is to reduce total energy intake. The larger the daily deficit in energy balance, the more rapid the weight loss. A deficit of 300–500 kcal/day will produce a weight loss of 300–500 grams/week, and a deficit of 500–1,000 kcal/day will produce a weight loss of 500–1,000 grams/week. Total energy expenditure declines and normalizes along with weight loss, and total energy intake should therefore gradually be reduced further to maintain the energy deficit. An alternative approach is to take advantage of the differences in the satiating power of the various dietary components in order to cause a spontaneous reduction in energy intake. This is the principle of the *ad libitum* higher-protein, low-GI (glycemic index) diet, and of the low-carbohydrate diets.

Choosing the Dietary Energy Deficit

Initially the target of a weight loss program should be to decrease body weight by 10%. Once this is achieved a new target can be set. Patients generally want to lose more weight, and greater initial weight loss is associated with better long-term success, but it should be remembered that even a 5% weight reduction improves risk factors and risk of comorbidities. However, several factors should be taken into consideration: the patient's degree of obesity, previous weight loss attempts, risk factors, comorbidities, and personal and social capacity to undertake the necessary lifestyle changes.

Theoretical versus Clinical Outcome

Translating the physiologically based considerations regarding energy balance and weight loss into clinical practice requires a high degree of compliance, which can be difficult to obtain. Adherence to the diet is the cornerstone of successful weight loss, and is the most complicated part of the dietary management. To improve adherence, consideration should be given to the patient's food preferences, as well as to personal, educational, and social factors. Great efforts should be made to see the patient frequently and regularly.

Furthermore, long-term weight reduction is unlikely to succeed unless the patient acquires changed eating and physical activity habits, and also can address other obesity-promoting lifestyles (too little or impaired sleep, mental stress, etc.).

Options for Weight Loss Diets

There are several recognized weight reduction regimens, discussed in the sections below.

Very-Low-Energy Diets

Starvation (less than 200 kcal/day), the ultimate dietary treatment of obesity, is no longer used because of the numerous and serious medical complications associated with prolonged starvation. Starvation has been replaced by very-low-energy diets (VLED; 200–800 kcal/day), which aim to supply very little energy but all essential nutrients. The safety of these diets has been questioned, and today the 800 kcal/day VLED is the only version recognized as being both effective and safe. These are usually provided in the form of nutrition powders, or in the form of protein, mineral, trace element, and vitamin-enriched meals or drinks. Table 78.1 shows the typical composition. VLED can induce very rapid weight loss over a 2- to 3-month period. However, VLED are not educational and do not facilitate the gradual modification of the patient's eating behavior, nutritional knowledge, and skills, which seems to be required for long-term weight maintenance.

TABLE 78.1. Typical Composition of a Low-Energy Diet

Nutrient	Recommended intake
Energy	800–1,500 kcal/day
Total fat	25–35% of total calories
Protein	20–30% of total calories
Carbohydrate	35–55% of total calories
Fiber	20–30 g/day
Calcium	1,000–1,500 mg/day
Other vitamins, minerals, and trace elements	Recommended dietary allowance (RDA): Full coverage should be ensured by a vitamin/mineral supplement daily

Low-Energy Diets

Low-energy diets (LED) usually provide 800–1,500 kcal/day and normally consist of natural, normal foods but may include 1–4/day meal replacement products (Table 78.1). Although macronutrient composition of the diet is of less importance for short-term weight loss, it is now usually modified to maximize the beneficial effect on cardiovascular risk factors and insulin resistance, and to prevent cancers, perhaps also promoting long-term weight maintenance. For practical reasons LED are moderate-fat, higher-protein diets, with reduced refined carbohydrates (high GI), with a fixed energetic allowance. A patient may choose an energy level of 1,000–1,200 kcal/day for women and 1,200–1,500 kcal/day for men. LED produce a lower rate of weight loss than VLED, but randomized clinical trials demonstrate that the long-term (>1 year) weight loss is not different from that of the VLED. Furthermore, using LED for weight loss induction introduces healthy eating habits early in the weight reduction program, giving a longer period in which to familiarize the patient with the dietary changes that are a central element in a weight maintenance program.

Higher-Protein Diets

The level of protein in the diet normally recommended is determined by the minimum required to maintain nitrogen balance, but there is evidence that higher levels of dietary protein could help prevent and treat disorders such as obesity, metabolic syndrome, and type 2 diabetes.

Differential Effects of Foods and Nutrients on Appetite

Changing diet composition is an effective tool for enhancing satiety and reducing spontaneous energy intake. Evidence of the effects on body weight of low-GI, higher-protein, and low-carbohydrate diets stems mainly from mechanistic studies and randomized controlled trials (RCTs), as it is difficult to get a true picture from longitudinal, observational studies.

Higher-Protein Diets

Short-term studies show the mechanisms by which higher protein intake promotes negative fat balance and reduction of body fat stores. Protein generally exerts a greater satiety effect than other macronutrients, whether in drinks or in solid foods. There is accumulating evidence that this is partly mediated by a synergistic effect of the satiety hormones glucagon-like peptide 1 (GLP-1) and peptide YY (PYY) released from the small intestine. The thermic effect of protein is also greater than that of carbohydrate or fat. During weight loss, higher-protein diets preserve lean body tissue, the major determinant of resting and 24-hour energy expenditure, curbing reduction in energy expenditure. This is particularly significant when higher-protein diets are combined with physical training.

In the Diet, Obesity and Genes (DioGenes) study, a randomized, controlled, multicenter trial investigating diets for prevention of weight (re)gain following weight loss, an initial 8 week VLED (800 kcal/day) inducing major weight loss (mean 11.0 kg) was followed by a 6-month dietary intervention testing the effect of *ad libitum* diets varying in dietary protein and GI, on weight maintenance and obesity-related risk factors: low-protein (LP)/low-GI (LGI); LP/high-GI (HGI); high-protein (HP)/LGI; HP/HGI. All diets were moderate in fat (25–30% of energy). The target was for 10–15% of energy intake to comprise protein in the LP and 23–28% in the HP. Weight regain was 0.93 kg less in the HP groups than in the NP group, and 0.95 kg less in the LGI groups than in the HGI groups. Figure 78.1 shows weight regain after an initial weight loss of ~11 kg achieved over 8 weeks in obese subjects on an 800 kcal/day diet. HP diets were more likely to produce an additional 5% weight loss after randomization than NP diets (odds ratio, 1.92), and LGI diets were more likely to result in an additional 5% weight loss than were HGI diets (odds ratio, 2.54). In conclusion, a slight increase in dietary protein and corresponding reduction in carbohydrate, together with lowering GI by 5 units, exerted an additive effect on body weight regulation. After 14 months, subjects on the HP diets regained 2–3 kg less than those in the NP group, and those on HP diets lost a total of 7.3 kg compared to 4.5 kg in the NP groups.

The HP/LGI diet produced a spontaneous 14.3% decline in the prevalence of overweight and obesity among the children ages 5–18 years who participated in the trial. Other studies also demonstrate the importance of higher-protein, lower-carbohydrate load/ LGI for weight control and comorbid conditions.

Acceptability of HP Diets

The acceptability of HP diets is high, provided that dishes and meals from the normal food culture are incorporated. HP diets were more acceptable than the normal protein diets. The significantly lower dropout rate in HP and LGI groups would normally be attributed to the greater weight loss and maintenance success, but it also suggests that the diets were easily incorporated into normal food culture, and that availability, cost, and taste were not barriers for adopting the diet.

GI and Glycemic Load

An appreciable body of evidence supports higher dietary protein, and correspondingly reduced carbohydrate intake, as a method to enhance weight loss. This does not mean that carbohydrates should be avoided. Carbohydrates present in different foods have distinct physiological effects, including differences in rate of digestion and absorption, thereby influencing appetite (hunger and satiety), fuel partitioning, metabolic rate, and postprandial glycemia and insulinemia. The glycemic qualities of carbohydrate—defined by their GI and glycemic load (GL)—are most relevant to individuals who are overweight and at increased risk of diabetes. The GI is a food classification derived from the postprandial blood glucose response relative to a reference food, gram for gram of carbohydrate. The GL—the mathematical product of the GI and the amount of carbohydrate per serving—encapsulates both the quality and quantity of carbohydrate, and is the single best predictor of postprandial glycemia.

In overweight and insulin-resistant individuals, glycemic spikes and insulin demand are excessively increased. A meta-analysis of 24 prospective cohort studies with 7.5 million person-years of follow-up indicated that high dietary GL was positively associated with a 1.45-fold higher relative risk of type 2 diabetes per 100 g increment in GL. In the Nurses Health Study II, women consuming high GL diets were 60% more likely

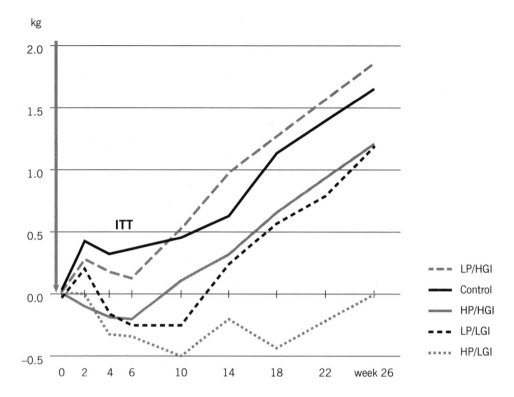

FIGURE 78.1. Weight regain after an initial weight loss of ~11 kg achieved over 8 weeks in obese subjects on a 800 kcal/day diet (arrow). After the initial weight loss, experimental subjects were randomized to four different *ad libitum* diets with no energy restriction ("Eat until you feel full"): LP (~16% protein), HP (~23% protein), and HGI and LGI (high- and low-GI diets). From Larsen et al. (2010). Copyright © 2010 Massachusetts Medical Society. Adapted by permission.

to be diagnosed with gestational diabetes during pregnancy. High dietary GI and GL also increase oxidative stress, inflammatory markers (C-reactive protein), and the risk of coronary heart disease events.

Meta-analyses of RCTs indicate that *ad libitum* low-GI and/or low-GL diets promote faster weight loss and greater loss of body fat than do conventional diets. Women following *ad libitum* low-GI or low-GL diets for 12 weeks lost 80% more fat mass than those on a conventional fiber-matched low-fat diet. Following a low-GL diet produced markedly greater decreases in weight (–5.8 vs. –1.2 kg) and body fat (–2.6% vs. –0.9%) at 18 months among obese adults ages 18–35 years with high 30-minute insulin concentration. Female sex, insulin resistance, and/or hyperinsulemia appear to increase the risk of poor outcomes on high-GI and/or GL diets.

Reduced energy expenditure following a period of weight loss is thought to contribute to weight regain. However, studies have shown that the drop in resting energy expenditure is greatest for conventional low-fat diets (205 kcal/day on average) and least for low-GI or low-GL diets (138–166 kcal/day). In the DioGenes study of overweight and obese individuals (discussed earlier), completion rate and maintenance of weight loss were highest among participants assigned to a combined HP–low-GI diet (23% of energy from protein, 30% from fat, and 47% from carbohydrate), whereas conventional dietary advice was associated with immediate weight regain (Figure 78.1). Taken together, the various studies demonstrate the importance of considering carbohydrate composition in weight management.

Added-Sugar and Sugar-Sweetened Beverages

A controversial and complex issue that continues to dominate the obesity debate is the role of sugar consumption in weight gain. The word *sugar* can refer to added or refined sugars, but scientifically, it covers both naturally occurring and added sugars because the body is unable to distinguish between different sources. Theoretically, a diet high in sugar(s) may result in the suppression of fat oxidation, creating a metabolic environment likely to promote obesity. However, this is also true of a diet high in starch, particularly, high-GI starch. When added sugars are substituted with other carbohydrates (e.g., starch with the same calories), there are no differences in BMI, weight, or body fat. While added sugars offer no nutritional benefits, their sweetness is an effective tool to increase enjoyment and consumption of nutrient-dense foods. The diets of children and adolescents do not need to be devoid of added sugars.

Meta-analyses of controlled feeding trials in which sugar-sweetened beverages (SSBs) were *added* to the diet showed a dose-dependent increase in weight. But studies that attempted to *reduce* SSB intake show equivocal effects. When limited to overweight participants only, a small amount of weight loss or less weight gain is evident. Two large RCTs in children and adolescents, with a high degree of compliance, provided convincing data that reducing consumption of SSB decreases weight gain and adiposity, although the effect size is small.

Replacement of caloric sweeteners with lower or zero-calorie alternatives may be a useful dietary tool to improve compliance and facilitate weight loss and weight loss maintenance by helping to reduce energy intake. In systematic reviews, low-calorie sweeteners modestly reduced BMI, fat mass, and waist circumference, but this is not evident in prospective cohort studies. Indeed, intense sweeteners are associated with a slightly higher BMI.

Fiber and Whole Grains

High intake of fiber and whole grains is recommended for the population at large because of their high micronutrient density, bulk, and satiating qualities. In large, prospective cohort studies, intake of cereal fiber and whole grain foods is strongly linked with decreased rates of weight gain, type 2 diabetes, ischemic heart disease, and hypertension. Unfortunately, the positive findings of observational studies have not been borne out in RCTs. Indeed, a *Cochrane Systematic Review* indicated that there were insufficient high-quality intervention studies to recommend whole grains. The positive effect of oat products may be ascribed to their slower digestion and absorption (low GI) rather than fiber content. Thus, ascribing an equal health value to all types of whole grain foods, without regard to the physical structure and type of cereal, may not be helpful. Thus, at the present time, the evidence to recommend whole grains in place of refined grains for weight loss per se is weak.

Low-Carbohydrate or Low-Fat Diets

Previously low-fat, high-protein diets were recommended as the optimal weight loss diet. However, along with several popular diet books promoting ketogenic, low-carbohydrate diets, numerous RCTs have been undertaken to assess efficacy and safety. Many low-carbohydrate diets restrict carbohydrate to <50 g/day, and there has been some safety concern. However, their efficacy to produce weight loss results in improvements in all cardiovascular and diabetes risk factors, and the major issue is whether the patient over the long-term can adhere to a diet that essentially eliminates all starchy and sugary carbohydrates. The low-carbohydrate intake depletes glycogen stores and the patient develops "anorexia of starvation," also seen in VLED. This is believed to be the mechanism behind the satiety effect, and the spontaneous reduction in energy intake that results from this diet.

A meta-analysis of RCTs that compared low-fat with low-carbohydrate diets, based on 17 studies, concluded that after 6 months, weight loss for participants on a low-carbohydrate diet was 1.4 kg greater than for those on a low-fat diet. At 12 months, the difference was only 0.8 kg.

Suggested Reading

Alexandraki, I., Palacio, C., & Mooradian, A. D. (2015). Relative merits of low-carbohydrate versus low-fat diet in managing obesity. *Southern Medical Journal, 108*(7), 401–416.—This systematic review and meta-analysis identified 17 studies of 6 months or longer duration showing a small but statistically significant difference in weight loss favoring lower-carbohydrate diets.

Astrup, A., & Brand-Miller, J. (2014). Obesity: Have new guidelines overlooked the role of diet composition? *Nature Reviews Endocrinology, 10*(3), 132–133.—Our Letter to the Editor cites evidence from intervention trials demonstrating the importance of dietary factors for weight control and disease prevention.

Clifton, P. M., Condo, D., & Keogh, J. B. (2014). Long term weight maintenance after advice to consume low carbohydrate, higher protein diets—a systematic review and meta analysis. *Nutrition, Metabolism and Cardiovascular Diseases, 24*(3), 224–235.—This systematic review and meta-analysis identified 32 studies of 12 months or longer. A difference of 5% or greater in percentage protein between diets at 12 months was associated with a threefold greater effect size compared with < 5%.

Larsen, T. M., Dalskov, S. M., van Baak, M., Jebb, S. A., Papadaki, A., Pfeiffer, A. F., et al. (2010). Diets with high or low protein content and glycemic index for weight-loss maintenance. *New England Journal of Medicine, 363*(22), 2102–2113.—In this large European study, a modest increase in protein content and a modest reduction in the GI led to an improvement in study completion and maintenance of weight loss.

Mozaffarian, D., Hao, T., Rimm, E. B., Willett, W. C., & Hu, F. B. (2011). Changes in diet and lifestyle and long-term weight gain in women and men. *New England Journal of Medicine, 364*(25), 2392–2404.—In three separate cohorts of American adults, 4-year weight change was positively associated with increased consumption of potatoes and potato products, and inversely associated with higher intake of yogurt and nuts.

Paddon-Jones, D., Westman, E., Mattes, R. D., Wolfe, R. R., Astrup, A., & Westerterp-Plantenga, M. (2008). Protein, weight management, and satiety. *American Journal of Clinical Nutrition, 87*(5), 1558S–1561S.—In this review, three mechanisms are suggested to explain a salutary effect of protein on weight control: increased satiety, higher thermogenesis, and better maintenance of fat-free mass.

Papadaki, A., Linardakis, M., Larsen, T. M., van Baak, M. A., Lindroos, A. K., Pfeiffer, A. F., et al. (2010). The effect of protein and glycemic index on children's body composition: The DiOGenes randomized study. *Pediatrics, 126*(5), 1143–1152.—In children whose parents were enrolled in the DiOGenes trial, the low protein–high GI diet increased body fat, whereas the high protein–low GI combination was protective against obesity.

79

Treatment of Obesity in Primary Care Practice

ADAM G. TSAI
THOMAS A. WADDEN

Primary care practitioners (PCPs) have been encouraged to become more active in the treatment of obesity given its enormous clinical burden and substantial economic costs. In 2003, the U.S. Preventive Services Task Force (USPSTF) recommended that PCPs screen all adults for obesity and offer affected individuals high-intensity behavioral weight loss counseling, either by providing such care themselves or referring patients to appropriate programs. In 2012, the USPSTF renewed this recommendation, specifying that programs should provide "intensive" (i.e., 12–26 counseling visits per year) comprehensive lifestyle modification, consisting of reduced energy intake, increased physical activity, and behavioral strategies to facilitate adherence to diet and exercise recommendations.

Historically, reimbursement of behavioral treatment of obesity has been limited or inconsistent. However, in 2011, the Centers for Medicare and Medicaid Services (CMS) approved the provision of intensive behavior therapy (i.e., lifestyle modification) for Medicare beneficiaries with a body mass index (BMI) ≥ 30 kg/m^2. The benefit provides 14 brief (10–15 minutes) visits in 6 months, followed by an additional six monthly visits if the patient loses at least 3 kg in the first half-year. While the uptake of this benefit has been modest to date, the CMS's actions were a critical first step in recognizing the treatment of obesity as part of routine medical care.

Interest in obesity management in primary care also has been stimulated by the recent publication of practice guidelines. In 2013, evidence-based behavioral and surgical treatments for obesity were reviewed by the American Heart Association, the American College of Cardiology, and The Obesity Society (AHA/ACC/TOS). These guidelines updated those originally developed in 1998 by the National Institutes of Health/National Heart, Lung, and Blood Institute. In 2015, the Endocrine Society published guidelines on pharmacotherapy for obesity. The establishment of the American Board of Obesity Medicine, which offers certification in obesity medicine as a subspecialty, also reflects growing interest in obesity management.

The Role of PCPs in Managing Obesity and Its Complications

Debate persists about the appropriate role of PCPs in treating obesity. Clearly, PCPs are responsible for diagnosing and treating health complications of excess weight. Numerous studies have demonstrated the health benefits of medical management (i.e., pharmacotherapy) for obesity-related diseases, including type 2 diabetes, hypertension, and hypercholesterolemia. Medical therapy is superior to weight reduction, in most cases, for treating cardiometabolic disorders and should be prescribed for patients with obesity as readily as it is for persons of average weight.

PCPs also are responsible for regularly monitoring their patients' weight and helping them understand how obesity affects health. Weight can be a sensitive topic (given patients' experiences with stigmatization), which PCPs must broach in a respectful, nonjudgmental manner. They might initiate such discussions by stating, "We haven't talked about your weight in a while. Would it be OK to discuss it? What are your thoughts about your weight and how it affects your health and daily functioning?" Patients often welcome the opportunity to share their weight-related concerns, particularly in lieu of being lectured about the need for weight reduction. This discussion may lead patients to volunteer that they would like to lose weight, in which case PCPs can inform them of the health benefits of a 5–10% reduction in initial weight and discuss options for achieving this goal. Alternatively, PCPs may inquire, "What are your goals for weight management at this time?" After listening carefully, practitioners can help patients clarify whether they wish to lose weight or instead focus on preventing further weight gain (with the opportunity to discuss weight reduction at a future time). In either case, PCPs should discuss specific treatment options and strategies available to meet patients' goals. They also should help patients set obtainable goals (i.e., 5–10% reduction), which often fall short of desired or expected weight losses.

The PCP's role in actually delivering high-intensity lifestyle counseling is less clear than that in providing medical therapy for obesity-related comorbidities. For example, if a patient meets the criteria for intensive behavioral treatment of obesity, should this care be provided within the office practice or health system in which the PCP works, or instead be "outsourced" to programs in the community? Similarly, should PCPs themselves provide intensive lifestyle counseling, as required by the new CMS benefit, or should another health care provider working under the PCP's supervision offer this care?

Figure 79.1 provides guidance on how PCPs can approach obesity management. Depending on the nature of their practice, PCPs can deliver lifestyle counseling and other interventions themselves, or they can treat obesity "collaboratively," working with staff in their immediate practices or with professionals (e.g., registered dietitians) potentially in their health system (see left-hand side of Figure 79.1). Evidence-based commercial or nonprofit weight loss programs in the community offer another option for PCPs unable to provide lifestyle counseling (right-hand side of Figure 79.1). In addition, patients may be referred to obesity specialists, who may be internal or external to the PCP's health system. We discuss each of these options below and summarize key research findings relevant to each, as determined from systematic reviews we published in 2009 and 2014. These reviews yielded two principal findings. The first was that lifestyle interventions that used "traditional" methods of behavioral treatment, including specific targets for caloric restriction, physical activity, and self-monitoring, produced greater weight loss than "alternative" behavioral counseling approaches, such as motivational interviewing or stages of change (and did not include specific energy intake and expenditure goals).

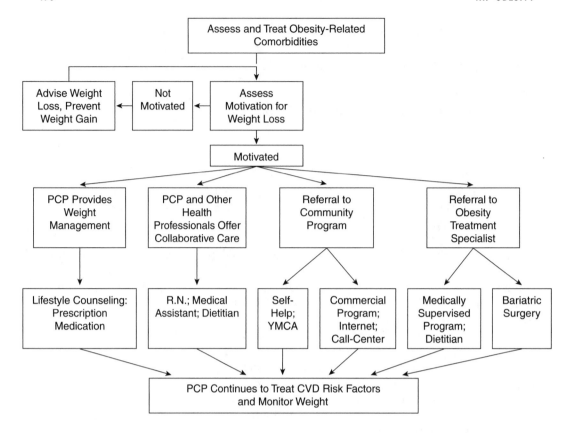

FIGURE 79.1. An algorithm for identifying an appropriate weight loss option. After treating cardio-vascular disease (CVD) risk factors and assessing patients' motivation for weight loss, PCPs may elect to offer intensive lifestyle counseling themselves (with or without pharmacotherapy) or to provide counseling in collaboration with other practice staff (e.g., medical assistant). Alternatively, PCPs may refer patients to community programs (e.g., Weight Watchers) or to obesity treatment specialists. From Tsai and Wadden (2009). Copyright © 2009 Springer. Reprinted by permission.

The second finding was that among studies that provided traditional behavioral treat-ment, high-intensity interventions (≥ 14 counseling sessions in 6 months) produced the largest weight losses.

PCPs' Options for Providing Obesity Management in Their Practice or Health System

PCPs Providing Lifestyle Counseling

PCPs may provide lifestyle counseling themselves (with or without the use of prescrip-tion medication). A majority, however, report that they do not have the time, training, or financial incentive to offer such care. Only a few studies have assessed the benefits of PCP-delivered counseling, which was limited in most cases to moderate- (1 session/ month) or low-intensity visits (< 1 session/month). These interventions produced mean losses of only 2–3 kg at 6–12 months, substantially less than the desired 5–10% reduction in initial weight. Physicians in the most successful intervention provided high-intensity, brief visits (i.e., 26, 10- to 15-minute sessions over 1 year) that produced a mean loss of 3.5 kg. However, participants in this trial were provided meal-replacement shakes, thus preventing assessment of the physician-delivered lifestyle counseling per se. To date, no controlled trials have assessed the efficacy or cost-effectiveness of the CMS model of high-intensity behavioral treatment, which mandates that counseling be provided by physicians, nurse practitioners, or physician assistants. There is a pressing need for evaluation.

PCPs Providing Collaborative Care

The approach most often used in trials of primary care treatment of obesity is the "collaborative" model, in which PCPs provide pharmacotherapy for patients' weight-related health conditions, and registered dietitians or other health counselors deliver lifestyle modification. Three recent interventions employed this approach. One used medical assistants (from the primary care office) as lifestyle coaches to provide monthly brief (10–15 minutes) counseling visits, which produced a mean weight loss of 2.9 kg after 2 years. Participants who received the same intervention enhanced by meal replacements or weight loss medication lost 4.7 kg. A second 2-year study compared traditional, group-based counseling, provided by registered dietitians, to a similarly high-intensity, individual intervention that was delivered by telephone from a centralized call center. Both interventions produced mean 2-year weight losses of 4.5–5.0 kg. In a third trial, a registered dietitian and an exercise physiologist were incorporated into a primary care office to provide high-intensity group lifestyle modification and achieved weight losses of 4.5–5.5 kg at 2 years. PCPs in these trials were informed regularly of patients' weight changes and congratulated them on their success during routine office visits.

PCPs' Options for Referring Patients for Obesity Management

PCPs without the time or resources to provide lifestyle counseling (or other interventions), or who believe that more aggressive intervention is needed (e.g., bariatric surgery), can refer patients to commercial weight loss programs or obesity specialists in the community. In all cases, PCPs will want to monitor patients' weight and health conditions regularly and adjust medications appropriately. Referral to the community should be viewed as another form of collaborative care.

Evidenced-Based Commercial Programs

For lifestyle modification, PCPs can refer patients to commercial or nonprofit weight loss programs that provide high-intensity behavioral treatment. As noted in the 2013 AHA/ACC/TOS guidelines, PCPs should recommend commercial programs that have published peer-reviewed evidence of their efficacy and safety. The efficacy of these programs was reviewed recently by Gudzune and colleagues (2015), who found that Weight Watchers and Jenny Craig provided the strongest evidence of their programs' success at 12 months, with mean weight losses of approximately 5–7% of initial weight. Outcomes also have been published for several medically supervised low-calorie diets (e.g., Health

Management Resources [HMR], OPTIFAST), as well as at least two self-directed meal plans (Atkins and SlimFast). Although not supported by randomized controlled trials, the Take Off Pounds Sensibly (TOPS) program is a low-cost nonprofit program that provides peer-led group sessions for weight loss and has been evaluated in several published studies.

Patients (and practitioners) must carefully review the costs of commercial programs and the services and products to be delivered. Programs that provide meals, whether as conventional foods or as liquid shakes and meal bars, can cost $100 or more per week, with additional charges for optional vitamins and supplements. Ideally, patients should pay about $15–25 per pound of weight loss during 4–6 months of intervention. (This price excludes the costs of conventional or prepared foods that must be purchased).

Referral to Obesity Specialists

An additional option is for PCPs to refer their patients to obesity specialists, who may be within or external to the PCP's health system. Referral should be considered for patients who have not benefited from lifestyle counseling or other interventions offered by the PCP, or for patients whose obesity and weight-related comorbid conditions are so severe as to require more aggressive intervention. A reasonable criterion for success in weight management is the achievement and maintenance of a 5–10% loss of initial weight. Some patients, however, require greater (long-term) weight loss to improve health complications and quality of life.

Among patients who meet BMI and other criteria, the most clear-cut referral may be for bariatric surgery. A large evidence base supports the safety and efficacy of Roux-en-Y gastric bypass and vertical sleeve gastrectomy in achieving long-term losses of 20–30% of initial weight, as well as improvements in comorbid conditions, particularly type 2 diabetes. PCPs play a critical role in ensuring that patients understand the risks and benefits of surgery, how the different operations alter the stomach and gastrointestinal system, and the extensive changes in eating behavior required postoperatively.

Patients who have never tried pharmacotherapy for obesity may wish to pursue this option before proceeding to bariatric surgery. Since 2012, four new drugs have been approved for chronic weight management. They include phentermine–topiramate, liraglutide (3.0 mg/day), lorcaserin, and bupropion–naltrexone (orlistat was approved for long-term use in 1999). The first two agents, as combined with moderate-intensity lifestyle counseling, induce mean weight loss of approximately 8–10% of initial weight in 6 months, while the latter two produce reductions of approximately 5–7%. Medications are nearly twice as effective when combined with a high-intensity program of lifestyle intervention.

Pharmacotherapy for obesity typically must be taken chronically to maintain weight loss. Due to inconsistent insurance coverage and the often high costs of medications, phentermine—approved in 1959 for the short-term treatment of obesity—remains the most commonly prescribed weight loss agent in the United States, principally because of its low cost and favorable efficacy. The Endocrine Society's guidelines on pharmacotherapy for obesity discuss the off-label use of this drug for chronic weight management.

Many PCPs are not comfortable prescribing weight loss medications, whether because of concerns with safety, modest long-term results, or other factors. Such practitioners may wish to refer their patients to specialists with greater expertise and comfort with pharmacological treatment, who also may provide high-intensity lifestyle modification.

Summary

Obesity is a highly prevalent and burdensome disease, but it is treatable. For decades, PCPs have played a critical role in assessing and managing obesity-related diseases, such as type 2 diabetes and hypertension. They have now been encouraged to facilitate the treatment of obesity itself, whether by directly providing high-intensity lifestyle modification (and other interventions) or by referring patients to appropriate resources and professionals in the community. Given the high costs of physicians, nurse practitioners, and other PCPs' time, as well as their limited training in weight management, we do not believe that most of these practitioners are well suited to deliver intensive lifestyle counseling. Instead, collaborative care appears to offer a more cost-efficient model, in which lifestyle counseling is provided by registered dietitians and other trained interventionists who work in concert with PCPs. The ever-expanding use of electronic health records, which potentially can link professionals in different physical settings, should facilitate collaborative care, whether the intervention selected is behavioral, pharmacological, or surgical. Similarly, the increased use of digital platforms to deliver weight management, which include devices for remotely monitoring patients' body weight, physical activity, and other variables, could greatly expand practitioners' abilities to support their patients' weight management efforts. These are the topics that will shape the next generation of research on the management of obesity in primary care practice.

Suggested Reading

Apovian, C. M., Aronne, L. J., Bessesen, D. H., McDonnell, M. E., Murad, M. H., Pagotto, U., et al. (2015). Pharmacological management of obesity: An Endocrine Society clinical practice guideline. *Journal of Clinical Endocrinology and Metabolism, 100*(2), 342–362.—These guidelines include discussion of the safety, efficacy, and clinical use of newly approved weight loss medications.

Appel, L. J., Clark, J. M., Yeh, H. C., Want, N. Y., Coughlin, J. W., Daumit, G., et al. (2011). Comparative effectiveness of weight-loss interventions in clinical practice. *New England Journal of Medicine, 365*(21), 1959–1968.—This 2-year randomized controlled trial found that a telephone-delivered, high-intensity lifestyle intervention was as effective as a traditional face-to-face program in patients recruited from primary care practices.

Centers for Medicare and Medicaid Services. (2011). Services and supplies incident to a physician's professional services: Conditions. 42 CFR § 410.26.—The Centers for Medicare and Medicaid Services cover 14 high-intensity lifestyle counseling session over 6 months for obese beneficiaries, when delivered by physicians, nurse practitioners, or physician assistants.

Gudzune, K. A., Doshi, R. S., Mehta, A. K., Chaudhry, Z. W., Jacobs, D. K., Vakil, R. M., et al. (2015). Efficacy of commercial weight-loss programs: An updated systematic review. *Annals of Internal Medicine, 162*(7), 501–512.—This article reviews the efficacy of evidenced-based commercial weight loss programs.

Jensen, M. D., Ryan, D. H., Apovian, C. M., Ard, J. D., Comuzzie, A. G., Donato, K. A., et al. (2014). Guidelines (2013) for the management of overweight and obesity in adults. *Obesity, 22*(Suppl. 2), S1–S410.—These guidelines review the assessment and risks of obesity, as well as the efficacy (as determined by randomized controlled trials) of dietary interventions, intensive lifestyle modification, and behavior therapy.

Leblanc, E. S., O'Connor, E., Whitlock, E. P., Patnode, C. D., & Kapka, T. (2011). Effectiveness of primary care-relevant treatments for obesity in adults: A systematic evidence review for the U.S. Preventive Services Task Force. *Annals of Internal Medicine, 155*(7), 434–447.—The CMS used the results of this systematic review to develop the high-intensity lifestyle intervention offered to obese beneficiaries.

Moyer, V. A., & U.S. Preventive Services Task Force. (2012). Screening for and management of obesity in adults: U.S. Preventive Services Task Force recommendation statement. *Annals of Internal Medicine, 157*(5), 373–378.—The USPSTF has played a leading role in getting primary care practitioners more involved in the management of obesity.

Tsai, A. G., & Wadden, T. A. (2009). Treatment of obesity in primary care practice in the United States: A systematic review. *Journal of General Internal Medicine, 24*(9), 1073–1079.—This review examines the effectiveness (in primary care practice) of different intensities of lifestyle counseling and the effects, in some studies, of combining counseling with pharmacotherapy.

Wadden, T. A., Butryn, M. L., Hong, P. S., & Tsai, A. G. (2014). Behavioral treatment of obesity in patients encountered in primary care settings: A systematic review. *Journal of the American Medical Association, 312*(17), 1779–1791.—Although increasingly popular with PCPs, motivational interviewing was not found to produce clinically meaningful weight loss unless combined with elements of traditional behavioral treatment including specific targets for caloric restriction and physical activity.

Treatments for Childhood Obesity

DENISE E. WILFLEY
DOROTHY J. VAN BUREN

Childhood is an important time to address the significant public health problem of obesity. Since children are still growing, slowing the rate of weight gain or achieving very modest weight losses can help children normalize their body weight. Although weight loss maintenance is challenging for adults, children have demonstrated good weight loss maintenance in response to treatment. Since obesity in childhood is a risk factor for the development of eating disorder psychopathology and for continued obesity through adolescence and adulthood, helping overweight or obese children achieve a healthier weight status represents a form of indicated or targeted prevention for these conditions in adulthood. Therefore, treating children who are overweight or obese results in improvements not only in the child's mental and physical health status but also in that child's future health.

Organizations and agencies such as the U.S. Preventive Services Task Force (USPSTF) and the American Academy of Pediatrics (AAP) have issued recommendations for the prevention and treatment of obesity in children. Additionally, numerous comprehensive reviews and meta-analyses have documented the effectiveness of multicomponent weight loss interventions for children that are of sufficient duration (i.e., greater than 25 hours of contact), that include a multicomponent focus on diet and physical activity, and that use behavioral change techniques. This chapter provides a brief overview of family-based behavioral weight control treatments (FBT) for childhood obesity. Current findings regarding factors impacting the effectiveness of these treatments, and directions for future research are also discussed.

Family-Based Behavioral Weight Control

FBT, developed and expanded upon by Leonard Epstein, Denise Wilfley, and colleagues, is a treatment approach consistent with USPSTF and AAP guidelines for treatment of childhood obesity and has demonstrated efficacy in both the short and the long term.

Modification of energy balance behaviors (i.e., decreasing caloric intake and increasing caloric expenditure) is the cornerstone of many weight loss interventions, including FBT. These goals are achieved through the use of behavioral treatment techniques and the active involvement of a parent or caregiver who is often also overweight or obese. The parent in FBT is encouraged to modify his or her own energy balance behaviors, provide support and encouragement for the child involved in treatment, and to engineer a home environment conducive to a healthy lifestyle for the entire family. It is this focus on change across the entire household that is a hallmark of FBT. Evidence suggests that extended treatment contact focusing on both the continued practice of self-regulatory behavioral skills and the use of family and social networks to support weight loss maintenance behaviors such as improved dietary intake and engagement in increased levels of physical activity is important to the long-term maintenance of weight loss during FBT.

Diet

Dietary targets of FBT include decreasing caloric intake, improving the nutritional quality of foods selected, and shifting food preferences. Decreases in caloric intake of approximately 500 calories per day from baseline, for a total of 1,000–1,200 calories/day for children and 1,200–1,400 calories/day for adults, are achieved by decreasing consumption of high-energy-dense, unhealthy foods, and increasing consumption of nutritious, low-energy-dense foods. A family-friendly method of categorizing foods according to traffic light colors is used in FBT to help families identify which foods to decrease (red foods—Stop and think; yellow foods—Proceed with caution by watching portion sizes), and which to increase (green foods—Go!). Red foods are calorically dense and/or have limited nutritional value (e.g., potato chips, candy, sugar-sweetened beverages). Yellow foods are more calorically dense than green foods but may be more nutritious than red foods (e.g., whole-grain bread), and most vegetables and fruits are considered green foods.

An important feature of FBT is that caloric restriction is not the only dietary goal; shifting taste preferences is also extremely important. To this end, foods that are modified to be lower in calories (e.g., foods with sugar substitutes such as diet soft drinks, low-fat cookies) are still considered red foods despite their lower caloric content. The goal of FBT is for families to make a shift to more nutritious foods and not to switch from one "junk" food to a lower-calorie version of the same food. In FBT, parental weight loss success predicts child weight loss, and this correlation can be explained, at least in part, by parental maintenance of lower red food intake over time.

Another method utilized in FBT for improving the nutritional quality of food and decreasing caloric intake is to encourage families to eat fewer meals away from the home. The average family in the United States eats approximately 35% of their meals away from home, and children who are overweight or obese eat a higher proportion of their meals away from home than do children who are not overweight or obese. FBT's focus on the reduction of the number of meals eaten away from home has a positive impact on not only participants' weight status but also the nutritional quality of the foods they eat.

Physical Activity

Physical activity targets in FBT include increasing moderate-to-vigorous physical activity, while decreasing time spent in sedentary nonschool- or nonwork-related pursuits. The colors of the traffic light again provide a family-friendly way of understanding an activity's intensity or metabolic equivalent (MET). For example, green activities (Go) are 5.0 METs or higher; yellow activities (Slow) are between 3.0 and 4.9 METs, while red activities (Stop) are less than 3.0 METs. Watching TV, playing video games, talking/texting on the phone, and playing games or "surfing" the Internet on the computer are all red activities. Any time spent on screentime activities for a purpose, for work or homework, are not counted as red activity time. Target goals for moderate-to-vigorous physical activity are 60–90 minutes/day for adults and children. However, FBT also emphasizes the importance of lifestyle physical activities as useful substitutes for sedentary pursuits. For example, walking to the store rather than driving not only involves more physical activity than driving but it is also more time consuming, leaving less time for engaging in computer games or TV watching. Since sedentary activities are often accompanied by eating, decreasing time spent in sedentary pursuits has the added benefit of decreasing caloric intake, in addition to increasing caloric output.

Behavioral Change Skills

FBT is a behavioral treatment, and the use of behavioral techniques for facilitating change is integral to its successful implementation. Self-monitoring, goal setting, successive approximation and shaping, modeling, and reward systems—the mainstays of good behavioral therapy—are utilized in FBT. Self-monitoring has been associated with better weight outcomes in children as well as in adults, and because of this association, it has long been considered one of the most important behavioral change techniques in weight loss interventions. Interestingly, a recent study of behavior change techniques used in a weight loss program for adults with type 2 diabetes concluded that the number of behavior change techniques participants reported utilizing was associated with weight loss success, more so than any one technique. Because of these findings, the authors of this study suggest that the more behavioral change tools we can offer to individuals engaging in weight loss interventions, the greater the likelihood that they will be successful in losing weight. To this end, recent research advances in the basic cognitive and behavioral sciences that have informed the development or refinement of additional behavioral change methods, such as training to enhance episodic future thinking skills to improve impulse control or strengthening goal setting skills by including implementation intention procedures to enhance prospective thinking or memory, show promise for inclusion in FBT's treatment armamentarium.

Family Involvement, Peer Support, and the Community

Parental involvement and parent training (e.g., praise, selective attention, positive reinforcement, modeling, and limit setting) are integral parts of FBT. Caregivers who are overweight or obese are encouraged to try actively to modify their own dietary and physical activity habits, while also supporting their child's weight loss efforts. Research into the social transmission of health behaviors suggests that childhood overweight/obesity is particularly sensitive to adult influence, highlighting the importance of focusing on parental weight loss in FBT.

Peer support for healthy energy-balance behaviors has also been found to enhance weight loss maintenance in children. Peer interactions are naturally reinforcing, so families are encouraged to help their children build positive peer networks, while simultaneously uncoupling socializing from unhealthful behaviors (e.g., unhealthy foods, watching television). However, for some children, peers are a source of distress due to weight-related teasing. Social problems do not seem to interfere with initial weight loss, but children with more social problems tend to have more difficulty maintaining their weight losses, highlighting the importance of helping children and their families acquire skills to address social problems (e.g., effective methods for coping with teasing). Not only does peer support help in the maintenance of healthy energy balance behaviors, but good peer relationships also improve a child's overall quality of life.

When children and their parents learn new weight control behaviors in FBT, these new behaviors coexist with the old behaviors associated with weight gain, and these old behaviors are easily activated in our obesogenic world. Therefore, current forms of FBT help families address these challenges by encouraging vigilance regarding the impact their community or built environment can have on eating and activity choices. Families are encouraged not only to identify the constraints or barriers to healthy lifestyle behaviors within their homes and communities, but also to identify and take advantage of the opportunities, resources, and interpersonal supports available to them within their communities to enhance their efforts to engage in and strengthen newly acquired energy balance behaviors. By encouraging families to consider all the environments in which they function (home, peer, school, community), FBT helps families build a culture of health to attenuate the influences of an obesogenic society.

Treatment Modality and Treatment Setting

While reviews and individual empirical studies support the importance of treatment duration for successful weight loss in pediatric populations, less is known about the impact of treatment modality. Efforts to "scale-up" weight loss treatment for children have often involved the use of groups. Although groups may provide opportunities for enhanced social support, it is difficult to effectively tailor the behavioral aspects of FBT when working strictly with groups. In fact, a recent review of the literature found that mixed-format pediatric weight loss interventions (i.e., programs that include both individual family sessions and group treatment sessions) have better treatment effect sizes than treatments delivered to groups only. Delivery of FBT to individual families allows interventionists to select the skills, treatment targets, and pacing most appropriate for each family's unique challenges and strengths. The result is a more efficient and robust treatment than can be achieved through group alone.

Most studies of pediatric weight management programs have taken place in specialty research or university settings. When weight management programs are initiated in community settings, they are often delivered through the schools and have been more successful at preventing overweight in children who are not yet overweight or obese than they have been in decreasing weight in children who enter the programs already overweight or obese. A community setting in which FBT has had some success is in primary care settings. The co-location of behavioral interventionists or mental health specialists within primary care settings are likely to become more common for the treatment of other childhood health and mental health issues, such as attention-deficit disorder, anxiety, or depression, and FBT is uniquely well suited for implementation within these emerging health care delivery systems (e.g., integrated behavioral health care or patient-centered medical care homes).

Conclusion

With its emphasis on the family, FBT is potentially a very cost-effective treatment for both adults and children, since the per unit cost of weight loss is lower for parents and children who are overweight or obese when treated together in FBT compared to being treated separately. Although families in FBT are encouraged to engineer the home environment to support healthy weight and lifestyle behaviors, certain individuals are genetically more vulnerable to our increasingly obesogenic environment than are others. Thus, continued research into individual, modifiable factors that affect treatment response is needed, particularly into the study of the cognitive and environmental factors that drive, constrain, or compete with an individual's energy balance choices (e.g., behavioral economics, the built environment).

Since severe obesity in childhood tracks into adulthood, and treatment is most successful when started at a young age, advocacy efforts must continue to ensure that access to screening, prevention, and reimbursement for quality care is made available to young children and their families. To meet this need for broader availability of affordable and effective care, research is urgently needed into how best to integrate FBT into existing and emerging health care systems. Several multisite trials have tested FBT, and in the process of conducting these trials, effective methods for training individuals to deliver treatment with a high degree of competency have been developed. With proper training, behavioral interventionists working within primary care, mental health centers, or school settings, could add FBT to their skills set. A central system for training or credentialing individuals to provide FBT is needed, so that this effective treatment may be made more widely available.

Suggested Reading

Altman, M., Holland, J. C., Lundeen, D., Kolko, R. P., Stein, R. I., Saelens, B. E., et al. (2015). Reduction in food away from home is associated with improved child relative weight and body composition outcomes and this relation is mediated by changes in diet quality. *Journal of the Academy of Nutrition and Dietetics, 115*(9), 1400–1407.—Experimental confirmation of the importance of targeting an increase in meals eaten at home in pediatric weight loss programs.

Best, J. R., Goldschmidt, A. B., Mockus-Valenzuela, D. S., Stein, R. I., Epstein, L. H., & Wilfley, D. E. (2016). Shared weight and dietary changes in parent–child dyads following family-based obesity treatment. *Health Psychology, 35*(1), 92–95.—This study sheds light on the contributions shared dietary changes make toward the long-established association that has been found between parent and child weight loss in FBT.

Best, J. R., Theim, K. R., Gredysa, D. M., Stein, R. I., Welch, R. R., Saelens, B. E., et al. (2012). Behavioral economic predictors of overweight children's weight loss. *Journal of Consulting and Clinical Psychology, 80*(6), 1086–1096.—This study provides a good example of the importance of assessing predictors of weight loss success in childhood weight loss programs and how these findings can be used to guide the development and inclusion of additional behavioral treatment components to potentiate weight loss outcomes.

Epstein, L. H., Paluch, R. A., Wrotniak, B. H., Daniel, T. O., Kilanowski, C., Wilfley, D., et al. (2014). Cost-effectiveness of family-based group treatment for child and parental obesity. *Childhood Obesity, 10*(2), 114–121.—Children who are overweight or obese often have parents who are also overweight or obese, and this study demonstrates the cost savings of FBT that targets weight changes in both the child and parent in one treatment, compared to intervening with children and adults separately.

Frerichs, L. M., Araz, O. M., & Huang, T. T. K. (2013). Modeling social transmission dynamics of unhealthy behaviors for evaluating prevention and treatment interventions on childhood obesity. *PLoS ONE, 8*(12), e82887.—A thought-provoking examination of the importance of expanding our focus from the individual to include their social ties, particularly the importance of taking into account the impact of adults in a child's life, when designing and evaluating efforts to prevent and treat childhood obesity.

Goldschmidt, A. B., Wilfley, D. E., Paluch, R. A., Roemmich, J. N., & Epstein, L. H. (2013). Indicated prevention of adult obesity: How much weight change is necessary for normalization of weight status in children? *JAMA Pediatrics, 167*(1), 21–26.—Excellent discussion of how small weight changes can have big effects on the weight trajectory of young children.

Hankonen, N., Sutton, S., Prevost, A. T., Simmons, R. K., Griffin, S. J., Kinmonth, A. L., et al. (2015). Which behavior change techniques are associated with changes in physical activity, diet and body mass index in people with recently diagnosed diabetes? *Annals of Behavioral Medicine, 49*(1), 7–17.—Although this study was conducted with adults, it is unique in its attempt to evaluate the role of behavior change techniques in weight loss outcomes.

Hayes, J. F., Altman, M., Coppock, J. H., Wilfley, D. E., & Goldschmidt, A. B. (2015). Recent updates on the efficacy of group-based treatments for pediatric obesity. *Current Cardiovascular Risk Report, 9*(4), 16.—This review provides preliminary evidence for the importance of using a mixed format rather than group-only format when designing and delivering FBT weight loss programs.

Whitlock, E. P., O'Connor, E. A., Williams, S. B., Beil, T. L., & Lutz, K. W. (2010). *Effectiveness of primary care interventions for weight management in children and adolescents: An updated, targeted systematic review for the USPSTF* (Evidence Synthesis No. 76, AHRQ Publication No. 10-05144-EF-1). Rockville, MD: Agency for Healthcare Research and Quality.—This review establishes the research basis for assessing and recommending treatment for childhood obesity.

Wilfley, D. E., Stein, R. I., Saelens, B. E., Mockus, D. S., Matt, G. E., Hayden-Wade, H. A., et al. (2007). Efficacy of maintenance treatment approaches for childhood overweight: A randomized controlled trial. *Journal of the American Medical Association, 298*(14), 1661–1673.—This well-constructed study demonstrates that continued contact improves weight loss outcomes in children and that continued use of behavioral and social facilitation skills have a positive impact on these outcomes.

Weight Loss Approaches for Black Populations

GARY G. BENNETT
BRYAN C. BATCH

The Problem of Obesity in Black Populations

The year 1955 ushered in many firsts: Rosa Parks refused to give up her seat, Disneyland opened its gates, and McDonald's launched a fast-food revolution. The year also marked the start of the impending obesity epidemic—at least for black women. It was in the mid-1950s that obesity rates among black women first diverged from those of white women, and at no time since has the divide come close to closing. In comparison, only in the past decade, as obesity rates rose among all men, have black men's waistlines grown larger than those of whites. The epidemic's proportions remain staggering for blacks: Obesity affects nearly half of all blacks, more than half of black women, and Grade 3 obesity is twice as common in blacks as in any other racial/ethnic group. As dire as these data are, their health implications are even more concerning. Obesity is a (and likely "the") leading preventable cause for many of the conditions that disproportionately affect blacks, including cardiovascular disease, type 2 diabetes, some cancers, and kidney disease.

Although obesity is popularly viewed as a problem of poverty, socioeconomic factors are not consistently associated with obesity among blacks. Among black women, there is an inverse relation between income and obesity, but for men, there is a long- and still-standing positive socioeconomic gradient, such that the highest obesity rates are found for men at the highest income levels. While these patterns differ somewhat when other measures (e.g., education) are used to proxy socioeconomic standing, it is clear that obesity has become a generalized epidemic for blacks.

It is challenging to identify the degree to which specific obesity determinants are unique to black populations. Indeed, the entire U.S. population has been exposed to obesogenic forces, particularly the widespread availability of fast, cheap, energy-dense foods, as well as secular shifts favoring sedentary time. What makes these determinants particularly impactful for blacks and other high-risk populations is their greater intensity and historical intractability. Arguably, less clear, although certainly implicated, are the genetic, epigenetic, and broader biological factors involved in the epidemic's rise.

When an abnormal condition becomes the norm for a population, impacts on socio-cultural norms, attitudes, and perspectives follow. Most studies show that black women tolerate heavier body weights, have a greater social acceptance of overweight, have less body weight dissatisfaction, and have heavier body weight ideals compared to whites. Blacks have less recognition of the health consequences of obesity compared to other groups, and are two to three times more likely to misperceive their weight, even after receiving a physician diagnosis of overweight. Women who misperceive are 65% less likely to have interest in losing weight, compared to those with accurate perceptions. Even when overweight black women are dissatisfied with their weight, there are negligible impacts on perceived attractiveness. While these sociocultural factors may protect black women against disordered eating, they may also reduce weight loss motivation.

What Works for Weight Loss?

After extensive review, consensus national guidelines for obesity treatment were released in 2013. The guidelines are based largely on evidence from "gold standard," often mul-tisite, behavioral weight loss trials (e.g., Diabetes Prevention Program, Look AHEAD, Premier). The tested interventions maintain unique designs but share common foundational elements. Behavioral weight loss treatment of this type generally produces up to 8 kg weight loss at 1 year. However, these approaches produce reliably smaller weight loss outcomes in blacks relative to other racial/ethnic groups. Moreover, the absolute magnitude of weight losses produced by these approaches is frequently moderate and inconsistently clinically meaningful. A recent systematic review of seven leading multisite trials reported that, on average, blacks lose 2–4 kg less than whites over 6–12 months. Nevertheless, findings from multisite trials represent our best evidence. Findings from non-multisite trials, although better tailored to local populations and contexts, produce outcomes of less than 4 kg over 6–12 months. Similarly, small outcomes are common in community-based translations of the Diabetes Prevention Program, trials conducted in primary care practice and faith-based settings, and those using digital health designs.

A few issues are worth mentioning to help contextualize these findings. First, until recently, blacks were underrepresented in efficacy trials of weight loss interventions. This proportional underrepresentation has been a concern, both in an absolute sense and relative to the epidemic's dimensions. Blacks in these trials have been disproportionately recruited in single sites, which may introduce biases, particularly considering regional food preferences, sociocultural considerations, and contextual barriers/facilitators. Second, irrespective of race/ethnicity, these trials comprise highly motivated individuals who are infrequently socioeconomically disadvantaged. So trial findings likely represent a ceiling of potential intervention effects, particularly in high-risk populations. Third, the operational complexity of these trials complicates their widespread dissemination in general, and especially into settings that serve high-risk populations. Fourth, nearly everything we know about weight loss in blacks is based on the experiences of women. Fewer than half of weight loss trials focused on blacks have included men, and when black men are recruited, their numbers are small. However, the 1-year weight losses of approximately 7% for black men reported by both the Look AHEAD and Diabetes Prevention Program trials were among the largest observed for black populations. These strong outcomes for black men have not been mirrored in smaller, largely community-based trials. While selection biases might be driving the positive effects for black men in larger efficacy trials, the results provide insight into strategies that might be leveraged to maximize outcomes in black populations. Finally, it might be insufficient to focus solely on kilograms lost to judge the utility of interventions in black populations. Even with moderate weight losses, interventions may confer benefit if they produce ongoing engagement, are sustainable, and improve key secondary and patient-centered outcomes. These are important areas for future investigation.

With nearly 20 million blacks affected by obesity, we should be cautious in how we extrapolate best practices from trials conducted in a small number of highly selected individuals. That said, the evidence base does provide some clear take-home messages. Research-tested behavioral weight loss interventions can produce modest weight loss, particularly among men. However, these weight loss interventions—even those the field deems "gold standard"—reliably produce smaller weight loss outcomes among blacks relative to other groups. Interventions tested in the published literature are unlikely to meaningfully impact existing disparities in obesity and related outcomes because of their relatively small effect size in controlled settings, and because these effects likely diminish in real-world practice.

The drivers of racial disparities in treatment outcomes are likely multifactorial and challenging to discern because too few studies have addressed the question. Nevertheless, we can speculate that many common obesogenic environmental risk factors, sociocultural perspectives, and social influences are also barriers to obesity treatment success. Impaired health literacy, and numeracy are disproportionately prevalent among racial/ethnic minorities and might affect treatment outcomes given the inherent quantitative complexity of traditional obesity interventions. Several studies have reported lower treatment adherence among blacks, but it appears that differences in adherence alone may not explain disparities in treatment outcomes. A common refrain is that disparities in treatment outcomes may emerge from the failure to culturally adapt intervention content for black populations.

Does Cultural Adaptation Improve Outcomes?

As we noted earlier, there are numerous distinct, if not unique, sociocultural considerations that characterize blacks' experience of obesity. Many have hypothesized that culturally adapting treatment content would better engage black adults, thus improving treatment outcomes. Part of the challenge in interpreting this literature is the varying operationalization of cultural adaptation. While several conceptual frameworks provide guidance, there is considerable variability in how they are operationalized. Outcomes have been similarly variable. A recent systematic review found that trials of culturally adapted weight loss interventions for blacks produced 6-month outcomes of approximately 2–6 kg. The most successful interventions used sociocultural elements, such as addressing traditional foods, food insecurity, faith/spirituality, and body image. However, the least effective trials also utilized the same approaches. Better-performing trials also invested in stakeholder engagement, during both the design and implementation of the intervention. Several caveats are worth noting. First, very few trials have compared culturally adapted approaches to more generic treatment approaches. Given that the absolute magnitude of outcomes produced by both treatment types is similar, it is possible, but unlikely, that relative differences are large. Second, we know very little about how such strategies work for men. Finally, some might consider racial concordance a very basic form of cultural adaptation, but there is no evidence that such matching produces larger outcomes. Thus, while there is strong conceptual appeal of cultural adaptation, we have little empirical evidence that it produces superior outcomes relative to generic treatments.

Moving toward Comprehensive Obesity Treatment

Obesity treatment and *weight loss* have become largely synonymous terms, but clinical practice guidelines also advise weight gain prevention for those who are not interested in, or ready for, weight loss. Prevention may be indicated for a large segment of the obese population. Up to one-half of obese individuals are uninterested in weight loss. Disinterest is more common among blacks than among whites, particularly those who are socioeconomically disadvantaged. Blacks also have less weight loss motivation compared to whites, including for culturally adapted interventions.

There is strong evidence that without treatment, many will gain weight. During midlife, black women gain weight more rapidly, and at a greater magnitude (at least .5 kg/year more), than do white women. Midlife weight gain has a pronounced effect on obesity prevalence and chronic disease risk in racial/ethnic minority groups. Maintaining one's weight might contain, or even attenuate, the adverse cardiometabolic risks associated with weight gain. Unfortunately, most women are unable to prevent weight gain on their own. In CARDIA, less than 10% of black women (and 20% of all women) maintained their weight over 15 years.

Bennett and colleagues tested a weight gain prevention intervention for overweight and Grade 1 obese black women who were patients in rural community health centers. After 12 months, a majority of intervention participants were twice as likely to be at or below their baseline weight, compared to those in usual care; these intervention effects persisted for up to 4 years. There is no question that weight loss should be the primary goal for obese patients, but for patients who are uninterested or unready, weight gain prevention may convey clinical benefits.

The obesity epidemic's impact on blacks and other high-risk populations remains one of the great public health challenges of our time. In addition to its severe health, social, and economic consequences, obesity drives the seemingly intractable disparities in a wide range of clinical conditions. Obesity's determinants emerge from multiple ecological levels, and effective treatment and prevention strategies likely should mirror this complexity. However, with 20 million blacks currently affected by obesity, we desperately need effective clinical obesity treatments today. Unfortunately, progress in treating obesity in black populations has been disappointing. The goals for the next generation of treatment research are clear. We must improve treatment outcomes, reduce disparities, and extend evidence-based treatments to new delivery channels and settings—even those that may be nontraditional homes for health interventions. Given the need for effective treatments to engage patients over time, we should involve stakeholders in the design and implementation of intervention activities. We should also be working with stakeholders to identify surrogate outcomes that are more patient-centered and perhaps more culturally relevant. In short, we need renewed urgency to contend with the epidemic because, at present, our best evidence is not evidence enough.

Suggested Reading

Bennett, G. G., Foley, P., Levine, E., Whiteley, J., Askew, S., Steinberg, D. M., et al. (2013). Behavioral treatment for weight gain prevention among black women in primary care practice: A randomized clinical trial. *JAMA Internal Medicine, 173*(19), 1770–1777.—This randomized clinical trial with black women showed that a "maintain, don't gain" approach could be a useful alternative treatment for reducing disease risk associated with obesity in this population.

Bennett, G. G., Steinberg, D. M., Stoute, C., Lanpher, M., Lane, I., Askew, S., et al. (2014). Electronic health (eHealth) interventions for weight management among racial/ethnic minority adults: A systematic review. *Obesity Reviews, 15*(Suppl. 4), 146–158.—This systematic review assessed the efficacy of eHealth interventions for weight management among racial and ethnic/minority adults with obesity. There is evidence suggesting that eHealth approaches can produce short-term weight loss outcomes of moderate magnitude.

Flynn, K. J., & Fitzgibbon, M. (1998). Body images and obesity risk among black females: A review of the literature. *Annals of Behavioral Medicine, 20*(1), 13–24.—This review found that a primary care-based intervention prevented weight gain over 12 months among socio-economically disadvantaged black women.

Kong, A., Tussing-Humphreys, L. M., Odoms-Young, A. M., Stolley, M. R., & Fitzgibbon, M. L. (2014). Systematic review of behavioural interventions with culturally adapted strategies to improve diet and weight outcomes in African American women. *Obesity Reviews, 15*(Suppl. 4), 62–92.—This article systematically reviewed trials of behavioral interventions that incorporated cultural adaptations to treat overweight and obesity among blacks. While there is evidence supporting the utility of cultural adaptation during formative work, there is little evidence detailing how these strategies impact outcomes.

Kumanyika, S., Whitt-Glover, M. C., Gary, T. L., Prewitt, T. E., Odoms-Young, A. M., Banks-Wallace, J., et al. (2007). Expanding the obesity research paradigm to reach African American communities. *Preventing Chronic Disease, 4*(4), A112.—The authors introduced an expanded research paradigm for developing obesity interventions for blacks. Community leaders and researchers contributed in order to provide an expanded knowledge base and promote an understanding of contexts beyond the traditional biomedical focus.

Lancaster, K. J., Carter-Edwards, L., Grilo, S., Shen, C., & Schoenthaler, A. M. (2014). Obesity interventions in African American faith-based organizations: A systematic review. *Obesity Reviews, 15*(Suppl. 4), 159–176.—The authors systematically reviewed trials of interventions targeting weight and related behaviors in predominantly black faith-based settings. Results suggest that interventions in these settings can reduce weight, and increase fruit and vegetable intake and physical activity.

Newton, R. L., Griffith, D. M., Kearney, W. B., & Bennett, G. G. (2014). A systematic review of weight loss, physical activity and dietary interventions involving African American men. *Obesity Reviews, 15*(Suppl. 4), 93–106.—This systematic review detailed the efficacy of behavioral lifestyle interventions targeting black men, designed to produce weight loss, increased physical activity, and healthful eating. Fewer than half of the 14 studies reviewed reported statistically significant improvements in the outcomes of interest.

Osei-Assibey, G., Kyrou, I., Adi, Y., Kumar, S., & Matyka, K. (2010). Dietary and lifestyle interventions for weight management in adults from minority ethnic/non-white groups: A systematic review. *Obesity Reviews, 11*(11), 769–776.—This article provides a systematic review of randomized controlled trials involving dietary and lifestyle interventions for weight management in racial/ethnic minority groups. It indicates support for minimal-to-moderate effect sizes for the studied interventions, but many trials had elevated risk of bias.

Samuel-Hodge, C. D., Johnson, C. M., Braxton, D. F., & Lackey, M. (2014). Effectiveness of diabetes prevention program translations among African Americans. *Obesity Reviews, 15*(Suppl. 4), 107–124.—This article systematically evaluates studies from 2003 to 2012 focused on translation of the Diabetes Prevention Program in black populations. Although intervention designs were varied, results suggested that average weight loss for black participants was half of that achieved in the original trial.

Wingo, B. C., Carson, T. L., & Ard, J. (2014). Differences in weight loss and health outcomes among African Americans and whites in multicentre trials. *Obesity Reviews, 15*(Suppl. 4), 46–61.—This review of multicenter weight loss trials found that compared to whites, blacks lost less weight over 6 months but had less or similar weight regain.

Portion Size and Energy Density

BARBARA J. ROLLS
SAMANTHA M. R. KLING

In an environment filled with large portions of energy-dense foods and beverages, it is challenging for people to consume appropriate amounts and avoid weight gain. Such foods and beverages are highly palatable, inexpensive, and dominate the choices available in many settings, including convenience stores, vending machines, and restaurants, making it difficult to shift people to healthier choices. This chapter focuses on the effects of portion size and energy density on energy intake, how these effects relate to obesity, and the implications of these findings for dietary recommendations and future research.

Portion Size, Energy Intake, and Obesity

Even though the trends toward higher rates of obesity and super-sized portions began in the 1970s, few studies had evaluated the effects of portion size on weight status and intake before 2000. Population-based studies have since shown that consumption of large portions of high-energy-dense foods is related to excess body weight, adiposity, and increased energy intake. Likewise, experimental studies have demonstrated that when adults and children are served larger portions, they consume more calories and a greater weight of food. This effect is seen for beverages, amorphous foods (e.g., pasta and casseroles), and unit foods (e.g., sandwiches and packaged snacks), and has been observed in many settings, including laboratories, restaurants, and child care centers.

With the widespread availability of large portion sizes, it is critical to determine whether overeating in response to larger portions is compensated for at later eating occasions or whether the effect is sustained over time. Several controlled studies have demonstrated that serving larger portions leads to increased intake over a day in children and over 11 days in adults. In a worksite setting, doubling the portion size of lunch significantly increased self-reported intake over periods of up to 6 months. These data demonstrate that larger portions can have persistent effects over multiple days, resulting in substantial increases in energy intake, thus overriding the regulation of energy balance over prolonged periods of time.

To determine whether the response to larger portions varies between individuals, research continues to investigate how characteristics such as age, body weight, disinhibition, or satiety responsiveness relate to these effects. However, the effect of portion size on intake is robust in most individuals and has been consistently found in children as young as 3 years of age, demonstrating that environmental factors affect eating behavior early in life. Studies are beginning to explore how eating behaviors develop, how consumption norms are established, and how information about portions appropriate for energy needs should be conveyed.

Strategies to Moderate the Effect of Portion Size

Several strategies to counter the effects of portion size have been proposed; however, their acceptability and long-term effectiveness have not been determined. Possible approaches include nutrition education, consumer awareness campaigns, nutrition and point-of-purchase labels that provide clear portion size information, incentives for the food industry to offer smaller and/or a greater variety of portions, and recently developed mobile technology, such as smartphone applications. Limited data are available on the long-term effects of these approaches on decisions about appropriate portions and long-term weight loss or maintenance. A number of randomized controlled trials have demonstrated the efficacy of both liquid meal replacements such as diet shakes, and solid preportioned foods such as frozen meals for weight loss and weight loss maintenance. The preportioned foods add structure to meals and minimize decisions around how much to eat, but it is not known whether they lead to a better understanding of appropriate portions and whether this knowledge is applied to other foods.

Portion control is important for weight management; however, urging people simply to "eat less" of all foods may not be the most effective or accepted approach, since high-energy-dense foods disproportionately increase energy intake compared with those lower in energy density. A more effective strategy may be to encourage people to increase the proportion of low-energy-dense foods in their diets, while limiting portions of high-energy-dense foods. If people lower the energy density of their diet, they can eat satisfying portions while managing their body weight.

Energy Density, Energy Intake, and Obesity

Energy density, or the amount of energy per gram of food, has been found consistently to influence satiety and energy intake. The combination of macronutrients and water in food determines the energy density; fat is the most influential macronutrient at 9 kcal/g, and carbohydrates and protein both contain 4 kcal/g. Water has the greatest influence on overall energy density, since it is the largest component of many foods and contributes weight and volume without supplying any energy (0 kcal/g). Foods can be divided into categories based on their energy density for purposes of meal planning and portion control. Very-low-energy-dense foods have an energy density less than 0.6 kcal/g, low-energy-dense foods have 0.6–1.5 kcal/g, medium-energy-dense foods have 1.6–3.9 kcal/g, and high-energy-dense foods have 4.0–9.0 kcal/g. Therefore, for the same amount of energy, a larger portion can be consumed when the energy density is low. For example, a 100-calorie snack of a very-low-energy-dense food such as strawberries is approximately 300 grams, while pretzels, a medium-energy-dense food, provide only 25 grams.

Diets higher in energy density have been shown to be related to energy intake, body weight, and weight gain in several population-based epidemiological and longitudinal studies. Free-living adults who reported a higher-energy-dense diet consumed more energy, were more likely to be obese, and gained more weight over 6–8 years compared to those reporting a diet lower in energy density. A diet higher in energy density was also found to be associated with higher fat mass, excess adiposity, and obesity in children.

The energy density of foods is a robust determinant of satiety and energy intake in experimental feeding studies. For example, in controlled studies, serving higher-energy-dense foods increased energy intake for up to 14 days in adults and over 2 days in children. In addition, the effects of energy density on energy intake persisted when the macronutrient content of foods was varied, suggesting that multiple methods can be used to lower energy density in order to lower energy intake. These include increasing the water content through the addition of vegetables or fruit, or decreasing the proportion of fat or sugar. In particular, modifying recipes by adding extra vegetables to reduce the energy density of a food has been found to be an effective strategy in both adults and children to increase vegetable intake and decrease energy intake while maintaining acceptance of the dish.

Strategies That Utilize the Effect of Energy Density

Both laboratory and clinical trial data indicate that reducing energy density can be an effective approach for weight management. For example, in a yearlong trial, women with obesity who were counseled to reduce dietary energy density by increasing intake of fruits and vegetables, along with reducing intake of fat, had greater weight loss than those who were advised to reduce only fat intake. In the multicenter PREMIER trial that included three different lifestyle interventions, dietary changes that reduced energy density were related to greater weight loss after 6 months. Additional clinical trials indicate that diets low in energy density can also help patients maintain their weight loss. In one trial, instruction on reducing dietary energy density led to sustained weight loss 36 months after the start of the intervention. Since the response to energy density emerges early in life, reductions in energy density could possibly be used strategically to prevent excess energy intake leading to overweight in children as well as in adults.

The 2010 U.S. Dietary Guidelines Advisory Committee Report found evidence to support "a relationship between energy density and body weight in adults and in children and adolescents such that consuming diets lower in energy density may be an effective strategy for managing body weight" (Perez-Escamilla et al., 2012, p. 671). A low-energy-dense diet meets the recommendations of most health organizations in that it is high in vegetables and fruits, whole grains, fish, and other sources of lean protein, and is low in unhealthy fats and refined carbohydrates. Additionally, choosing low-energy-dense foods can help individuals not only eat satisfying amounts that will help control hunger and manage weight but also a diet rich in nutrients. However, foods high in energy density are palatable, inexpensive, and widely available compared to foods lower in energy density, suggesting the need to change the food environment to help consumers to make healthier choices.

Strategies That Utilize the Combined Effects of Portion Size and Energy Density

Since individuals have ready access to foods that vary both in portion size and energy density, it is important to understand how these factors work together to affect energy intake. Experimental studies that simultaneously varied portion size and energy density found that these effects were independent and combined to affect satiation or *ad libitum* consumption in both children and adults. Serving larger portions of higher-energy-dense foods led to a sustained increase in energy intake over several days compared to when smaller portions of lower-energy-dense foods were served. Furthermore, varying energy density had a stronger effect on energy intake than manipulating portion size, and participants often did not notice the changes in energy density and accepted the lower- and higher-energy-density versions of food similarly. This suggests that reductions in energy density can be combined with decreases in portion size to produce foods that would be accepted by consumers, while helping them eat fewer calories.

In a food environment shaped by consumer preferences and expectations, meals are often composed of small portions of low-energy-dense fruits and vegetables, along with large portions of energy-dense meats, starches, and grains. This meal pattern is problematic in that it promotes excess energy intake, hence the 2010 Dietary Guidelines recommendation to "make half your plate fruits and vegetables" (U.S. Department of Agriculture and Department of Health and Human Services, 2011, p. 1). In support of this recommendation, experimental studies have demonstrated that *substituting* larger portions of foods lower in energy density for more energy-dense meal components can lead to increased intake of the lower-energy-dense foods and reductions in meal energy intake. Another effective strategy to enhance satiety and reduce overall meal intake is to serve large portions of low-energy-dense foods such as soup, salad, or fruit as a first course, without other competing foods.

Recommendations

In recent years, significant advances have been made in understanding how characteristics of the food environment influence energy intake and body weight, and how they can be varied strategically to improve nutritional status. Changes in the portion size and energy density of foods can be used either independently or in combination to counter overconsumption.

1. Strategies, such as use of preportioned foods, that promote consumption of portions that are appropriate for an individual's energy needs are recommended, but there has been little research on the effectiveness or sustainability of other portion control strategies for weight management.
2. To manage weight, individuals should choose lower-energy-dense options to help them improve their diet and feel full on fewer calories. The energy density of food can be lowered by increasing the water content through the addition of vegetables or fruit, or by decreasing the proportion of fat or sugar.
3. The effects of portion size and energy density can be used strategically to improve diet quality and reduce energy intake. Individuals should aim to increase the

proportion of lower-energy-dense foods in their diet by serving them in larger portions and moderating portions of foods higher in energy density.

Further research is needed to determine the best ways to encourage consumers to adapt and sustain these healthy choices; however, their effectiveness will depend on altering the current food environment, so that lower-energy-dense choices are easily accessible, appealing, and affordable.

Acknowledgments

This research was supported by the National Institute of Diabetes and Digestive and Kidney Diseases (Grant Nos. DK039177, DK059853, and DK082580) and by the U.S. Department of Agriculture, National Institute of Food and Agriculture (Grant No. 2011-67001-30117).

Suggested Reading

Birch, L. L., Savage J. S., & Fisher J. O. (2015). Right sizing prevention: Food portion size effects on children's eating and weight. *Appetite, 88,* 11–16.—This article provides an overview of the research pertaining to the effect of portion size on preschool children's eating behavior and weight status, and highlights unanwered questions and gaps in the literature.

English, L., Lasschuijt, M., & Keller, K. L. (2015). Mechanisms of the portion size effect: What is known and where do we go from here? *Appetite, 88,* 39–49.—This review summarizes the influence of visual cues, meal microstructure (e.g., bite size), postingestive effects, and cognitive processes on the portion size effect.

Herman, C. P., Polivy, J., Pliner, P., & Vartanian, L. R. (2015). Mechanisms underlying the portion-size effect. *Physiology and Behavior, 144,* 129–136.—The authors discuss possible mechanisms driving the portion size effect, in particular, the perceived "appropriateness" of the amount served.

Perez-Escamilla, R., Obbagy, J. E., Altman, J. M., Essery, E. V., McGrane, M. M., Wong, Y. P., et al. (2012). Dietary energy density and body weight in adults and children: A systematic review. *Journal of the Academy of Nutrition and Dietetics, 112,* 671–684.—The relationship between energy density and body weight in adults, children, and adolescents was systematically reviewed by the 2010 Dietary Guidelines Advisory Committee, and the results are described in this article.

Pourshahidi, L. K., Kerr, M. A., McCaffrey, T. A., & Livingstone, M. B. (2014). Influencing and modifying children's energy intake: The role of portion size and energy density. *Proceedings of the Nutrition Society, 73,* 397–406.—This article summarizes both observational and experimental research on the effects of portion size and energy density on children's energy intake and risk for overweight and obesity.

Rolls, B. J. (2010). Plenary Lecture 1: Dietary strategies for the prevention and treatment of obesity. *Proceedings of the Nutrition Society, 69,* 70–79.—This review focuses on the effects of portion size and energy density on intake and the implications for the prevention and treatment of obesity.

Rolls, B. J. (2012). *The ultimate volumetrics diet.* New York: Morrow.—This book is a guide to strategically using portion size and energy density to manage weight, while eating satisfying amounts of nutritious foods.

Rolls, B. J. (2014). What is the role of portion control in weight management? *International Journal of Obesity, 38,* S1–S8.—This article reviews the research on the effect of portion size on energy intake, stratgies to moderate this effect, and how these strategies have been applied to weight management.

Steenhuis, I. H., & Vermeer, W. M. (2009). Portion size: Review and framework for interventions. *International Journal of Behavioral Nutrition and Physical Activity, 6,* 58.—This review summarizes the research on the effects of portion size on energy intake, possible mechanisms for this relationship, and the effectiveness of interventions targeting portion control.

U.S. Department of Agriculture & Department of Health and Human Services. (2011). Dietary Guidelines 2010: Selected messages for consumers. Retrieved from *www.cnpp.usda.gov/ sites/default/files/dietary_guidelines_for_americans/SelectedMessages.pdf.*

Behavioral Treatment of Obesity

MEGHAN L. BUTRYN
THOMAS A. WADDEN

Behavior therapy for obesity consists of a set of principles and techniques that promote changes in eating patterns, physical activity, and other aspects of weight control. This approach, which is now typically referred to as behavioral weight control or lifestyle modification, has become the first line of treatment for obesity, as recommended by several organizations, including the joint recommendations of the American Heart Association, American College of Cardiology, and the Obesity Society. Behavioral weight control has three key components: a low-calorie diet; increased physical activity; and use of behavioral strategies to facilitate adherence to diet and exercise goals. This chapter describes the components and effectiveness of behavioral weight control and considers future directions for research, treatment development, and dissemination.

Primary Components and Structure of Treatment

Calorie Intake

Behavioral weight loss programs typically prescribe a daily calorie target to induce an energy deficit. This target is usually between 1,200 and 1,500 kcal/day for women and between 1,500 and 1,800 kcal/day for men. It may take a few weeks of calibration for each participant to identify the calorie level that produces the desired loss of 0.5–1 kg/week. Prescribing a diet that restricts certain types of foods, such as a low-carbohydrate diet, also can be effective in reducing calorie intake.

Physical Activity

Participants are instructed to increase their physical activity gradually to approximately 150–180 minutes/week over the first 6 months. Higher levels often are prescribed during weight loss maintenance given findings that approximately 60 minutes/day of physical activity are needed to reduce the risk of weight regain. Activity usually consists of brisk walking or other forms of moderate-intensity aerobic exercise.

Self-Monitoring

Recording the type and amount of all foods and beverages consumed, along with their calorie content, is a critical component of treatment. Self-monitoring helps participants identify patterns in their eating behavior, select targets for reducing calorie intake, and track progress in meeting a calorie goal. Self-monitoring of physical activity is encouraged, either through a chart, log, or use of a device such as a pedometer or other sensor. Participants keep a record of weight change and weigh themselves at home regularly, usually once or twice per week during active weight loss, and as often as daily during weight loss maintenance.

Goal Setting

Treatment focuses on making objective, measurable changes in eating, activity, and related behaviors. Participants set specific targets for calorie intake, minutes of physical activity, and frequency of self-monitoring in order to lose 0.5–1 kg/week, with an ultimate goal of a 5–10% reduction in initial weight. After each treatment session (described later), participants also may set a short-term goal for changing a related weight control behavior, such as making a grocery list or asking a friend to go for a walk. Treatment helps participants make specific plans for implementing the behaviors selected. Participants are encouraged to set goals that represent sustainable changes to their lifestyles.

Stimulus Control

Participants learn to reengineer their environments using stimulus control strategies. They create cues that prompt positive eating and exercise behaviors, making healthier choices easier and more automatic. They also modify cues that are associated with overeating (or sedentary behavior), such as reducing the availability of tempting foods in the home.

Other Components

Behavioral programs usually include additional components such as problem solving and skills for increasing social support. Participants also learn cognitive restructuring skills, such as identifying cognitive distortions (e.g., "I'll never be able to lose weight since I ate that dessert") and replacing them with rational responses. Relapse prevention training teaches participants to anticipate and respond to lapses and high-risk situations.

Structure and Frequency of Sessions

Treatment sessions are typically delivered by a psychologist, dietitian, or other health professional, in individual or group format. Sessions are usually held weekly for 12–24 weeks, followed by every-other-week or monthly meetings. Sessions begin with each participant being weighed in private, which provides an important opportunity for accountability and reinforcement, and prompts the participant to reflect on the relationship between weight change and key behaviors from the previous week. After the weigh-in, participants report on their progress in meeting goals from the previous session. The remainder of the meeting focuses on acquiring a new weight management skill, as designated in the curriculum, using ingroup activities and discussion. The session concludes with setting goals and assignments. Group sessions usually last 60–90 minutes, with individual meetings about half that time.

Efficacy and Benefits of Behavioral Weight Control

Structured behavioral weight loss programs, as described earlier, produce an average loss of 7–10 kg in the first 6 months, equal to a reduction of 7–10% of initial weight. Weight losses are largest when at least 14 sessions are provided during this time; lower-intensity interventions are not as effective. Within any given program, variability in weight loss is notable, with as many as 20–30% of participants failing to achieve even a 5% weight loss, and with some participants losing 15–20% of their body weight. Individuals with the best attendance and greatest consistency in keeping self-monitoring records achieve the largest weight losses. The use of portion-controlled diets, including meal replacements, reliably increases short-term weight loss.

Long-Term Weight Loss

Gradual weight regain is common after initial weight loss. In the absence of further treatment, participants typically regain 3–4 kg in the first year following weight loss, with 1–2 kg/year thereafter. Five years after treatment, about half of the participants have returned to their baseline weight (or above), with the other half maintaining some weight loss. Decreased adherence to diet and exercise prescriptions and a return to previous habits contribute to weight regain, as do unfavorable changes in appetite hormones (e.g., ghrelin, leptin) and energy expenditure (both resting and nonresting), which are precipitated by caloric restriction and weight loss. These compensatory biological responses regrettably "defend" the body against weight reduction.

The most effective method for preventing or slowing weight regain is to continue behavioral treatment on an every-other-week or monthly basis after initial treatment. Sessions during this time are an important source of support and accountability. They provide an opportunity to address weight regain early and maintain motivation for the substantial effort required for weight loss maintenance. The most successful individuals usually engage in high levels of physical activity (e.g., 225–300 minutes/week), eat a low-calorie diet, and self-monitor weight regularly. Long-term weight losses also are typically largest in individuals who achieved the largest short-term losses, revealing their persistent adherence and motivation.

Health Benefits

As described in Chapter 75, behavioral weight loss programs produce many health benefits. Even a modest loss of 3–5% of initial weight can improve triglycerides, blood glucose, hemoglobin A1c, and diabetes risk. Weight loss of 5–10% improves blood pressure and high-density lipoprotein (HDL) cholesterol. Greater weight losses generally produce greater changes in risk factors. The Diabetes Prevention Program (DPP) demonstrated a clear reduction in the risk of developing type 2 diabetes in the overweight or obese adults with impaired glucose tolerance who were assigned to a lifestyle intervention, lost an average of 7 kg, and exercised for 150 minutes/week. Onset of diabetes over the initial follow-up period (which averaged 2.8 years) was 58% lower in participants assigned to the lifestyle intervention, compared to placebo. After 10 years of follow-up, lifestyle participants had regained to within 2 kg of their baseline weight, but their incidence of type 2 diabetes remained 34% lower than in the placebo group.

Look AHEAD, another landmark study that examined health outcomes of weight loss, enrolled over 5,000 overweight or obese adults with type 2 diabetes and randomly assigned them to long-term lifestyle intervention or a support and education control group. After an average of 9.6 years, approximately 50% of lifestyle intervention participants maintained a clinically meaningful weight loss (i.e., $\geq$ 5%) and experienced significant improvements in mood, quality of life, and physical function, and reduction of sleep apnea. However, there was no difference between groups in cardiovascular morbidity or mortality (the study's primary outcome), possibly because the comparison group lost more weight than expected during extended follow-up, and both groups had excellent control of traditional cardiovascular risk factors (i.e., blood pressure, blood glucose, lipids) because of extensive use of medications (antihypertensive agents, etc.).

Dissemination

Dissemination of behavioral weight loss treatment is a high priority for the field. The DPP, for instance, has been disseminated successfully in settings such as the Young Men's Christian Association (YMCA), cooperative extensions services, churches, and military bases. Several lessons have been learned from DPP dissemination efforts. First, programs should include new training materials that meet the needs of a wider-than-usual array of treatment providers. Training that includes a scientific rationale for the intervention, interactive education and evaluations, and continued support is particularly effective. Second, retaining a sufficient dose and duration of treatment contacts in community settings is necessary for continued efficacy. In instances in which the original DPP was adapted to have fewer sessions and delivered in a briefer period, it was less effective. Stakeholders in various areas will need to work together to determine how to maintain long-term contact between participants and providers in a cost-effective and feasible manner.

Remotely delivered and digitally based treatment approaches will likely be critical components of dissemination. Phone-delivered interventions, for instance, have the potential to be as effective as in-person contact for inducing weight loss or promoting weight loss maintenance. Phone calls may be conducted individually or as group conference calls. The use of digital tools for behavioral weight loss delivery also is developing rapidly, as described in Chapter 91. Web-based programs, for instance, may be available to many individuals who cannot attend face-to-face behavioral weight loss programs, and the cost of such programs is typically lower. In general, Web-based programs produce a loss of 1–5 kg, which is superior to no intervention but significantly less than that achieved in face-to-face programs. However, there is marked variability in Web-based program components and efficacy. Efficacy improves when programs include components that promote engagement, provide personalized feedback, and emphasize self-monitoring and skills training. One of the most promising ways of using Web-based programs may be to supplement, rather than replace, face-to-face contact. Using a hybrid approach (i.e., face-to-face plus Web-based) to extend treatment contact improves weight outcomes and may make continued contact more feasible.

Developments in the mobile health (i.e., mHealth) field also are creating opportunities to integrate smartphones, text messages, and apps into face-to-face behavioral weight loss programs or to use these tools for remote program delivery. Tools such as barcode scanners, physical activity sensors, and wireless scales allow data to be collected in real time with automated, immediate feedback. Research must evaluate the optimal use of such tools with regard to timing, frequency, and content.

New Theoretical Approaches

Efforts to improve short- and long-term weight loss with behavioral weight control have included supplementing this therapy with other theoretical approaches. *Motivational interviewing (MI),* which has received extensive attention, is a patient-centered approach to counseling that emphasizes participants' choosing treatment goals and strategies that are personally relevant to them. MI-trained interventionists use empathy and reflective listening to help participants explore their desire for behavior change and potential ambivalence about it (e.g., "You seem to want to lose weight to improve your health, but you're worried about having to give up some of your favorite foods"). They similarly encourage participants to select changes in diet and physically activity that are consistent with their preferences. In this regard, MI typically is less prescriptive and directive than traditional behavioral weight control. When used as a primary approach to weight reduction, MI generally has not induced clinically meaningful weight loss, most likely because participants have not had clear targets for caloric restriction. MI, however, has been shown in some (but not all) studies to improve weight loss when added to traditional behavioral weight control. Its addition is probably most useful with patients who appear ambivalent or unmotivated to adhere to recommended diet and physical activity plans.

The "third generation" or "third wave" of behavior therapies includes mindfulness-based cognitive therapy, dialectical behavior therapy, and acceptance and commitment therapy (ACT). Research on the application of these approaches to obesity is ongoing, particularly the use of acceptance-based behavioral treatment, in which ACT is integrated with traditional behavioral weight control. Acceptance-based strategies foster the ability to tolerate uncomfortable internal experiences in the service of goal-directed behavior. These strategies are designed to facilitate the identification and internalization of values and lasting commitment to behavior consistent with these values. Mindful decision making also is emphasized. Future trials will determine whether these approaches ultimately improve average weight loss. Clinical experience suggests that they may potentially meet the needs of particular participants, such as those who do not respond well to traditional behavioral treatment.

The Future of Behavioral Weight Control

Despite nearly 50 years of research on behavioral weight control, many challenges remain to be addressed. There is substantial variability in weight loss during the first few months of treatment, and more must be learned about factors responsible for suboptimal response and how treatment might be tailored to meet the needs of nonresponders. Emerging neuropsychological and psychobiological research in areas such as delay discounting, reward perception, and appetite regulation also may lead to a greater understanding of the difficulty of weight loss maintenance, as well as new ideas about how behavioral treatment can address such challenges. Providing greater access to behavioral weight loss treatment, and doing so in a way that allows for continued contact over the long term, is a key priority. Effective training programs for providers who operate in a variety of settings must be created, and funding for such programs must be available. Technology will undoubtedly be a component of dissemination efforts, and it will be critical to determine the optimal balance between device-based and clinician-based interactions. Finally, obesity prevention efforts must be expanded greatly to decrease the number of individuals who require behavioral weight control in the first place.

Acknowledgments

Preparation of this chapter was supported, in part, by Grant No. R01DK92374 from the National Institutes of Health (to Meghan L. Butryn). We thank Zayna Bakizada for her editorial assistance.

Suggested Reading

Diabetes Prevention Program Research Group. (2009). 10-year follow-up of diabetes incidence and weight loss in the Diabetes Prevention Program Outcomes Study. *Lancet, 374,* 1677–1686.—Participants' loss of 7 kg at 1 year protected them from developing type 2 diabetes at 10 years, despite their regaining most of the weight lost at follow-up.

Forman, E., Butryn, M., Juarascio, A., Bradley, L., Lowe, M., Herbert, J., et al. (2013). The mind your health project: A randomized controlled trial of an innovative behavioral treatment for obesity. *Obesity, 21,* 1119–1126.—This article describes an acceptance-based form of behavioral treatment and identifies moderators that determined which participants lost more weight with this approach than with traditional behavioral treatment.

Jensen, M. D., Ryan, D. H., Apovian, C. M., Ard, J. D., Comuzzie, A. G., Donato, K. A., et al. (2014). 2013 AHA/ACC/TOS guideline for the management of overweight and obesity in adults: a report of the American College of Cardiology/American Heart Association Task Force on Practice Guidelines and the Obesity Society. *Circulation, 129*(25, Suppl. 2), S102–S138.—These treatment guidelines provide a systematic review of the behavioral treatment of obesity, of the effects of different diets on weight loss, and related topics.

Look AHEAD Research Group. (2006). The Look AHEAD study: A description of the lifestyle intervention and the evidence supporting it. *Obesity, 14,* 737–752. This article describes the lifestyle intervention provided in the Look AHEAD study and examines the research that led to its development.

Look AHEAD Research Group. (2013). Cardiovascular effects of intensive lifestyle intervention in type 2 diabetes. *New England Journal of Medicine, 369*(2), 145–154.—The Look AHEAD study failed to find that a loss of 8.6% of initial weight decreased the occurrence of cardiovascular morbidity and mortality, although the intervention was associated with numerous other health benefits.

MacLean, P. S., Wing, R. R., Davidson, T., Epstein, L., Goodpaster, B., Hall, K. D., et al. (2015). NIH working group report: Innovative research to improve maintenance of weight loss. *Obesity, 23*(1), 7–15.—This article provides an excellent analysis of the key behavioral, genetic, and physiological factors that make maintaining weight loss so challenging.

Wadden, T., Webb, V., Moran, C., & Bailer, B. (2012). Lifestyle modification for obesity: New developments in diet, physical activity, and behavior therapy. *Circulation, 125,* 1157–1170.—This narrative review provides more detailed examination of many of the topics covered in our chapter.

West, D., DiLillo, V., Bursac, Z., Gore, S., & Greene, P. (2007). Motivational interviewing improves weight loss in women with type 2 diabetes. *Diabetes Care, 30,* 1081–1087.—Participants who received behavioral weight control combined with motivation interviewing lost approximately 2 kg more than those who received behavioral weight control alone, although weight losses in both groups were smaller than expected.

84

Pharmacological Treatments for Obesity

REKHA B. KUMAR
LOUIS J. ARONNE

Body weight/fat mass is subject to homeostatic control, and there is disruption of this homeostasis in the disease of obesity. There are two bodies of neurons in the hypothalamus that integrate information from peripheral signals coming from the fat cell, gut, and pancreas, in order to regulate appetite and energy expenditure through thermogenesis. Various areas from the periphery to the hypothalamic nuclei are targets of the current medicines for obesity.

Lifestyle interventions including a calorie-restricted diet, and increased physical activity remain the cornerstone of treatment for patients who are overweight and obese. However, lifestyle modifications have not been effective in producing long-term weight loss. Counterregulatory neurohormonal mechanisms aimed at maintaining fat mass as a survival measure, as well as several environmental obstacles, have been identified as promoting weight regain after diet-induced weight loss. The National Heart, Lung, and Blood Institute of the National Institutes of Health, recommends that for individuals who fail to respond to lifestyle interventions after 6 months of treatment, or have a body mass index (BMI) > 30 kg/m^2, or a BMI > 27 kg/m^2 along with weight-induced comorbidity, may have weight loss medication added to their treatment plan.

The goal of pharmacotherapy is not only to reduce weight, but also, more importantly, to improve the comorbid conditions associated with obesity, such as hyperglycemia, hyperlipidemia, and atherosclerotic heart disease. Patients and physicians should appreciate that obesity is a chronic disease that will require long-term treatment. They should also understand that the efficacy of the current medication options is limited to 5–10% body weight loss in the majority of successful patients. Medications should only be used as an adjunct to healthy lifestyle changes, including an increase in daily activity and adherence to a calorie-deficit diet.

Impressive advances in the pharmacological management of obesity have been made over the past few years. There are now five medicines for chronic weight management available in the Unites States: orlistat, phentermine–topiramate, lorcaserin, buproprion–naltrexone, and liraglutide. These five agents have separate mechanisms of action and varying adverse effect profiles, as well as a range in therapeutic efficacy. There are also two agents approved for short-term use in obesity: phentermine and diethylpropion.

Orlistat

Prior to 2012, the only weight loss medicine for long-term use was orlistat (Xenical), which was approved by the U.S. Food and Drug Administration (FDA) in 1999. Orlistat promotes weight loss by inhibiting gastrointestinal lipases, thereby decreasing the absorption of fat from the gastrointestinal tract. On average, 120 mg of orlistat taken three times per day will decrease fat absorption by 30%. Orlistat at a lower dose of 60 mg three times daily, called Alli, is approved for over-the-counter use in the United States. Several trials have supported orlistat's efficacy as an aid to weight loss and maintenance. In the Xenical in the Prevention of Diabetes in Obese Subjects (XENDOS) trial, after 4 years, the orlistat-treated patients (120 mg three times daily) had lost 5.8 kg compared with 3.0 kg in the placebo group ($p < .001$). In patients who had impaired glucose tolerance, the 4-year weight reductions were 5.7 kg and 3.0 kg, respectively. Over the entire study period, a significantly higher proportion of patients treated with orlistat compared with those treated with placebo achieved weight losses > 5% and 10% of total body weight. After 4 years, 52.8% of the orlistat patients had lost 5%, and 26.2% had lost 10% of their initial body weight. In addition to promoting weight loss and maintaining lost weight, orlistat has been shown to improve insulin sensitivity and lower serum glucose levels. In the XENDOS study, the cumulative incidence of diabetes was 9.0% in the placebo plus diet and lifestyle group, and 6.2% in the subjects receiving orlistat. This outcome corresponds to a risk reduction of 37.3% ($p = .0032$).

Phentermine–Topiramate

Low-dose, controlled-release phentermine plus topiramate (as one capsule) was approved by the FDA in 2012 as a long-term treatment for obesity in adults with a BMI $\geq$ 30 kg/m^2 or a BMI $\geq$ 27 kg/m^2 with at least one weight-related comorbidity. Phentermine is an adrenergic agonist that promotes weight loss by activation of the sympathetic nervous system and release of norepinephrine and dopamine, with a subsequent decrease in food intake and increased resting energy expenditure. This occurs by modulating activity of anorectic or orexigenic peptides in hypothalamic nuclei. Topiramate, an FDA-approved medicine for epilepsy and migraine prophylaxis, has been shown to reduce body weight by reducing appetite and decreasing caloric intake. Phentermine–topiramate is available in four doses: 3.75/23 mg (starting dose), 7.5/46 mg (lowest treatment dose), 11.25/69 mg, or 15/92 mg (maximum treatment dose).

The 52-week CONQUER trial randomized 2,487 patients who were obese with a mean BMI of 36.6 kg/m^2 and comorbidities including hypertension, dyslipidemia, diabetes or prediabetes, or abdominal obesity to either placebo, midtreatment dose (7.5/46 mg), or maximum treatment dose (15/92 mg), with results showing 6.6 and 8.6% placebo subtracted weight loss in the lower dose and maximum dose arms, respectively. In the CONQUER trial, 70% of patients who took the top dose (15/92 mg) and 62% who took the recommended dose (7.5/46 mg) achieved 5% or greater weight loss after 1 year versus 21% of those who took placebo ($p < .0001$).

Improvement in systolic and diastolic blood pressure and triglycerides, and greater increases in high-density lipoprotein (HDL) were seen in subjects treated with phentermine–topiramate compared with placebo in the CONQUER trials. Improvements in fasting glucose and insulin levels were seen, and a 54 and 76% reduction in progression to type 2 diabetes in the two treatment groups, respectively, was noted in patients without diabetes at baseline.

Lorcaserin

Lorcaserin, a selective serotonin (5-HT_{2C}) receptor agonist, was approved by the FDA in 2012 as a long-term treatment for obesity. Lorcaserin selectively activates the central 5-HT_{2C} receptor over the 2A and 2B receptors. Lorcaserin reduces appetite by binding to the 5-HT_{2C} receptors on anorexigenic pro-opiomelanocortin (POMC) neurons in the hypothalamus. The nonselective serotonergic agonists, fenfluramine and dexfenfluramine, also caused weight loss but increased the risk of serotonin-associated cardiac valvular disease, potentially mediated through the 5-HT_{2B} receptor. Due to its selective agonism of the 5-HT_{2C} receptor, lorcaserin should not have cardiac valvular effects. The development program has focused on excluding that possibility, but long-term data will be necessary. Lorcaserin, a 10-mg tablet, is meant to be taken twice daily.

The Phase III double-blind placebo controlled BLOOM trial included 3,182 overweight or obese adults who received lorcaserin 10 mg twice daily (bid) or placebo for 52 weeks, in conjunction with diet and exercise. At Week 52, all subjects were rerandomized to either placebo or lorcaserin for an additional year. At 1 year, the average placebo subtracted weight loss was 3.6%, and 47% of the subjects taking lorcaserin lost > 5% of weight as compared to 20.5% in the control group. Subjects who showed a weight loss of > 5% in Year 1 and were maintained on lorcaserin treatment in Year 2 were able to maintain their weight loss better than those who had been switched to placebo.

The Behavioral Modification and Lorcaserin for Overweight and Obesity Management (BLOOM) study results also showed significant changes in hemoglobin A1c (HbA1c), total cholesterol, blood pressure, triglycerides, and heart rate in the lorcaserin versus placebo group. The BLOOM-DM study was conducted in obese subjects with type 2 diabetes. This trial showed that at 52 weeks, 37.5% of patients treated with lorcaserin 10 mg bid showed a weight loss > 5%, which was more than twice the percentage in the placebo group. There was a reduction of HbA1c of 0.9% in those on lorcaserin as compared to 0.4% reduction in the placebo group.

Bupropion–Naltrexone

Bupropion–naltrexone (Contrave) was approved by the FDA for weight loss in September 2014. Bupropion's primary mechanism of action is via dopaminergic and noradrenergic stimuli, without inhibition of monoamine oxidase (MAO) or reuptake of serotonin. Inhibiting reuptake of dopamine and/or norepinephrine decreases the "reward pathway" that various foods can induce. The second component of Contrave is naltrexone, a pure opioid antagonist that blocks an opioid pathway that may slow weight loss.

Four 56-week multicenter, double-blind, placebo-controlled trials (CONTRAVE Obesity Research, or COR-I, COR-II, COR-BMOD, and COR-Diabetes) were conducted to evaluate the effect of bupropion–naltrexone in conjunction with lifestyle modification in a placebo-controlled cohort of 4,536 patients. The COR-I, COR-II, and COR-BMOD trials enrolled patients with a BMI ≥ 30 kg/m² or overweight (BMI ≥ 27 kg/m²) and at least one comorbidity. The COR-Diabetes trial enrolled patients with BMI > 27 kg/m² with type 2 diabetes, with or without hypertension and/or dyslipidemia. The primary end points were percent change from baseline body weight and the proportion of patients achieving at least a 5% reduction in body weight. In the 56-week COR-I trial, the mean change in body weight was –5.4% in patients assigned to bupropion–naltrexone 360/32 mg compared with –1.3% in the placebo group. The clinically significant cutoff of 5% reduction in body weight from baseline occurred in 42% of treatment group patients versus 17% of placebo patients.

In the COR-Diabetes trial, 44.5% of patients receiving bupropion–naltrexone lost ≥ 5% of their body weight after 56 weeks versus 18.9% of patients on placebo ($p < .001$). Patients using bupropion–naltrexone also showed a 0.6% reduction in HbA1c from baseline, compared to a 0.1% reduction in placebo. In all of the COR trials, secondary cardiovascular end points were met, including statistically significant improvements in waist circumference, visceral fat, HDL cholesterol, and triglycerides.

Liraglutide

Liraglutide 3.0 mg was approved by the FDA in December 2014. Liraglutide is a glucagon-like peptide 1 (GLP-1) receptor agonist. Liraglutide has been used for type 2 diabetes in doses up to 1.8 mg. In animal studies, peripheral administration of liraglutide results in uptake in specific brain regions regulating appetite, including the hypothalamus. A study involving obese individuals without diabetes demonstrated that liraglutide 3.0 mg/day suppressed acute food intake and subjective hunger, and delayed gastric emptying. Conversely, energy expenditure in subjects treated with liraglutide 3.0 mg/day decreased, even when corrected for weight loss, which was probably reflective of metabolic adaptation to weight loss.

Liraglutide Phase III studies included populations with overweight and obesity, including those with comorbidities such as prediabetes , hypertension, hyperlipidemia, type 2 diabetes, and sleep apnea. In these studies, liraglutide 3.0 mg was associated with a greater weight loss of approximately –5%, compared with placebo and identical lifestyle intervention. Total mean weight loss from baseline in these studies is in the range of –6 to –8% with liraglutide 3.0 mg. Significantly more patients taking liraglutide lost 5% or more of their body weight versus those taking placebo (63.5 vs. 26.6%). In addition to weight loss, there was a decrease in waist circumference, systolic and diastolic blood pressure, LDL and HDL cholesterol, and triglycerides.

Phentermine and Diethylpropion

Phentermine (separate from the phentermine–topiramate combination) was the first FDA approved short-term medication for weight loss, and it is still available today. Phentermine is a sympathomimetic anorexogenic agent. A study from 1968 is the only longer-term controlled trial of phentermine. In this study, 64 patients completed 36 weeks of placebo, phentermine, or placebo and phentermine on alternating days. Both phentermine groups lost approximately 13% of their initial weight, while the placebo group lost only 5%. Phentermine's main side effects are related to its sympathomimetic properties, such as elevation in blood pressure and pulse, insomnia, constipation, and dry mouth. Diethylpropion, another symphatomimetic and a derivative of bupropion, is also an approved short-term drug for treating obesity. It acts through modulation of norepinephrine action.

Summary

For the first time, patients who are obese are able to benefit from five different FDA-approved pharmacological agents for chronic weight management and two agents for short-term use. Although mean weight loss in Phase III trials is generally 5–10%, those who will lose more on any medicine can often be identified as those who lose at least 5% of body weight after 3 months of treatment. While a higher percentage of total body weight is lost with use of combination phentermine–topiramate compared to bupropion–naltrexone, orlistat, and lorcaserin, there are more contraindications to its use and potential adverse effects. Lorcaserin and bupropion–naltrexone carry different adverse effect profiles, and interactions with other psychiatric medications may preclude use of one or the other. When choosing a medication for obesity, several factors need to be considered, such as comorbidities, medication interactions, and risk of potential adverse effects and insurance costs.

Suggested Reading

DeFronzo, R. A., Bergenstal, R. M., Bode, B., Kushner, R., Lewin, A. J., Skjøth, T. V., et al. (2014). *Effects of liraglutide 3.0 mg and 1.8 mg on body weight and cardiometabolic risk factors in overweight and obese adults with type 2 diabetes mellitus (T2DM): The scale diabetes randomized, double-blind, placebo-controlled, 56-week trial.* Presentation at the 96th annual meeting of the Endocrine Society, Chicago.—This study evaluates the effect of higher doses beyond 1.8 mg of the FDA-approved diabetes medicine liraglutide as a treatment for obesity.

Gadde, K. M., Allison, D. B., Ryan, D. H., Peterson, C. A., Troupin, B., Schwiers, M. L., et al. (2011). Effects of low-dose, controlled-release, phentermine plus topiramate combination on weight and associated comorbidities in overweight and obese adults (CONQUER): A randomised, placebo-controlled, phase 3 trial. *Lancet, 377,* 1341–1352.—This article describes a phase 3 clinical trial for the medication combination of phentermine–topiramate for the treatment of obesity.

Greenway, F. L., Fujioka, K., Plodkowski, R. A., Mudaliar, S., Guttadauria, M., Erickson, J., et al. (2010). Effect of naltrexone plus bupropion on weight loss in overweight and obese adults (COR-I): A multicenter, randomized, double-blind, placebo-controlled, phase 3 trial. *Lancet, 376,* 595–605.—The COR studies were multicenter trials evaluating efficacy of the combination medicines bupropion–naltrexone for the treatment of obesity.

Korner, J., & Aronne, L. J. (2003). The emerging science of body weight regulation and its impact on obesity treatment. *Journal of Clinical Investigation, 111*(5), 565–570.—The authors discuss the physiology of body weight regulation and outline pathophysiology of the obese patient.

NHLBI Obesity Education Initiative, National Heart, Blood Institute, North American Association for the Study of Obesity, Expert Panel on the Identification, Treatment of Overweight, & Obesity in Adults (U.S.). (2002). *The practical guide: Identification, evaluation, and treatment of overweight and obesity in adults* (No. 2-4084). Bethesda, MD: National Heart, Lung, and Blood Institute.—This National Institutes of Health handbook outlines principles about diagnosing overweight and obesity in patients. This guide includes information on epidemiology of obesity, complications patients experience, as well as treatment options.

Smith, S. R., Weissman, N. J., Anderson, C. M., Sanchez, M., Chuang, E., Stubbe, S., et al. (2010). Multicenter, placebo-controlled trial of lorcaserin for weight management. *New England Journal of Medicine, 363*(3), 245–256.—This study is a Phase III trial on the use of lorcaserin for obesity treatment.

Surgery for Obesity

Roux-en-Y Gastric Bypass and Sleeve Gastrectomy Procedures

CHRISTOPHER R. DAIGLE
PHILIP R. SCHAUER

Multiple studies have demonstrated that bariatric (or metabolic) surgery is associated with significant and durable weight loss, and is associated with remarkable improvement of obesity-related comorbidities. In contrast, lifestyle intervention (diet and exercise) and pharmacotherapy have largely been ineffective in producing significant quantity and durability of weight loss in patients with severe obesity. Furthermore, the beneficial effects of bariatric surgery on disease-specific risk reduction, long-term quality-of-life improvement, and overall mortality are well documented.

The degree of weight loss and the effect on obesity-related comorbid conditions depend on the bariatric surgical approach, whose classification typically is based on the procedure's restrictive and/or malabsorptive effect. There are numerous factors a multidisciplinary team must consider before offering bariatric surgery, and not all patients are appropriate candidates. Based on widely adopted 1991 National Institutes of Health guidelines, patients are potential candidates for bariatric surgery if they have chronic severe obesity (body mass index [BMI] ≥ 40 kg/m^2) or BMI ≥ 35 kg/m^2 with obesity-related comorbidity. International Diabetes Federation guidelines consider patients with a BMI of 30–35 kg/m^2 and poorly controlled type 2 diabetes as potential candidates as well. The various bariatric surgical approaches differ with respect to morbidity profiles and expected efficacy; thus, a tailored approach is needed for each and every patient considering bariatric surgery.

Recent data from the International Federation for the Surgery of Obesity and Metabolic Diseases summarize results of a questionnaire-based study assessing worldwide trends in bariatric surgery. Based on their survey of 2013, they reported that the most commonly performed procedure in the world is the Roux-en-Y gastric bypass (RYGB; 45%), followed by sleeve gastrectomy (SG; 37%), adjustable gastric banding (AGB; 10%) and biliopancreatic diversion (BPD), with or without duodenal switch (DS) (2.5%). RYGB has long since been the cornerstone of this rapidly evolving field, but recently the popularity of SG has risen dramatically for several reasons beyond the scope of this chapter. In fact, recent trends suggest that SG has overtaken RYGB as the most common bariatric operation worldwide. It is important to note the key differences between RYGB and SG anatomical alterations. Our aim in this chapter is to summarize those differences, along with an evidenced-based summary of comparative outcomes of the various bariatric surgical approaches.

Anatomical Considerations

From the standpoint of an anatomical definition, the SG procedure is primarily restrictive, in that it reduces gastric volume by 75%, whereas RYGB is a combination of restriction and malabsorption. However, categorizing procedures as restrictive or malabsorptive is an oversimplistic way of conceptualizing the profound weight loss and metabolic effects these procedures bestow. For example, patients often experience normalization of metabolic parameters (e.g., blood sugar) before any appreciable weight loss has occurred, which suggests that far more complex mechanisms are at play (e.g., neuroendocrine, bile acids, and gut microbiome theories). Nevertheless, it is important to understand the anatomic differences between bariatric procedures such as SG and RYGB.

The two major anatomical alterations in RYGB are creation of a 15–30 ml gastric pouch via surgical stapling/transection and "rewiring" of the small intestine (in a Roux-en-Y configuration), such that a significant portion of proximal small intestine receives gastric contents before biliary secretions are added, thus reducing absorption (Figure 85.1). This creates three distinct small intestinal channels (or limbs): (1) the *alimentary limb* originating from the gastric pouch; (2) the *biliopancreatic limb* carrying biliopancreatic secretions to the small intestinal anastomosis; and (3) the *common channel,* where biliopancreatic secretions and ingested food finally meet. This constellation of changes ultimately promotes smaller meals, decreased absorption, and complex physiological alterations that we do not yet understand fully.

The SG procedure (Figure 85.2) also achieves weight-independent changes (i.e., neuroendocrine) that are not simply explained by restriction alone. In this procedure, a gastroscope or Bougie is classically placed orally after the patient is under anesthesia, and this is used to guide the surgeon in surgically stapling the stomach into an almost banana shape, reducing the volume by around 75%. There are no intestinal rearrangements in this procedure, and the transected stomach is removed before the end of the case.

Weight Loss Outcomes

Unfortunately, there is a relative paucity of randomized controlled trials with long-term results comparing weight loss outcomes between the various bariatric procedures; however, there are several excellent large observational studies that address weight loss. Overall, the percent excess weight loss (%EWL = [initial weight kg – final weight kg]/[initial weight kg – ideal body weight kg] at BMI 25 × 100%) after bariatric surgery has been reported to be 47–70% in long-term series. In 2011, Hutter and colleagues published the first report from the American College of Surgeons Bariatric Surgery Center Network (ACS-BSCN) based on its large, multicenter longitudinal database. This study positioned

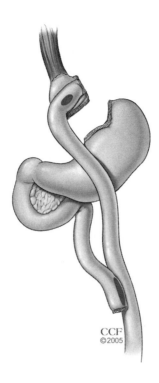

FIGURE 85.1. Roux-en-Y gastric bypass procedure. Reprinted with permission, Cleveland Clinic Center for Medical Art and Photography, © 2005–2016. All rights reserved.

laparoscopic SG in between AGB and RYGB with respect to morbidity (AGB has the lowest) and effectiveness (RYGB has the highest). In total, 28,616 patients from 109 hospitals were analyzed: 944 laparoscopic sleeve cases, 12,193 adjustable bands, 14,491 laparoscopic RYGB, and 988 open RYGB. The mean absolute BMI reduction after laparoscopic SG (11.87 kg/m²) was found to be less than the weight loss achieved by laparoscopic (or open) gastric bypass (15.34 kg/m²), but greater than that seen with LAGB (7.05 kg/m²) at 1-year follow-up. Similarly, the Michigan Bariatric Surgery Collective recently published its prospective statewide study, which matched 2,949 laparoscopic SG patients to equal numbers of laparoscopic RYGB and AGB patients. At 1-year follow-up, the mean %EWL for the SG group was 60%, which was significantly lower than that for RYGB (69%, $p < .0001$, but higher than AGB (34%, $p < .0001$). The Swedish Obesity Study and nine other observational studies (nonrandomized) have shown that bariatric surgery leads to durable weight loss and reduced overall morbidity and mortality in severely obese people. Long-term randomized controlled trials (RCTs) have yet to confirm this mortality reduction with bariatric surgery.

Complications of Bariatric Surgery

In 2004, Buckwald and colleagues published their systematic review and meta-analysis (the most cited article in bariatric surgery) addressing outcomes after bariatric surgery,

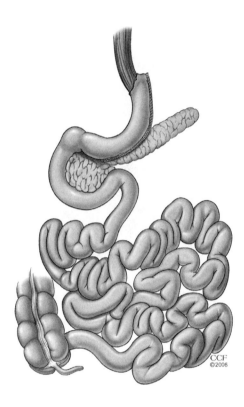

FIGURE 85.2. Sleeve gastrectomy procedure. Reprinted with permission, Cleveland Clinic Center for Medical Art and Photography, © 2005–2016. All rights reserved.

and they reported low overall early and late mortality rates after bariatric operations (0.28 and 0.35%, respectively). Not surprisingly, mortality was noted to be higher in open and conversion cases (conversion from the laparoscopic approach to laparotomy). Similarly, in 2009, the Longitudinal Assessment of Bariatric Surgery Consortium (LABS) published prospective multicenter observational outcomes of 4,776 patients who had bariatric surgery and reported a comparable mortality rate of 0.3%. Postoperatively, cardiopulmonary complications (myocardial infarction, pulmonary embolism) are by far the leading cause of mortality after bariatric surgery. For cases performed at Centers of Excellence, the overall mortality rate for RYGB, as reported by the LABS study, was 0.4%. After RYGB, the most serious procedure-specific early complication is anasto-motic leakage, with an incidence ranging from 0.1 to 5.6%. Increasing age, higher BMI, multiple comorbidities, male gender, smoking, and/or a history of prior bariatric surgery are all associated with higher leak rates after RYGB.

As previously stated, the first report from the ACS-BSCN is frequently quoted when discussing where SG falls on the perioperative adverse outcome and efficacy spectrum. In this study, laparoscopic SG had a higher 30-day morbidity (5.61 vs. 1.44%, $p < .05$), reoperative rate (2.97 vs. 0.92%, $p < .05$) and readmission rate (5.4% vs. 1.17%, $p < .05$) when compared to AGB; however, reoperation and intervention rates were lower for SG when compared to RYGB. Importantly, there was no statistical difference in mortality rates between SG (0.11% at 30 days, 0.21% at 1 year) and RYGB (0.14 and 0.34%).

Perioperative adverse outcomes encountered after SG are similar to those seen after RYGB; however, there are surgery-specific complications (both early and late) related to SG, including strictures (narrowing of the sleeve), staple line leaks, and intractable acid reflux.

It is imperative that health care workers who deal with postoperative bariatric surgery patients be aware of the potential late complications that can arise after surgery. One should be concerned about a patient with a history of RYGB who presents with signs or symptoms of bowel obstruction, as this can represent an internal hernia (small bowel herniating through nonanatomical defects arising from the Roux-en-Y configuration) or gastrojejunal anastomotic stricture (anastomotic narrowing that prevents emptying of the gastric pouch). Importantly, internal hernias are more common after laparoscopic cases, and the incidence ranges from 0.5 to 5.0%. Abdominal pain, with or without signs of small bowel obstruction, is the most common presentation for internal hernias, and diagnostic laparoscopy is the diagnostic method of choice (high false-negative rates are associated with computed tomography scans). The incidence of anastomotic stricture can vary depending on the operative approach but can occur in 2–10% of cases. The etiology of a stricture is not always clear but it may be related to ischemia, recurrent marginal ulcers, scarring, and/or technical considerations, such as excessive tension on the anastomosis. Strictures are diagnosed by upper intestinal contrast study or endoscopy, and they can often be therapeutically dilated at the time of endoscopy. Marginal ulcers occur in 2% of RYGB patients within the first year, then in 0.5% for up to 5 years. Some marginal ulcerations arise for unknown reasons but most are associated with smoking and/or nonsteroidal anti-inflammatory drug (NSAID) usage.

Nutritional complications are classically associated with malabsorptive procedures and are typically seen after procedures such as BPD or RYGB. However, nutritional deficiencies can still occur after restrictive procedures (e.g., laparoscopic sleeve gastrectomy [LSG]), and these patients should also be monitored. Anemia, usually mild, is common after RYGB, and iron deficiency ranges from 17 to 30%. Deficiencies in other trace minerals (i.e., copper, zinc) and vitamins (A, B_1, B_{12}, E, D, and K) can also occur after bariatric surgery. It is also important to monitor for vitamin D and calcium deficiencies, which can lead to osteopenia or osteoporosis, and these patients will also need lifelong monitoring for protein malnutrition.

Metabolic Effects of RYGB and SG

Bariatric surgery is associated with remarkable improvement of obesity-related comorbid conditions such as type 2 diabetes mellitus (T2DM), hypertension, dyslipidemias, obstructive sleep apnea, and fatty liver disease, to only name a few. However, it is the profound effect on T2DM that has brought bariatric surgery into the spotlight and has helped transform the field into a bona fide metabolic specialty. In 2012, two RCTs were published (both in the *New England Journal of Medicine*) comparing bariatric surgery to conventional or intensive medical therapy for T2DM. Mingrone's study was a single-center trial that included 60 patients (20 BPD, 20 RYGB, and 20 conventional medical therapy) ages 30–60 years with BMI ≥ 35 and T2DM for at least 5 years. Their primary end point was diabetes remission at 2 years postintervention, defined as fasting glucose level < 100 mg and HbA1c < 6.5%. They reported diabetes remission in 95% of BPD patients and 75% of RYGB patients, whereas none of the medical therapy subjects achieved remission (p < .001). Our group simultaneously published an RCT (STAM-PEDE) with 150 morbidly obese subjects with poorly controlled T2DM (mean age, 49 ± 8 years) randomized to intensive medical therapy alone, medical therapy plus RYGB, or medical therapy plus SG. Our study had a more stringent primary end point (HbA1c < 6.0%, with or without medications) at 1-year follow-up and we found that 12% of medical therapy patients achieved primary end point, compared to 42% (p = .002) in the RYGB plus medical therapy group and 37% (p = .008) in the SG plus medical therapy arm. We concluded that 12 months of bariatric surgery plus medical therapy was superior to intensive medical therapy alone in achieving glycemic control in morbidly obese patients with uncontrolled T2DM. The 3-year follow-up of STAMPEDE showed continued superiority of surgery plus medical therapy versus medical therapy alone.

Conclusion

The significant weight loss and metabolic effects of bariatric surgery in severely obese patients, as well as a relatively good safety profile, are well supported by recent observational studies and RCTs. Lifestyle intervention and pharmacotherapy, while relatively low risk, have been ineffective in treating severe obesity. Nonrandomized studies such as the Swedish Obese Subjects (SOS) study suggest that bariatric surgery may result in significant long-term reduction in mortality associated with severe obesity. For severely obese patients not responding to lifestyle intervention or pharmacotherapy, bariatric surgery should be considered the standard of care for treating severe obesity.

Suggested Reading

Aminian, A., Daigle, C. R., Brethauer, S. A., & Schauer, P. R. (2014). Citation classics: Top 50 cited articles in bariatric and metabolic surgery. *Surgery for Obesity and Related Diseases, 10*(5), 898–905.—Excellent review of the most cited articles in bariatric surgery.

Buchwald, H., Avidor, Y., Braunwald, E., Jensen, M. D., Pories, W., Fahrbach, K., et al. (2004). Bariatric surgery: A systematic review and meta-analysis. *Journal of the American Medical Association, 292*(14), 1724–1737.—The most cited article in the field of bariatric surgery; an absolute "must read" systematic review and meta-analysis of bariatric surgery outcomes.

Carlin, A. M., Zeni, T. M., English, W. J., Hawasli, A. A., Genaw, J. A., Krause, K. R., et al. (2013). The comparative effectiveness of sleeve gastrectomy, gastric bypass, and adjustable gastric banding procedures for the treatment of morbid obesity. *Annals of Surgery, 257*(5), 791–797.—Large, statewide observational study (Michigan Bariatric Surgery Collaborative) comparing outcomes of AGB, SG, and RYGB.

Hutter, M. M., Schirmer, B. D., Jones, D. B., Ko, C. Y., Cohen, M. E., Merkow, R. P., et al. (2011). First report from the American College of Surgeons—Bariatric Surgery Center Network: Laparoscopic sleeve gastrectomy has morbidity and effectiveness positioned between the band and the bypass. *Annals of Surgery, 254*(3), 410–422.—The famous study that placed SG between adjustable banding and gastric bypass with respect to morbidity and efficacy.

Longitudinal Assessment of Bariatric Surgery (LABS) Consortium. (2009). Perioperative safety in the longitudinal assessment of bariatric surgery. *New England Journal of Medicine, 361*(5), 445–454.—Another large, multicenter observational study assessing 30-day outcomes in patients undergoing bariatric surgery.

Mingrone, G., Panunzi, S., De Gaetano, A., Guidone, C., Iaconelli, A., Leccesi, L., et al. (2012). Bariatric surgery versus conventional medical therapy for type 2 diabetes. *New England*

Journal of Medicine, 366(17), 1577–1585.—RCT comparing RYBG and BPD to intensive medical therapy for T2D in morbidly obese subjects.

Schauer, P. R., Bhatt, D. L., Kirwan, J. P., Wolski, K., Brethauer, S. A., Navaneethan, S. D., et al. (2014). Bariatric surgery versus intensive medical therapy for diabetes—3-year outcomes. *New England Journal of Medicine, 370*(21), 2002–2013.—Recently published 3-year outcomes from the STAMPEDE study.

Schauer, P. R., Kashyap, S. R., Wolski, K., Brethauer, S. A., Kirwan, J. P., Pothier, C. E., et al. (2012). Bariatric surgery versus intensive medical therapy in obese patients with diabetes. *New England Journal of Medicine, 366*(17), 1567–1576.—The STAMPEDE trial—RCT comparing intensive medical therapy alone, medical therapy plus RYGB, or medical therapy plus SG for the treatment of T2D.

Sjöström, L., Narbro, K., Sjöström, C. D., Karason, K., Larsson, B., Wedel, H., et al. (2007). Effects of bariatric surgery on mortality in Swedish obese subjects. *New England Journal of Medicine, 357*(8), 741–752.—This large, prospective, controlled study from Sweden is the second most cited article in bariatric surgery and the foundation of several important studies in the field.

86

Surgical Devices for Obesity

BRUCE M. WOLFE
ELIZAVETA WALKER

The adverse effects of obesity on health are highly variable among individuals but, in general, are progressively more common and severe as the severity of obesity increases. The approaches and benefits of weight loss are detailed elsewhere in this volume. The Look AHEAD trial demonstrated that sustained weight loss of approximately 5% is maintained by intensive lifestyle intervention over a period of several years, with many persons sustaining considerably more weight loss. Roux-en-Y gastric bypass and similar interventions, in contrast, accomplish average weight loss in the range of 30% or more, with apparently greater impact on health among people with severe obesity and related comorbidities. Specifically, induction of remission of type 2 diabetes, diminished incidence, and related mortality of various cancers and survival are associated with gastric bypass.

Despite these demonstrated benefits of alterations of gastrointestinal anatomy for the purpose of weight loss, the number of people with severe obesity who undergo such procedures in any given year is exceedingly low, in the range of 1–2% per year of people with severe obesity. Factors involved in this incomplete application of what appears to be a safe and effective intervention include a fear of serious complications, hesitancy to undergo major irreversible alterations of gastrointestinal anatomy, and cost. Thus, there is a need for intermediate approaches to the treatment of obesity for persons who fail to maintain desired weight loss with lifestyle intervention, with or without pharmacotherapy, that are less invasive, that present less perioperative and long-term risk, and are available at lower cost. The application of prosthetic materials and devices has emerged as an important option for accomplishing weight loss to address the treatment gap between intensive lifestyle intervention, with or without medication, and major surgical alteration of gastrointestinal anatomy.

Experience with all of these interventions has consistently demonstrated that whatever the intervention for the treatment of obesity may be, it must be ongoing. Although exceptions occur, in general, when the weight loss intervention is discontinued, be it lifestyle intervention, medication, or surgical procedure, regain of weight typically occurs.

Jaw Wiring

Weight loss among patients with severe obesity following intestinal bypass led to a search for interventions that may achieve weight loss without producing the frequent and life-threatening complications of intestinal bypass. One such approach, jaw wiring, was reported in several small series. These and other trials demonstrated that average weight loss of 25–30 kg could be accomplished. The jaw wires could not remain in place permanently, however, and weight was gradually regained after removal of the wires. Attempts to maintain the weight loss, such as application of an abdominal nylon cord, were attempted but, similarly, were not practical for long-term use and led to abandonment of jaw wiring and related procedures to accomplish weight loss.

Devices Placed or Done by Gastrointestinal Endoscopy

Devices placed or procedures done for weight loss by flexible luminal gastrointestinal (GI) endoscopy are attractive to patients and providers, as they represent "incisionless surgery." Such procedures are commonly done on an outpatient (same-day) basis and have low complication rates, two components that tend to minimize cost. Such procedures may not have to produce weight loss comparable to gastric bypass to take their place as weight loss procedures.

The extension of GI endoscopy technology includes the capacity to perform full-thickness GI suturing and incisions, and other procedures commonly done by laparoscopic or open surgical methods. Plication of the stomach has been performed, and techniques for performance of gastric bypass are under development. As these developments of technology and techniques evolve, it will be critical to consider the lessons of the past such as the transient benefit of open or laparoscopic partial gastric plication. Increased rates of complications that are particularly serious or life threatening following GI endoscopic procedures will not be acceptable.

Intragastric Balloons

The induction of a perception of fullness and satiety following gastric distention, thought to result from activation of vagal afferents, has been demonstrated by several investigators. The first gastric balloon, or bubble, approved for clinical use in the United States was introduced in 1985. The Garen–Edwards gastric bubble (GEGB®) was placed by an endoscopic procedure. Initial reports of weight loss led to early enthusiasm for this procedure. A subsequent sham controlled crossover study, however, questioned the efficacy of this prosthetic device in achieving weight loss. In addition, complications including premature deflation of the bubble with transit into the small intestine, where obstruction, perforation, and in rare cases death occurred, led to abandonment of this device.

A subsequent intragastric balloon, the BioEnterics intragastric balloon (BIB®), is a larger balloon, constructed to minimize premature deflation. Filling the balloon with methylene blue was added to give the patient a signal that deflation of the balloon had occurred, indicating prompt endoscopic removal. Complications among 2,515 patients in a multicenter Italian experience included gastric perforation in 0.19%, premature balloon rupture in 0.36%, esophagitis in 1.27%, and gastric ulcer in 0.2%. There were two fatalities among patients who had undergone previous gastric surgery. Body mass index (BMI) was reduced from 44.4 to 35.4, or 20% over the 6 months the balloon was in place. Most recently, a device comprising two intragastric balloons has been demonstrated to accomplish similar weight loss. This study by Ponce and colleagues was a sham controlled clinical trial in which 13.9% excess of weight was lost at 24 weeks.

This increasing experience with intragastric balloons indicates that the present iterations of these devices are associated with initial weight loss that is intermediate between lifestyle intervention, with or without medication, and gastric bypass. This weight loss is associated with the identification of apparent health benefits associated with weight loss that is also intermediate. The relative safety has been improved, such that major or life-threatening complications are exceedingly rare. The primary unresolved issues are the duration that a single balloon can be safely left in place, as well as sustainability of weight loss. The application of serial intragastric balloons as weight regain occurs following scheduled balloon removal has been proposed. The practicality and safety of this approach remains to be determined.

The Duodenal–Jejunal Bypass Liner

The duodenal–jejunal bypass liner is a long plastic tube that is implanted by flexible GI endoscopy. The liner or sleeve is anchored in the proximal duodenum, immediately distal to the pylorus. It extends to the promixal jejunum when fully placed. The concept is that by directing the ingested nutrients and related GI secretions into the lumen of the sleeve, the nutrients will not be exposed to the duodenal and proximal jejunal mucosa. This is intended to avoid secretion of hormones or peptides that may adversely affect glucose metabolism. It is also possible the duodenal–jejunal bypass liner will shift digestion and absorption of nutrients somewhat distally in the GI tract, thereby stimulating a greater release of glucagon-like peptide 1 (GLP-1), which is enhanced as exposure of nutrients to the GI mucosa is extended distally. Outcomes from two randomized controlled trials (RCTs) show percent total weight loss in the range of 5–6%, which is not statistically significantly greater than that in controls. Modest improvement in the status of diabetes management was reported, such as discontinuation of insulin in 13%, and similar reductions in requirement for other diabetes medications. Safety concerns have raised definite questions as to the future clinical role of this device. Premature removal of the device prior to study completion at 24 weeks occurred in 15–20% of subjects. These removals were required due to device or anchor migration, abdominal pain, food impaction in the sleeve, and other symptoms. Recently, several reported cases of multiple hepatic abscesses have been associated with the application of this device. It is therefore unclear what the clinical use of this intervention will be in the future.

Gastric Banding

The application of prosthetic bands has been a conceptually attractive procedure for many years. The vertical banded gastroplasty is a procedure in which a partial plication of the stomach is done and the communication between the small partitioned gastric pouch and body of the stomach is reinforced with a mesh or silastic ring. The vertical banded gastroplasty procedure gained widespread popularity as it replaced intestinal bypass as the weight loss operation of choice, when intestinal bypass was abandoned due to unacceptable complications. This was the predominant procedure utilized in the Swedish Obese Subjects (SOS) controlled trial, which demonstrated long-term weight loss of approximately 15% of total body weight and was associated with numerous health benefits, including improved survival, as noted earlier. Complications of gastric and esophageal dilatation, gastroesophageal reflux, band erosion, and weight regain, however, led to its replacement by adjustable gastric banding.

The development of the adjustable gastric band, the tightness of which can be adjusted by inflation or deflation percutaneously, achieved widespread popularity due to its perioperative safety compared to gastric bypass and its encouraging early weight losses, in the range of 20% on average. Recent studies have demonstrated that the weight loss, initially described as similar to that of gastric bypass, at 3 years and beyond is, on average, in the range of 15%. In addition, the necessity for frequent interventions to adjust band tightness, late complications of gastric and/or esophageal dilation, gastroesophageal reflux disease (GERD) with complications such as aspiration, and band erosion have led to a substantial reduction in the application of this procedure.

Neural Modulation

The concept of peripheral or central neural modulation by electrical stimulation or ablation has been considered for centuries and is the subject of increasing research for a variety of conditions. Initial neural modulation as a treatment for obesity was applied as gastric stimulation, which was done by placing leads on the stomach. Early enthusiasm for this approach was stimulated by the relative simplicity of the laparoscopic procedure required to place the leads and its high degree of safety. Initial weight loss was modest, but it improved when a preoperative screening algorithm was applied in an effort to select patients more likely to be successful. In this population, excess weight lost over 1–2 years approached 40% (approximately 16–20% total weight loss). The safety record for this procedure was excellent, but sustained weight loss was disappointing, such that efforts to develop this technology further have been suspended.

Vagal Nerve Blocking

Truncal vagotomy was undertaken in many patients as treatment for peptic ulcer disease in the past. An observation that persistent satiety, as well as little, if any, regain of weight lost prior to vagotomy led to the hypothesis that vagotomy could be used as a primary intervention to accomplish weight loss. This hypothesis is supported by experimental studies demonstrating a relationship between vagal innervation and the secretion and function of gut hormones, including ghrelin, involved in the regulating of energy balance. Two clinical trials of truncal vagotomy for weight loss, one as a primary surgical procedure and the other as an adjunct to vertical banded gastroplasty, produced encouraging early weight loss that was not sustained. The hypothesis developed that intermittent vagal blockade would avoid the accommodation to vagotomy, which presumably explained the transient nature of vagotomy-induced weight loss. An implantable device was then developed to deliver intermittent vagal blockade by electrical signaling to the vagal trunks at the diaphragm and was confirmed in animal models.

Early experience with this device demonstrated mean 14.2% excess weight loss at 6 months. An excellent safety record was observed. A subsequent sham-controlled RCT showed 24.4% loss of excess weight in the treated group versus 15.9% excess weight lost in the sham group (9.2% total body weight loss and 6.0% in the sham group). Serious adverse events reported in 3.7% of the vagal nerve block group included a need to reposition the neuroregulator or prolonged hospitalization for 1–2 days. No mortality or life-threatening complications were observed. While longer-term follow-up is needed to determine the sustainability and longer-term complication rates of vagal nerve blockade, these early results suggest that vagal nerve blockade may offer an intermediate procedure for weight loss, as well as risk and alteration of GI anatomy, proving attractive to patients hesitant to undergo GI-altering procedures such as gastric bypass and sleeve gastrectomy.

Other Devices

Several other devices have been proposed, some of which are under evaluation, whereas others are not. Examples include an intraperitoneal balloon intended to compress the stomach externally, oral appliances, partially obstructing appliances placed at the gastroesophageal junction, and gastrostomy tube placement for aspiration of ingested nutrients, among others. The search for procedures involving lesser invasion, or alteration, of GI anatomy, to lower risk and possibly lower cost is a research priority. Further research will be required before any of these investigational procedures take their place in the clinical armamentarium for the treatment of obesity.

Conclusion

Research is in progress to develop weight loss procedures utilizing devices that require lesser operative procedures than gastric bypass or sleeve gastrectomy, produce fewer complications, and compete economically. Such procedures may fill a gap between nonsurgical weight loss treatment and established bariatric surgical procedures despite intermediate weight loss. Short- and long-term complications must be minimized for this goal to be achieved.

Suggested Reading

Alfredo, G., Roberta, M., Massimiliano, C., Michele, L., Nicola, B., & Adriano, R. (2014). Long-term multiple intragastric balloon treatment—a new strategy to treat morbid obese patients refusing surgery: Prospective 6-year follow-up study. *Surgery for Obesity and Related Diseases, 10*(2), 307–311.—This article examines the efficacy of intragastric balloon treatment in 83 patients with obesity (BMI > 40) who refused surgery. The 6-year study measured weight loss, quality of life, and comorbid conditions of obesity.

Busetto, L., Segato, G., De Marchi, F., Foletto, M., De Luca, M., Caniato, D., et al. (2002). Outcome predictors in morbidly obese recipients of an adjustable gastric band. *Obesity Surgery, 12*(1), 83–92.—This study describes 260 morbidly obese patients enrolled in a 3-year study that measured the success rate of laparoscopic adjustable banding with Lap-Band®. With a success rate of 35.7%, the study provided both failure and success predictors in the effectiveness of this device.

Courcoulas, A. P., Christian, N. J., Belle, S. H., Berk, P. D., Flum, D. R., Garcia, L., et al. (2013). Weight change and health outcomes at 3 years after bariatric surgery among individuals with severe obesity. *Journal of the American Medical Association, 310*(22), 2416–2425.—This 3-year study examined weight loss, among other health parameters, after bariatric surgery utilizing the LABS Consortium, a national multicenter observational cohort study. Sophisticated parsing of outcomes reveals maximum weight change during the first postoperative year, with variability as time after surgery increases.

Dixon, J. B., O'Brien, P. E., Playfair, J., Chapman, L., Schachter, L. M., Skinner, S., et al. (2008). Adjustable gastric banding and conventional therapy for type 2 diabetes: A randomized controlled trial. *Journal of the American Medical Association, 299*(3), 316–323.— A 4-year unblinded RCT measured whether surgically induced weight loss resulted in better glycemic control/remission of type 2 diabetes than conventional diabetes therapy in 60 participants.

Ikramuddin, S., Blackstone, R. P., Brancatisano, A., Toouli, J., Shah, S. N., Wolfe, B. M., et al. (2014). Effect of reversible intermittent intra-abdominal vagal nerve blockade on morbid obesity: The ReCharge randomized clinical trial. *Journal of the American Medical Association, 312*(9), 915–922.—This 5-year RCT examined vagal nerve blockade therapy compared with a sham control device to test for efficacy among 239 morbidly obese participants with concurrent weight management education.

O'Brien, P. E., Dixon, J. B., Brown, W., Schachter, L. M., Chapman, L., Burn, A. J., et al. (2002). The laparoscopic adjustable gastric band (Lap-Band®): A prospective study of medium-term effects on weight, health and quality of life. *Obesity Surgery, 12*(5), 652–660.—In this prospective study enrolling 709 patients with severe obesity, a device was surgically placed to control the level of gastric restriction in order to measure comorbid conditions and manage overweight status over a period of 6 years.

Ponce, J., Woodman, G., Swain, J., Wilson, E., English, W., Ikramuddin, S., et al. (2015). The REDUCE pivotal trial: A prospective, randomized controlled pivotal trial of a dual intragastric balloon for the treatment of obesity. *Surgery for Obesity and Related Diseases, 11*(4), 874–881.—This article examined the efficacy of a dual balloon system with diet and exercise versus a placebo with diet and exercise in the treatment of obesity. In this prospective RCT, the two groups were observed and their adverse event profiles were compared.

Shikora, S. A. (2004). "What are the yanks doing?": The U.S. experience with implantable gastric stimulation (IGS) for the treatment of obesity—update on the ongoing clinical trials. *Obesity Surgery, 14*(Suppl. 1), S40–S48.—A secondary review on the safety and effectiveness of implantable gastric stimulation (IGS) trials in the United States concludes that IGS is a safe treatment of obesity, with technical improvements and patient selection amplifying effectiveness.

Sjöström, L. (2013). Review of the key results from the Swedish Obese Subjects (SOS) trial—a prospective controlled intervention study of bariatric surgery. *Journal of Internal Medicine, 273*(3), 219–234.—Compared to nonsurgical care, bariatric surgery was associated with a long-term reduction in overall mortality in this long-term, prospective, controlled trial. Objective study measures and follow-up for 8 years is provided.

Sjöström, L., Peltonen, M., Jacobson, P., Sjöström, C. D., Karason, K., Wedel, H., et al. (2012). Bariatric surgery and long-term cardiovascular events. *Journal of the American Medical Association, 307*(1), 56–65.—Compared with conventional nonsurgical care, bariatric surgery was associated with reduced number of cardiovascular deaths and lower incidence of cardiovascular events in obese adults in this 15-year prospective, controlled study.

The Role of Scalable, Community-Based Weight Management Programs

GARY D. FOSTER
ANGELA MAKRIS
ALEXIS C. WOJTANOWSKI

Given the prevalence of obesity and its associated medical, psychosocial, and economic consequences, it is imperative to provide weight loss treatments that are both effective for sustained weight loss and accessible. Behavioral treatments, either alone or in combination, are the cornerstone of any effective obesity treatment. This chapter reviews guidelines for effective treatment, with a focus on making empirically based treatments accessible.

Addressing the Need for Treatment

The U.S. Preventive Services Task Force (USPSTF) and the most recent obesity management guidelines from the American Heart Association (AHA), the American College of Cardiology (ACC), and The Obesity Society (TOS) have directed clinicians to screen all adults for overweight/obesity, and offer or refer individuals to behavioral weight loss interventions. To aid health care providers in developing and identifying quality weight loss interventions, delivered in primary care or a community-based setting, these panels have provided specific criteria for behavioral lifestyle interventions (see Table 87.1).

Evidence Base for Behavioral Treatment

The behavioral treatment of obesity is an approach that helps individuals develop a set of skills to achieve a healthier weight. It includes multiple components, commonly referred to as the "behavioral package," such as self-monitoring (of intake, activity and weight), goal setting, problem solving, cognitive restructuring, and relapse prevention. Since its

TABLE 87.1. Criteria for Behavioral Lifestyle Interventions for Weight Loss

	2012 USPSTF[a] recommendations	2013 AHA/ACC/TOS[b] guidelines
Longer-term duration (minimum of 12 sessions,[a] ≥ 6 months[b])	X	X
High-intensity (12–26 sessions/year,[a] ≥ 14 sessions/6 months[b])	X	X
Multicomponent/comprehensive	X	X
Behavioral counseling to facilitate adherence to diet and activity recommendations (portions, stimulus control, addressing barriers to change, etc.)	X	X
Goal setting (weight loss of 5–10% within 6 months,[a,b] daily dietary intake,[b] weekly physical activity minutes[b])	X	X
Improving diet or nutrition[a]/prescription of a moderately reduced diet (energy deficit of ≥ 500 kcal/day)[b]	X	X
Increased physical activity[a]/physical activity goal (≥ 150 minutes/week)[b]	X	X
Regular self-monitoring (intake, activity, weight)	X	X
Strategies for maintained lifestyle changes and weight loss	X	X
Onsite, in-person, individual, or group sessions	X	X
Sessions provided by a clinican[a]/trained interventionist[b]	X	X
When lifestyle interventions are not possible in primary care offices or available by referral, the following are alternate modes of delivery:		
Community-based[a]/commercial programs using counseling (provided peer-reviewed published evidence of safety and efficacy)[b]	X	X
Electronically delivered weight loss programs (Internet or telephone) with personalized feedback (may result in smaller weight losses than face-to-face)		X

first evaluation in 1967, behavioral treatment has been perhaps the most rigorously evaluated of all approaches for the management of obesity. Behavioral treatments produce an average weight loss of approximately 5–10% (5–10 kg) of initial weight over 6–12 months. Interventions that persist beyond 1 year generally report gradual weight regain of 1–2 kg/year. For example, the Look AHEAD trial, a large multicenter study of individuals with type 2 diabetes that used state-of-the-art behavioral treatment (known as an "intensive lifestyle intervention"), reported average weight losses of 8.6, 6.2, and 4.7%, respectively, of initial weight after 1, 4, and 8 years of treatment (vs. 0.7, 0.9, and 2.1% in the minimal contact control group). Participants in the intensive behavioral group practiced several key weight control behaviors (e.g., goal setting around daily energy intake and weekly physical activity minutes, portion control, self-monitoring). Additionally, participants who lost ≥ 10%, and kept it off, practiced weight-control behaviors more consistently than those who lost but regained weight. These findings not only show that behavioral treatment is effective and superior to minimal care despite weight regain over time, but they also underscore the need for continuous implementation of weight control strategies and recurring, long-term support.

The Need for Broader Implementation

Enthusiasm about the efficacy (and minimal adverse effects) of the behavioral approach is dampened by its limited availability and high cost. A preponderance of the research on behavioral approaches has been conducted in specialized clinics, typically academic medical centers. A global public health problem such as obesity cannot be adequately addressed by a relatively small number of tertiary care centers. Even in the primary care setting, many physicians and other health care providers lack the training and time required for successful weight management. As such, scalable, community-based weight loss programs may play a role in providing effective treatment to large numbers of persons with overweight and obesity. While community-based programs are suggested for referral, there are no specific program recommendations, which leaves clinicians uncertain about where to send their patients, and consumers confused about the myriad options.

The Landscape and Benefits of Community-Based Weight Management Programs

The wide variety of nationwide weight loss programs can be loosely categorized on the following factors: facilitation (interventionist or self-directed), intensity (number of sessions per year, ranging from high with > 12 sessions/year to low with < 12 sessions/year or self-directed), support (group sessions, online coaching, one-on-one counseling, online community), and program-provided resources (tracking tool, books, printed materials, meal replacements).

This variety permits individuals to choose a program that provides the best fit, including proximity, engagement level, dietary and activity preferences, and cost. National programs have an expansive reach, both to geographically sparse areas and to different segments of the population, and are able to reach people through a variety of modalities (face-to-face, digital, virtual) and locations (worksite, retail centers, churches). The programs are typically standardized, allowing for replication and dissemination through training on intervention protocols and procedures. Weight loss programs that can be easily accessed and resumed at any time ensure long-term access to treatment, with its inevitable stops and starts; such an approach provides consistency for a chronic condition such as obesity.

Efficacy of Scalable Commercial Weight Loss Programs

While the variety and sheer volume of community-based commercial weight loss programs provide many benefits, few programs meet the criteria outlined by the USPSTF and expert panels (Table 87.1). The programs vary greatly in their efficacy, safety, and acceptability (cost, difficulty of adherence, level of support). Clinicians, policymakers, health insurers, employers, and individuals need help evaluating available programs, so they can determine which programs merit provider referral, patient engagement, and third-party payment.

A 2015 review in the *Annals of Internal Medicine* has provided that guidance. The review gathered all of the long-term randomized controlled trials (RCTs ≥ 12 weeks) and prospective case studies (≥ 12 months) published on existing commercial and proprietary weight loss programs and examined the efficacy and safety of each, compared to control/ education or behavioral counseling. The list of 141 "weight loss" programs was narrowed to the 32 programs that contained dietary intervention and behavioral support. Among those 32, only 11 programs had published data across 42 RCTs. The programs were divided into three categories: market leaders (Weight Watchers [WW], Jenny Craig [JC], and Nutrisystem [NS]), very-low-calorie programs (VLCPs; Health Management Resources, Medifast, OPTIFAST), and self-directed programs (Atkins, The Biggest Loser Club, eDiets, Lose It!, SlimFast). Of the 11 programs, only six, the market leaders and VLCPs, met USPSTF criteria, and are the focus here. Table 87.2 details the main components of each of these programs.

Weight Watchers, Jenny Craig, and Nutrisystem

Compared to control/education, WW resulted in approximately 3% greater weight loss at 12 months. JC resulted in approximately 5% greater weight loss than control/education and counseling at 12 months. NS showed a 4% greater weight loss compared to control/ education and counseling at 3 months, but there were no trials longer than 6 months. Taken together, these findings suggest that these weight loss programs successfully facilitate clinically meaningful weight loss and are superior to providing minimal or no care.

Health Management Resources, Medifast, and OPTIFAST

Compared to counseling, Health Management Resources (HMR) produces 13% greater weight loss at 6 months; Medifast produces a 6% greater weight loss at 4 months, with no significant difference at 9 months; and OPTIFAST produces a 4–9% greater weight loss at 4–5 months, with no difference at 12 months. Combining findings from case series with those of RCTs, there were losses of 15–25% of initial weight over 3–6 months of treatment with HMR and OPTIFAST. While weight regain is common, there are still losses of approximately 8–9%, 7%, and 5% at 1, 3, and 4 years after treatment, respectively, suggesting that these programs are comparable or even more effective than academic-based, intensive behavioral interventions.

Recommendations

Based on the available evidence, the review provided referral recommendations for each category of programs. The market leaders were all found to be high-intensity and to have few adverse effects; however, only WW and JC produced sustained (1 year) weight loss, and WW was the most cost-effective and had the lowest monthly cost. Therefore, the authors concluded that WW and JC should be the primary targets of referrals. The VLCPs were also high-intensity, but had high program costs and higher risk for adverse events, such as gallstones. The AHA/ACC/TOS guidelines recommend that very-low-calorie diets should only be suggested in limited cases, and under strict medical supervision. The five self-directed programs, while affordable, were low-intensity and did not meet

TABLE 87.2. Key Components and Costs of Commercial Weight Loss Programs That Meet USPSTF Criteria

Program[a]	Diet	Physical activity	Support	Monthly cost	RCTs	Duration of RCTs (months)
Weight Watchers: monthly pass (meetings and etools)	Conventional food, Intake tracking	Encouraged, Activity tracking	Weekly group counseling sessions, In-person (WW trained alumnus)[d], Unlimited one-on-one counseling, Online (WW trained alumnus)[d], Online community forum	$45[e]	8	3–24
Nutrisystem: core or uniquely yours	Meal replacements[b], Intake tracking	Encouraged, Exercise plans, Activity tracking	Unlimited one-on-one counseling, Online/telephone (dietitians or NS-trained weight loss counselors)[g], Online community forum	$280–340[f]	3	3–6
Jenny Craig: in center or anywhere	Meal replacements[b], Intake tracking	Encouraged, Activity tracking	Unlimited one-on-one counseling, In-person (In center only)/telephone/video chat (JC-trained counselor), Online community forum	$469–709[e,f]	3	12–24
HMR: clinic or at home	Meal replacements[c], Intake tracking (select programs)	Encouraged, Activity tracking (select programs)	Medical supervision (clinic only), Weekly group counseling sessions, in person (clinic),[g] telephone (at home) (HMR-trained health educator), Unlimited one-on-one counseling, telephone[g] (HMR-trained consultants)[d], Online community forum	$240–600[f]	4	3–6
Medifast: center[b]	Meal replacements[c], Intake tracking	Encouraged, Activity tracking	Medical supervision, Frequency dependent on center one-on-one counseling, in-person (center-trained nutritionists)[d], Unlimited nutrition support, telephone (MediFast nutritionist), Online community forum	$300–400[f,h]	1	9

(continued)

TABLE 87.2. (*continued*)

OPTIFAST[b]	Meal replacements[c] Intake tracking	Encouraged Activity tracking	Medical supervision, frequency dependent on center one-on-one/group counseling, in person (center health care professionals)[d] Online community forum	$665[e,f]	4	5–15

Note. From Gudzune et al. (2015). Copyright © 2015 American College of Physicians. Adapted by permission. Costs and support updated based on information taken from program website and calls to program customer service as of October 2015.

[a]If the program has multiple versions (home, in clinic, online), the version(s) with behavioral support that was/were tested in the RCTs is/are detailed. HMR, Health Management Resources; USPSTF, U.S. Preventive Services Task Force.

[b]Low calorie.

[c]Low calorie or very low calorie.

[d]Note about counselors: WW: Sessions led by an individual who successfully completed the WW program and have been trained by WW in behavioral principles. HMR: consultant who uses HMR foods. Medifast: centers are independently owned franchises, counselor training determined by center. OPTIFAST: providers are medical professionals who become OPTIFAST product providers and have access to training resources, protocols for medical monitoring, and behavioral education.

[e]Some health insurance companies or employers offer discounts and/or other options to assist in covering costs.

[f]Includes costs of meal replacements, consumer needs to supplement with fresh produce and dairy.

[g]Study intervention differed from what is available to the general public. Nutrisystem: Two of the three studies involved weekly, in-person group sessions with highly trained practitioners from the University (not NS trained), and the third study did not involve any counseling at all. The general public only has access to one-on-one online or telephone support from NS trained counselors. HMR: For the three studies that utilized in-person groups and telephone calls, it is unclear whether the counselors were HMR trained, and for one study, the intervention included one-on-one in-person meetings and organized exercise sessions. The general public has access only to in-person group meetings and no exercise sessions.

[h]Centers vary. Medifast: Centers are independently owned franchises, and vary in frequency of in-person visits, counselor training, and costs ($300–400 is for cost of the food only, there are additional membership fees). OPTIFAST: Centers are medical professionals who become product providers and vary in counselor credentials and costs.

543

USPSTF criteria. In addition, the results were hard to interpret, as many of the interventions tested altered versions of the programs not generally available (e.g., book plus counseling sessions with a dietitian). The overarching message for clinicians, providers, and those affected by overweight and obesity was to focus on programs that meet USPSTF criteria (Table 87.1), and within that group of programs, prioritize programs that have a substantial evidence base and proven longer-term efficacy (Table 87.2). WW and JC were identified as the strongest programs.

Conclusions

The USPSTF recommends that clinicians screen all adults for overweight/obesity and provide or refer them to behavioral weight loss treatment. Expert panels, including the USPSTF and the AHA/ACC/TOS, have identified the criteria of recommended behavioral interventions (Table 87.1), given the strong evidence for producing clinically meaningful weight losses of 5–10% in 6–12 months. However, given that more than one-third of U.S. adults have obesity, the volume of screenings, referrals, and treatment greatly exceed the limited capacities of primary care providers and specialized programs.

Accessible, community-based weight loss programs can play a significant role in providing evidence-based treatment of overweight and obesity. In order for this potential to be fully realized, policy efforts should be directed to providing full or partial reimbursement for empirically validated treatments. Currently, while physicians are paid to screen and refer, most patients are left to incur the cost of treatment, which poses a significant barrier for many.

Nationally available weight management programs can help address the epidemic in a variety of ways that meet consumers' needs and preferences. While there are many positives to having choices when it comes to weight loss treatments (online or in-person, meal replacement or conventional foods, self-directed or facilitated), not all programs meet the USPSTF guidelines, and there is risk that effort and money will be spent on programs of lower quality. Expert panels have provided criteria to distinguish high-intensity programs and clinicians; individuals, insurers, and employers should consider these criteria when choosing a program. Even among these programs, however, greater emphasis should be placed on programs that have proven efficacy and lower cost.

Suggested Reading

Gudzune, K. A., Doshi, R. S., Mehta, A. K., Chaudhry, Z. W., Jacobs, D. K., Vakil, R. M., et al. (2015). Efficacy of commercial weight-loss programs: An updated systematic review. *Annals of Internal Medicine, 162*(7), 501–512.—This article provides a current and thorough review of the efficacy of the commercial weight loss programs based on studies published from October 2002 until November 2014. Most of the findings and summary statements in this chapter are based on this review.

Jensen, M. D., Ryan, D. H., Apovian, C. M., Ard, J. D., Comuzzie, A. G., Donato, K. A., et al. (2014). 2013 AHA/ACC/TOS guideline for the management of overweight and obesity in adults: A report of the American College of Cardiology/American Heart Association Task Force on Practice Guidelines and the Obesity Society. *Circulation, 129*(25, Suppl. 2), S102–S138.—This article provides guidelines for the management of overweight and obesity in adults from the AHA/ACC/TOS.

Look AHEAD Research Group. (2014). Eight-year weight losses with an intensive lifestyle intervention: The look AHEAD study. *Obesity (Silver Spring), 22*(1), 5–13.—This article describes the long-term outcomes of a behavioral intervention.

Moyer, V. A. (2012). Screening for and management of obesity in adults: U.S. Preventive Services Task Force recommendation statement. *Annals of Internal Medicine, 157*(5), 373–378.—This article provides the recommendations of the USPSTF on screening and management of obesity.

Tsai, A. G., & Wadden, T. A. (2005). Systematic review: An evaluation of major commercial weight loss programs in the United States. *Annals of Internal Medicine, 142*(1), 56–66.—This article provides a review of the efficacy of commercial weight loss programs based on studies published from January 1, 1966, until October 1, 2003. Some of the findings and summary statements in this chapter are based on this review.

Wadden, T. A., Webb, V. L., Moran, C. H., & Bailer, B. A. (2012). Lifestyle modification for obesity new developments in diet, physical activity, and behavior therapy. *Circulation, 125*(9), 1157–1170.—This article provides an overview of research regarding behavioral lifestyle intervention.

88

Exercise in the Management of Obesity

JOHN M. JAKICIC
RENEE J. ROGERS

Overweight and obesity are significant public health problems in the United States and other countries throughout the world. Excess body weight is associated with numerous chronic conditions that include cardiovascular disease, diabetes, some forms of cancer, musculoskeletal disorders, and others, along with related intermediate risk factors. The increasing prevalence of excess body weight, referred to as overweight and obesity, has resulted in numerous approaches to be developed and implemented in an attempt to prevent and successfully treat this health condition and related comorbidities. At the cornerstone of many of these approaches is lifestyle modification, with exercise being a key component. However, these approaches no longer focus specifically on exercise, but rather on the broader scope of physical activity that includes but is not limited to structured periods of exercise.

Physical Activity without Dietary Counseling on Weight Loss

Physical activity has been shown to be an important behavior that impacts numerous health-related outcomes. These health benefits were highlighted in the 1996 Surgeon General's Report on Physical Activity and Health, and more recently in the 2008 Physical Activity Guidelines for Americans. Many of these health benefits of physical activity have been observed independent of body weight or in the absence of significant weight loss. Thus, it appears that adults with excess body weight can realize health benefits from engagement in physical activity irrespective of weight change.

Physical activity without dietary counseling or a recommendation to reduce energy intake can also result in weight loss, but the average magnitude of weight loss appears to be modest, in the range of approximately 1–3 kg. However, in the review of the literature conducted for the 2008 Physical Activity Guidelines Advisory Committee Report, this magnitude of weight loss was only observed in response to at least 180 minutes/week of physical activity. Moreover, there may be a dose–response effect, with the magnitude of weight loss increasing as dose of physical activity increases. For example, a review of the literature conducted for the 2009 Position Stand of the American College of Sports Medicine (ACSM) showed no change in body weight in response to <150 minutes/week of physical activity, whereas there were graded increases in weight loss as physical activity also increased.

The majority of data to support the effect of physical activity on weight loss has primarily included aerobic forms of physical activity (e.g., walking, cycling). However, other forms of physical activity have also been examined, with the most common form being resistance exercise. Resistance exercise has been shown to increase lean body mass, muscular strength and function, and to have a favorable effect on many cardiometabolic risk factors. However, resistance exercise has been shown to have a modest influence on weight loss in studies that are typically 3–6 months in length, with similar findings observed in the limited number of studies that have had a longer duration. While this lack of a significant effect on weight loss may be blunted by any concomitant increase in lean mass that may be observed with resistance exercise, clinicians and health-fitness professionals may want to consider using resistance exercise in combination with other forms of physical activity to enhance the likelihood of reducing body weight.

Another physical activity strategy that may contribute to weight loss has been the recommendation to increase nonexercise forms of physical activity. These approaches usually include recommendations to increase the number of steps walked through lifestyle forms of physical activity. The average increase resulting from this type of approach has been 2,000–3,000 steps per day, and when examined over a period of 3 months, this has resulted in a modest reduction in body weight of approximately 1–2 kg. Thus, it may be necessary to combine these lifestyle approaches to physical activity with structured forms of activity (exercise) to allow for an adequate increase energy expenditure that results in significant weight loss.

Physical Activity Combined with Dietary Counseling on Weight Loss

Clinical guidelines recommend that physical activity be implemented in combination with a reduction in energy intake to elicit the greatest short-term and long-term effects on body weight. There are numerous studies with consistent findings to show that, on average, an additional 1–3 kg of weight loss is achieved when physical activity is combined with an energy-restricted diet compared to the energy-restricted diet alone. These findings have been reported in adults who are overweight, obese, or severely obese, with interventions ranging from 3 to 12 months or longer in duration. While 1–3 kg of additional weight loss may appear to be modest, this actually results in approximately 20% more weight loss than what can be achieved with a reduction in energy intake alone. Thus, lifestyle intervention programs for weight loss should include physical activity as a key component to allow for maximal weight loss.

It appears that physical activity becomes even more important for enhancing long-term weight loss and for prevention of weight regain. Numerous cross-sectional and observational studies have shown an association between physical activity participation and improved long-term weight loss. Moreover, primary and secondary analyses of data from randomized trials also support the association between long-term weight loss and greater participation in physical activity. A consistent finding in many of these studies is that a relatively high level of moderate-to-vigorous physical activity, equivalent to approximately 200–300 minutes/week, is associated with improved long-term weight loss and less weight regain. This has led many professional medical and health-related organizations to recommend that this magnitude of physical activity be prescribed within the context of comprehensive weight loss programs.

More recent evidence from clinical intervention studies appears to suggest that the pattern of moderate-to-vigorous physical activity combined with engagement in light intensity physical activity may also be key considerations for improving long-term weight loss and the prevention of weight regain. A comprehensive behavioral intervention that included both diet and physical activity showed that both moderate-to-vigorous intensity physical activity performed in bouts of at least 10 minutes and total minutes of light intensity physical activity were significantly greater in individuals achieving at least 10% weight loss at 18 months compared to those achieving less weight loss. Moreover, a similar pattern was observed when examining individuals who lost at least 10% of their initial body weight at 6 months and were able to sustain this magnitude of weight loss at 18 months. Key to these findings is that the moderate-to-vigorous physical activity performed in bouts of at least 10 continuous minutes totaled 200–300 minutes/week. Thus, this may suggest that clinical interventions for weight loss that focus on reducing energy intake also include a prescription for moderate-to-vigorous physical activity performed in bouts of at least 10 minutes to be increased to 200–300 minutes/week, while also sustaining or increasing participation in light intensity physical activity.

The Role of Physical Activity in Medical Approaches for Weight Loss

Bariatric surgery and other medical procedures have become more commonplace for the treatment for obesity. A variety of procedures have been implemented, such as gastric bypass, gastric sleeve, gastric banding, and, more recently, nonsurgical procedures such as the gastric balloon. While the role of physical activity within the context of all of these procedures has not been thoroughly examined, there is a growing literature to support the inclusion of physical activity in the treatment plan for patients who undergo many of these procedures. While recent evidence does not conclusively indicate that inclusion of physical activity with bariatric surgery procedures will enhance weight loss within the initial 6 months following surgery, there is greater evidence to support the importance of physical activity for improving surgically induced weight loss at 12 months and beyond. Thus, the current evidence suggests that a comprehensive treatment plan for patients undergoing bariatric surgery should include a recommendation to engage in physical activity.

Physical Activity Associated with Other Weight Loss Behaviors

A key pathway by which physical activity influences body weight is through its impact on energy expenditure. However, there is evidence that physical activity may also influence body weight, and therefore weight loss, through its associated influences on other key weight control behaviors that include energy intake and eating behaviors. Results from weight loss intervention studies have shown that higher levels of physical activity are associated with better compliance to dietary change and engagement in eating behaviors that have been shown to be important for weight loss. Moreover, there is some evidence that physical activity may influence biological pathways, such as appetite-regulating hormones, which may also influence eating behavior and energy intake. However, despite the influence of physical activity on these biological pathways, results do not consistently demonstrate that this ultimately results in reduced energy intake, as studies have shown that for some individuals, physical activity may increase energy intake. Thus, from a clinical intervention perspective, the importance of physical activity in the treatment of obesity may involve increased energy expenditure combined with enhanced dietary compliance and reduced energy intake. However, attention must also be given to those individuals who are engaging in sufficient amounts of physical activity but not losing weight, as this may suggest a compensatory increase in energy intake that warrants dietary counseling.

Safety of Physical Activity and Structured Exercise for Adults with Obesity

Engagement in physical activity or structured exercise can be associated with some degree of health risk; however, this risk is relatively low when it progresses in an appropriate manner and when appropriate screening occurs prior to initiation of such a program. Moreover, not all individuals need to obtain clearance from their physician or undergo a diagnostic exercise test prior to initiating a light-to-moderate physical activity program. Guidelines published by the ACSM indicate that individuals with multiple risk factors, but without symptoms or known cardiovascular, pulmonary, metabolic, or kidney problems, can initiate a program that includes activities similar to walking without the need for medical clearance. This suggests that the vast majority of adults with obesity who meet these criteria should be able to engage in light-to-moderate intensity forms of physical activity safely. However, for adults with obesity who are symptomatic or who have known cardiovascular, pulmonary, metabolic, or kidney disease, a medical evaluation is recommended prior to initiating such a program of physical activity.

Recommendations

Our research group has been involved in clinical approaches for weight loss that involve physical activity for the past 20 years. This research and our experience lead us to the following conclusions:

1. For the average adult seeking to lose weight, physical activity alone, without a concomitant reduction in energy intake, will result in modest weight loss. Moreover, weight loss that includes a reduction in energy intake but does not also include physical activity will have a blunted effective compared to when these approaches are used in combination. Thus, for adults seeking to lose weight, the most effective behavioral approach should include a recommendation to appropriately reduce energy intake appropriately in combination with adequately increasing physical activity.

2. For the average adult, progressing to a level of physical activity that is equivalent to 200–300 minutes/week of moderate-to-vigorous intensity physical activity (e.g., brisk walking) that is completed in bouts of at least 10 minutes, in combination with an appropriate reduction in energy intake, will result in enhance long-term weight loss and reduce the risk of weight regain.

3. In addition to aerobic forms of physical activity (e.g., walking, cycling), adults seeking weight loss may also benefit from resistance exercise and other forms of lighter intensity physical activity that can increase steps walked each day.

4. Physical activity appears to be beneficial for individuals who undergo surgical and nonsurgical medical approaches to weight loss; therefore, physical activity should be a component of their treatment plan.

5. Regardless of magnitude of weight loss, adults with excess body weight can realize significant health benefits by being physically active.

Suggested Reading

Donnelly, J. E., Blair, S. N., Jakicic, J. M., Manore, M. M., Rankin, J. W., & Smith, B. K. (2009). American College of Sports Medicine Position Stand: Appropriate physical activity intervention strategies for weight loss and prevention of weight regain for adults. *Medicine and Science in Sports and Exercise, 41*(2), 459–471.—This article describes the results of a systematic review regarding the influence of physical activity on the prevention and treatment of overweight and obesity.

Eckel, R. H., Jakicic, J. M., Ard, J. D., de Jesus, J. M., Miller, N. H., Hubbard, V. S., et al. (2014). 2013 AHA/ACC guideline on lifestyle management to reduce cardiovascular risk: A report of the American College of Cardiology/American Heart Association Task Force on Practice Guidelines. *Circulation, 129*(25, Suppl. 2), S76–S99.—This systematic review and resulting clinical practice guideline includes information on the cardiometabolic effects of physical activity in the absence of weight loss.

Jakicic, J. M., Marcus, B. H., Lang, W., & Janney, C. (2008). Effect of exercise on 24-month weight loss maintenance in overweight women. *Archives of Internal Medicine, 168*(14), 1550–1559.—A secondary analysis of data from this randomized intervention trial demonstrated the association between greater levels of physical activity and improved 24-month weight loss in adults.

Jakicic, J. M., Tate, D. F., Lang, W., Davis, K. K., Polzien, K., Neiberg, R. H., et al. (2014). Objective physical activity and weight loss in adults: The step-up randomized clinical trial. *Obesity, 22*(11), 2284–2292.—This report on a secondary analysis of data from a randomized intervention trial shows that objectively measured moderate-to-vigorous physical activity performed in bouts of at least 10 minutes and total light-intensity physical activity are associated with improved 18-month weight loss and maintenance of at least 10% weight loss in adults.

Jakicic, J. M., Winters, C., Lang, W., & Wing, R. R. (1999). Effects of intermittent exercise and use of home exercise equipment on adherence, weight loss, and fitness in overweight women: A randomized trial. *Journal of the American Medical Association, 282*(16), 1554–1560.—A secondary analysis of data from this randomized intervention trial demonstrated the association between greater levels of physical activity and improved 18-month weight loss in adults.

Jensen, M. D., Ryan, D. H., Hu, F. B., Stevens, F. J., Hubbard, V. S., Stevens, V. J., et al. (2013). 2013 AHA/ACC/TOS guideline for the management of overweight and obesity in adults. *Circulation, 129*(25, Suppl. 2), S102–S138.—This systematic review and resulting clinical practice guideline includes information on the effects of lifestyle approaches, including physical activity, on weight loss.

Physical Activity Guidelines Advisory Committee. (2008). *Physical Activity Guidelines Advisory Committee Report, 2008.* Washington, DC: U.S. Department of Health and Human Services.—This report includes a review of the literature for the effects of physical activity on weight loss in the absense of dietary recommendations to reduce energy intake.

U.S. Department of Health and Human Services. (1996). *Physical activity and health: A report of the Surgeon General.* Collingdale, PA: Diane Publishing.—This report includes a comprehensive review of the scientific evidence to support the health benefits, including weight control, of physical activity.

Body Image Issues in Obesity

DAVID B. SARWER

Obesity is associated with a significant psychosocial burden. Excess body weight is associated with impairments in quality of life, including a particularly salient aspect of quality of life for many individuals—body image. This chapter provides an overview on the relationship between obesity and body image. Excess body weight is associated with increased body image dissatisfaction, whereas weight loss in all of its forms typically results in improvements in body image for many individuals.

A Brief History of Body Image

Interest in and scholarship about the psychological construct of body image has existed for the past century. Much of the earliest work was undertaken by physicians working to uncover the basic elements of the mind–body relationship. In the early to mid-1900s, plastic surgeons and other medical professionals began to write about the significant impact of disfiguring wounds of war on psychological functioning. In the 1950s and 1960s, physicians and surgeons were joined by mental health professionals in the exploration of the association between one's external physical appearance and the subjective appraisal of it. Beginning in the 1970s, social-psychological research began to provide a new perspective on the psychological aspects of physical appearance. This now sizable body of research shows clearly that individuals who are more physically attractive are judged or perceived in more favorable light than those who are less attractive. A great many studies also show that more attractive individuals receive preferential treatment in a variety of social situations across the lifespan.

On the heels of this research, interest in the "internal" view of physical appearance—body image—exploded in the early 1990s. Scholars in this area developed theoretical models of body image (typically from a cognitive-behavioral perspective) and conducted high-quality empirical research that rapidly advanced scholarship in the area.

Much of early body image theory was modeled around the weight and shape concerns of individuals with eating disorders. As research into the global obesity problem flourished in the 1990s, the body image concerns of overweight and obese individuals garnered more attention.

Definitions and Theoretical Models of Body Image

Body image has been defined in several ways. Cash and Pruzinsky defined body image as those perceptions, thoughts, and feelings associated with the body and bodily experience. This definition captures the multidimensional nature of body image, starting with an individual's perception of the physical reality of appearance. These physical perceptions subsequently interact with standards for one's appearance, as well as the resulting cognitions and emotions. Unfortunately, the definition does not specifically highlight body image behaviors that may result from these perceptions, thoughts, and feelings. More recently, Cash and Smolak (2011) described body image as "the psychological experience of embodiment." This is a concise yet encompassing description that, although not as detailed as other characterizations, leaves the reader with a sense of the important role that body image plays in the overall human experience.

A number of theoretical models of body image also have been described. The cognitive-behavioral model is perhaps most widely used in research and clinical applications. In addition to including the perceptual, cognitive, affective, and behavioral aspects noted earlier, the model also focuses on historical and proximal influences on body image. In brief, historical influences include an individual's physical characteristics, personality traits (these may place an individual "at risk" to be overly concerned about his or her external appearance), interpersonal experiences (e.g., modeling and appearance-focused teasing), and cultural socialization. Proximal influences include appearance schematic processing that, along with more general cognitive processes, lends "meaning" to activating situations and events in daily life. These historical and proximal variables influence two fundamental body image attitudes—body image investment and body image evaluation (i.e., the degree to which an individual is satisfied or dissatisfied with his or her appearance). The interaction of the degree of investment in one's appearance and the degree of (dis)satisfaction influences subsequent behavior.

The Etiology of Body Image Dissatisfaction

Prevalence

More than half of women and slightly less than half of men are believed to be dissatisfied with their overall appearance. Two-thirds of women and more than half of men report dissatisfaction with their body weight. As almost 70% of Americans are now overweight or obese, and the rates of overweight and obesity of other westernized countries are comparable, these results are more intuitive than surprising.

Although body image dissatisfaction is somewhat universal, it varies across different groups of individuals. Women are typically far more dissatisfied with their body image than are men. Differences also exist across ethnic groups. African American women, compared to European American women, typically report less body image dissatisfaction. Among other ethnic groups, body image dissatisfaction appears to be related to the degree of acculturation.

Specificity

Body image concerns can be global and/or specific. Clinicians often hear the global complaint, "I just can't stand my body." This may be particularly common for those suffering with obesity. A number of studies have suggested that body image dissatisfaction is associated with degree of excess body weight. The strength of this association, however, is modest. This finding is consistent with theories of body image suggesting that there may be little association between what one thinks about one's body and the objective reality of one's appearance. At the same time, many individuals report some specific concerns with their appearance. Slightly less than 50% of women report dissatisfaction with their waist and abdomen, irrespective of actual body weight. Perhaps this finding is not all that surprising given the mass media and the fashion industry's fascination with thinness as a hallmark trait in their depictions of physical beauty.

Severity

Another issue to consider is the severity of the body image dissatisfaction. Some degree of body image dissatisfaction appears to be "normative" in contemporary society. This dissatisfaction is believed to motivate a number of appearance-enhancing behaviors, including cosmetics and fashion purchases, cosmetic surgery, and weight loss. Some women report an excessive degree of dissatisfaction with their weight and shape that may negatively impact behavior. For example, some may camouflage their bodies with clothing, change their posture or body movements, and avoid looking at their bodies. Others report embarrassment in social situations because of their weight.

Clinical Significance

Another issue to consider is whether body image dissatisfaction is associated with clinically significant distress. Studies of women with obesity have found a relation between decreased body image satisfaction, low self-esteem, and increased self-reported depressive symptoms. A small minority of women with obesity also appear to experience extreme body image dissatisfaction, consistent with the diagnosis of *body dysmorphic disorder,* defined as a preoccupation with an imagined or slight defect in appearance that causes clinically significant distress or impairment in social, occupational, or other important areas of functioning.

Risk Factors

There appear to be a number of risk factors associated with the development of body image dissatisfaction secondary to obesity. These include both current weight status and recent weight trajectory, as well as gender, race, sexual orientation, disordered eating, appearance-related teasing, and increased investment in appearance.

Body Image and Reasons for Seeking Weight Loss

Body image dissatisfaction is believed to play a significant role in motivating weight loss. Weight reduction, in fact, may be the most popular form of body image therapy, contributing tens of billions of dollars to the American economy each year. While some individuals may engage in weight loss to improve their health and fitness, the majority do so to improve their physical appearance and body image, even among those who suffer with extreme obesity.

Improvements in Body Image with Weight Loss

Several studies have documented improvements in body image with weight loss, whether through lifestyle modification, pharmacotherapy, or bariatric surgery. Patients typically report statistically significant improvements in both general and weight-specific aspects of body image with modest weight losses of even 5–10% of initial body weight. The improvements in body image seen with bariatric surgery are often larger in magnitude. Interestingly, individuals who undergo bariatric surgery report these improvements within the first 6 months of surgery, and before they have reached their maximum weight losses. These self-reported improvements in body image are well maintained within the first several years after surgery and when some individuals experience some modest weight regain.

Nevertheless, some individuals report substantial dissatisfaction with their bodies after losing massive weight through bariatric surgery. This dissatisfaction typically is attributed to excess, loose skin of the abdomen, thighs, and arms, and leads more than 50,000 American annually to undergo body contouring surgery with a plastic surgeon. The most common of these procedures is breast reduction surgery, although plastic surgeons can perform procedures on most areas of the body to improve their appearance following weight reduction. Although little research has examined the influence of these body contouring procedures on persons with obesity specifically, a more general body of literature suggests that plastic surgery patients experience significant improvements in their body image postoperatively.

Conclusions

Obesity is associated with a significant psychosocial burden for many individuals. Most individuals report substantial impairments in quality of life, including more specific domains of quality of life, such as body image. Women and men with obesity report heightened levels of body image dissatisfaction, but it is encouraging that weight loss is associated with improvements in body image for most individuals. However, some persons with extreme obesity who undergo bariatric surgery eventually turn to body contouring procedures to ultimately improve their appearance and body image.

Suggested Reading

Cash, T. F. (2008). *The body image workbook: An eight-step program for learning to like your looks* (2nd ed.). Oakland, CA: New Harbinger.—A self-help workbook that is a valuable tool for individuals looking to improve their body image.

Cash, T. F., & Smolak, L. (Eds.). (2011). *Body image: A handbook of science, practice, and prevention* (2nd ed.). New York: Guilford Press.—The second edition of this seminal handbook provides a comprehensive overview of the body image literature across multiple perspectives.

Foster, G. D., Wadden, T. A., & Vogt, R. A. (1997). Body image before, during, and after weight loss treatment. *Health Psychology, 16,* 226–229.—One of the earliest investigations of the body image concerns of women who seek weight loss treatment and the improvements that come with weight reduction.

Hatfield, E., & Sprecher, S. (1986). *Mirror, mirror: The importance of looks in everyday life.* Stony Brook: State University of New York Press.—This classic text summarizes the social psychological research on the impact of physical appearance on daily life.

Jarry, J. L., & Cash, T. F. (2011). Cognitive-behavioral approaches to body image change. In T. F. Cash & L. Smolak (Eds.), *Body image: A handbook of science, practice, and prevention* (2nd ed., pp. 415–423). New York: Guilford Press.—This chapter provides a detailed description of a cognitive-behavioral model of body image.

Rosen, J. C., Orosan, P., & Reiter, J. (1995). Cognitive behavior therapy for negative body image in obese women. *Behavior Therapy, 26,* 25–42.—One of the first empirical studies of cognitive-behavioral therapy to improve body image in women with obesity and independent of weight loss.

Sarwer, D. B., Dilks, R. J., & Spitzer, J. C. (2011). Weight loss and changes in body image. In T. F. Cash & L. Smolak (Eds.), *Body image: A handbook of science, practice, and prevention* (2nd ed., pp. 369–377). New York: Guilford Press.—This chapter provides a detailed review of the relationship between weight loss and changes in body image.

Sarwer, D. B., Thompson, J. K., & Cash, T. F. (2005). Body image in obesity in adulthood. *Psychiatric Clinics of North America, 28,* 69–87.—This article summarizes the literature on the body image concerns of women and men before and after weight loss.

Sarwer, D. B., Wadden, T. A., & Foster, G. D. (1998). Assessment of body image dissatisfaction in obese women: Specificity, severity, and clinical significance. *Journal of Consulting and Clinical Psychology, 66,* 651–654.—An early empirical article documenting the specificity, severity, and clinical significance of body image concerns in women with obesity who received lifestyle modification for weight loss.

Schwartz, M. B., & Brownell, K. D. (2004). Obesity and body image. *Body Image, 1,* 43–56.—This widely cited review article summarizes the literature on obesity and body image.

Improving Maintenance of Weight Loss

DELIA SMITH WEST

Sustained weight loss is arguably the greatest challenge currently facing the obesity treatment field. Researchers have developed behavioral interventions that consistently achieve average weight losses of 7–9% of initial body weight, and weight losses of this magnitude produce a wide range of health benefits. However, those health improvements attenuate and even disappear in the face of weight regain.

Clinical lore and early research indicate that individuals tend to regain about one-third of the weight they lost within the first year following treatment, and that within 3–5 years the majority will have returned to their initial weight. Recent clinical studies offer a more optimistic pattern of weight maintenance. The Look AHEAD (Action for Health in Diabetes) study, a multisite, controlled trial, randomized over 2,500 adults with type 2 diabetes to an intensive lifestyle intervention arm. Among the 825 lifestyle participants who achieved weight losses of 10% or greater at the end of the first year, 39% had sustained weight losses of 10% or higher a full 8 years later. An additional 26% had maintained at least a 5% weight loss at 8 years. These data on the possibility of meaningful weight maintenance are far more promising than earlier assumptions. What remains to be determined is how best to achieve these sustained weight losses outside the confines of a highly-controlled clinical trial.

Other indications that long-term weight maintenance is possible can be seen among participants in the National Weight Control Registry (NWCR), which enrolls individuals who have sustained weight losses of at least 30 pounds for at least 1 year, with a goal of identifying factors associated with long-term weight maintenance among successful dieters. The NWCR has enrolled over 10,000 successful dieters and is following these individuals prospectively to determine weight change trajectory and predictors of weight maintenance. Among those who have 10 years of follow-up data available ($N = 2,886$), an impressive majority of them (87%) have sustained weight losses of at least 10% of their initial weight. Although some weight regain was evident over this period, the cohort has maintained average estimated weight losses of 23.1 kg (74% of their initial weight loss) after a decade.

Recent studies of weight maintenance interventions provide a fairly consistent picture of weight patterns, despite the use of two different research designs and slightly different ways of operationalizing weight maintenance. Researchers tend to either solicit individuals who have previously lost a benchmark amount of weight on their own (by various means) and randomize these recruits to different maintenance approaches, or enroll participants and provide them with a standardized weight loss program prior to initiating the different maintenance approaches. Outcomes are measured as (1) weight regain from the point of entry into the maintenance intervention, (2) the proportion maintaining study entry weight (or close to entry weight), and/or (3) total weight loss over the observation period, with clinically meaningful weight thresholds (e.g., $\geq 5\%$ or $\geq 10\%$) often used to classify success. These different approaches to examining the important research questions surrounding weight maintenance make cross-study comparisons challenging and may contribute to a slower path to clarity on best practices.

Nonetheless, it appears that even with maintenance programs in place, individuals who have achieved a sizable weight loss (8–10% of initial body weight) experience some modest weight regain, with regains ranging from 2.5–3.1 kg over 1–2 years among individuals offered in-person maintenance programs. Phone-based maintenance interventions also have support, with outcomes comparable to face-to-face programs and a favorable cost-efficiency profile. Utilizing phone-based maintenance programs is particularly attractive in populations for which travel to a central location might be problematic (rural areas, populations with travel limitations, etc.).

Internet-delivered maintenance programs appear less effective in preventing regain than face-to-face maintenance programs. However, there may be a special role for Internet-based weight regain prevention as an initial maintenance tactic within a stepped-care approach, whereby individuals receive an initial Internet-based treatment, with the more intensive in-person program reserved for those who fail to remain weight stable with the Internet-based treatment. Other stepped-care approaches to weight regulation have demonstrated that reserving the more intensive (and often more expensive) interventions for those who do not respond to the lower-intensity interventions is feasible, efficacious, and cost-effective, suggesting that such an approach may be appropriate for the current cost-conscious health care environment.

Identification of specific individual variables that are consistently associated with successful weight maintenance has proven elusive. Although age, race, and gender are often associated with weight losses during intensive behavioral interventions, these variables do not typically distinguish between those who regain after significant weight loss and those who do not. Initial weight loss is a fairly robust predictor of ultimate weight suppression, although the duration of follow-up may impact the nature of the relationship. Specifically, in some studies, individuals with larger initial weight losses demonstrate greater regain early on, but over extended time periods (i.e., 10 years), they ultimately experience greater weight losses. This has led to a focus on increasing initial weight losses as a strategy to promote greater long-term weight losses.

Strategies that are reported by successful weight maintainers include engaging in high levels of physical activity, regular self-weighing, and maintaining a low-calorie dietary pattern. Because the sustained implementation of these self-regulation behaviors is so consistently associated with weight maintenance, interventions often extend treatment to include a weight-maintenance component that focuses on behavioral strategies to sustain exercise and dietary habits. The average effect of an 18-month behavioral weight-maintenance program is 3.2 kg greater weight loss than that seen among individuals provided with an educational control program or no contact over that maintenance period. Extending contact with individuals without offering behavioral strategies targeting diet and activity does not appear to facilitate weight maintenance.

Maintenance programs appear to forestall weight regain by promoting greater adherence to recommended physical activity and calorie levels; individuals who remain actively engaged in the treatment program experience the best weight loss outcomes. However, a consistent finding across studies is that engagement in extended treatment diminishes over time, with attendance at intervention sessions decreasing dramatically after 6–12 months. It is hard to know whether those who are successful stay engaged or whether staying engaged produces greater success. Nonetheless, strategies to reduce barriers to remaining engaged and to reinforce sustained engagement represent a promising direction for improving weight maintenance.

Emerging technologies may play a significant role in these efforts. Technology can be used to implement core weight maintenance strategies in real time, including self-monitoring, tracking of objective data, and provision of meaningful feedback and personalized messaging. Such an approach can inform effective self-regulation strategies, maintain motivation, and reinforce continued engagement in weight-maintenance-promoting behaviors. Smartphone apps facilitate self-monitoring of physical activity and dietary intake, as can "wearable" devices (e.g., physical activity trackers). Digitally connected scales can interface with smartphones to graph body weight over time and prompt self-regulation if regain is noted, and can even transmit weight data to elicit a response from treatment providers. Likely these will not be panaceas, and motivating individuals to remain vigilant about dietary intake and promoting high levels of physical activity will continue to present challenges. However, these technologies open up frontiers in personalization that offer promise for more effective long-term weight management.

Current weight maintenance programs tend to apply the same strategies as weight loss induction programs, and some have argued that an individual's initiation of weight loss efforts may be driven by different decision criteria and supported by different behaviors than are sustained weight-maintenance actions. Specifically, individuals initiating weight loss behaviors may be motivated by the desire to achieve positive future goals (e.g., improved health or increased mobility), whereas maintenance of these behaviors may be motivated more by their desire to avoid returning to an unfavorable baseline state (e.g., poor health or reduced mobility). A weight-maintenance approach focused on sustaining motivation, by strengthening satisfaction with progress, and supporting autonomous self-regulation, by eliciting personal motivations for engaging in long-term behavior change, has been demonstrated to be as effective as a more traditional skills-based maintenance program. A similar motivation-based approach delivered by phone was also demonstrated to be effective. Finally, there is emerging evidence that behaviors that help individuals effectively maintain weight loss may be different from those that help them actually lose weight (and those that help with weight loss may not be particularly useful for weight maintenance).

Other novel approaches to weight maintenance suggest that the skills to sustain a stable weight should be the focus of initial treatment, and only after that should individuals be counseled in weight loss. This effectively turns weight maintenance into the primary focus rather than the afterthought. Using a "maintenance-first" approach can double the long-term weight losses achieved over 18 months and merits further examination. Other investigators have shown that providing some additional behavioral supports later in the course of treatment may provide better long-term outcomes than offering all the behavior change aids early in the intervention. Extended obesity treatment programs such as the Look AHEAD trial, which have impressive long-term weight outcomes, offer a series of annual campaigns and refreshers that are short "bursts" of more intensive intervention embedded within minimal ongoing individual contact; these periodic bouts of intervention provide a more continuous care model of obesity treatment, without the burden of a rigorous meeting schedule, and they merit further investigation to determine the parameters associated with the most effective campaigns and refreshers.

A further consideration in identifying strategies to enhance weight maintenance is how best to incorporate exercise. Controlled trials indicate that interventions that target both diet and physical activity produce better long-term weight losses than those that target diet alone. Current recommendations are to engage in 200–300 minutes/week of moderate-to-vigorous structured exercise to prevent weight regain. Studies indicate that those who engage in higher levels of exercise are among the most successful weight maintainers. There appears to be a special role for exercise above and beyond that of energy expenditure alone; those who are more active have better adherence to dietary goals, and exercise may neutralize some of the biological pressures to regain weight. Questions remain about the optimal exercise prescription for sustained weight control, with uncertainties about how the combination of exercise type (e.g., walking, aerobic, and/or resistance) and timing (during weight loss induction and/or maintenance) influence weight maintenance. Home-based exercise (as compared to gym- or office-based), prescription of short bouts of activity that accumulate over the day, and provision of exercise equipment for the home have all been shown to increase adherence and contribute to greater weight losses. Sustaining adherence to physical activity prescriptions long-term is perhaps the greatest challenge associated with effective weight maintenance.

Enhancing social support for weight-maintaining behaviors is another dimension that offers promise for improving weight maintenance. Capitalizing on existing social support networks or engineering social support within treatment groups can increase weight maintenance, at least in some studies. Emerging evidence suggests that interventions that incorporate online social networks may be effective at promoting weight loss; however, the role of social media in weight maintenance remains to be explored in greater detail.

Finally, determining which maintenance approach is best for which individuals may be a worthwhile direction to explore. There are a range of evidence-based approaches to maintenance that have distinct underlying elements that translated into different intervention methods, and there are diverse dietary and exercise prescriptions that have empirical support. Furthermore, there is substantial variability in maintenance intervention outcomes. Taken together, this suggests that matching a person's preferences, biology, or previous experiences (or some other dimension) to an appropriate maintenance program may be more effective than assuming that one intervention will be effective for all people. The limited data available on matching personal preferences and treatment approaches do not always support enhanced weight outcomes, but the concept continues to have appeal and warrants further study, particularly as new matching parameters begin to emerge.

In summary, long-term weight maintenance is clearly possible. However, maintenance remains a challenging undertaking for the majority of individuals who have successfully lost weight, and innovative approaches to facilitate sustained weight loss are needed.

Suggested Reading

Kiernan, M., Brown, S. D., Schoffman, D. E., Lee, K., King, A. C., Taylor, C. B., et al. (2013). Promoting healthy weight with "stability skills first": A randomized trial. *Journal of Consulting and Clinical Psychology, 81*(2), 336–346.—An innovative approach to behavioral weight control that started with learning skills to maintain weight, then transitioned into a focus on weight loss induction produced greater long-term weight loss than the more common weight management program sequence that starts with weight loss and is then followed by weight maintenance skills.

Look AHEAD Research Group. (2014). Eight-year weight losses with an intensive lifestyle intervention: The Look AHEAD study. *Obesity (Silver Spring), 22*(1), 5–13.—This randomized controlled trial of a behavioral weight control intervention offers the best and most sustained weight loss outcomes for obese individuals with type 2 diabetes mellitus, demonstrating that sustained weight control is possible among individuals from diverse ethnic backgrounds who engage in specific behavioral strategies.

MacLean, P. S., Wing, R. R., Davidson, T., Epstein, L., Goodpaster, B., Hall, K. D., et al. (2015). NIH working group report: Innovative research to improve maintenance of weight loss. *Obesity, 23*(1), 7–15.—Report of an National Institutes of Health working group of experts from multiple disciplines addressing the challenges associated with preventing weight regain following weight loss, including poor adherence to behavioral regimens and physiological adaptations that promote weight regain.

Sciamanna, C. N., Kiernan, M., Rolls, B. J., Boan, J., Stuckey, H., Kephart, D., et al. (2011). Practices associated with weight loss versus weight-loss maintenance: Results of a national survey. *American Journal of Preventive Medicine, 41*(2), 159–166.—Practices associated with successful weight loss may be different than those that produce successful weight maintenance according to this cross-sectional strategy of a large number of U.S. adults, suggesting that those behaviors identified as beneficial for weight maintenance may need to be more strongly emphasized in behavioral weight control programs.

Thomas, J. G., Bond, D. S., Phelan, S., Hill, J. O., & Wing, R. R. (2014). Weight-loss maintenance for 10 years in the National Weight Control Registry. *American Journal of Preventive Medicine, 46*(1), 17–23.—The NWCR enrolled individuals who had lost at least 30 pounds and kept it off for at least a year, and followed them for a decade and identified the behaviors associated with sustained weight loss.

West, D. S., Gorin, A. A., Subak, L. L., Foster, G., Bragg, C., Hecht, J., et al. (2011). A motivation-focused weight loss maintenance program is an effective alternative to a skill-based approach. *International Journal of Obesity, 35,* 259–269.—A novel weight loss maintenance intervention specifically targeting motivational factors was found to be as effective in producing long-term weight control as the more standard skills-based approach; therefore, it offers an alternative program that can be considered for individuals with dwindling motivation for continued implementation of self-regulation behaviors.

Wing, R. R., Tate, D. F., Gorin, A. A., Raynor, H. A., & Fava, J. L. (2006). A self-regulation program for maintenance of weight loss. *New England Journal of Medicine, 355*(15), 1563–1571.—This self-regulation program featuring daily self-weighing and traffic light "zone" (green, yellow, and red) feedback that signaled the need for initiation of weight management behaviors was effective in producing weight maintenance, particularly when delivered face-to-face.

Using Digital Media to Address Obesity

DEBORAH F. TATE

It is hard to imagine obesity prevention or treatment approaches that would not take advantage of some form of technology. Since 2000, when the first Internet-delivered approaches to obesity treatment were developed and evaluated, access to the Internet has steadily grown, across age, race, and income levels. This chapter provides an overview on ways in which technology is used in obesity treatment, the evidence on digital media approaches, and suggestions for future directions that capitalize on the advantages technology confers for patients, practitioners, and researchers.

Overview

Internet access among adults has remained at about 84% since 2012. The digital divide has narrowed, but as of 2015, older adults and those with lower income still have less access, currently estimated at around 60–75%. More adults (90%) own a cellular phone, and over 65% are smartphone users. Smartphones are cell phones that have many of the capabilities of computers, including Internet access, e-mail, and touchscreens; also, they are mobile, which enhances their appeal. For some adults, namely, younger, lower income, and nonwhite individuals, the smartphone is the only means of Internet access.

The terms "digital media" or "digital health interventions" are umbrella terms to capture those interventions that use technology in health promotion or health care. Many other terms have been used to describe interventions with computers or devices connected to the Internet, including "eHealth," "interactive health communication applications," "Internet interventions," and "Web-based," "technology-based," "mobile health," or "mHealth" approaches. Internet or eHealth interventions are distinct from information delivered digitally and should contain key behavioral techniques that underlie effective interventions delivered via other channels. Internet interventions are often based on evidence-based behavioral, or cognitive-behavioral, treatment approaches, are highly structured, and include important elements, such as behavioral assessment, feedback, peer support, and decision support.

The earliest evaluations of digital obesity treatments were published in the 1980s, before Internet connectivity. They used portable computer software that included self-monitoring, goal setting, prompts, feedback, and reinforcement on weight loss progress. Though these early digital treatment packages were not rich with dynamic content, images, video, or social networking, the underlying functionality of these early programs included elements that are still fundamental today.

Evidence for Digital Treatment Approaches

Most systematic reviews and meta-analyses suggest that Internet-delivered interventions are more effective than controls across a range of outcomes, including weight loss. The preponderance of evidence show that digital interventions have been superior to no-intervention and minimal-intervention control groups in producing short-term, modest weight loss. A systematic review and meta-analysis published in 2015 showed that out of 84 randomized controlled trials, over half have been published since 2010, most studies have been short interventions of less than 6 months, and most have studied weight loss as opposed to weight gain prevention or weight loss maintenance. Average weight losses are relatively small, 2–3 kg; however, effects range across the literature, with some more intensive eHealth interventions achieving average weight losses of 5–8 kg at 6 months.

When compared with state-of-the-art behavioral treatments delivered in person, technology-based treatments have been less effective in producing weight loss. Estimates vary, but the average effect across digital studies appears to be at least 2 kg less weight loss in digital versus in-person treatment. Similarly, weight loss maintenance interventions that are delivered in person or via phone have achieved better prevention of weight regain than digital interventions. In one large study of weight loss maintenance, an Internet intervention was better than a control at reducing the proportion of participants who regained weight, but only the in-person treatment substantially reduced the magnitude of weight regained.

Hybrid programs combine use of the Internet or digital tools with either in-person visits or phone calls. Fewer studies have evaluated the efficacy of hybrid programs by adding (1) in-person visits to enhance Internet programs or (2) digital tools to enhance face-to-face programs. Generally, when an Internet or digital program has been comprehensive and include online weight management counseling, studies have not shown additive benefit to additional face-to-face treatment. Similarly, phone-based counseling in conjunction with Internet tools has been similar to face-to-face treatment with Internet tools. Studies have most commonly examined whether digital self-monitoring improves the efficacy of standard behavioral in-person treatment. Results have generally been positive, suggesting the importance of feedback on self-monitoring, and that as a potential mechanism, counselors receive more detailed self-monitoring data that enhance accountability and adherence to both self-monitoring and the behaviors needed for weight loss.

Important Components of Digital Interventions

E-Counseling and Social Support

Researchers are increasingly aware of the need to identify the specific techniques, or strategies within our interventions, whether digital or otherwise, that are used to change behavior. Early digital approaches to obesity management included the core elements of face-to-face behavioral treatment and transformed them for Internet delivery. These components included education or instruction, weekly reporting of weight and other self-monitoring behaviors, guidance and recommendations for weekly goal selection, and message boards, so participants could communicate with other members of the treatment group. Several studies in the early 2000s demonstrated that self-help-oriented approaches using the Internet produced weight losses of approximately 1–3 kg. Ongoing assistance from a weight loss counselor or group leader, either through weekly e-mail or through online chat groups has reliably improved these outcomes. Weight losses of about 4–8 kg, or approximately 5–7% of initial body weight, are achievable when weekly behavioral feedback and counseling support (via e-mail or online chats) are included as components of online programs.

Identifying that weekly e-counseling contributes to program efficacy is helpful; however, this component can involve multiple self-regulatory techniques that counselors encourage to support behavior change, including prompting, providing instruction, reinforcing, shaping, goal setting, problem solving, and feedback. Identifying exactly what techniques e-counselors are using or functions they serve for behavior change might enable future digital tools to better mimic those functions without the need for, or with less, human counseling. Several studies have attempted to create "digital counselors" or provide tailored feedback that mimics the behavioral support function of the counselor. Short-term studies have shown benefits to this approach over digital self-help alone, but more evidence is needed to determine the longer-term efficacy of the approach. It will be critical to determine ways to maintain motivation and promote adherence without the accountability of the e-counseling relationship.

Researchers have been increasingly interested in popular social networking or social media approaches to promote peer support or to utilize existing platforms to provide professional weight loss support. In 2015, over 60% of American adults reported using at least one social media platform, the most popular being Facebook. Consistent with the literature on social support for weight loss in general, there have been mixed or null results when the additive effects of online social networks have been compared with basic Internet weight loss programs, and few studies have provided insights into using these tools most effectively. Given their popularity, more research is needed to determine how they can best be used to support weight loss.

Digital Self-Monitoring

Self-monitoring is recognized as one of the core elements of behavioral treatment approaches and myriad digital tools, including online databases, apps, digital photography, and wearable devices, have been developed to capture dietary intake and physical activity. Historically, self-monitoring of diet was achieved with paper diaries and printed calorie books. Participants were also encouraged to record minutes of exercise or pedometer steps to track physical activity. Widespread use of the Internet, personal digital assistants (PDAs) and now smartphones has put extensive food databases and recording of activity at users' fingertips. A handful of studies have shown that adherence to monitoring is improved with mobile devices compared with paper diaries; although, over time, monitoring rates decline, and mobile monitoring with feedback still appears most useful for weight loss.

Simple pedometers or step counters have been available for activity tracking in the United States since the mid-1960s, but they have been replaced by ever-more affordable wearable accelerometers. These wearable devices offer objective tracking of physical movement and acceleration so that time and intensity of different activities are recorded with less participant burden. These data can be integrated with online programs and apps, or reviewed by providers as part of behavioral counseling activities.

In recent years, cellular and Internet connected scales offer seamless transfer of weight data to apps, online programs, or treatment providers. Frequent or daily weighing is gaining attention as a powerful self-regulatory tool and may be particularly useful if participants are nonadherent to traditional diet-monitoring approaches. One recent study used cellular-connected smart scales to promote daily weighing, with weekly e-mailed lessons and semiautomated feedback. Adherence to daily weighing using the smart scale was high; participants in the daily weighing intervention lost 6% of their initial body weight at 6 months, significantly more than the waiting-list control group, which suggests promise for this form of self-monitoring.

Dose, Frequency, and Intensity of Contacts

The early format of online treatments for obesity were modeled after traditional face-to-face programs and adopted similar frequency of contact and duration of care. Few studies have been conducted specifically to determine the frequency of contact needed to produce adequate weight loss using digital approaches; however, like in-person treatment, studies with at least weekly contact for 4–6 months have shown better outcomes. The way people engage with mobile technologies suggests that frequent, shorter-duration intervention "touches" may be needed; however, important intervention content or components may not lend themselves to this format. More research is needed to inform recommendations in this area.

One of the as yet unmet promises of digital health is delivering help not on a predetermined schedule but "just in time," or when help or intervention is needed. Furthermore, the "just-in-time" intervention is delivered in a manner that is "adaptive" or adjusted to the progress and needs of specific participants. Thus, interventions or messages to help facilitate behavior change are delivered at the moment they might be most useful to the participant. Messages are sent in response to a set of criteria that tailor the recommendations or message based on the needs of the participant, and the phase of weight loss. These interventions can be thought of as "super" tailored and adapted to the user's progress or behaviors over frequent time intervals. Capitalizing on these techniques may allow us to deliver on the early promise that digital tools will put a therapist in everyone's back pocket.

These unprecedented capabilities may allow us to overcome one of the shortcomings of digital interventions—declining engagement over time. Little is known about the optimal engagement with digital tools. Much of the early research on engagement was limited because participants needed to self-report progress at specific intervals to drive other intervention features (e.g., weekly feedback requires user input at least weekly). We are better able to monitor data automatically from smart scales, phones, and wearables now. There are also numerous ways to "touch" participants with intervention—e-mail, text messages, websites, social media, and so forth. Participants may be best engaged if they choose how to receive an intervention, or how to report their information. More research is needed to determine the best way to consider engagement given the changing technology landscape.

Summary and Recommendations

In summary, the widespread adoption of technology and our ability to use an array of technologies, and to frequently assess adherence to the behaviors needed for weight loss, afford great opportunities for digital treatment of obesity. After 15 years of research on digital tools for obesity management, and as the field moves forward, several recommendations may be made:

1. The efficacy of comprehensive Internet-delivered approaches in the short term (< 6 months) compared to no treatment has been well established. Future studies should focus on ways to enhance weight losses achieved with digital approaches and their efficacy for weight gain prevention and weight loss maintenance.
2. Research is needed on engagement, in particular, on what level of engagement is necessary, and how best to promote engagement with digital interventions.
3. The field will advance more rapidly if we begin to identify core functions or active ingredients needed to produce weight loss, then apply the best available technology or technologies to serve those functions rather than focus on the technology itself.
4. Studies using automated messaging, and just-in-time adaptive interventions that do not rely on human-participant interactions or those that use human counselors in a stepped-care manner are needed to identify more cost-effective ways to support behavior change using digital media.

Suggested Reading

Burke, L. E., Conroy, M. B., Sereika, S. M., Elci, O. U., Styn, M. A., Acharya, S. D., et al. (2011). The effect of electronic self-monitoring on weight loss and dietary intake: A randomized behavioral weight loss trial. *Obesity, 19*(2), 338–344.—Randomized trial showing that mobile monitoring improves adherence to monitoring over paper and when combined with feedback improves weight loss.

Harvey-Berino, J., West, D., Krukowski, R., Prewitt, E., VanBiervliet, A., Ashikaga, T., et al. (2010). Internet delivered behavioral obesity treatment. *Preventive Medicine, 51*(2), 123–128.—Randomized trial comparing an Internet intervention with in-person treatment and a hybrid intervention and demonstrates the benefit of in-person treatment over Internet and hybrid conditions, but no additional benefit of hybrid over Internet.

Hutchesson, M. J., Rollo, M. E., Krukowski, R., Ells, L., Harvey, J., Morgan, P. J., et al. (2015). eHealth interventions for the prevention and treatment of overweight and obesity in adults: A systematic review with meta-analysis. *Obesity Reviews, 16*(5), 376–392.—Recent systematic review of 84 randomized trials using eHealth and mHealth approaches.

Jensen, M. D., Ryan, D. H., Apovian, C. M., Ard, J. D., Comuzzie, A. G., Donato, K. A., et al. (2014). 2013 AHA/ACC/TOS guideline for the management of overweight and obesity in adults: A report of the American College of Cardiology/American Heart Association Task Force on Practice Guidelines and the Obesity Society. *Circulation, 129*(25, Suppl. 2), S102–S138.—Provides joint task force review of the evidence for Internet delivered interventions and recommendations for its use in the treatment of obesity.

Steinberg, D. M., Tate, D. F., Bennett, G. G., Ennett, S., Samuel-Hodge, C., & Ward, D. S. (2013). The efficacy of a daily self-weighing weight loss intervention using smart scales and e-mail. *Obesity, 21*(9), 1789–1797.—Randomized trial demonstrating the efficacy and use of cellular connected scales and e-mail feedback to promote daily weighing and weight loss.

Tate, D. F., Jackvony, E. H., & Wing, R. R. (2006). A randomized trial comparing human e-mail counseling, computer-automated tailored counseling, and no counseling in an Internet weight loss program. *Archives of Internal Medicine, 166*(15), 1620–1625.—Randomized trial demonstrating that weight loss is improved with both automated feedback messages and human e-counseling at 3 months but that human e-counselors are better 6 months.

Valle, C. G., & Tate, D. F. (2014). Technology-based interventions to promote diet, exercise, and weight control. In L. A. Marsch, S. E. Lord, & J. Dallery (Eds.), *Behavioral health care and technology: Using science-based innovations to transform practice* (pp. 113–138). New York: Oxford University Press.—Provides a comprehensive review of different functions of technology for weight loss, diet, and exercise promotion.

Wing, R. R., Tate, D. F., Gorin, A. A., Raynor, H. A., & Fava, J. L. (2006). A self-regulation program for maintenance of weight loss. *New England Journal of Medicine, 355*(15), 1563–1571.—Randomized trial of weight loss maintenance shows that Internet and in-person are helpful in reducing the number of participants who regain weight, but only the in-person treatment reduces the magnitude of regain.

OBESITY PREVENTION AND POLICY

The Role of Government in Contributing to and Addressing the Obesity Epidemic

THOMAS A. FARLEY

The obesity epidemic is characterized by not only a rise in the number of people who are extremely overweight but also an increase in adiposity across the entire U.S. population. By 2010 more than two-thirds of U.S. adults were overweight or obese. This kind of population shift cannot be explained by genetic factors or a lack of individual willpower; it represents normal people living in an altered and abnormal environment. If we want to change the trajectory of the obesity epidemic, we must identify and change the features in our modern environment that are responsible.

The environment that we inhabit is not natural; it is man-made. It is shaped by the policies and actions of organizations, such as businesses, nonprofit organizations, and government. But even the actions of nongovernmental organizations take place within the framework set by government policies. For example, government has many policies on agriculture and food retailing that influence whether the food industry produces and markets healthy or unhealthy food. The question for those who wish to reverse the obesity epidemic, then, is not whether the government should have a role, but rather whether governments—at federal, state, and local levels—should update their current policies to address this new public health crisis. This chapter summarizes current government policies that influence obesity and policy changes that should be considered to address obesity at the population level.

Physical Activity

Levels of physical activity in the United States are far below those recommended for health, and lower levels of physical activity are associated with greater weight gain. Physical activity as a means of transportation (primarily walking) is influenced by whether residences are close to destinations such as retail stores and workplaces, and whether there are safe pedestrian routes to those destinations, which are determined by government

569

policies for land use and transportation. After World War II, federal, state, and local government land use policies favored segregation of residential, commercial, and industrial areas, and government transportation policies favored automobiles at the expense of public transit or pedestrians. As a result, many people now live in places where it is impractical or unsafe to walk for transportation. Physical activity for recreation or health is influenced by proximity to parks and other recreational facilities. Where local governments have not invested in parks, residents have insufficient access to facilities for recreational physical activity.

These policies can be changed. Creating "active living" neighborhoods is often dependent on changes in rules regarding land use, transportation, and recreation. Zoning should encourage high-density, mixed-use development, so that people live within walking distance of retail stores and workplaces. Transportation planning should incorporate a full range of transportation modes, including public transit, walking, and bicycling (e.g., through "complete streets" rules). Local government policies should emphasize parks and other recreational facilities that are within walking distance of residences, not only by building more parks but also by encouraging shared use of recreational facilities at schools. Cities should adopt policies facilitating transportation by bicycle, such as installing bicycle racks, requiring bicycle accommodation within buildings, and assisting bike-share programs. Cities should also write building and fire codes for multistory buildings that encourage open, prominent, accessible stairways to encourage stair use.

Food Consumption

Even more important for obesity prevention are changes in government rules to create a healthier food environment.

Food is highly regulated by all levels of government, from the farm to the grocery checkout counter. Federal agriculture policies subsidize and provide other incentives for farmers to grow commodity crops (especially corn, wheat, soybeans, and sugar). These incentives, by removing the risk of growing these commodities, encourage overproduction. By contrast, it is a risky endeavor for farmers to grow fruits and vegetables (which have lower energy densities). These policies have had a profound effect on U.S. agriculture. According to federal statistics, between 1970 and 2000, during the steepest increase in obesity rates in the United States, per-capita corn production more than doubled. In 2014, approximately 50 times as many acres in the United States were planted with corn as were planted with the top 34 vegetables combined.

Other policies come into play as food is processed and marketed. The U.S. Department of Agriculture (USDA) regulates the production of meat, not for nutritional purposes but to reduce bacterial contamination. Likewise, state and local governments, following the guidance of the U.S. Food and Drug Administration (FDA), regulate food stores and restaurants to reduce the risk of infectious diseases but not chronic diseases. The FDA also mandates the labeling of food for consumers, but the current labeling system communicates little about foods' health risks.

The federal government has several multibillion dollar nutrition programs that effectively purchase and distribute large quantities of food to tens of millions of Americans at no cost to consumers, thereby shaping the entire food market. The largest is the Supplemental Nutrition Assistance Program (SNAP, formerly Food Stamps), which currently serves approximately 1 in 7 Americans. While the National School Lunch Program and the Special Supplemental Nutrition Program for Women, Infants, and Children (known as WIC) now have meaningful nutrition standards, SNAP has no nutrition standards, which means that it distributes huge quantities of unhealthy food. Together, these agricultural and food policies and programs have created a food environment that is rich in energy-dense, highly-processed "food products" made from commodity crops. These products are largely free of bacterial pathogens, but they promote obesity and the chronic diseases that are today's leading causes of death.

An important example is sugary drinks. Since the 1970s, soft drinks have been sweetened with high-fructose corn syrup (HFCS), which became very plentiful and inexpensive because of government incentives to overproduce corn. As corn production surged, from 1980 to the 2000s, domestic production of HFCS more than quadrupled. The abundance and low cost of the sweetener gave the soft drink industry an incentive to increase the portion sizes of their beverages. With SNAP, the government pays the cost when tens of millions of consumers purchase sugary drinks. As a result of these government policies and industry actions taken in response, between 1977 and 2001, Americans more than doubled their consumption of sugary drinks.

All of these problems can be addressed by changing government food policies. To start, federal government agricultural support programs should offer incentives to farmers to grow fruits and vegetables rather than corn, wheat, sugar, and other energy-dense commodity crops. Applying policies and programs that reduce the inherent risk of farming to vegetables would increase their production and stimulate the food industry to be just as creative in marketing vegetables as they are now in marketing corn and sugar.

State and local government regulation of the food distribution system should update its century-old focus on food safety for the era of chronic diseases. These rules designate foods at risk of bacterial contamination (e.g., milk and meat) as "potentially hazardous" and limit the sales of those foods to licensed grocery stores. Today, the greatest health hazards from food are development of chronic diseases such as diabetes and heart disease, so energy-dense snack foods should be seen as hazardous and appropriate for regulation. For example, in New York City, the Board of Health used its authority over food safety in restaurants to limit the portion size of sugary drinks to 16 ounces. While courts blocked this specific action, government authority for a rule of this sort does exist. Similar rules could prohibit sales of energy-dense snack foods at retailers such as pharmacies and general merchandise stores that are not licensed for the sale of groceries. Local zoning rules could limit the number, density, or location of convenience stores that sell little besides unhealthy snack foods.

The FDA's food-labeling scheme could be vastly improved. As has been proposed elsewhere, food labels could communicate about the health risks of foods using simple "traffic light" colors on the front of packages. Alternatively or in addition, the packages could bear warnings about particularly hazardous foods, such as those delivering large quantities of sugar or salt. Labeling such as this has two potential benefits: (1) It could educate or dissuade consumers from buying the products, and (2) it might persuade food companies to reformulate their items to be less hazardous as a way of avoiding the red light or warning label requirement.

Federal food programs offer great potential for addressing the obesity problem. When these programs have incorporated nutrition standards, program beneficiaries' diets have improved. In 2009, the WIC program strengthened its nutrition requirements, which changed the foods that participating retail stores must stock. Nearly all small stores chose to meet the healthier standards rather than drop out of the program, and as stores offered healthier items, the diets of people receiving WIC improved. Nutrition standards for the National School Lunch Program, which feeds 30 million children, were strengthened with the Healthy Hunger-Free Kids Act of 2010, with minimum amounts of fruits, vegetables, and whole grains to be served at meals, and new nutrition standards for competitive snack foods sold in school snack bars and vending machines (including a prohibition on sugary drinks). In early evaluations, after the new standards were implemented, students ate healthier foods rather than throwing them out. Unfortunately, as of this writing, the companies that supply food to schools, working with some members of Congress, are pushing to weaken these standards.

The largest federal program—SNAP—offers the greatest opportunity. Three policy options to consider for SNAP are incentives for purchasing healthier items, restrictions on unhealthy items, and enhanced requirements for participating retail stores. Financial incentives for purchasing fruits and vegetables have been shown by the USDA to be effective; when they were tested in a rigorous study, families on SNAP purchased and consumed substantially more produce. These incentives could be combined with restrictions on the use of SNAP benefits to purchase items that are particularly unhealthy. Currently, beneficiaries cannot use SNAP benefits to buy tobacco products, alcoholic beverages, or prepared food (e.g., deli sandwiches). Given the strong association between consumption of sugary drinks and obesity, the USDA should add a restriction on sugary drinks from SNAP purchases. Other items to consider for restriction are grain-based desserts (e.g., cookies and snack cakes), which are energy-dense and high in sugar, refined grains, and fats.

Currently, food stores must meet modest requirements to participate in the SNAP program. Strengthening these requirements could substantially alter the food environment, especially for low-income people. For example, the USDA could specify a minimum amount of shelf space for fresh fruits and vegetables and maximum shelf space for energy-dense snack foods and beverages. Shelf space allocation has a strong influence on food purchases, so reducing the space for energy-dense snack foods would reduce sales (and consumption) of those items, and increasing the shelf space for fresh fruits and vegetables would increase sales (and consumption) of those items. Because SNAP serves such a large fraction of households in low-income neighborhoods, most stores will meet enhanced criteria rather than forego the SNAP revenue. If they did make those changes, all consumers in those neighborhoods, and not just SNAP beneficiaries, would benefit from shopping in stores displaying a healthier mix of products.

Finally, taxation is a widely used government policy that can be applied to prevent obesity. Any tax structure that raises the price of unhealthy foods or lowers the price of healthy foods will promote healthier eating. Sales taxes can be used for this; for example, in some states, food is exempt from sales taxes, but unhealthy foods are nonexempt and therefore taxable. Alternatively, excise taxes on particularly obesity-promoting items such as sugary drinks have been proposed. Early indications from Mexico, where a sugary drink tax took effect in 2014, are that it is reducing sales as expected.

Conclusion

Increasingly, obesity experts and advocates recognize the obesity crisis as originating in our everyday environment. Government officials write the rules that ultimately shape that environment. Modest changes in current government policies and programs offer many solutions to the epidemic. Those seeking solutions should use the democratic process to advocate for those changes.

Suggested Reading

Center for the Study of the Presidency and Congress. (2012). SNAP to Health: A fresh approach to improving nutrition in the Supplemental Nutrition Assistance Program. Available at *www.snaptohealth.org*.—This report from an expert group includes several recommendations for how SNAP rules could be changed to promote health.

Cohen, J. F. W., Richardson, S., Parker, E., Catalano, P. J. & Rimm, E. B. (2014). Impact of the new U.S. Department of Agriculture school meal standards on food selection, consumption, and waste. *American Journal of Preventive Medicine, 46*, 388–394.—This early evaluation of the strengthened nutrition standards in the National School Food Program shows a beneficial impact on the diets of children and refutes claims that children would refuse to eat healthier food.

Economic Research Service, U.S. Department of Agriculture. (2016). Sugar and sweeteners. Available at *www.ers.usda.gov/topics/crops/sugar-sweeteners/background.aspx#hfcs*.—This gives background and data on the production and prices of sweeteners, including sugar and HFCS.

Gleason, S., Morgan, R., Bell, L., & Pooler, J. (2011). *Impact of the revised WIC food package on small WIC vendors: Insight from a four-state evaluation*. Portland, ME: Altarum Institute.—This study demonstrates that small retailers chose to meet the strengthened nutrition standards of the WIC program rather than drop out, showing the potential for strengthened nutrition standards for SNAP.

National Agricultural Statistics Service, U.S. Department of Agriculture. (2014). Crop Production Historical Track Records, April 2014. Available at *www.nass.usda.gov/publications/todays_reports/reports/croptr14.pdf*.—This data report shows the rapid and disproportionate rise in corn production in recent decades.

Nielsen, S. J., & Popkin, B. M. (2004). Changes in beverage intake between 1977 and 2001. *American Journal of Preventive Medicine, 27*, 205–210.—This documents the large increase in consumption in sugary drinks during the period of the most rapid rise in obesity.

Sallis, J. F., Floyd, M. F., Rodríguez, D. A., & Saelens, B. E. (2012). Role of built environments in physical activity, obesity, and cardiovascular disease. *Circulation, 125*(5), 729–737.—This is a comprehensive review of the research on the relationship between features of the built environment and physical activity.

Silver, L., & Bassett, M. T. (2008). Food safety for the 21st century. *Journal of the American Medical Association, 300*(8), 957–959.—This explains the rationale for applying the concept of food safety to chronic disease prevention.

U.S. Department of Agriculture. (2014). Summary of crop commodity programs. Retrieved from *www.ers.usda.gov/agricultural-act-of-2014-highlights-and-implications/crop-commodity-programs.aspx*.—This page and the links on it include information on the various federal support programs and incentives for growth of commodity crops.

Whaley, S. E., Ritchie, L. D., Spector, P., & Gomez, J. (2012). Revised WIC food package improves diets of WIC families. *Journal of Nutrition Education and Behavior, 44*(3), 204–209.—This is an example of studies demonstrating the positive impact of strengthened nutrition standards in WIC on diet.

Closing the Energy Gap to Address Obesity

Y. CLAIRE WANG

With more than one-third of U.S. children and adolescents and over two-thirds of adults being overweight or obese, clinical and public health interventions to address obesity by focusing on promoting physical activity, healthy eating, or both, have gained traction at the local, state, and federal levels. While weight regulation and energy balance drive weight change of individuals, preventive efforts aim to address the prevailing phenomenon of caloric surplus across a large population. A major challenge for these larger-scale obesity prevention efforts targeting not a person, but a community, lies in the lack of common metrics to compare the potential effectiveness of programs to alter diet and physical activity to reduce excess energy intake.

To meet this need, the concept of a population-level "energy gap" and its applications in far-reaching prevention efforts uses the mean daily caloric surplus (energy in minus energy out) over a long period of time as a way to (1) gauge the scale of the excess calories underlying the historic shift in the body mass index (BMI) distribution; (2) set population-level goals for action in order to close the energy gap; and (3) compare the potential impact of interventions with varied population reach, intensity, and behavioral targets. These applications are described below.

Historic data since the 1970s indicate that U.S. adults put on an average of 2 extra pounds a year, a net result of consuming readily available, energy-dense foods and beverages, while expending fewer calories. It is more complex in children, for whom weight (and height) gain are part of normal growth. Accounting for normal weight gain during child growth, in 2006, Wang and colleagues estimated that U.S. children on average gained an excess of 1 pound/year over the period of 1988–1994 and 1999–2002 (a period with minimal changes in average height among U.S. youth). This translated to 110–165 kcal/day of a positive energy gap, depending on assumed activity levels. When only considering children at baseline who became overweight adolescents, the average energy imbalance was estimated to be 600–1,100 kcal/day over the 10- year period, fueling an excess weight gain of 26.5 ± 9.7 kg, substantially larger than the population average (4.3 kg). Several other researchers have also attempted to quantify the energy gap during a specific time period, with similar assumptions on the efficiency of converting energy to weight gain.

These estimates corrected the "small energy gap" views proposed in earlier studies (see Figure 93.1), but have been shown to remain a slight underestimate. Updated analyses have applied more sophisticated models to account for changes in body composition in both adults and children, suggesting that the energy gap responsible for the rise in U.S. obesity since the late 1970s was more in the range of 200–300 kcal/day. In 2011, Hall and colleagues estimated that the energy gap accounting for the mean BMI shift between 1978 and 2005 was approximately 220 kcal/day. It is similar in order of magnitude when compared to the reported increase in per-capita energy intake in the United States over that period (190 kcal/day), suggesting that high caloric intake may have played a larger role in energy imbalance than did low physical activity. Further addressing changes in body composition and assuming more realistic energy-conversion efficiency during healthy growth among children and youth, Hall and colleagues estimated that the energy gap between 1976–980 and 2003–2006 periods is in the range of 210 kcal/day in boys and 190 kcal/day in girls.

Setting Population Goals for Prevention

The energy gap calculations from the works by Hall and colleagues (2012) and Wang and colleagues shed light on the difference in caloric balance at the present time and before the rise of the obesity epidemic. The Hall and colleagues findings suggest that reducing energy intake in a cohort of children by around 200 kcal on average would return the mean body weight to levels characteristic of the late 1970s. These estimates provide a framework to translate population-level obesity reduction goals, such as those of the U.S. Healthy People objectives.

Healthy People 2020 set the goal of reducing the prevalence of obesity by 10% from 2005–2008 levels among children and youth ages 2–19 years—to bring overall prevalence down to 14.6% by 2020. The energy gap that must be closed in order to achieve this goal was estimated to be approximately 64 kcal/day, using 2007–2008 population data as the baseline. The energy gap targets are greater for adolescents, and there is a substantial variability by race/ethnicity because non-Hispanic black and Mexican American youth are farther from achieving Healthy People goals than are non-Hispanic whites. Among adolescents ages 12–19 years, reaching the Healthy People 2020 goal would require narrowing their current energy gap by an estimated 64 kcal/day (non-Hispanic white), 230

FIGURE 93.1. Converting calories to pounds: The erroneous 3,500-kcal Rule.

It is worth noting that assumptions applied in estimating the energy gap matters a great deal. In early studies, researchers were misguided by the applying a simple rule of thumb for converting weight change to calories: 3,500 calories equals 1 pound of body weight gained. Using this assumption, researchers concluded that the obesity epidemic was caused by a small energy imbalance—about 30 calories a day on average, a miniscule estimate that led to an overoptimistic view that small changes (e.g., taking fewer bites of food) are all that is needed to reverse obesity. Such calculation is misleading because, for an individual to continue to gain weight, it requires an energy gap large enough to not only deposit fat mass but also to overcome the additional energy expenditure from a higher body weight, as well as a compensatory metabolic slowdown.

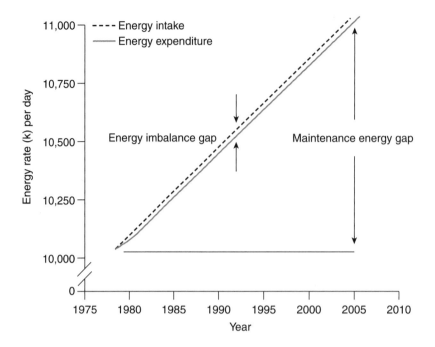

FIGURE 93.2. The energy gap underlying the observed increase in average body weight of a popula-tion has two main components: A smaller, energy imbalance gap is the small difference between energy intake (top line) and expenditure rates (bottom line) on the daily basis, while the mainte-nance energy gap is the change of energy intake required to maintain the final body weight com-pared with the initial weight. From Hall et al. (2011). Copyright © 2011 Elsevier Ltd. Adapted by permission.

kcal/day (non-Hispanic black), and 123 kcal/day (Mexican American), respectively. By building links between prevalence-based goals (e.g., 10% less obesity) and energy gap goals, community- and policy-based efforts are one step closer to gauging the degree of intensity required to meet their goals.

The Impact of Interventions on Closing the Energy Gap to Address Obesity

How can the energy gap framework inform efforts to tip the energy balance in the right direction? By calculating the net, average impact on energy balance of a policy or inter-vention, stakeholders can deploy this common metric as a springboard for prioritizing and comparing the wide range of possible interventions. The average caloric impact (ACI) measure can summarize a program's impact on the population's energy balance by esti-mating the difference it would make on calories consumed or calories expended for an average individual on a daily basis. In order for an intervention to have a large impact on obesity at the population level, it has to have a wide reach, long enough duration, good intensity (e.g., the vigor of physical activity), and strong evidence of effectiveness.

As an example, an intervention to cut television viewing time in children reduced energy intake by nearly 106 kcal/day. Imposing a competitive food standard in California middle schools was associated with 78 kcal/day ACI. In comparison, adding 10 minutes of physical education a day, while certainly helpful, would only impact children during the ~180 days of school in a year. For middle school students, this translates to an average of 14 kcal/day impact on energy balance. To sufficiently address energy imbalance across communities with varied demographic composition and sociocultural backdrops, comprehensive, multicomponent approaches to foster a supportive environment and to engage, enable, and empower people to adopt healthy eating and active living norms will be necessary.

Implications for Prevention

Use of the energy gap provides an analytic framework to inform clinical societies and public health agencies in setting realistic expectations and establishing science-based guidelines to guide obesity prevention efforts. In addition, insight from existing estimates also underlines the importance of early prevention because the energy gap becomes bigger and harder to close as individuals accumulate more excess weight over time, and after the weight-gaining pattern has been established for many years. Closing the energy gap and reversing the childhood and adult obesity epidemic, especially for individuals who are already overweight or for those with the highest risk of becoming overweight, will require more than a single intervention. Far greater caloric deficits will be required to return obese individuals to a healthy weight than those required to reverse the average weight gained by the population.

Suggested Reading

Butte, N. F., Christiansen, E., & Sørensen, T. I. (2007). Energy imbalance underlying the development of childhood obesity. *Obesity, 15*(12), 3056–3066.—This study was among the first to use empirical data to quantify the total energy cost of weight gain and increase in energy intake and/or decrease in physical activity associated with weight gain in children and adolescents. The results indicated that halting obesity by counteracting the energy surplus requires a sizable decrease in intake or increase in activity, which rebutted the notion of "small changes."

Hall, K. D., Butte, N. F., Swinburn, B. A., & Chow, C. C. (2013). Dynamics of childhood growth and obesity: Development and validation of a quantitative mathematical model. *Lancet Diabetes and Endocrinology, 1*(2), 97–105.—This study quantified the relationship between excess weight gain and energy balance during childhood growth, by developing a mathematical model calibrated to body composition data in children. This model also provided the most up-to-date energy gap estimates for U.S. children and youth.

Hall, K. D., Sacks, G., Chandramohan, D., Chow, C. C., Wang, Y. C., Gortmaker, S. L., et al. (2011). Quantification of the effect of energy imbalance on bodyweight. *Lancet, 378*, 826–837.—This study provides a quantification of the relationship between changes in energy intake, body weight, and energy expenditure in adults, and includes an interactive, Web-based tool that allows the user to simulate how diet and physical activity changes impact body weight and composition over time. Available at *http://bwsimulator.niddk.nih.gov.*

Hill, J. O., Wyatt, H. R., Reed, G. W., & Peters, J. C. (2003). Obesity and the environment: Where do we go from here?. *Science, 299*, 853–855.—This widely cited study popularized the idea that a "small changes" approach is sufficient to close the energy gap and reverse the obesity epidemic, based on the 3,500 kcal/lb rule. The underestimation was later acknowledged by the authors in subsequent studies, though they also stressed the role of small behavioral changes, such as walking, in weight gain prevention.

Swinburn, B. A., Sacks, G., Lo, S. K., Westerterp, K. R., Rush, E. C., Rosenbaum, M., et al. (2009). Estimating the changes in energy flux that characterize the rise in obesity prevalence. *American Journal of Clinical Nutrition, 89*(6), 1723–1728.—This study developed an equation relating energy flux (total energy intake and total energy expenditure at steady state) to body weight in adults associated with the obesity epidemic. The authors characterized the small "energy imbalance gap" in the context of daily life and the larger energy flux associated with higher body weight that accumulates over time.

Wang, Y. C., Gortmaker, S. L., Sobol, A. M., & Kuntz, K. M. (2006). Estimating the energy gap among US children: A counterfactual approach. *Pediatrics, 118*(6), e1721–e1733.—This study was among the first to quantify the magnitude of energy imbalance underlying the shift in body size among U.S. children and adolescents, accounting for normal weight gain during growth.

Wang, Y. C., Orleans, C. T., & Gortmaker, S. L. (2012). Reaching the healthy people goals for reducing childhood obesity: Closing the energy gap. *American Journal of Preventive Medicine, 42*(5), 437–444.—This study quantified how much the energy gap needs to close in order to reach the childhood obesity target of 10% lower than 2005–2008 levels at the population level. These estimates were then benchmarked with key energy balance behaviors to inform preventive efforts.

Global Efforts to Address Obesity

CORINNA HAWKES

This chapter focuses on efforts around the world to prevent obesity through population-based policies to improve food environments and, therefore, diets. These policies are recommended in strategies and action plans of the World Health Organization (WHO) and regional and national strategies. They take the form of laws, mandatory regulations, official guidelines for voluntary adoption, or structured incentives to encourage actions by other stakeholders. They are typically developed and implemented at not only the national level but also at regional and local levels.

Actions Around the World

In 2004, the Member States of the WHO adopted a Global Strategy on Diet, Physical Activity and Health. The strategy emphasized population-based approaches to making "healthier choices the easier choices." This population-based approach was reaffirmed in the United Nations Political Declaration on the Prevention and Control of Noncommunicable Diseases (NCDs) in 2011. The WHO's Global Action Plan for the Prevention and Control of NCDs 2013–2020 then adopted a clear list of population-based recommendations to address unhealthy diets. These actions are also highlighted in WHO regional plans for the Americas and Europe.

Coincident with the development of global recommendations, countries around the world stepped up their actions to improve food environments. Table 94.1 lists the core set of obesity-focused food policy actions taken since 2004 and exemplifies the different actions countries have taken. As shown, policy actions take many different forms. For example, countries in Latin America, Central America, and Europe mandate nutrient labels on all packaged foods with limited exceptions, while nutrient lists must be provided only on select categories of packaged foods in Malaysia. Countries have taken different approaches to front-of-pack labels. Australia has voluntary guidelines for a "Health Star Rating," while Ecuador is the only country to date to have mandated that all packaged foods carry a "traffic light" label. An increasing number of countries in Europe, Latin America, and the Middle East have developed mandatory standards on foods served in schools. For example, in Costa Rica, an Executive Decree permits schools to sell only foods and drinks that meet specific nutritional criteria; in France, regulations also cover the diversity and composition of meals, water provision, and portion size, while South Korea also restricts certain foods from being provided within a 200-meter radius of schools. In Europe, fruit and vegetable schemes have become part of the school landscape in large part as a result of the European Union School Fruit Scheme, which provides financing to distribute fruits and vegetables to children ages 6–10 years in schools and requires "accompanying measures" such as educational programs.

One of the most significant steps countries—notably middle-income countries—have taken is health-related food taxes. In Mexico, for example, an excise duty of 1 peso ($0.80) per liter is applied on sugary drinks and an ad valorem excise duty of 8% applies to foods with high caloric density. In Hungary a "public health tax," adopted in 2012, is applied on the salt, sugar, and caffeine content of various categories of ready-to-eat foods, including soft drinks (both sugar-sweetened and artificially sweetened) and energy drinks. Countries do not, however, appear to have implemented subsidies for healthier foods; even targeted programs that subsidize healthy food for vulnerable groups appear to be rare.

Despite the adoption of the WHO Set of Recommendations on the Marketing of Food and Nonalcoholic Beverages to Children in 2010, a very small number of countries restrict advertising to children. All of the restrictions take different forms, and none is comprehensive. Although Ireland, Mexico, South Korea, and the United Kingdom all restrict TV advertising of high-fat, sugary, and salty foods, children are still exposed to advertising on family programming and other communications channels. Select channels and products have been targeted by specific countries: Mexico's regulation includes restrictions in cinema; South Korea includes one aspect of Internet advertising; and Iran focuses on soft drinks.

A considerable number of countries have engaged with industry to improve the nutrient quality of the whole food supply. However, these focus on trans fats and salt rather than more obesity-related factors, such as calories, sugars, or portion size. Two exceptions are the French Charter of Engagement with the food industry and the U.K. Responsibility Deal, which both involve efforts to reduce sugar and calories. Several Pacific Island countries, which rely heavily on imports for their food supply, have changed import tariffs in order to increase availability of fruits, vegetables, and fish, and to reduce the supply of sugary foods.

Policy actions at the level of retailing have been notably fewer, with the United States leading the way with the Healthy Food Financing Initiative to incentivize stores to locate in underserved areas. A small number of countries have taken actions to increase the availability of healthier foods in specific outlets. In Singapore, a government program provides incentives for the widely and commonly patronized street food vendors to serve healthier ingredients and foods such as fiber-enriched noodles, low-fat milk, and and drinks with lower sugar content. In Brazil, the Market Modernization Program engages fruit and vegetable supply centers to increase the availability and promotion of fruits and vegetables. A small number of local areas have imposed planning restrictions on fast-food outlets in the United Kingdom and the United States.

TABLE 94.1. Examples of Implemented Policy Actions Around the World to Improve Food Environments (2004–2015)

Example of specific policy actions	Example of countries with implemented action[a]
Setting nutrition label standards and regulations on the use of claims and implied claims on foods	
Mandatory nutrient list on all packaged foods	China, Central American countries, EU-28, Israel, MERCOSUR countries, United States
Mandatory nutrient list on select categories of packaged foods (e.g., breads, soft drinks)	Malaysia
Mandatory front-of-pack labeling	Ecuador, Thailand (snack foods only)
Government-approved voluntary front-of-pack labeling	Australia, England, Singapore
Mandatory calorie labeling on menus	Some Australian states, Canadian provinces, and U.S. states
No health claims on "unhealthy" foods	Australia, New Zealand
Offering healthy foods and setting standards in public institutions and other specific settings	
Mandatory standards for foods available in schools	Bermuda, Brazil, Chile, Costa Rica, Fiji, Finland, France, Hungary, Jordan, Kuwait, Lithuania, Mauritius, Mexico, Slovenia, United Kingdom, Uruguay, United States
Mandatory standards for foods in and around schools	South Korea
Ban on vending machines in educational institutions	France
Fruit and vegetable initiatives in schools	Some Canadian provinces, EU-28, Norway, United States
Using economic tools to address food affordability and purchase	
Health-related taxes on specified foods	Berkeley (California, United States), France, Hungary, Mexico, Samoa
Targeted subsidies for healthy foods for vulnerable groups	United Kingdom, United States
Restricting food advertising and other forms of commercial promotion	
Mandatory restrictions of TV advertising to children of foods high in fat, sugar, and salt	Ireland, Mexico, South Korea, United Kingdom
Mandatory restrictions on select films advertising in cinemas	Mexico
Mandatory restrictions on the use of specific marketing techniques for foods high in fat, sugar, and salt	South Korea (Internet advertising with incentives to purchase); Ireland (use of celebrities); United Kingdom (product placement and sponsorship of TV programs)
Mandatory restriction of broadcast advertising of soft drinks	Iran
Mandatory health message on advertisements	France

(continued)

TABLE 94.1. *(continued)*

Improving the quality of the food supply[b]	
Government–industry initiatives with voluntary commitments by food industry to reduce calories sugars, portion size	England, France
Import tariffs to enhance healthiness of the food supply	Pacific Island countries (e.g., Cook Islands, Fiji, French Polynesia, Nauru, Samoa, Tonga)

Setting incentives and rules to create a healthy retail	
Incentives for stores to locate in underserved neighborhoods	United States
Initiatives to increase the availability of healthier foods/reduce the availability of unhealthy foods in select food outlets	Brazil, France, Singapore, United Kingdom
Planning restrictions on food outlets	United Kingdom, United States

Note. Data from *www.wcrf.org/nourishing.* Only implemented policies are included; excludes policies in place in the past but since repealed.

[a]For a full list of countries, *see www.wcrf.org/nourishing.*

[b]Excludes policies on salt and trans fats.

The Need for Further Progress

Though there has been significant progress, there remains a long way to go to increase the global coverage of food policy actions to improve food environments. As already indicated, there has been very little progress in key policy areas, such as restrictions on marketing to children. There are also notably fewer actions in lower-income countries, with implementation of actions declining directly with national income level. A review of 180 implemented actions found that 68% were from high-income countries, 27% were from upper-middle-income countries, 5% from lower-middle-income countries, and none were from low-income countries.

Another key issue is lack of implementation. A review of national strategy documents between 2004 and 2013 revealed a plethora of planned policy actions in low- and middle-income countries to address the intake of fat, fruits, and vegetables—including legislation on marketing, school food, labeling, and the location of fast food outlets—but with little evidence of implementation.

There are also numerous examples of failures to pass laws in the first place. New York City's failure on portion size restrictions for soda presents one much-reported example. Globally, it is most evident in the case of commercial food promotion to children; proposed laws have failed to pass in at least 12 countries. Similar to other policy areas, this reflects fierce lobbying. The result has been either no action or weaker actions. For example, in France, the mandating of health-oriented messages on advertising (Table 94.1) reflected a weakening of a proposed ban on unhealthy food advertising. In place of legislation, governments have looked to the private sector for voluntary action. For example, internationally, there are now more industry-led "pledges" on food advertising to children than government regulations. These approaches neither adopt stringent criteria nor take a comprehensive approach.

Another quality issue is that countries have taken actions in the field of behavior change communication (e.g., education, public awareness), without accompanying actions to improve food environments. In China, for example, there is a relatively extensive range of educational campaigns and programs in different settings, but the only implemented action on the food environment is the requirement to list nutrients on food packages (Table 94.1).

Another gap is the lack of a truly comprehensive, intersectoral approach. Numerous countries have developed comprehensive, multisectoral plans—such as the Brazilian *Intersectoral Strategy for Obesity Prevention and Control* (2014–present), the *Healthy Weight, Healthy Lives* childhood obesity strategy in England (2008–2011), the Israeli *National Program to Promote Activity, Healthy Lifestyle* (2011/2012–present), and the *National Agreement for Nutritional Health: A Strategy Against Overweight and Obesity* in Mexico (2010–2014). Yet truly systemic implementation of this "in all policies" type of approach at the national level appears to be very limited, with France appearing to have taken the most comprehensive approach to date. In practice, the local level has proved a more fertile ground for testing out more comprehensive approaches. New York City is often cited as having undertaken the most comprehensive regulatory approach to improve the healthiness of food environments. Another example is *Healthy Together Victoria*, a policy in Australia that took an explicit "systems" approach to the prevention of ill health, including obesity.

Moving Forward

Furthering the progress of global efforts to address obesity by improving food environments will take new alliances demanding change. Policy actions to improve food environments have much in common all around the world. Yet a voice for a global, civil society to push for the greater adoption of actions to address obesity has yet to emerge. Funding is also needed to create capacity in countries to develop and implement actions, and enable them to evaluate the actions they have taken. Such research will help the United States and countries around the world to understand better what works and how to design more effective actions to prevent unhealthy diets and obesity.

Suggested Reading

Hawkes, C., Jewell, J., & Allen, K. (2013). A food policy package for healthy diets and the prevention of obesity and diet-related non-communicable diseases: The NOURISHING framework. *Obesity Reviews, 14*(S2), 159–168.—This article explains the rationale for the World Cancer Research Fund International NOURISHING Framework, which is the source of the material in Table 94.1.

Hawkes, C., & Sassi, F. (2015). Improving the quality of nutrition. In D. McDaid, F. Sassi, & S. Merkur (Eds.), *Promoting health, preventing disease: The economic case.* Copenhagen: WHO.—This book chapter sets out the evidence for the main policy actions taken around the world, including the evidence on cost-effectiveness.

Hawkes, C., Smith, T. G., Jewell, J., Wardle, J., Hammond, R. A., Friel, S., et al. (2015). Smart food policies for obesity prevention. *Lancet, 385,* 2410–2421.—This article sets out how food policy actions to address obesity could be more effectively designed.

Lachat, C., Otchere, S., Roberfroid, D., Abdulai, A., Seret, F. M. A., Milesevic, J., et al. (2013).

Diet and physical activity for the prevention of noncommunicable diseases in low- and middle-income countries: A systematic policy review. *PLoS Medicine, 10*(6), e1001465.—This article provides an overview of strategies in low- and middle-income countries to promote fruit and vegetable consumption and reduce saturated fat and salt intake.

Roberto, C. A., Swinburn, B., Hawkes, C., Huang, T. T., Costa, S. A., Ashe, M., et al. (2015). Patchy progress on obesity prevention: Emerging examples, entrenched barriers, and new thinking. *Lancet, 385,* 2400–2409.—This article summarizes the state of play of national actions on obesity around the world and provides insights into the barriers facing implementation.

WCRF International. (2014). *Food policy highlights from around the world.* London: WCRF International.—This brief from the nongovernmental organization World Cancer Research Fund International highlights national examples of policy actions that have been implemented around the world and show particular promise.

World Health Organization. (2012). *Assessing national capacity for the prevention and control of noncommunicable diseases: Report of the 2010 global survey.* Geneva: Author.—This report provides an overview of the capacity countries have to implement policies to promote healthy eating.

World Health Organization. (2013). *Global nutrition policy review.* Geneva: Author.—This document presents the results of a survey of policies taken by WHO member states to address obesity and other forms of malnutrition.

Are National Food Policies Helping or Hurting Obesity Prevention?

MARION NESTLE

Health advocates increasingly recognize that national food policies are essential for reversing current trends in obesity prevalence. In 2000, Michael Jacobson and I argued in *Public Health Reports* that then-current recommendations for preventing obesity invariably focused on the need for educating individuals to decrease energy intake and increase energy expenditure but failed to consider the many factors in society and in the food environment that acted as barriers to individual actions. Those factors included, and still include, cultural, social, and economic aspects of current food systems that make high-calorie, inexpensive food available for consumption everywhere, at all times of day, and in very large portions.

We noted that although the deleterious health effects of obesity had been observed since the mid-1950s, national action plans to reverse its increasing prevalence had consisted mostly of wishful thinking and admonitions to individuals rather than well-thought-out public health strategies to promote more healthful dietary choices. Our article suggested a broad range of policies in education, food labeling, food marketing, health care, and transportation to make it easier for individuals to eat more healthfully and to be more active. To pay for such policies, we suggested small taxes on food items that provide "empty" calories, such as soft drinks, or on products that reduce physical activity, such as automobiles.

Even so, we were not the first to invoke the need for policy approaches aimed at obesity prevention, as well as educational strategies aimed at individuals. In the late 1970s, Albert J. Stunkard made similar suggestions, but these were ignored in favor of views of obesity and its health consequences as matters of personal responsibility. But the sharp increase in obesity prevalence in the years just prior to 2000 was enough to convince us and others that attempts to change individual behavior were ineffective; furthermore, they could only be effective if accompanied by supportive changes in the food environment.

585

Benefits of Obesity Prevention Policies

As the high personal and economic cost of obesity to individuals and to society became more evident, health advocates increasingly called on governments to enact policies to improve the environment of food choice. By now, local and state governments, and even the federal government, have enacted one or more of a broad range of policies aimed at preventing obesity in children and adults, especially those of low income, or at restricting the production or marketing practices of food companies. Table 95.1 lists examples of policies that have been tried, implemented, or are under serious consideration by advocates.

Several observations argue in favor of policy approaches. Educating individuals is demonstrably ineffective. Policies that have been implemented tend to show benefits. And the degree of food industry opposition to anti-obesity measures strongly suggests that these measures are likely to work. The evidence in favor of policy interventions is substantial. Studies show that teaching children about healthy eating improves their attitude toward eating healthier foods, especially when accompanied by garden programs. Children in schools serving healthier meals tend to have healthier weights. Removing

TABLE 95.1. Policy Interventions to Reduce the Prevalence of Obesity

Children

- School gardens
- Nutrition education
- Nutrition standards for school and child care meals
- Elimination of sodas from fast-food meals
- Restrictions on toys with fast-food meals
- Restrictions on television advertising of unhealthful foods
- Restrictions on junk food sales near schools
- Nutrition standards for food marketing

Adults

- Community garden projects
- Fruit and vegetable incentive programs
- Nutrition education
- Calorie labels on fast-food items ("menu" labels)
- Restrictions on misleading health claims
- Nutrition standards for federal food assistance programs
- Warning labels on unhealthful foods

Food companies

- Incentives for healthier food retail environments
- Nutrition standards for foods served in public institutions
- Nutrition standards for product reformulation
- Size caps on unhealthful foods
- Taxes on unhealthful foods
- Elimination of tax deduction for business expenses related to marketing unhealthful foods to children

The political system

- Incentives for corporate social goals, as well as growth
- Restrictions on corporate contributions to election campaigns (repeal *Citizens United*)

toys from fast-food meals decreases children's desire for those meals. The less time children spend watching television, the less likely they are to be overweight. Supporting the purchase of fruits and vegetables in low-income communities increases the supply and purchase of those foods.

Although most studies of calorie labels on fast-food meals show small, if any, effects on purchase patterns, the effects are greater among the subset of customers who pay attention to the postings. Like trans-fat labeling, menu labeling has induced food manufacturers to reformulate their products with healthier ingredients. The most impressive evidence of policy efficacy derives from studies of taxes on sugar-sweetened beverages. In its first 6 months, the Mexican tax was associated with a 6% reduction in soda sales. In its first month, the Berkeley, California, tax decreased sales while generating more than $100,000 to be used for child health programs. A more recent analysis documented a 21% decrease in soda consumption in Berkeley's low-income communities. Taxes do modify dietary choices and their benefits are even greater in low-income groups most at risk for chronic disease.

Food Industry Opposition

Preventing obesity requires people to eat less, move more, or both, but eating less reduces food industry profits. Thus, no anti-obesity measure that might decrease purchases of foods and beverages should be expected to be free of political opposition. Indeed, the greater the likelihood that an intervention will succeed in reducing purchases, the more strongly the food industry is likely to oppose it. Within each of its sections, Table 95.1 lists policies roughly in order of political expediency. Although on principle they oppose every measure that might reduce sales, companies making food products targeted by "eat less" messages are especially vigorous in doing everything they can to delay, weaken, or eliminate measures that might restrict their ability to market to children, cap portion sizes, or tax their products.

Marketing to children is the food industry's line in the sand. Although major food and beverage companies have voluntarily agreed not to advertise unhealthful products to children under the age of 12, they forcefully oppose government attempts to set nutrition standards for marketing food products to children, even when such standards are voluntary. When an Interagency Working Group (IWG) representing four government agencies attempted to set voluntary standards for food marketing to children, food trade associations complained to Congress. In response, Congress required the IWG to conduct a cost–benefit analysis, thereby killing this *voluntary* measure.

Food companies opposing the U.S. Department of Agriculture (USDA) school nutrition standards also used Congress to get what they wanted. The potato and pizza industries, for example, were affected by the new standards. They induced Congress to use the appropriations process to overturn two regulations, one restricting the number of times potatoes could be served in school lunches during a week and the other affecting the volume of tomato paste used on pizza.

In 2015, the food industry succeeded in getting Congress to use the appropriations process again, this time to delay implementation of menu labeling in chain restaurants for a year. The industry also induced Congress to use the appropriations process to block the USDA from allowing federal dietary guidelines to say anything about the environmental impact and unsustainability of diets high in meat.

Drawing on lessons learned from the tobacco industry, beverage companies use every trick in that industry's "playbook" to oppose nutrition standards for food assistance programs, warning labels, size caps, and taxes. The playbook involves casting doubt on the science, discrediting critics, framing government interventions as indications of nanny-statism, coopting community and health professional groups, and, of course, lobbying and contributing to election campaigns; these last playbook items were made easier by recent Supreme Court decisions. Use of the playbook was especially visible in New York City's attempt to remove sodas from eligibility for purchase with benefits from the Supplemental Nutrition Assistance Program (SNAP, formerly Food Stamps). Antihunger organizations funded by soda companies publicly opposed the city's attempt, even though the prevalence of obesity is higher among SNAP recipients than in other low-income groups. To oppose the city's proposed soda cap rule, which would restrict the size of sugary drinks sold in places under city jurisdiction to 16 ounces or less, soda companies and their trade association funded "front" groups and community organizations to oppose the measure, took the city to court, and eventually won. The soda industry has contributed tens of millions of dollars to front groups to fight soda taxes, successfully, with two exceptions to date: Berkeley, California, which framed the debate as "Berkeley vs. Big Soda," and Philadelphia, which framed the tax as a method to generate revenues to support prekindergarten programs.

Future Directions for Policy Advocacy

Although it is well established that to be effective, policies must lead to environmental changes that support healthier food choices, not one of the policies listed in Table 95.1 can reverse obesity prevalence on its own. All of them are needed to support a vision of obesity not so much as a matter of personal responsibility but as a personal consequence of a food system focused far more on selling products than on promoting nutrition and public health. Because the purpose of food companies is to sell products and generate profits for stockholders, changing this environment comes up against corporate business imperatives and is only possible through government intervention. In this situation, governments need to establish a level playing field for food industry marketing, so that restrictions apply equally to all companies. A key part of a vision for obesity prevention is to align agricultural policies with health policies, so that the kinds of foods that receive subsidies, for example, are those that best promote health. The goal of all policy interventions must be to make the healthful choice the easy choice and, even better, to make it the *preferred* choice.

How do we get from here to there in the current political climate? Despite the need for substantive improvements in the food environment, existing obesity prevention policies tend to be fragmented, uncoordinated, and lacking in overall vision. This is understandable given the level of food industry opposition to any measure that might reduce demand, decrease availability, or increase prices. Therefore, changing the food environment requires an understanding that obesity prevention is both a political and a health goal. Health advocates must engage the political system and use it to promote health for individuals and for society.

Engagement means learning how the political system works: how bills are passed, how elections are funded, and how lobbying is accomplished. It means visiting local, state, and federal representatives and talking to them about how healthier food environments will benefit constituents and society. It means educating and organizing communities to support public health interventions, recruiting allies, and developing evidence-based arguments to counter those of critics. It means writing opinion pieces and letters to editors as well as editorials in professional journals. For many health professionals, political engagement seems remote from the day-to-day demands of helping overweight patients deal with our current, toxic food environment.

But detoxifying this environment can only be accomplished by advocates willing to take on the challenges of reducing the impact of money on politics. The goal must be to elect political representatives who are more responsive to concerns about the health of the citizens they represent than to the food corporations that, as part of the normal course of doing business, put profits over public health.

Suggested Reading

Center for Science in the Public Interest. (2015). *Congressional catering: How big food and agricultural special interests wield influence in Congress and undermine public health.* Washington, DC: Center for Science in the Public Interest.—Analyzes food industry lobbying methods and expenditures to oppose dietary guidelines, school nutrition standards, restrictions on trans fat, and sodium reduction.

Falbe, J., Thompson H. R., Becker, C. M., Rojas, N., McCulloch, C. E., & Madsen, K. A. (2016). Impact of the Berkeley excise tax on sugar-sweetened beverage consumption. *American Journal of Public Health* [Epub ahead of print].—Pre- and posttax surveys document a 21% decline in soda consumption in Berkeley's low-income communities as compared to a 4% increase in neighboring cities without soda taxes.

Gortmaker, S. L., Long, M. W., Resch, S. C., Ward, Z. J., Cradock, A. L., Barrett, J. L., et al. (2015). Cost effectiveness of childhood obesity interventions: Evidence and methods for CHOICES. *American Journal of Preventive Medicine, 49*(1), 102–111.—Demonstrates substantial cost savings from excise taxes on sugar-sweetened beverages, elimination of tax subsidies on television advertising to children, educational initiatives, and efforts to promote physical activity.

Hawkes, C., Smith, T. G., Jewell, J, Wardle, J., Hammond, R. A., Friel, S., et al. (2015). Smart food policies for obesity prevention. *Lancet, 385,* 2410–2421.—Describes the principal components of policies effective in improving the food environment and choices of individuals.

Huang, T. T.-K., Cawley, J. H., Ashe, M., Costa, S. A., Frerichs, L. M., Zwicker, L., et al. (2015). Mobilisation of public support for policy actions to prevent obesity. *Lancet, 385,* 2422–2431.—Focuses on the need to mobilize popular support for obesity prevention policies; calls on the public health community to make community engagement a priority.

Mozaffarian, D., Afshin, A., Benowitz, N. L., Bittner, V., Daniels, S. R., Franch, H. A., et al. (2012). Population approaches to improve diet, physical activity, and smoking habits a scientific statement from the American Heart Association. *Circulation, 126*(12), 1514–1563.—Describes policies that have achieved some success in promoting healthier weights.

Nestle, M. (2015). *Soda politics: Taking on big soda (and winning).* New York: Oxford University Press.—Documents the methods used by health advocates in the United States and internationally to reduce consumption of sugar-sweetened beverages and to counter the marketing practices of companies that make them.

Nestle, M., & Jacobson, M. F. (2000). Halting the obesity epidemic: A public health policy approach. *Public Health Reports, 115,* 12–24.—Reviews history and suggests broad range of policy approaches to obesity prevention.

Roberto, C. A., Swinburn, B., Hawkes, C., Huang, T. T.-K., Costa, S. A., Ashe, M., et al. (2015). Patchy progress on obesity prevention: Emerging examples, entrenched barriers, and new thinking. *Lancet, 385,* 2400–2409.—Suggests the need for policies to address and counter environmental influences on the food choices of individuals.

Stunkard, A. J. (1980). The social environment and the control of obesity. In A. J. Stunkard (Ed.), *Obesity* (pp. 438–462). Philadelphia: Saunders.—Early in the rise in prevalence of obesity, Stunkard recognized the critical need for policy interventions to improve the environment of food choice.

Thow, A. M., Downs, S., & Jan, S. (2014). A systematic review of the effectiveness of food taxes and subsidies to improve diets: Understanding the recent evidence. *Nutrition Reviews, 72*(9), 551–565.—Reviews 43 studies; concludes that tax strategies are effective in reducing intake of targeted products over a broad range of rates.

The Role of Advocacy in Preventing Obesity

ROBERTA R. FRIEDMAN

Since the publication of the previous edition of this book, the nation has made significant progress in passing obesity prevention policies at the national, state, and local levels. Victories include improved nutrition standards for federally funded nutrition programs such as the National School Lunch Program and the Women, Infants, and Children (WIC) program, state "complete streets" legislation to improve access and safety for bicyclists and pedestrians on roadways, local procurement policies prohibiting the use of government funds to purchase foods and beverages of minimal nutritional value, and a penny-per-ounce tax on sugary drinks in Berkeley, California, to name a few. These hard-won successes are the products of advocacy by community groups, nonprofit organizations, and medical and public health professionals, among others. But the defeats suffered by obesity prevention advocates—failing to pass legislation or to shepherd strong standards through the regulatory process—were the result of successful advocacy as well, by those who prefer to maintain the status quo for financial, political, or other reasons.

No matter what the outcome, public policy is always influenced by advocacy. The country's continued high rates of overweight, obesity, and related chronic diseases, and the power of those who would stymie progress, necessitate continued advocacy, including advocacy by those reading this book, the professionals from the public health, medical, mental health, and other fields. This chapter defines advocacy's role in obesity prevention and describes how individuals, including professionals, can make crucial contributions to the process.

Advocacy Defined

Advocacy is the act of publicly supporting or recommending a cause or proposal, in order to influence legislative or regulatory decisions concerning it. Obesity prevention advocacy, then, is the act of publicly supporting recommendations that have the potential to reduce and/or prevent obesity. This discussion focuses on governmental advocacy, but advocacy can also occur in nongovernmental spheres, to encourage the implementation of health-promoting policies in corporate, nonprofit, and other work settings. The ultimate goal is the adoption of policy that improves access to good nutrition and physical activity opportunities, but there are intermediate goals as well. These can include capacity-building shifts in the public's and decision makers' awareness of, and attitudes toward, an issue and its severity; the building of public and political will to support appropriate solutions; the creation or strengthening of ad hoc or long-term alliances focused on solutions and composed of individuals, community groups, opinion leaders, and decision makers; and the implementation, enforcement, and evaluation of policy. No matter what the goal, advocacy is a dynamic process involving short- and long-term strategies, wins and losses, and shifting contexts, "players," and objectives.

Many people assume that advocacy always involves lobbying, which they cannot or do not want to do, but lobbying is just one of many tools available to advocates. Advocacy involves a variety of other activities. Many of them can fit into a busy professional's work life and advance, rather than conflict with, the principles to which health care and public health professionals are committed.

The Advocate's Role

Successful advocacy involves persuading decision makers and other interested people of the urgency of the problem and the benefits of the proposed solutions, using science and data; appealing to the emotions of the decision makers to reinforce the need for change, using stories and anecdotes; and engaging in discussion and negotiation to find a mutually agreed-upon solution. Anyone who has a personal or professional interest in, or knowledge about, an issue can play a role in advocacy. Advocacy works best when a diverse group of interested parties (often including unlikely allies) forms a coalition to influence decisions about policymaking. Members bring to the coalition their diverse knowledge of, perspectives on, and experiences with the issue, so that, collectively, the group gains the deepest understanding of the issue and is then best equipped to present it to decision makers.

Coalitions should include those people who have a personal interest in obesity prevention, such as parents, youth, and grassroots groups that are disparately affected by obesity and its related chronic illnesses. It is important that decision makers hear their personal stories about the psychological, physical, and economic toll that obesity and related diseases take. Coalitions should also include professionals, such as public health and medical experts; social scientists; lawyers; economists; community organizers; advocates for youth, poor people, and people of color; and teachers, among others. Their role is to complement the personal stories with the objective knowledge and information gained through experience in the field.

Another role for advocates is to counterbalance the influence of the food and beverage industries, which have regularly opposed campaigns to pass commonsense obesity prevention policies that could affect their bottom line, or have attempted to reverse advocacy victories already in place. These industries use their considerable resources to persuade the public and decision makers that they are part of the solution to obesity, not the problem, and that legislation or regulation is not necessary. For example, in their well-funded response to current state and local public health campaigns to reduce consumption of sugar-sweetened beverages (through warning label measures, taxes, procurement policies, etc.), industry lobbyists claim to offer reliable, practical, and scientific knowledge and information about the effect of these beverages on health, and assert the key role of physical inactivity in high obesity rates. Experienced professionals, such as the readers of this volume, have the credibility, as well as the knowledge, to ensure that the public and decision makers do not simply take industry arguments at face value.

Key Elements of Policy

The most effective obesity prevention policies will contain these key elements: optimal defaults to change environments, a focus on health equity, solutions based on science, and an evaluation component. Advocates should work to incorporate as many of these as possible into their proposed solutions.

Changing the Default in Environments

Effective obesity prevention policies make our "environments"—the places in which we live, work, and play—more healthful. We make many decisions every day about diet and exercise. These decisions may be large, small, intentional or unintentional, but they are almost always influenced by what is most readily available, by default, in our environment. Advocates should promote policies that change environments by creating optimal defaults, which make it easier for individuals to make healthful choices. Examples include making water or low-fat milk (rather than soda) the beverage offered by default in a fast-food kid's meal, making it easier to feed children more healthfully, or mandating the inclusion of bike lanes and sidewalks when building new roadways, making it easier for people to exercise.

Health Equity

Disparities in rates of obesity and related diseases in people of color and in low-income groups are well documented, and of great concern. There is a long-overdue and growing call to focus on how health equity is addressed in health policy. Equity is achieved when those groups that, historically, have been disadvantaged are given the means to achieve their highest level of health. Obesity prevention policy must take into account disparate access to the solutions proposed. For example, legislation to improve the safety and accessibility of parks must take into account that parks in high-income neighborhoods may require a smaller allocation in order to improve safety than do parks in low-income neighborhoods. Advocates should discuss the proposed solutions with those who will be affected by their implementation, to gauge the impact. Together, they can analyze proposed legislation for both intended and unintended consequences, using a health equity lens, and suggest language that ensures that the populations most affected will be given special consideration.

Science-Based Solutions

The solutions proposed to prevent obesity should be evidence-based ones. Health care and public health professionals can play a critical role here, by providing decision makers with the science that documents the problem, supports the proposed solutions, and analyzes the intended and unintended consequences.

Evaluation

Advocates should reinforce the need for evaluation provisions in legislative language, to advance the understanding of what does and does not work in obesity prevention. Outcomes will have an impact on future obesity prevention proposals.

Steps and Activities

Campaigns to pass obesity prevention legislation often follow the basic steps outlined below, many of which offer opportunities for busy professionals to contribute to the advocacy process at different times.

Advocacy usually begins with *defining the problem* and *determining a set of solutions*. This includes conducting literature searches for reviews of research to gather data on the scope of the problem; its causes; the populations affected; and the social and economic impacts, including health care costs, evaluations of experiments or interventions, and other information that supports solutions. Health care and public health professionals can help write this information in accessible forms (e.g., policy briefs and fact sheets) for the public and decision makers, who may not have the skills to translate the science or the time to read about the issue in depth.

Forming a coalition, or joining an existing one, as noted earlier, is another important step in advocacy. Professionals can work with a coalition in a variety of large and small roles: Serve as the groups' issue experts and consultants, help write campaign strategy, translate the science, or simply add their signatures to a coalition letter in support of legislation.

With materials in hand, advocates can begin to *educate the public and decision makers* about the problem's severity, costs, and potential solutions. This is called "ground softening," and it is an important precursor to introducing legislation. Decision makers and the public may be more likely to support legislation if they understand the problem and its potential solutions.

When the coalition members are in agreement about the policy solutions to advocate, they must *identify the key decision makers* to target. Who has the power to make the desired change? At the state or federal level, the most important targets are usually the Speaker of the House, the Senate president, and the chairs of the committees that will hold hearings on bills. Professionals who have already established relationships with legislators can use their connections to introduce the issue and discuss possible solutions. Activities include researching the targets to find out (among many other things) whether health and public health in general have been among their interests or whether obesity prevention in particular has been a goal for them.

It is critical to every advocacy campaign to *understand the opposition*. Rarely does a proposed obesity solution go unopposed. The more novel (and perhaps the more potentially effective) the proposal, the more opposition there will be. Advocates can prepare for it by learning as much as possible about who the opposition is, who funds them, what tactics they use to influence key decision makers, and what their main arguments are. Advocates can then prepare counterarguments for use in the media, by legislative sponsors, in hearings, and for informational materials. If the coalition has the resources, *public polling* to gauge the public's support for a proposal can be extremely useful in understanding how it might be received by both the public and decision makers.

Devising a strategy to *work with the media* is an essential step in advocacy, to gain the support of the public and key decision makers. There are many ways for advocates to engage the media, involving varying levels of commitment. They include conducting radio or TV interviews; pitching a news story to a local, state, or national newspaper; writing an opinion editorial or letter to the editor; or meeting with members of a newspaper's editorial board to convince them to publicly support a proposal. Using social media such as Facebook, Twitter, or YouTube, and blogging are increasingly effective ways to reach and educate or influence the public and decision makers.

When the goal is passage of legislation, *lobbying* is always a step in the process. There are two types of lobbying: direct and grassroots. *Direct lobbying* involves communicating with a legislator in order to influence his or her vote on specific legislation. *Grassroots lobbying* involves contacting voters about specific legislation, and includes a "call to action," in which voters are asked to contact their own legislators in order to influence their vote on a bill. Advocates can call, write to, or meet with legislators to talk about the merits of the bill and why it should be passed, submit written and/or oral testimony before committees, or write a call to action to grassroots constituents, asking them to urge their legislators to vote for legislation.

Summary

Advocacy is essential for obesity prevention. Victories are achievable, but only if advocates from a wide variety of backgrounds contribute their skills, knowledge, and stories. A health care or public health professional can choose where, when, and how often to participate in the process, by translating research for, and educating decision makers and the public, and using his or her credibility to influence the adoption of policies that will be effective in preventing obesity.

Suggested Reading

Brownell, K. D., & Warner, K. E. (2009). The perils of ignoring history: Big Tobacco played dirty and millions died. How similar is Big Food? *Milbank Quarterly, 87,* 259–294.—Compares and contrasts the script used by the tobacco industry to fight government antitobacco action, to the one used by the food industry to influence public opinion, legislation and regulation, litigation, and the conduct of science.

Brownson, R. C., Fielding, J. E., & Maylahn, C. M. (2009). Evidence-based public health: A fundamental concept for public health practice. *Annual Review of Public Health, 30,* 175–201.—A discussion of the concept of evidence-based public health and its benefits, which includes a higher likelihood of successful policies being implemented.

Dodson, E. A., Fleming, C., Boehmer, T. K., Haire-Joshu, D., Luke, D. A., & Brownson, R. C. (2009). Preventing childhood obesity through state policy: Qualitative assessment of enablers and barriers. *Journal of Public Health Policy, 30,* S161–S176.—Interviews with legislators and staffers reveal the factors that positively influence the passage of childhood obesity prevention legislation, and the barriers, giving advocates valuable insights when considering state-level policy.

Farrer, L., Marinetti, C., Cavaco, Y. K., & Costongs, C. (2015). Advocacy for health equity: A synthesis review. *Milbank Quarterly, 93,* 392–437.—A synthesis of the evidence in the literature on advocacy for health equity, which provides a body of knowledge to inform practice.

Friedman, R. R., & Schwartz, M. B. (2008). Public policy to prevent childhood obesity, and the role of pediatric endocrinologists. *Journal of Pediatric Endocrinology and Metabolism, 21,* 717–725.—An overview of types of proposed public policy to overcome childhood obesity and a discussion of the professional's role in advocacy.

Goldstein, H. (2009). Commentary: Translating research into public policy. *Journal of Public Health Policy, 30,* S16–S20.—Describes four steps using research in the policy development process, and highlights ways researchers and advocates can work together to achieve policy objectives.

Huang, T. T., Cawley, J. H., Ashe, M., Costa, S. A., Frerichs, L. M., Zwicker, L., et al. (2015). Mobilisation of public support for policy actions to prevent obesity. *Lancet, 385,* 2422–2431.—Discusses strategies to build popular demand for obesity prevention policies, and the contributions a diverse coalition can make.

Lesser, L. I., Ebbeling, C. B., Goozner, M., Wypij, D., & Ludwig, D. S. (2007). Relationship between funding source and conclusion among nutrition-related scientific articles. *PLoS Medicine, 4* (1), e5.—An examination of industry funding of nutrition-related scientific articles and possible bias of conclusions in favor of sponsors' products.

Radnitz, C., Loeb, K. L., DiMatteo, J., Keller, K. L., Zucker, N., & Schwartz, M. B. (2013). Optimal defaults in the prevention of pediatric obesity: From platform to practice. *Journal of Food and Nutritional Disorders, 2,* 1–8.—A discussion of the concept of optimal defaults and its application to pediatric obesity prevention in several domains.

Strategies for Creating Obesity Policy Change

MARGO G. WOOTAN

The food environment in the United States makes it difficult for Americans to eat well and maintain a healthy weight. Though not impossible, all too often, healthy eating is like swimming upstream.

People's food choices are affected by what food is available, its price, how it is packaged, portion sizes, convenience, its attractiveness and presentation, information and claims, marketing, and politics. For example, food availability affects how often and what people eat. In the present time, food is everywhere; it is in vending machines, at gas stations, ball games, shopping malls, bus stations, airports, highway rest stops, and schools. Even buying printer cartridges at an electronics store or towels at a home goods store involves exposure to candy promotions.

Companies know that just seeing that food makes people feel hungry. Often, people purchase food when they are not physiologically hungry and are not thinking of a snack before getting to checkout.

Portion sizes are often large, and studies show that people eat more food when they are served more. What restaurants serve or the package size of a snack helps set the context for what people think is a reasonable amount to eat, and that regularly results in eating too much.

Soda and other sugary drinks have gone from being an occasional treat to the standard beverage offering. Sugary drinks are the single biggest source of calories for U.S. adults and children; people get more calories from soft drinks than from bread, hamburgers, french fries, or other foods. Also, sugary soft drinks are the only individual food that is directly linked to obesity.

Furthermore, people are bombarded with messages to eat. Unfortunately, most of those messages come from the food industry, not health professionals. The United States underfunds public health at the national, state, and local levels. Meanwhile, the food industry spends $33 billion a year to promote mostly fatty, salty, sugary, high-calorie, low-nutrition foods.

Individuals are, of course, ultimately responsible for what they eat, and parents are responsible for what they feed their children. But although obesity rates have increased over the last 30 years in both adults and children, there is no evidence to show that over this same time period willpower has declined or that parents love their children any less.

During the recent recession, many people recognized that their financial situation was not solely their own doing; clearly, the economy (e.g., availability of jobs, cost of housing) and federal and state policy (e.g., taxes, credits) shape people's financial situations. Like the economy affects our personal finances, so too does the food environment in which we live, work, and shop affect the foods we buy and eat.

Most Americans want to eat well—not all, but the majority—and people are not actively choosing to be overweight. Yet two-thirds of U.S. adults are either overweight or obese. In fact, Americans spend more than $60 billion a year for weight-loss products, programs, and gym memberships, and 84% report actively trying to maintain or lose weight.

To achieve a healthy weight and consistently eat well, Americans need a food environment that supports their efforts. They not only need help from health professionals, but also support from workplaces, schools, food companies, restaurants, and policymakers. But to transform our obesogenic food system into one that supports healthy eating and healthy weights will require advocacy, not only by organizations but also by health professionals, researchers, parents, and other concerned citizens.

The number of national organizations that work on nutrition has grown over the last decade. Still, many organizations that work on nutrition cannot afford a lobbyist (public health groups are often underfunded); they cover a large number of issues of which nutrition is only a small part; or they have lobbying restrictions due to their nonprofit status or because their funding comes from foundations that cannot support lobbying activities.

Even if there were a stronger nutrition lobby in Washington, D.C., and every state capitol, we would still need the involvement of individuals to succeed. Constituents are influential. Most Congressional and state legislative offices are responsive to constituents—after all, "constituent" is another term for voter. It cannot be overstated how much individuals can make a difference to the success of nutrition policy outcomes.

Advocacy is a core public health function, and individuals cannot count on someone else to do it. For those who are new to advocacy, it may seem a bit daunting—speaking up and using strategies that are unfamiliar. This chapter reviews some of the basics of advocacy and describes how even people who are busy with their "real job" can get involved and help support nutrition and obesity prevention policies.

Who Are the Targets of Nutrition and Health Advocacy?

Advocacy can take place at the federal, state, or local level. Though some say all politics is local, nutrition policy is important at all levels, as is nutrition advocacy. Overall, no one level of government or policy is more important than the other for supporting healthy eating and healthy weights. Which level of policy or environmental change to focus on depends on what issue is of greatest interest and where an individual feels the greatest influence is possible. For example, a person interested in reducing unhealthy food marketing on television or urging major companies to reformulate their products might choose a national focus. A father may choose to work on healthier school lunches in his child's local school or school district, or an employee might choose to advocate for healthier food and beverage options in her own worksite cafeteria.

Advocates often try to persuade government officials, who are therefore the targets of their advocacy efforts. Legislative targets include the U.S. Congress, state legislatures, city councils, and county commissions—both the elected officials themselves, and just as importantly, their staff members. Congressional staff members and those in state legislatures are decision makers. Legislative staff members write legislation, budgets, and appropriations bills, and shepherd bills through the legislative process.

Federal, state, and local government agencies implement nutrition and obesity policies, including departments of health, agriculture, education, transportation, human services, parks and recreation, and others. In some cases, these same agencies may have the authority to develop nutrition policies themselves, independent of the legislature under their existing authority. People who work for executive branch agencies may work on nutrition policy through not only their own agency but also cross-agency work or advocacy. For example, health department officials work on healthy school foods with the Department of Education or collaborate with the corrections department to improve the nutritional quality of food in prisons.

Advocating for positive changes in food and nutrition policy should not just include government officials; advocacy efforts should also focus on organizations; institutions; and food, beverage, entertainment, or other companies. Examples include:

- Urging a worksite to change the pricing in its cafeteria to increase the costs of the unhealthy options and use those funds to subsidize vegetables and other healthy foods (e.g., price the french fries four times higher than the side vegetable).
- Working with the PTA to urge a local school to use only healthy fund-raisers (those that do not involve food or include only healthy food).
- Urging the state chapter of the American Heart Association or American Cancer Society to work on a specific policy.
- Encouraging local restaurants to offer fruit and vegetables instead of french fries and to supply low-fat milk or water instead of soda with kids' meals.
- Asking local retailers to stop marketing candy and soda at checkout and instead offer nonfood merchandise or healthy options, such as fruit, nuts, and water.

Tools of the Trade

A decade ago, advocates focused their energy on educating decision makers about the importance of nutrition and physical activity. However these days, most policymakers and the public recognize the seriousness of poor nutrition and obesity. Obesity is front-page news, and many policymakers are interested in addressing it. Nevertheless, there is still the need to convey to legislators and other policymakers the major impact that poor diet and inactivity have on health and health care costs. In all advocacy efforts, it is important to identify key messages needed to cultivate interest in and support for a policy.

Influencing nutrition and obesity policy can occur through approaches people associate with advocacy, such as calling, writing, or tweeting at an elected official; organizing health professionals, colleagues, parents, or concerned citizens to write letters, e-mails, or sign petitions (anyone can set up a petition via websites such as Care2 or *Change. org*); meeting with policymakers; testifying at hearings or listening sessions; or writing comments on regulations. Advocacy also occurs informally, for example, by urging a business or university official to adopt a healthy meeting policy; forwarding to fellow members of a professional society a model letter addressed to a state legislator; speaking to a colleague in a sister agency about a policy idea; or conducting a study that lays the groundwork for a policy change.

Some people may feel unsure about how to advocate or lobby. Few health professionals or researchers are trained in advocacy and public policy. However, health professionals and researchers should not worry that they do not know all the ins and outs of legislative or regulatory processes. Legislative staff members or agency representatives are expert in doing this. Legislative staff members often cover a wide range of issues and are unlikely to have as much expertise in nutrition or public health as researchers or health professionals. Policymakers are the process experts; health professionals and researchers can be the content expert. Expertise as a health professional, educator, or researcher will be appreciated and respected.

The basic *tools* for advocacy are familiar—letters, e-mails, phone calls, meetings, and social media. E-mails or phone calls from health professionals or citizens, either in an official capacity or as private citizens, are valuable. Another key tool in advocacy is meeting with policymakers or their staff members.

When a local, state, or national organization works on a policy, it can be influential. Still, hearing a similar message from a constituent can reinforce the message and increase the chance of gaining the legislator's support. Many organizations try to make it easy for individuals to engage in advocacy by providing model e-mails, model talking points for phone calls and meetings, and model social media posts, and other background documents to their members or followers. Finding an organization whose policy priorities you support can be a time-efficient and effective way to support local, state, or national policy. Groups such as the Center for Science in the Public Interest keep people updated on nutrition policies, provide contact information for key officials, and model messages that can be adapted and shared with policy makers through e-mails, phone calls, meetings, or tweeting (see *cspinet.org/actnow*). Taking action through such networks has a strong track record of successfully influencing policy, for example, helping to strengthen school nutrition standards, ensuring that chain supermarkets and convenience stores provide calorie information for their prepared foods, and pressuring food companies to reduce marketing of candy and other junk food to children.

Advocacy versus Lobbying

The types of advocacy and approaches a person uses may vary depending on his or her employer. For government employees, how much and the types of advocacy in which they can engage differs from state to state and depend on the views of each governor, state, or county health officer, or other supervisor. Within the same state or locality, staff members' ability to advocate changes as administrations change, depending on the governor, state health officer, or department chair's interpretation of the law, personality, and willingness to push the envelope. One state health official relayed that he liked to push right up against the line between advocacy and lobbying and peer over it. If he did not get his hand slapped from time to time, he felt he was not being a strong enough advocate. Others are more conservative in their approach.

The ability to act as an advocate might also depend on an individual's position within an organization, as well as the organization's official position, if any, on the policy. For example, once a state health department has a position in support of more funding for Centers for Disease Control and Prevention (CDC) chronic disease programs, department of health staff members might be able to advocate for the program.

In general, state and local government employees are allowed to contact elected officials in their capacity as private citizens; the right to free speech is protected by the Constitution. However, a person should conduct such independent actions outside of work time, using a personal e-mail account or phone. In some organizations, people can do education and advocacy, but cannot lobby. One rule of thumb is that advocacy becomes lobbying when action is requested on a specific bill or legislative matter. It is important for individuals to check with their own agency/institution policy for guidance to make clear what is permissible, and, if necessary, to push for greater ability to advocate.

One way to address barriers to acting as an advocate is to work with others in coalition, with each coalition member fulfilling roles that he or she is skilled at and able to do. Organizations come together in local, state, and national coalitions to share information, combine resources, and enhance their effectiveness. Each organization in a coalition can participate in ways allowed by their institution, bringing different skills, resources, and grassroots constituencies in support of policies and food system changes. If, for example, a person is restricted from lobbying in his or her job, it might still be possible to educate elected officials and to provide information about diet-related diseases in the state but leave it to other coalition partners to follow up with details about a specific bill.

The National Alliance for Nutrition and Activity (NANA; *nanacoalition.org*) is the largest nutrition and obesity prevention coalition in the country, with more than 500 local, state, and national member organizations. Together, NANA members have worked together to successfully increase by 20-fold funding for the CDC's nutrition, physical activity, and obesity division; pass a national law to get soda, candy, and other unhealthy snacks and drinks out of vending machines, school stores, à la carte in cafeterias, and in-school fund-raisers; improve school lunches; and pass a national law to ensure labeling of caloric content of items on menus in chain restaurants.

Conclusions

The basic skills of advocacy are ones that many health professionals already have. Much of it is education, but instead of counseling a patient or teaching a student, an individual might talk to a local school board member, a colleague in the state agriculture department, or a state legislative staffer. As in consumer education, how the case is made for a policy depends on who the audience is.

Advocacy can be easier if done with partners. Finding an organization that has common interests can help guide individuals through the process, provide materials, and support efforts. The engagement of many more health professionals, researchers, and other concerned citizens is essential to enact the nutrition policies and food system changes that will make it possible for more Americans to eat well, be active, and maintain a healthy weight.

Suggested Reading

Cohen, D. A., & Babey, S. H. (2012). Contextual influences on eating behaviors: Heuristic processing and dietary choices. *Obesity Reviews, 13,* 766–779.—This review examines how automatic responses to contextual food cues, such as portions, packaging, and food availability, encourage overeating and poor nutrition.

International Food Information Council (IFIC) Foundation. (2015). Food and health survey. Retrieved June 1, 2015, from *www.foodinsight.org/sites/default/files/2015%20food%20 and%20health%20survey-%20executive%20summary%20-%20final.pdf.*—This annual survey assesses food and nutrition beliefs and behaviors in the United States.

Malik, V. S., Schulze, M. B., & Hu, F. B. (2006). Intake of sugar-sweetened beverages and weight gain: A systematic review. *American Journal of Clinical Nutrition, 84,* 274–288.—This review of epidemiological and experimental evidence found that greater consumption of sugar-sweetened beverages is associated with weight gain and obesity.

Ogden, C. L., Carroll, M. D., Kit, B. K., & Flegal, K. M. (2014). Prevalence of childhood and adult obesity in the United States, 2011–2012. *Journal of the American Medical Association, 311,* 806–814.—This study provides national estimates of childhood and adult obesity rates and how they have changed over time.

U.S. Department of Agriculture. (2013). Food dollar series: Documentation. Washington, DC: Author. Retrieved from *www.ers.usda.gov/data-products/food-dollar-series/documentation.aspx#.U0RLIqhdU3l.*—The USDA's food dollar series measures annual domestic food expenditures and describes the percentage of those expenditures paid to farmers for product versus the amount that goes toward processing, packaging, transportation, retail, food service, energy, advertising, and other costs.

U.S. Department of Agriculture, U.S. Department of Health and Human Services. (2010). *Dietary guidelines for Americans 2010.* Washington, DC: U.S. Government Printing Office.—These guidelines provide authoritative advice about healthy eating and maintaining a healthy weight, and serve as the basis for federal nutrition advice, policy, and programs.

Young, L., & Nestle, M. (2002). The contribution of expanding portion sizes to the U.S. obesity epidemic. *American Journal of Public Health, 92,* 246–249.—This study found that food portions' increasing size parallels individuals' increasing body weights.

Legal Approaches to Addressing Obesity

JENNIFER L. POMERANZ

Government Authorities and Limitations

The law is a powerful tool to address obesity. The U.S. Constitution grants the federal government specific enumerated powers and reserves the remaining authorities for states. Local governments are a creation of the states and can only act to the extent permitted by the state. Federal authorities have the power to regulate interstate commerce, tax, spend, and disseminate information. States have the concurrent powers to tax, spend, and inform; however, states, and to the extent permitted, locales, also have a unique ability to address public health, safety, and welfare through what is known as "police power." Classic examples of states' use of police power include sanitation and restaurant inspection laws, but states can use this power to address the obesogenic food environment.

The Constitution also sets limits on the ability of government to act. In the realm of public health, there is sometimes tension between government and private interests. Private rights are protected by the first 10 amendments to the Constitution, the Bill of Rights. The First Amendment's protection of speech has become highly relevant to obesity prevention and control strategies because food companies argue that any restriction on their ability to market goods to consumers violates their right to free speech. The U.S. Supreme Court has held that the First Amendment does protect advertising and labeling, called "commercial speech," from unwarranted government interference. This protection hinders the government's ability to restrict unhealthy food and beverage (collectively, food) communications.

Another constitutional barrier to the passage of effective laws aimed at preventing obesity stems from the legal concept of preemption. The Supremacy Clause of the Constitution declares that federal law is the supreme law of the land; this enables the federal government to preempt, or trump, state and local law. States have a similar ability to preempt local action. For example, after the Metropolitan Board of Health of Nashville and Davidson County, Tennessee, passed the first menu labeling law in the South, the state legislature preempted local boards of health from enacting such regulations. This nullified the previously passed law and preempted all other boards of health in Tennessee from enacting menu labeling requirements.

There are several evidence-based strategies that support the government's role in enacting laws to address obesity. These include increased information on food labels, reducing unhealthy food marketing, improving the school food environment, increasing the price of unhealthy food, and increasing access to healthy food. The legal approaches to address these policies are discussed below, along with expectations for future directions.

Food Labels

The U.S. Food and Drug Administration (FDA) is the federal agency responsible for overseeing and enforcing the labeling requirements for the vast majority of food products and for the calorie labels on covered vending machines and restaurant menus. Although the First Amendment protects commercial actors' right to communicate with potential consumers, the Supreme Court confirmed that this does not translate into a right to sell products without providing consumers truthful information about one's goods. Thus, the government may legally require that companies disclose factual information about the products available for sale in the marketplace. This authorization underlies many labeling requirements such as the Nutrition Facts Panel (NFP), ingredient lists, and the disclosure of common allergens.

The FDA is also responsible for regulating health and nutrition claims permitted on food packaging. When a company makes false or deceptive claims, or claims that do not abide by FDA regulations, the agency sends a Warning Letter to the business, noting its violations and seeking correction. These letters may not lead to specific or global changes, so aggrieved consumers and consumer advocacy groups pursue litigation against food companies in an effort to address questionable claims. These lawsuits have had mixed success in court, but some led manufacturers to make fewer controversial claims, such as the claim "natural," for instance, on food of questionable naturalness.

Although information alone rarely changes behavior, increased labeling requirements provide consumers with information they need to make informed decisions and may lead to food industry reformulation. For example, after the FDA required food manufacturers to disclose *trans fat* on the NFP due to its association with heart disease, food companies reformulated products to reduce or eliminate the ingredient. In 2014, the FDA proposed regulations to update the NFP with an added sugar disclosure, among other changes. It is likely that food companies may similarly reformulate products when final regulations become effective. In the future, the FDA may increase added sugar labeling requirements due to the ingredient's link with poor nutrition; for example, it might limit the ability of manufacturers to make health or nutrition claims on highly sugared products.

Food Marketing

Evidence indicates that food marketing impacts the food preferences of people of all ages. There is widespread interest in addressing food marketing that is especially directed at children; however, legally, this is a challenging topic to address. As mentioned, the First

Amendment protects commercial actors from government interference with their right to advertise their products, including to children. However, false, deceptive, and misleading commercial speech is not protected by the First Amendment, so government may regulate these communications. The Federal Trade Commission (FTC) is the federal agency responsible for truthful advertising in all venues except product packaging (regulated by the FDA), and it brings individual cases against food marketers for false, deceptive, and misleading communications. The FTC may also bring a case when it deems an advertisement to be "unfair," for example, if it encourages unsafe behaviors. However, this authority has not translated into a comprehensive legal mechanism to address unhealthy food marketing. Rather, the government relies on the food industry to self-regulate due to First Amendment barriers.

It is noteworthy that even when the government seeks to protect children in the context of products that they cannot legally purchase, such as tobacco, the Supreme Court has struck down restrictions that interfere with the right of adults to access such speech. But when a product is illegal for a child to purchase, restrictions in child-oriented spaces, such as playgrounds, are easier to pass and more likely to be upheld by courts.

One exception to this line of commercial speech jurisprudence is that the government can limit speech in schools. The Supreme Court recognizes that schools are dedicated to an education mission in which children are a captive audience and courts therefore defer to school officials to determine which speech is appropriate for students. The First Amendment analysis is therefore different because schools are considered a nonpublic forums so officials may limit marketing on school property by enacting what are called "viewpoint-neutral" guidelines. This means that officials cannot choose among viewpoints within a subject area, but they can ban all food marketing altogether or prohibit the marketing of foods not permitted to be sold on school grounds. In fact, the U.S. Department of Agriculture (USDA) proposed a rule that would require education agencies to include in their wellness policies a plan that limits permissible marketing to only those foods that may be sold under the Smart Snacks rule (or more restrictive standards). Therefore, the imposition of stronger nutrition requirements for school foods can support stricter food marketing prohibitions.

As an important aside, Congress passed the Healthy, Hunger-Free Kids Act in 2010 to improve the quality of school food. This is an evidenced-based strategy to address poor nutrition in children, especially those from low-income families, who rely on school meals. The federal government provides funding to states conditioned on the schools abiding by federal nutrition guidelines. The law is straightforward that government can regulate school food programs in this manner.

Food Taxes

Although the federal and state governments share the power to tax, states are the primary taxing authority over food through sales tax provisions. Approximately a dozen states tax all food at general sales tax rates; many more states tax specific food products usually deemed non-necessities. Sales taxes have not been shown to decrease consumption, nor is that their intent. Excise taxes, on the other hand, are assessed at the producer or distributor level and have proven to decrease the purchase of taxed products such as cigarettes.

Excise taxes result in an increase in the base price of the product, and the revenue stream can be earmarked, or dedicated, to a specific purpose. Public health experts support imposing an excise tax on sugary beverages to address obesity and diabetes, with the revenue stream dedicated to other public health programs. Berkeley, California, was the first jurisdiction to successfully implement a sizable excise tax on sugary beverages for the purpose of reducing consumption. Not all local jurisdictions have the authority to enact taxes, which is a legal barrier for those locations. State legislators nationwide have proposed sugary beverage excise tax bills; politics and industry opposition are the primary barriers to the imposition of these laws. It is likely that a state will pass such a tax in the future, which may lead to increased acceptance of this policy nationally.

Police Power

The police power affords state governments the discretion to determine the method to regulate unhealthy practices to protect public health. Public health laws are generally legally valid if they have a rational basis, which means that they are not unreasonable, arbitrary, or capricious, and do not violate the Constitution. States can use this power to address the modern food environment through various strategies, ranging from well-established mechanisms, such as zoning and licensing, to more innovative legal solutions to obesity, such as a sugary beverage serving size restriction.

Zoning ordinances are generally used to regulate land use and the built environment, whereas licensing is a method to regulate persons, and existing and new business operations. States generally delegate these powers to local governments, which can use them to improve access to healthier food or discourage access to unhealthy food. For example, local governments have used their zoning authority to establish quotas on the number of fast-food outlets permitted in a district, regulate outlet density in the community, and restrict their distance from other uses, such as schools. Zoning can also be used to attract full-service supermarkets and farmers' markets to locate within an area specifically zoned for such uses.

The government can also require a business to obtain a license in order to operate, and it may place specific conditions on the license to ensure compliance with government prerogatives. For example, Minneapolis, Minnesota, has a conditional licensing program that only grants licenses to grocery stores that sell healthy food on a continuous basis. Conditional licensing has been recognized as an effective public health tool in the context of tobacco control, but it is less common in food retail. However, this may change in the future as the benefits of government control and the flexibility to change the terms of the license are realized by more government entities seeking to shape the food environment.

Preemption

State and local governments have been the primary innovators of unique legal solutions to address obesity and improve the food supply. Local governments were the first to enact menu labeling laws, ban trans fat in restaurant food, pass ordinances regarding toys in fast-food meals, and try to restrict the sale of large servings of sugary beverages. The food industry lobbies against such measures; part of its strategy is to pursue preemptive legislation withdrawing the ability of local governments to act on an issue. Sometimes preemption can be practical. For example, Congress preempted states from enacting certain food-labeling requirements that differ from those of the FDA. Other times, legislators pursue preemption to concentrate power at the higher level of government or to support business interests instead of public health. For instance, at the urging of the Mississippi Hospitality and Restaurant Association, the state passed a law preempting all local governments from passing laws like those mentioned earlier. In order to avoid limiting local self-determination, states could alternatively enact minimum standards upon which locales can build.

Future Action and Conclusion

Legislators and health departments have attempted policy changes that have been successful in some cases and unsuccessful in others; these will likely resurface again on the policy agenda. For example, federal, state, and local legislators have unsuccessfully urged the USDA to pilot a program to test food-purchasing limitations for the Supplemental Nutrition Assistance Program (SNAP), which is the nation's largest food assistance program. Policymakers have proposed that sugary beverages should be removed from the definition of eligible food under SNAP. Although the USDA has rejected all such proposals, there is broad public support and increasing momentum for such a change.

The most promising government policies to address obesity stem from a convergence of valid legal authorities, strong leaders, and evidence-based strategies. However, due to the pressing nature of obesity, legal approaches must sometimes be attempted in the face of uncertainty. Gaining public support is important, especially for innovative legal solutions, so effective advocacy campaigns are crucial. There is a need for strong leaders who are willing to pursue public health interests despite opposition, in order to address obesity and the obesogenic food environment successfully.

Suggested Reading

Dietz, W. H., Benken, D. E., & Hunter, A. S. (2009). Public health law and the prevention and control of obesity. *Milbank Quarterly, 87*(1), 215–227.—Reviews the National Summit on Legal Preparedness for Obesity Prevention and Control convened by the CDC in 2008, and discusses the use of a systematic legal framework—the use of legislation, regulation, and policy—to address the multiple factors that contribute to obesogenic environments.

Gostin, L. O. (2007). Law as a tool to facilitate healthier lifestyles and prevent obesity. *Journal of the American Medical Association, 297*(1), 87–90.—Discusses how law can be used as a tool to prevent overweight and obesity.

Gostin, L. O., Pomeranz, J. L., Jacobson, P. D., & Gottfried, R. N. (2009). Assessing laws and legal authorities for obesity prevention and control. *Journal of Law, Medicine and Ethics, 37*(Suppl. 1), 28–36.—Highlights the progressive use of laws at every level of government and the interaction of these laws as they relate to obesity prevention and control. The discussion considers the status of legal interventions in three domains—Healthy Lifestyles, Healthy Places, and Healthy Societies—and identifies gaps in the use of law for obesity prevention and control.

Institute of Medicine. (2011). *Legal strategies in childhood obesity prevention: Workshop summary*. Washington, DC: National Academies Press.—Summarizes the workshop that the Institute of Medicine held in 2010, during which stakeholders discussed current and future legal strategies to combat childhood obesity.

Mello, M. M., Studdert, D. M., & Brennan, T. A. (2006). Obesity—the new frontier of public health law. *New England Journal of Medicine, 354*(24), 2601–2610.—Reviews the rationale for regulatory action to combat obesity, examines legal issues raised by early initiatives, and comments on the prospects for public health law in this area.

Pertschuk, M., Pomeranz, J. L., Aoki, J. R., Larkin, M. A., & Paloma, M. (2013). Assessing the impact of federal and state preemption in public health: A framework for decision makers. *Journal of Public Health Management and Practice, 19*(3), 213–219.—Reviews the consequences of preemption, including its potential impact on grassroots public health movements, and proposes practical questions and considerations to assist decision makers in responding to preemptive proposals. The preemption framework is a tool to support effective decision making by helping the public health field anticipate, assess, and, if necessary, counter preemptive policy proposals.

Pomeranz, J. L. (2016). *Food law for public health.* New York: Oxford University Press.—Provides a comprehensive look at food law in the United States from a public health perspective, exploring topics such as federal, state, and local government authorities and limitations; food marketing, labeling, and safety; federal nutrition programs; and litigation.

Pomeranz, J. L., & Gostin, L. O. (2009). Improving laws and legal authorities for obesity prevention and control. *Journal of Law, Medicine and Ethics, 37*(Suppl. 1), 62–75.—This is the companion article to "Assessment of Laws and Legal Authorities for Obesity Prevention and Control," by Gostin et al. (2009), which identified gaps in the law for obesity prevention and control. It addresses methods to close those gaps by presenting legal action items for policymakers and public health practitioners at the federal, tribal, state, local, and community levels to consider when developing, implementing, and evaluating obesity prevention and control strategies and interventions.

Pomeranz, J. L., Teret, S. P., Sugarman, S. D., Rutkow, L., & Brownell, K. D. (2009). Innovative legal approaches to address obesity. *Milbank Quarterly, 87*(1), 185–213.—Provides legal solutions available to the government to address obesity at the federal, state, and local levels; discusses preemption, limiting children's food marketing, confronting potential addictive properties of food, compelling industry speech, increasing government speech, regulating conduct, using tort litigation, and considering performance-based regulation as an alternative to typical regulatory actions.

Wooten, H., McLaughlin, I., Chen, L., & Fry, C. (2013). Zoning and licensing to regulate the retail environment and achieve public health goals. *Duke Forum for Law and Social Change, 5,* 65–96.—Discusses two policy approaches—zoning and licensing—that communities can take to improve the impact of food retailers' achievement of public health goals, such as limiting the location or density of retailers who sell unhealthy products, regulating the mix and types of products sold by retailers, leveraging participation in federal food assistance programs, and introducing incentives to encourage retailer to adopt additional measures to improve health.

Stealth Interventions for Obesity

Strategies for Behavioral, Social, and Policy Changes

THOMAS N. ROBINSON

Process Motivators and Outcome Motivators

Motivation is considered a key factor in behavior change. One often hears lack of motivation invoked by patients, health professionals, and policymakers to explain their failures to change behavior—for example, "I am just not motivated enough to get up an hour early to exercise," "My patients aren't motivated to follow my recommendations," or "The school board was more motivated by saving money than improving school lunches."

One may consider two types of motivators when designing behavior change interventions for individuals, families, groups, and populations: outcome motivators and process motivators. We define *outcome motivators* as motivators that focus on the anticipated outcomes of behavior change, such as weight loss or improved health. These types of incentives dominate in health counseling and public health messaging—for example, "If you don't lose weight, you may end up with diabetes," "If I can lose 10 pounds, I will look great in that dress," or "If we tax sugary drinks, we can improve the health of our community." Outcome motivators appeal to our desire to link our actions today with future benefits (or to avoid future harms).

Outcome motivators are often at the root of initial decisions to adopt a new behavior. For obesity, these may include trying to avoid or reverse the associated health and social consequences, such as perceived physical appearance, not being teased, obesity-related medical complications, and risks of future medical problems. While outcome motivators may be sufficient to impact intentions to change behavior and, in some cases, initiate action, they are rarely sufficient to change and sustain the behaviors required to lose weight, prevent excess weight gain, and support policies to promote population healthy weight. A large body of research in cognitive psychology supports this; humans discount the importance of future costs and benefits compared to immediate costs and benefits. Many people can point to family, friends, or acquaintances who have been unable to change their behaviors and lose weight even after having personal experiences

609

with severe consequences, such as surviving a heart attack, having a lower leg amputated due to complications of diabetes, or having lost a close family member or friend from an obesity-related complication. How could the salience of those experiences be insufficient to motivate action to prevent them from repeating? Clearly, outcome motivation alone is insufficient for many.

In contrast, *process motivators* are focused on participation in the behavior change process itself, rather than the outcomes of change. Process motivators are the often immediate rewards associated with going for a walk or run, resisting the vending machine, or sparring with beverage lobbyists about a sugary drink tax. These rewards can be the feeling of pride in accomplishing the next incremental goal, social interactions at the gym, competing with a friend, or the thankful e-mail an elected official receives from a constituent. They are short-term incentives that help individuals stay engaged in the change process at the moment. Because these rewards are so proximal to the activities themselves, they also help one persist at the process of change hour to hour, day after day, month after month, and year after year. As a result, process motivators are more likely to be sufficient to help individuals initiate and persist at behavior change over time. Unfortunately, when you look at many health education and clinical, public health, and policy interventions to prevent, treat, and control obesity, they tend to strongly highlight outcome motivators and mostly ignore process motivators.

Stealth Interventions

Interventions emphasizing process motivators over outcome motivators are referred to as *stealth interventions* because, from the perspective of participants, they do not necessarily look and feel like health interventions. Rather than emphasizing health-related messaging, stealth interventions incorporate design elements to increase the intrinsic motivation of the intervention activities themselves. *Intrinsic motivation* refers to inherently or internally rewarding behavior and contrasts with behavior for which one receives extrinsic rewards. Intrinsic motivation is often functionally measured by increased attention, effort, and persistence at a task or activity. Intrinsically motivating design elements can include adding fantasy or context to an activity. In an afterschool sports intervention, for example, a drill to dribble soccer balls around cones as fast as possible becomes navigation of a raft around sharks in the ocean. Offering perceived choice and control over parts of an activity can also result in greater, more sustained effort, even if the choices are inconsequential for the purpose of the activity. In the soccer ball dribbling activity, this might be choosing between navigating a raft around sharks in the ocean or avoiding planets in a spaceship. Without changing the basic underlying activity, participants are empowered by choosing the way the activity is framed. Individualization can also be used, such as addressing a participant by name at the beginning of an activity or referring to some personal characteristic (e.g., age, gender, birthdate). Curiosity, goals, challenge, discovery, problem solving, competition with oneself, and cooperation with others are yet other factors that can be incorporated into interventions. While not exhaustive, these examples illustrate how specific intervention design characteristics that are independent of the content or purpose of the activity itself can serve as process motivators to drive attention, effort, and persistence.

These features have played a key role in the design of effective interventions to reduce children's screen time and to increase moderate and vigorous activity in an afterschool sports program. Spending less time watching television and more time engaging in vigorous exercise training are not activities that one might expect children to find motivating. However, by designing activities that emphasize the rewards of engaging in the activity itself, one can create greater levels of participation in health behavior change activities and outcomes.

As illustrated by the previous examples, if one focuses on the process of change, it may be possible to engage individuals in health behavior change interventions without focusing on the health outcomes at all. From the point of view of participants, their participation is driven by the intrinsically motivating features of the activity—the process of participation. The health outcomes that motivated the clinician, the public health programmer, or the policymaker who designed the intervention (e.g., weight loss, diabetes prevention, vending regulation) are more of a long-term side-effect of participation from the participant's perspective.

In addition to making less attractive activities more intrinsically motivating, this understanding leads one to consider exploring activities that themselves are not only intrinsically motivating but also may produce health benefits as side effects. Dance and team sports are two examples that many find enjoyable but that also may involve high levels of physical activity and reduce opportunities for snacking and screen time. Thus, one can design dance classes or a sports league to engage individuals in vigorous levels of activity without referring to them as exercise or weight control activities. Randomized controlled trials of ethnic dance classes for girls, such as hip-hop, traditional African, and step dance for African American girls and Mexican Ballet Folklorico for Latina girls have demonstrated improved lipid profiles, less prediabetes, less depressive symptoms, and greater cultural identity in high-risk girls, compared to more traditional health and nutrition education. These activities may already be characterized by many process motivators and may be enhanced to include more, such as choreography and storytelling, costumes or uniforms, team membership, performing in front of family and friends, learning about one's ethnic heritage, and so forth. Others have suggested examples such as dog walking, birdwatching, or nature hikes as similar stealth interventions to increase physical activity as a side effect of participation.

Social and Ideological Movements as Stealth Interventions

Can stealth interventions help create even greater effects? When looking for examples in which individuals and/or groups make large and sustained changes in their health behaviors, many involve social and ideological movements. Conveniently, a relatively large number of existing social and ideological movements have goals that overlap with the goals of obesity prevention, treatment, and control. Movements to fight climate change and promote environmental sustainability are one example because efforts to slow climate change endorse eating less meat and replacing automobile rides with more active forms of transportation. Similarly, the animal protection movement emphasizes eating a plant-based diet. Social justice and workers' rights campaigns may also turn people away from meat and fast-food because of the low pay and poor working conditions of workers in those industries. Efforts to promote community safety and raise property values may also focus on sidewalks, bike lanes, traffic calming, and the creation of additional parks to increase walkability. Movements to promote national security and energy independence endorse less automobile use. National security also demands a physically fit military, and retired military leaders have brought attention to the need for improving fitness in the population. Efforts to raise money for a charitable cause may involve training for and participating in a walking, running, or biking event. Political action in support of social and ideological movements can, itself, be a stealth intervention to increase physical activity because it may involve neighborhood canvassing, collecting signatures, or marching in public demonstrations. Initial studies have started to explore these approaches, and two recent randomized controlled trials in children and young adults suggest the potential promise of this approach.

Participating in social and ideological movements often taps into deeper process motivators related to self-identity, values, beliefs, and emotions. Participation also usually provides opportunities for social interaction, social support, behavioral modeling, and experiences that may boost perceived collective efficacy and self-efficacy. Mere participation also becomes a short-term win. Because the ultimate goals of movements are often very large, long-term, and illusive (e.g., reversing climate change, increasing community safety, achieving breakthroughs in cancer research), short-term failures to achieve these goals do not necessarily undermine perceived self-efficacy for participation in the process of change. Thus, the benefits of participation itself reinforce continued participation. In contrast, interventions focusing on weight loss or short-term eating and activity changes allow for lapses or plateaus to be more readily interpreted as personal failures, potentially threatening self-efficacy and deterring continued participation in the process of change. This, of course, is an important feature that distinguishes stealth interventions from standard approaches that focus on health outcomes. By focusing on process motivators, it is possible to reduce perceived risk of failure and instead focus on the motivating aspects of participation, in and of itself.

In addition, social and ideological movements usually focus on producing group- and/or societal-level changes by shaping public opinion, norms, and policies that in turn may create feedback loops that further reinforce their goals. For example, a movement to improve humane treatment of livestock may lead to regulations that drive up the cost of meat to consumers, decreasing its consumption and triggering increased availability of plant-based options, creating a social environment that helps the participating members and others succeed in their attempts to further reduce their meat consumption.

Finally, while many existing social and ideological movements have goals that can potentially contribute to obesity prevention, treatment, and control, the same process motivators can strengthen movements more directly linked to health and obesity. Like the anti-tobacco movements that continue to play an important role in reducing tobacco-related diseases, movements to build parks in high-risk urban communities, improve the quality of school lunches, label added sugar, or tax sugary beverages, for example, also may be strengthened if they can emphasize salient process motivators for participation.

Summary

Stealth interventions may increase and sustain behavior change by focusing on the inherent rewards of the process of change itself, or process motivators. This paradigm contrasts with the standard approach of attempting to motivate behavior change by focusing on health-related outcomes. Interventions can incorporate process motivators by utilizing design characteristics to increase intrinsic motivation. Stealth interventions can also be focused around activities that are already highly motivating for participants and promote healthful behaviors as side effects, such as dance classes and team sports. Finally, stealth interventions in the form of social and ideological movements may represent strategies to achieve larger and more sustained behavior changes. Many existing social and ideological movements overlap in their goals with obesity prevention, treatment, and control, and may represent effective alternative approaches to addressing obesity in individuals, groups, and society.

Suggested Reading

Hekler, E. B., Gardner, C. B., & Robinson, T. N. (2010). Effects of a college course about food and society on students' eating behaviors. *American Journal of Preventive Medicine, 38,* 543–547.—University students in a course on social and ideological aspects of food and agriculture changed their eating behaviors more favorably than students in courses focusing on obesity and public health courses.

Institute of Medicine, Standing Committee on Childhood Obesity Prevention. (2012). *Alliances for Obesity Prevention: Finding common ground: Workshop summary.* Washington, DC: National Academies Press.—Summary of a workshop exploring possible alliances with other non–health organizations, sectors, and movements whose efforts might also support goals for obesity prevention.

Lepper, M. R., Master, A., & Yow, W. Q. (2008). Intrinsic motivation in education. In M. L. Maehr, S. Karabinick, & T. Urdan (Eds.), *Advances in motivation and achievement: Vol. 15. Social psychological perspectives* (pp. 521–555). New York: Macmillan.—A review of the effects of increasing intrinsic motivation on children's learning and a model of conceptually distinct goals and strategies to increase intrinsic motivation in education.

Robinson, T. N. (2010). Stealth interventions for obesity prevention and control: Motivating behavior change. In L. Dube, A. Bechara, A. Dagher, A. Drewnowski, J. LeBel, P. James, et al. (Eds.), *Obesity prevention: The role of brain and society on individual behavior* (pp. 319–327). New York: Elsevier.—Description of the conceptual model for stealth interventions.

Robinson, T. N. (2010). Save the world, prevent obesity: Piggybacking on existing social and ideological movements. *Obesity, 18*(Suppl. 1), S17–S22.—Description of the potential use of existing social and ideological movements as stealth interventions to prevent and treat obesity.

Robinson, T. N., & Borzekowski, D. L. G. (2006). Effects of the SMART classroom curriculum to reduce child and family screen time. *Journal of Communication, 56,* 1–26.—Effects of a screen time reduction intervention on child and family screen time, with a description of incorporating intrinsically motivating features into intervention design.

Robinson, T. N., Matheson, D. M., Kraemer, H. C., Wilson, D. M., Obarzanek, E., Thompson, N. S., et al. (2010). A randomized controlled trial of culturally-tailored dance and reducing screen time to prevent weight gain in low-income African-American girls: Stanford GEMS. *Archives of Pediatrics and Adolescent Medicine, 164,* 995–1004.—In a randomized controlled trial, African American girls randomized to participate in an ethnic dance and screen time reduction intervention significantly reduced their total cholesterol, low-density lipoprotein (LDL) cholesterol, and rate of prediabetes and depressive symptoms, and increased their cultural identity over 2 years compared to girls randomized to health education.

Weintraub, D. L., Tirumalai, E. C., Haydel, K. F., Fujimoto, M., Fulton, J. E., & Robinson, T. N. (2008). Team sports for overweight children: The Stanford Sports to Prevent Obesity Randomized Trial (SPORT). *Archives of Pediatrics and Adolescent Medicine, 162,* 232–237.—In a small randomized controlled trial, overweight and obese children randomized to an after-school soccer program had significant decreases in body mass index z-scores and increases in total daily moderate and vigorous physical activity compared to children randomized to health education.

Slim by Design

Using the CAN Approach to Develop Effective Obesity Policies

BRIAN WANSINK

Introduction: Small and Large Policies

Policy solutions to obesity can be tremendously more powerful—and broad—than we currently imagine. Unfortunately, we often handicap ourselves by only thinking about government policies that start with a capital *P*. Instead, every person in every place has food policies—these are policies with a small *p*. They are the habits and daily patterns, such as the policy to keep a fruit bowl on the counter at home or to keep soft drinks off the counter. It might be a policy to say a word of thanks before dinner, clean our plates, or not let our children eat dessert unless they have finished their vegetables—or not have dessert at all. These policies can either work for us or against us.

Importantly, just as we have personal policies, so do restaurants, schools, grocers, and workplaces. While some might be standard operating procedures (SOPs) that are written down, others are simply rules of thumb, such as "The customer is always right," or "Always suggest coffee after a meal if there isn't a waiting line." These policies are fluid and flexible. If a policy causes a company to lose money or customers, it can be changed immediately.

There are two key questions to answer when creating workable policies to help reduce obesity: (1) Who can most easily solve the problem? and (2) What policy can help them do this? To illustrate an approach to answering the first question, I use three new findings about the overeating of breakfast cereals to show how three different problems can be effectively addressed by different parties. To illustrate how to answer the second question, I then outline the CAN approach (making healthy foods more "convenient, attractive, and normal") and show how it is being effectively implemented in schools and elsewhere to help make consumers slim by design. As stated earlier, for any eating-related situation, once we know who should be most responsible for enacting change, we can use the CAN approach to develop the solution or policy to make it happen.

Who Can Most Easily Solve This Problem?

Many efforts to change eating behavior focus on nutrition education or restrictive policy changes. For instance, if we want children to drink less chocolate milk and more white milk at school, one approach would be to ban chocolate milk. Unfortunately, this does not always seem to work. When 11 elementary schools in Oregon did this, milk sales dropped by 11%, milk cost went up 10%, milk waste went up 30%, and 8% fewer children ate school lunch. The unsuccessful ban lasted less than a year.

A successful alternative approach would have been to simply make white milk more convenient, attractive, and normal to drink than chocolate milk. When white milk is made more convenient by moving it to the front of the cooler, sales typically increase by 30–40%. If at least one-third of all milk is white, sales increase another 35%. No complaints. No dropouts. No price increases.

When looking for a solution to an eating problem, when should we ask the government, when should we ask institutions, and when should ask consumers? The answer has to do with the extent to which consumers or institutions can control the relevant drivers of eating, the evidence of success, and the possibility of an unintended consequence.

As an illustration, consider three new discoveries of why we overeat breakfast cereal. Figure 100.1 provides graphic summaries of these three articles' findings. The first shows that the average cereal box pictures a serving size that is 74% larger than what their nutrition facts panel recommends. This causes an 11% overserving of cereal. The second shows that the shelf height level of children's cereals and the gaze of the characters on the boxes (51 of 59 cereals) look down and meet the eyes of children. This increases sales and feelings of trust by 18%. The third is a correlational study that shows that 210 Syracuse, New York, mothers who had cereal visible on their kitchen counters weighed 9.8 kg (21 pounds) more than their neighbors who did not.

If we think the behavioral consequences (overbuying or overeating) of these packaging or placement actions should be addressed, we would first want to determine which group (government, industry, or consumers) can most effectively address it. We would then want to determine whether the strength of the evidence is strong enough and the effect size is large enough to be compelling, then determine whether there might be unintended negative consequences to asking government, industry, or consumers to act on these findings. Since unintended negative consequences are often unforeseen, running field tests—when possible—could give confidence and avoid the regrets of a bad law (e.g., Prohibition) that is difficult to eliminate.

In the case of cereal, each of these three troubling problems should be addressed by a different group. As indicated in Table 100.1, if cereal boxes picture excessive portions, consumers cannot do anything about this, but these packaging photos can be changed by companies. These depictions are widespread, and the impact on serving sizes is robust. It appears to be the appropriate venue for a government policy solution that the company picture the stated serving size on the box, or state that what is depicted is an exaggerated serving size (and perhaps state calories).

Now consider the case of cereal boxes being placed at the eye-level of a child and the gaze of the character on the box being directed down (e.g., toward children's eyes). Although this is something consumers cannot control (other than having their children wait at the end of the cereal aisle), it would also be difficult for companies or retailers to control. Everything cannot be placed on a 6-foot shelf, and dictating the level of eye gaze of characters on a box would be a difficult fight to win. Nor is it evident that much would

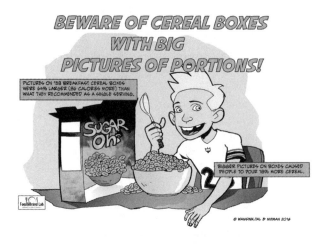

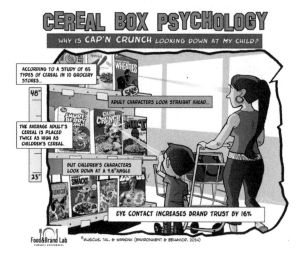

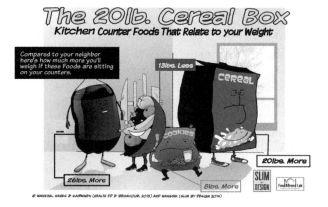

FIGURE 100.1. How cereal packaging and shelf placement lead to overconsumption. Copyright © Brian Wansink. Reprinted by permission.

TABLE 100.1. Policy Solutions to How Cereal Packaging and Placement Leads to Overconsumption

Three recent findings	Can consumers or institutions control this?	Strength of evidence and possibility of unintended consequence	Best possible solutions: government policy, company policy, or consumer policy
Cereal boxes picture serving sizes that are 74% larger than what their nutrition facts panel recommends. This causes an 11% overserving of cereal (Wansink et al., 2017).	• Consumers cannot control this. • Packaging changes can be made by companies.	• Exaggerated depictions are widespread. • The impact on serving is robust.	Government policy solution • Picture the stated serving size on the box. • State that what is depicted is an exaggerated serving size (and perhaps state calories).
The gaze of the characters on children's cereal looks down and meets the eyes of children. This increases sales and feelings of trust by 18% (Musicus et al., 2015).	• Consumers cannot control this. • Coordination and logistics make placement changes and box modifications difficult.	• Downward eye gaze occurs in 85% of children's cereals. • Choice evidence is lab-based with college students, not field-based with children.	Company policy solution • Strength of evidence and difficulty of implementation make government policy infeasible. • Encourage companies or retailers to adjust placement and promote as a public service.
Women who have cereal visible on their kitchen counter weight 9.8 kg (21 pounds) more than a neighbor who does not (Wansink et al., 2015).	• Consumers can control whether they place cereal on counter if they are aware of its consequences. • Companies have little control over consumers in their homes.	• Correlational evidence only. • Significant with women but not men. • Strongest with people who work at home.	Consumer policy solution • Public health campaigns, nutrition counseling, and training can emphasize keeping cereal off counters. • Dietary guidelines can emphasize only having fruit visible on the counter.

change. There is no evidence that any less cereal would be consumed or that the shoppers would buy anything healthier. As a result, it would be best to encourage a company- or industry-based solution. Companies could adjust placement (or change boxes) and promote it as a public service or evidence that they help shoppers shop better. Although the evidence is not overly compelling, a consumer-related movement could encourage this if enough people thought it to be a burning issue.

Last, consider the research from the Syracuse Study that shows that 210 Syracuse mothers with cereal visible on the kitchen counter weighed 9.8 kg (21 pounds) more than their neighbors who did not. This is something consumers could easily control (by putting the cereal away). Even though the evidence is correlational and only women were studied, there is seemingly no risk or unintended consequence in recommending that people simply keep their counters clear of any food other than a fruit bowl. As a result, this would entail a consumer policy solution, and the plan would then focus on consumer education. This could be done through public health campaigns, nutrition counseling, training that emphasizes keeping cereal off counters, and recommendations on implementing the Dietary Guidelines to have only having fruit visible on the counter.

The CAN Approach: Expanding the Policy Toolbox

Our food environment has evolved to provide food that is highly available, attractive, and especially affordable. Although this has helped to make us overweight, the solution is not to make food less available, less affordable, and less attractive. No one wants to have to hunt or grow their own food and to pay five times more for bread or ice cream so that they eat less. There needs to be another solution.

In dozens of different eating behavior studies in homes, grocery stores, restaurants, and schools, using the CAN approach has been shown to be much more effective than taking favorite foods away or artificially restricting what someone can order. Doing this creatively and effectively alters not only a person's food choice but also taste evaluations, perhaps leading to habitually healthier choices. Although these downstream ripples of one's food choices are critical to changing habits and health, the CAN approach is immediately effective in changing choice. Details about this are briefly summarized below.

Increasing Convenience

First, healthy foods need to be the convenient choice—convenient to see, to order, to pick up, and to consume. Consider what happens in schools that have adopted a behavior change program called the Smarter Lunchroom Movement. In one study, when one of the food lines in a school cafeteria was redesigned to be a convenient line that only offered prepackaged healthy entrées and foods (e.g., salads), sales of these healthy foods increased 77% within 2 weeks.

Convenience can relate to the way food is offered. If one were to ask children why they do not eat more apples or pears, 5- to 9-year-old children say an apple is too big for their mouths or it gets stuck in their braces. Adolescent girls say they do not eat more fruit because it is messy, and it looks unbecoming or unlady-like. One solution to both problems would be to provide children with cut fruit. Indeed, when we put fruit sectionizers in school lunchrooms, children ate 70% more fruit.

Increasing Attractiveness

The second principle of the CAN approach is that the healthy choice needs to be made to be more attractive relative to what else is available. This includes more attractive names, appearance, prices, and expectations. Fruit that is served in a steel chafer pan or stored in the bottom drawer of a refrigerator is not as attractive as fruit in a colorful bowl. Even simply giving food a descriptive name makes it more attractive and increases a person's taste expectations and enjoyment of it. For instance, Dinosaur Trees are more exciting to a child and taste better than broccoli, and a Big Bad Bean Burrito tastes better and is more exciting than a vegetarian burrito. Even putting an Elmo sticker on apples led 46% more day-care children to take and eat an apple instead of a cookie. Putting fruit in a nicer bowl leads children to take more, and putting garnishes near a salad makes people rate the taste as better.

Increasing Normality

Many consumers prefer what is popular—what they think is normal to order and eat. This includes choices that are more normal to order, to purchase, to serve, and to eat (see Table 100.1). Efforts that make the healthy choice seem more normal appear to make it so. For instance, when 50% of the milk in a cooler is white (vs. chocolate), middle school students are nearly three times as likely to take a white milk than when only 10% of the milk is white. It seems like the normal choice. The same applies at home. When healthier food is placed on the front or middle shelf in a cupboard or refrigerator, it is more frequently taken and is rated as the more normal food to take; otherwise, it would not be so convenient.

Consumption norms—particularly those resulting from implicit visual cues coming from physical dimensions (Table 100.2)—hold tremendous promise for researchers for three reasons: (1) their reach is farther than has been appreciated; (2) they can be found in an endless number of forms; and (3) their perceptual nature makes consumers more vulnerable than they believe. From an intervention standpoint, changing the size of a cafeteria tray or the size of a label on a restaurant menu can change consumption in an automatic way that does not necessitate willpower or an expensive public health

TABLE 100.2. The CAN Approach to Changing Behavior in One's Food Radius

	Make it more convenient.	Make it more attractive.	Make it more normal.
A grocery store manager who wants to sell more fish at full price . . .	Places fish in a center cooler at the end of the vegetable section.	Offers easy, appealing fish recipe ideas on notecards next to the fish that people can take with them.	Puts floor decals near the fish that has a green dashed line pointing toward the fish.
A restaurant owner who wants to sell more high-margin shrimp salads . . .	Makes it easy to find on the menu by putting it on the first page and in a bold font.	Gives it a catchy name or one that appeals to the senses—"Scrumptious Savory Shrimp Salad Bonanza, anyone?"	Describes it as a special or a manager's favorite.
An office manager who wants her workers to leave their desk and eat in the new healthy cafeteria . . .	Adds a $5 "grab and go" line filled with healthier foods, and maybe an honor system cash box.	Has a more attractive cafeteria, break room, or brown bag series.	Posts notices and news on bulletin boards in the cafeteria, break room, or fitness room, and not in the work area.
A school lunch manager who wants to get more kids to take and eat fruit . . .	Puts it within easy reach in two different parts of the line— beginning and end.	Puts it in a colorful bowl and/or gives it a colorful sign.	Puts it in front of the cash register with a sign: "Take an extra one for a snack."
A mother who wants to eat better at home . . .	Puts precut vegetables on the middle shelf of the fridge and the bread out of sight.	Buys more tempting salad dressings with cool names and less tempting bread.	Sets salad bowls on the dinner table every day, even if they aren't being used, and gets rid of the butter dish.

Note. From Wansink (2014). Copyright © 2014 Brian Wansink. Adapted by permission.

education campaign. One area in which this is particularly important is when dealing with nutrition and children—getting children to eat their vegetables.

The Smarter Lunchroom Movement: Getting Kids to Eat Their Vegetables

To illustrate how behavioral science is a tool that can change choices and eating behavior, consider the challenge of encouraging children to make smarter choices in school cafeterias. Rising obesity rates among children have led to pressure to drop higher-calorie items such as cookies and french fries from the menu. Proponents believe that if children cannot buy it, they will not consume it. But children have many other eating options: They can skip lunch, bring potato chips from home, or walk or drive to a fast-food place. Introducing ultrahealthy foods into the lunchroom requires more money, and probably will not entice a disenfranchised student back to the lunchroom. Suppose, however, that rearranging, repositioning, and reframing the currently offered food items could instead encourage children to buy more of the healthy foods and less of the rest. This strategy costs little and could improve meal quality, as well as retain patronage.

To help schools in this regard, we have designed a do-it-yourself Scorecard that food service personnel, parents, or students can use. Figure 100.2 displays this tool, and there is also a free app (Smarter Lunchroom scorecard). Each lunchroom can get as many as 100 points because there are 100 tasks or changes that help kids choose and eat better. Most schools first score around 20–30 points, but they can quickly move up to 50 points within a couple weeks if they really focus.

Conclusion

There is a German word, *Verschlimmbesserung*, that resonates with many well-intended but inexperienced handymen. It roughly translates to "trying to fix something but making it worse." Public policy is a well-intended but inexperienced handyman in the food environment. Although some success has been achieved in the tobacco environment, the food environment is different—just as fixing your car requires different tools than fixing your home.

Institutions across the world are pulling together to create new policies that are healthier for consumers and can save money (by reducing food waste) or make more money (attracting more customers). Grocery stores and convenience stores in the United States and Norway are adopting a Slim by Design scorecard to help them set up stores to help consumers shop better. One of the largest hotel chains in Scandinavia (Nordic Choice Hotels) is setting up buffets to help guests take less food and waste less food.

The solution for many eating-related behavior problems is to broaden our view of the types of policies that can empower consumers. As the illustration with new breakfast cereal findings indicated, sometimes we can encourage consumers to develop a new personal policy; in other cases we can help institutions develop win–win policies that they can profitably use to help consumers eat healthier. There are blueprints to help. It is important to realize that effective policies can take many different forms.

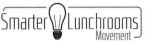 **Smarter Lunchrooms Self-Assessment** | Scorecard

Since its founding in 2009 the Smarter Lunchrooms Movement has championed the use of evidence-based, simple low and no-cost changes to lunchrooms which can simultaneously improve participation and profits while decreasing waste. This tool can help you to evaluate your lunchroom, congratulate yourself for things you are doing well and and identify areas of opportunity for improvement.

Instructions

Read each of the statements below. Visualize your cafeteria, your service areas and your school building. Indicate whether the statement is true for your school by checking the box to the left. If you believe that your school does not reflect the statement 100% do not check the box on the left. After you have completed the checklist, tally all boxes with check marks and write this number in the designated area on the back of the form. This number represents your school's baseline score. The boxes which are not checked are areas of opportunity for you to consider implementing in the future. We recommend completing this checklist annually to measure your improvements!

It's not nutrition ...until it's eaten!

Important Words

Service areas: Any location where students can purchase or are provided with food

Dining areas: Any location where students can consume the food purchased or provided

Grab and Go Meals: Any meal with components pre-packaged together for ease and convenience – such as a brown bag lunch or "Fun Lunch" etc.

Designated Line: Any foodservice line which has been specified for particular food items or concepts – such as a pizza line, deli line, salad line etc.

Alternative entrée options: Any meal component which could also be considered an entrée for students - such as the salad bar, yogurt parfait, vegetarian/vegan or meatless options etc.

Reimbursable "Combo Meal" pairings: Any reimbursable components available independently on your foodservice lines which you have identified as a part of a promotional complete meal – For example you decided your beef taco, seasoned beans, frozen strawberries and 1% milk are part of a promotional meal called the, "Mi Amigo Meal!" etc.

Non-functional lunchroom equipment: Any items which are either broken, awaiting repair or are simply not used during meal service – such as empty or broken steam tables, coolers, registers etc.

Good Rapport: Communication is completed in a friendly and polite manner

Focusing on Fruit

☐ Fruit is available in all food service areas

☐ Daily fruit options are available in two or more locations on the service lines

☐ At least one daily fruit option is available near all registers (If there are concerns regarding edible peel, fruit can be bagged or wrapped)

☐ At least two types of fruit are available daily

☐ Whole fruit options are displayed in attractive bowls or baskets (instead of chaffing/hotel pans)

☐ A mixed variety of whole fruits are displayed together in bowls in all service areas

☐ Sliced or cut fruit is available daily

☐ Daily fruit options are displayed in a location in the line of sight and reach of students (Consider the average height of your students when determining line of sight)

☐ Daily fruit options are bundled into all grab and go meals available to students

☐ All available fruit options have been given creative or descriptive names

☐ All fruit names are highlighted on all serving lines with name-cards or product IDs daily

☐ All fruit names are highlighted and legible on menu boards in all service and dining areas

☐ Fruit options are not browning, bruised or otherwise damaged

☐ All fruit options are replenished so displays appear "full" continually throughout meal service and after each lunch period

☐ All staff members, especially those serving, have been trained to politely prompt students to select and consume the daily fruit options with their meal

Promoting Vegetables & Salad

☐ Vegetables are available in all food service areas

☐ Daily vegetable options are available in two or more locations in all service areas

☐ At least two types of vegetable are available daily

☐ Daily vegetable options are displayed in a location in the line of sight and reach of students (Consider the average height of your students when determining line of sight)

☐ Daily vegetable options are bundled into all grab and go meals available to students

☐ A salad bar is available to all students

☐ All available vegetable options have been given creative or descriptive names

☐ All vegetable names are highlighted on all serving lines with name-cards or product IDs daily

☐ All vegetable names are highlighted and legible on menu boards in the service and dining areas

☐ Vegetables are not wilted, browning, or otherwise damaged

☐ All vegetable options are replenished so displays appear "full" continually throughout meal service and after each lunch period

☐ All staff members, especially those serving, have been trained to politely prompt students to select and consume the daily vegetable options with their meal

Moving More White Milk

☐ White milk is available in all service areas

☐ White milk is in two or more locations in all service areas

☐ All beverage coolers have white milk available

☐ White milk represents 1/3 of all visible milk in the lunchroom

☐ White milk is placed in front of other beverages in all coolers

☐ White milk is eye-level and within reach of the students (Consider the average height of your students when determining eye-level)

☐ White milk crates are placed so that they are the first beverage option seen in all milk coolers

☐ White milk is bundled into all grab and go meals available to students as the default beverage

☐ White milk is highlighted on all serving lines with a name-card or product ID daily

☐ White milk is highlighted and legible on the menu boards in all service and dining areas

☐ White milk is replenished so all displays appear "full" continually throughout meal service and after each lunch period

Entrée of the Day

☐ A daily entrée option has been identified to promote - a targeted entrée in each service area and for each designated line (deli-line, pizza-line etc.)

(continued on next page)

FIGURE 100.2. Smarter Lunchrooms self-assessment scorecard. Copyright © Brian Wansink. Reprinted by permission.

☐ Alternative entrée options (salad bar, yogurt parfaits etc.) are highlighted on posters or signs within all service and dining areas

☐ Daily targeted entrée is visible to students of average height for your school in all service areas and on each designated line

☐ Daily targeted entrée is placed as the first entrée option available in all service areas and on each designated line

☐ Daily targeted entrées have been provided with creative or descriptive names

☐ Targeted entrée name is highlighted on each respective serving line with a name-card or product ID daily

☐ Targeted entrée names are highlighted and legible on menu boards within all service and dining areas

☐ Daily targeted entrees are replenished so all displays appear "full" continually throughout meal service and after each lunch period

☐ A reimbursable meal can be created in any service area available to students (salad bars, snack rooms, speed lines, speed windows, dedicated service lines etc.)

Increasing Sales Reimbursable Meals

☐ Reimbursable "Combo Meal" pairings have been determined for each service area (i.e. - a targeted entrée, fruit, vegetable and milk or targeted entrée, milk and fruit etc.)

☐ All components of a reimbursable meal are available in two or more locations in the service areas

☐ A reimbursable meal has been bundled into a grab and go meal available to students

☐ Grab and go reimbursable meals are available in all service and dining areas (al a carte windows etc.)

☐ Grab and go reimbursable meals are available by all registers

☐ Grab and go reimbursable meals are within reach of students of average height for your school in all service areas

☐ Grab and go reimbursable meals are replenished so all displays appear "full" continually throughout meal service and after each lunch period

☐ Reimbursable meals can be created using alternative entrees (salad bar, yogurt parfait etc.)

☐ Reimbursable "Combo Meal" pairings have been provided creative or descriptive age-appropriate names (i.e. – Hungry Kid Meal, Meal Deal, Athlete's Meal, Bobcat Meal etc.)

☐ Names for reimbursable "Combo Meal" pairings are highlighted on serving lines with name-cards or product IDs daily (i.e. – "Crunchy Carrots – part of the Hungry Kid Meal!)

☐ Names for reimbursable "Combo Meal" pairings are highlighted and legible on menu boards within the service and dining areas

☐ Reimbursable "Combo Meal" pairings are promoted on posters or signs within the lunchroom, along the lunch-line and within the school building

☐ All components for reimbursable "Combo Meal" pairings are replenished so all displays appear "full" continually throughout meal service and after each lunch period

Creating School Synergies

☐ Posters displaying healthful foods are visible and readable from all points in the service and dining space

☐ Menu boards featuring today's meal components are visible and readable from all points in the service and dining space

☐ A dedicated space/menu board is visible and readable from 5ft away within the service and dining area where students can see tomorrow's menu items

☐ Signage/posters/floor decals are available to direct students toward all service areas

☐ Trash on the floors, in, or near garbage cans is removed between each lunch period

☐ Cleaning supplies and utensils are returned to a cleaning closet or are not visible during service and dining

☐ Compost/recycling/tray return and garbage cans are tidied between lunch periods

☐ Compost/recycling/tray return and garbage cans are at least 5 feet away from dining students

☐ Dining and service areas are clear of any non-functional lunchroom equipment or tables during service

☐ Sneeze guards in all service areas are clean

☐ Trays and cutlery are within arm's reach to the student of average height within your school

☐ Obstacles and barriers to enter service and dining areas have been removed (i.e. – garbage cans, mop buckets, cones, lost and found etc.)

☐ Clutter is removed from service and dining areas promptly (i.e. – empty boxes, shipments of foods, empty crates, pans, lost and found etc.)

☐ Self-serve salad bar utensils are at the appropriate portion size or larger

☐ Student artwork is displayed in the service and/or dining areas

☐ All lights in dining and service areas are currently functional and on

☐ Dining space is branded to reflect student body or school (i.e. – school lunchroom is named for a school mascot or local hero/celebrity

☐ Milk coolers and service lines are decorated with decals/magnets etc. wherever possible

☐ Students must ask to purchase al a carte items from staff members

☐ Students must use cash to purchase al a carte items which are not reimbursable

☐ Half portions are available for at least two dessert options

☐ A monthly menu is provided to all student families, teachers, and administrators

☐ A monthly menu is visible and readable within all communal spaces within the school building

☐ The monthly menu highlights creative and descriptive names which were provided for the menu items

☐ Posters or signs highlighting the creative and descriptive names and respective menu items are visible in the service and dining areas

☐ Student groups are involved in the development of creative, descriptive and names for menu items

☐ Student groups are involved in the creation of artwork promoting menu items within the dining space and school building

☐ Student groups are involved in modeling good behavior to others (i.e. – high school students eating in the middle school lunchroom once a month) at least quarterly

☐ Student surveys are used to inform menu development, dining space décor and promotional ideas

☐ Teachers and administrators are involved in the development and implementation of promotional ideas

☐ Teachers and administrators dine in the lunchroom with students at least quarterly

☐ Cafeteria monitors have good rapport with students and lunchroom staff

☐ The dining space is used for other learning activities beyond meal service (i.e. – measuring, cooking or school garden activities) at least quarterly

☐ Students, teachers, and or administrators announce daily meal deals or targeted items in daily announcements

☐ The school participates in other food program promotions such as: Farm to School, Chefs Move to School, Fuel Up to Play 60, Share our Strength etc.

☐ The school has applied or been selected for in the Healthier US School Challenge

☐ Staff is trained to smile and greet students upon their entering the service line

☐ Staff is encouraged to eat in the lunchroom with students when on break quarterly

☐ All promotional signs and posters are rotated, updated or changed at least quarterly

☐ All creative and descriptive names are rotated, updated or changed at least quarterly

It's not nutrition ...until it's eaten!

Total Checked: _____

FIGURE 100.2. (*continued*)

Suggested Reading

Chandon, P., & Wansink, B. (2012). Does food marketing need to make us fat?: A review and solutions. *Nutrition Reviews, 70*(10), 571–593.—This shows the mechanisms that make the four P's of marketing (product, place, promotion, and price) effective in some cases and ineffective in others. Furthermore, it shows the profitable win–win solutions that marketers can use to improve how consumers shop.

Wansink, B. (2005). *Marketing nutrition: Soy, functional foods, biotechnology, and obesity.* Champaign: University of Illinois Press.—To successfully demarket obesity, we have to give people an alternative. Marketing nutrition is the flip side of demarketing obesity. This book provides 14 unique insights and tools on what this means for labeling, targeting, accelerating adoption, prototyping, and laddering. The techniques are useful to a mother encouraging her children to eat vegetables, to a company exporting a high-protein tofu, and to a government trying to encourage children to drink more milk and fewer soft drinks.

Wansink, B. (2007). *Mindless eating: Why we eat more than we think.* New York: Bantam.—We make over 200 unconscious eating decisions about food every day. This shows what they are and how we can guide them to help us eat "mindlessly" better, without thinking about it, dieting, or depriving ourselves.

Wansink, B. (2014). *Slim by design: Mindless eating solutions for everyday life.* New York: Morrow.—This is the most comprehensive blueprint for how to battle obesity successfully and change eating behaviors among consumers, communities, and countries. It has been the prime force behind new eating systems in the United Kingdom and Scandinavia, and it also outlines the powerful use of win–win diagnostic and prescriptive scorecards in the five principal areas where we eat: our homes, restaurants, supermarkets, workplaces, and schools.

Wansink, B. (2015). Change their choice!: Changing behavior using the CAN approach and activism research. *Psychology and Marketing, 32*(5), 486–500.—This offers a simple but powerful social-science and consumer-behavior-based framework (often called behavioral economics) that can be used to change behavior in any context. It is adopted from the book *Slim by Design,* and is the backbone of the Smarter Lunchroom approach.

Wansink, B., & Pope, L. (2015). When do gain-framed health messages work better than fear appeals? *Nutrition Reviews, 73*(1), 4–11.—Public health messages are often fear appeals, but they are usually ineffective. By answering four questions about a target audience, this review contends that one can predict whether a gain-framed health message will be more effective than a loss-framed message. The resulting framework helps predict which type of nutrition-related health message will be most effective with a given audience target.

Wansink, B., & van Ittersum, K. (2016). Boundary research: Tools and rules for impactful research in emerging fields. *Journal of Consumer Behaviour, 15*(5), 390–410.—For graduate students and junior faculty with nontraditional (boundary) research areas, this article describes new tools that boundary researchers can use to get started, published, and promoted. These include writing for surprising impact, positioning their research against a larger theme, developing a research impact matrix for promotion, and estimating a 10-year citation record.

Behavioral Economics and Obesity

LIZZY POPE
STEPHEN T. HIGGINS
LEONARD H. EPSTEIN

Neoclassical economic theories are based on several assumptions, namely, that (1) humans make rational decisions, (2) humans have all of the information needed to make decisions, and (3) a person making a wrong decision quickly learns from mistakes to maximize utility. Unfortunately, human decision making (i.e., behavioral choice) often does not conform to these assumptions. Research has repeatedly shown that we humans have difficulty making decisions in areas in which we are inexperienced, uninformed, or emotional, and when feedback is slow or infrequent, such as choices surrounding weight control. Behavioral economic theory acknowledges that humans do not always behave rationally and are often influenced by factors in their immediate environments that contribute to self-control problems and shortsightedness. To combat irrationality, behavioral economists advocate for a model wherein healthier choices are made more attractive, yet the ability to choose less healthy options is preserved.

Decision-Making Biases

Behavioral economists have identified biases in decision making, such as present-biased preferences, anchoring, and loss aversion, that commonly push preferences in unhealthy directions. Present-biased preferences cause us to procrastinate when actions involve immediate costs, and to make hasty choices toward options that include smaller but more immediate rewards even when alternatives involving larger but more delayed rewards are available. This bias in how we make choices can become a substantive obstacle for those trying to manage their weight, as they must continually deny themselves immediate pleasure in the form of favorite foods or sedentary activities, while aiming for a longer-term reward such as weight loss/maintenance, which is not guaranteed. Anchors influence decision making by serving as reference points and include social norms, habits, framing, and other contextual factors, many of which support food and exercise choices that are less beneficial to our long-term health. The premise of loss aversion is that humans prefer avoiding losses even more than experiencing gains. Loss aversion coupled with status quo bias (the desire to continue with the familiar) likely contributes to common difficulties in giving up certain preferred but relatively unhealthy foods or activities when trying to eat better or exercise more.

Incentives

Behavioral economic theory predicts that providing opportunities to earn short-term material incentives will increase the frequency of otherwise low-probability behaviors such as exercising or achieving weight loss goals. Furthermore, by underscoring the potential immediate benefits of a healthy choice, incentives can increase motivation for healthier options by leveraging the same bias for the present discussed earlier that often underpins unhealthy choices. Of course, incentives involve the operant learning principle of reinforcement, wherein positive environmental consequences increase the future probability of the behavior, that precedes them. Also important to note is that financial incentives activate the same neurobiological mesolimbic reward systems as do fatty, salty, and sweet foods, and drugs of abuse. Again, they allow one to leverage the same processes that often drive unhealthy choices to instead promote health. Last, incentives increase activity in the prefrontal cortex, the brain area underpinning executive functions involved in goal seeking, including inhibition of well-learned responses occasioned by visceral factors such as drug cravings or hunger pangs.

Interventions using financial incentives for weight-related behavior change date back to initial behavior therapy studies in the 1960s, but there has been a recent resurgence of interest in incentive interventions for weight control and wellness to address the obesity epidemic. The results obtained from these studies clearly demonstrate the efficacy of financial incentives in promoting weight loss over the first 6 months of treatment, although, as with other behavioral weight loss programs, weight regain is common. While incentive schemes to reliably promote and maintain longer-term weight loss remain an important priority, results from a recent trial demonstrated that participants in a 12-week behavioral weight loss intervention plus incentives achieved 3.1% body weight loss 9 months after treatment versus participants in the behavioral weight loss intervention alone, who achieved 1.2% body weight loss. Twelve weeks of adjuvant group therapy sessions were also efficacious in sustaining weight loss.

Incentive Intervention Design Considerations

Many different incentive schemes have been effective for weight management. Research has yet to distinguish definitively whether reinforcing program attendance/adherence (process incentives) or weight loss outcomes (outcome incentives) is consistently more effective, although one of the few studies to experimentally examine the topic demonstrated approximately twofold greater weight loss when the incentive targeted predetermined weight loss or caloric intake goals compared to attendance at weight loss treatment sessions.

In addition to whether process or outcomes should be targeted, another consideration with incentive interventions is how to identify an effective incentive value for promoting or sustaining weight loss (i.e., reinforcement magnitude). Studies providing payment for weight loss have varied widely in the magnitude of the incentive given, with some providing as little as $1/day for walking, while others have provided as much as $6/day to meet weight loss goals. In general, larger incentive amounts produce larger effect sizes than smaller payments. For example, in a study comparing the efficacy of $7 or $14 per 1% weight loss, both incentives resulted in weight loss, but only the $14 incentive produced effects that differed significantly from the no-incentive controls.

Based on the basic learning literature, and research on incentives in the area of addictions, reinforcing as frequently as is practicable, especially early in the change effort, and minimizing delays between documenting a targeted outcome and delivering the incentive can be expected to increase treatment effect size. While some weight management studies using incentives have provided daily or weekly opportunities for reinforcement, others providing reinforcement only monthly or quarterly have nevertheless shown efficacy. No experimental research that we are aware of has compared these parameters.

A further consideration with incentive programs is who pays for the incentives. As discussed earlier, deposit contracts in which participants initially make a deposit of their own money, then have it returned upon goal completion, have led to successful weight loss. In a recent trial, deposit contract participants lost 8.7 pounds over 32 weeks, a significantly greater weight loss than that in the no-incentive control condition. Importantly, this model plays on our bias toward loss aversion. Deposit contracts also largely pay for themselves, which makes them attractive in settings in which funds to finance an incentive program are limited. However, deposit contracts are likely to exclude the participation of lower-income people who may particularly benefit from weight management interventions, as obesity becomes more overrepresented among lower socioeconomic populations. This same association with lower socioeconomic status is even more pronounced with cigarette smoking, and recent research in that area clearly demonstrated that smokers are reluctant to accept voluntarily an incentive condition involving a deposit contract, raising substantive questions about the utility of that model for reaching economically disadvantaged populations. Nevertheless, emerging, innovative commercial Internet sites allow individuals to place financial deposits that can be earned back, contingent on exercising, or achieving weight loss or other behavior-change goals.

Successful interventions have also used incentives funded by the interventionists in the form of lottery systems or direct payments. Interventionist-provided incentives often fall into two schedules of reinforcement—variable or fixed. Lottery systems provide variable-ratio reinforcement, which can be a very effective way to promote behavior change, as people cannot predict reinforcement availability and may therefore lose a reward opportunity if they fail to adhere continuously. In one 16-week incentive trial, participants in a lottery-incentive condition lost 13.1 pounds and remained significantly lighter than controls at 3-month follow-up.

A fixed-incentive scheme reinforces behavior on a predictable schedule. When using a fixed-incentive schedule, a specific payment pattern of escalating reinforcement magnitude for consecutive instances of goal achievement, with a reset contingency when the goal is not met, is commonly used in the substance abuse literature. This type of incentive delivery reduces the likelihood of clients taking "holidays" from the behavior change effort when they decide it is acceptable to "skip" 1 week because they will be losing minimal rewards for one-time nonadherence. Despite its success in substance abuse treatment, few weight management interventions have examined the escalating reinforcement magnitude with a reset contingency schedule, although it seems likely that its benefits would extend to this area as well.

Cost and Cost-Effectiveness

Interest in the cost-effectiveness of using incentives to promote weight loss has grown in the past several years, as incentive researchers have faced cost-related program criticisms. Although the visible costs of carrying out an incentive program may be larger than those for other types of interventions, overall program costs may actually be lower. For example, econometric results in a trial by Leahey and colleagues (2015) indicated that incentives ($64/kg lost) are a more cost-effective adjuvant intervention than group therapy ($113/kg lost) in promoting and sustaining weight loss. Future investigations of the cost-effectiveness of incentives will be important in determining their place in weight control efforts.

Other Behavioral Economic Strategies to Reduce Obesity

While incentives have been one of the most investigated behavioral economic strategies in the area of obesity, other types of interventions are of interest as well. Rearranging the *choice architecture*—the physical or environmental arrangement surrounding people's food and exercise decisions—is one way investigators can nudge people into making better long-term choices. Examples of choice architecture interventions include rearranging the school lunchroom to make fruit, vegetable, or white milk options more salient by placing them at eye level or within easier reach, or promoting physical activity by making stairs the more convenient and attractive option. Providing additional information, such as calorie labeling in restaurants or front-of-package labeling on foods, is another behavioral economic strategy investigators have employed to address obesity on a population level. Last, there has been a surge of interest in using excise taxes on sugar-sweetened beverages or junk food to dissuade purchasing. Several countries and the city of Berkeley, California, have enacted excise taxes (taxes per ounce of product), but evaluations of impact are not yet available. Behavioral economics would predict that excise taxes would be more effective than sales taxes, as excise taxes increase the salience of the tax to consumers, tying the price increase directly to the taxed food item. Excise taxes have been quite effective in curbing cigarette smoking over the past 40 years, especially among young people and those of lower socioeconomic status.

Conclusions

A multitude of successful controlled studies have demonstrated the efficacy of using behavioral economic strategies such as financial incentives to promote weight-related behavior change. While the range of weight loss has varied depending on study duration and design, clinically meaningful weight reductions with incentives have been achieved reliably. Although successful, there are still challenges around how to employ incentives most efficaciously and cost-effectively. More research, possibly using discrete-choice modeling, is needed to identify optimal intervention parameters such as incentive magnitude, schedule, and duration. Questions regarding possible differential impact of incentives among those of varying socioeconomic, racial, and ethnic backgrounds remain open, although such differences have not been evident in the addiction literature.

Also important is to continue examining how to sustain incentivized behavior change. This challenge is not unique to incentive interventions and applies to all weight control programs. Incentivizing behavior change without altering the surrounding environment is unlikely to result in long-term maintenance of behavior change or weight loss. Combining incentive interventions with choice architecture interventions, or actually incentivizing environmental alterations, as well as individual behavior change, may be necessary to create the type of supportive environments that can sustain weight loss. Using financial incentives to initiate change, then sustaining longer-term change with nonfinancial and less costly incentives merits investigation. Testing the efficacy of nonfinancial incentives only, such as social media tie-ins or access only to favorite items at the gym, is also important to examine given that they may be more scalable. Last, when financial incentives are an option, such as with the majority of employers currently offering wellness programs, it is important to encourage use of evidence-based incentive models. While there is still much to learn about how to optimize incentives in promoting healthy weight control, when done well, they represent an important evidence-based strategy for reducing obesity.

Acknowledgments

Preparation of this chapter was supported in part by National Institutes of Health Center of Biomedical Research Excellence Award No. P20GM103644 from the National Institute of General Medical Sciences.

Suggested Reading

Higgins, S., Silverman, K., Sigmon, S., & Naito, N. (2012). Incentives and health: An introduction. *Preventive Medicine, 55,* S2–S6.—A helpful overview of research on incentives for health behaviors. Situates the current climate in historical context and summarizes areas for future inquiry. Also introduces interested readers to further references for overviews on incentives in both the substance abuse literature and the obesity literature in a supplemental issue of *Preventive Medicine* devoted exclusively to the topic of incentives and health.

Jeffery, R. W. (2012). Financial incentives and weight control. *Preventive Medicine, 55*(Suppl.), S61–S67.—Recent review of incentives for weight loss. Incentives for weight loss resulted in twofold greater weight losses than incentives for attendance can be found in this source. Also details the Jeffery et al. (1978) study, the study by Finkelstein et al. (2007) using $7 or $14 incentives, and the study by Volpp et al. (2008) using a lottery incentive scheme to induce weight loss of 13.1 pounds, as referenced in the chapter.

John, L. K., Loewenstein, G., Troxel, A. B., Norton, L., Fassbender, J. E., & Volpp, K. G. (2011). Financial incentives for extended weight loss: A randomized, controlled trial. *Journal of General Internal Medicine, 26*(6), 621–626.—This trial of deposit contracts for weight loss over 32 weeks found that deposit contract participants lost 8.7 pounds compared to 1.2 pounds for the control condition.

Leahey, T. M., Subak, L. L., Fava, J., Schembri, M., Thomas, G., Xu, X., et al. (2015). Benefits of adding small financial incentives or optional group meetings to a Web-based statewide obesity initiative. *Obesity, 23*(1), 70–76.—One of the only studies to address cost-effectiveness of incentives for weight management. The authors found that incentives were more cost-effective than optional group sessions in a community-based Internet behavioral weight management program. This study also provides some support for the effiacy of incentives for long-term weight loss.

Liu, P., Wisdom, J., Roberto, C. A., Liu, L. J., & Ubel, P. A. (2013). Using behavioral economics to design more effective food policies to address obesity. *Applied Economic Perspectives and Policy, 36*(1), 6–24.—Examines the use of behavioral economic strategies, including choice architecture and information provision interventions, to address our decision-making biases.

Lussier, J. P., Heil, S. H., Mongeon, J. A., Badger, G. J., & Higgins, S. T. (2006). A meta-analysis of voucher-based reinforcement therapy for substance use disorders. *Addiction, 101,* 192–203.—A meta-analysis of the effects of financial incentives in reducing a wide range of different types of substance abuse.

Paul-Ebhohimhen, V., & Avenell, A. (2008). Systematic review of the use of financial incentives in treatments for obesity and overweight. *Obesity Reviews, 9*(4), 355–367.—Systematic review of incentives for obesity treatment. Examines various treatment parameters, such as duration, amount, frequency, and total weight loss achieved.

Purnell, J. Q., Gernes, R., Stein, R., Sherraden, M. S., & Knoblock-Hahn, A. (2014). A systematic review of financial incentives for dietary behavior change. *Journal of the Academy of Nutrition and Dietetics, 114,* 1023–1035.—A review of various study designs from 2006 to 2012 using incentives to promote dietary change. Suggests that incentives need to be theory based, and that more research is needed to deterrmine optimal amount, design, and type of incentives used.

RAND Health. (2013). *Workplace Wellness Programs Study.* Arlington, VA: RAND Corporation.—Overview of the prevalence of incentives in employer wellness programs, types of incentives being used, and the need for future research on best practices.

Thaler, R., & Sunstein, C. (2008). *Nudge: Improving decisions about health, wealth, and happiness.* New Haven, CT: Yale University Press.—Introduction to behavioral economic strategy and the use of nudges for healthy behaviors.

102

Taxes as a Means for Addressing Obesity

TATIANA ANDREYEVA
FRANK J. CHALOUPKA
JAMIE F. CHRIQUI

As the prevalence of obesity and diet-related noncommunicable diseases (NCDs) has reached epidemic proportions in the United States and globally, economic tools to incentivize behavior changes have become commonplace on the obesity-focused policy menu. Price changes through fiscal interventions, including taxes and subsidies, are central to these discussions. The economic theory behind the proposed fiscal approaches is the sensitivity of consumer demand to price changes and the predictable nature of price–demand shifts, which is a negative correlation for virtually all goods and services. Price promotions are routinely used by retailers and manufacturers to increase sales of their products by making them cheaper compared to alternatives. Raising prices works in the opposite way by increasing the relative cost of the targeted products and shifting consumers toward purchases of less expensive substitutes or other goods. Fiscal policy can encourage behavior changes by shifting relative prices up (through taxation) or down (through subsidies).

Taxation of products known to cause public health problems, such as tobacco or alcohol, has long been an effective strategy to discourage unhealthy behaviors. Many cities, states, and countries around the globe have seen significant declines in tobacco use as a result of increasing tobacco taxes. The body of evidence on the success of tobacco taxes has encouraged public health advocates and policymakers to consider taxation as a tool to discourage consumption of foods and beverages known as major contributors to obesity and many NCDs. Dietary factors, which are all modifiable, are estimated to account for about 40% of NCD-related mortality that in turn accounts for over 60% of deaths worldwide. Millions of premature deaths and billions of health care dollars can be avoided by addressing the major dietary deficiencies, namely, low intake of fruits, vegetables, and whole grains, and excessive consumption of added sugars, saturated fats, and sodium. Improving the diet of the population has become a key public health objective.

As with tobacco taxation, several economic considerations support government intervention in response to the obesity crisis. These are known as market failures to economists and include, at a minimum, externalities, asymmetric information, and time-inconsistent preferences. *Externalities* are costs to parties who did not choose to incur those costs; another person's or company's choices impose a cost on a third party. Well-known examples of externalities in public health include secondhand smoke, air pollution, and drunk driving. For obesity, there are significant external costs of individual decisions to manufacture and/or consume excessive amounts of unhealthy foods that lead to weight gain. These costs are in the form of the publicly financed health care costs, disability payments due to obesity, and fitness of military recruits, among others.

Another market failure, *information asymmetry,* is observed because companies have an incentive to present consumers only with beneficial information about their products or services. Thousands of marketing experts work creatively to influence consumer choices by advertising the positive features of their products, while withholding potentially unfavorable information, unless required by law to disclose it. For example, drug advertising has to include information about adverse effects of the drugs. All packaged foods in the United States are required to have a standard Nutrition Facts Panel and list ingredients. Menu labeling in chain restaurants is another example of the government trying to respond to information asymmetry in the food market and help consumers make informed decisions.

Finally, *time-inconsistent preferences* are choices or decisions made at different points in time that may be inconsistent with each other. A person's choice could be very satisfying in the short term but have negative consequences in a more distant future. With food, people often make choices based on their liking at the moment (tasty, convenient, affordable), with relatively little consideration for health outcomes years later.

Targets for Taxation

Taxation of calorie-dense, nutrient-poor foods and beverages is a promising strategy to encourage healthier diets and improve public health. The economics of higher prices would encourage consumers to switch away from taxable items to healthier options and ultimately healthier diets. In the long run, healthier eating habits would be expected to translate into reduced incidence of obesity and other NCDs, namely, heart disease and type 2 diabetes, as well as savings in health care costs and productivity gains. Earmarking of tax revenues toward effective health promotion and nutrition education programs could lead to additional behavior shifts and greater dietary and health benefits. Potential for promoting healthier food choices is further enhanced when taxes are implemented with other policies, as in the case of tobacco, with indoor smoking restrictions and minimum age limits on purchases. Implementing taxes in tandem with evidence-based nonfiscal policies is likely to be most effective in achieving public health gains.

The most publicized and potentially promising economic response to the obesity epidemic in the United States is taxation of sugary drinks, or beverages with added caloric sweeteners. Sugary drinks are the leading source of added sugar in the American diet, which makes them a straightforward choice in consideration of tax strategies to reduce excessive sugar intake and improve diet quality. Despite recent declines in consumption of sugary drinks among children and adults, Americans still consume twice as many calories from sugary drinks as several decades ago. In a variety of observational and randomized controlled trials (RCTs), excessive consumption of sugary drinks has been linked to weight gain, increased risk of type 2 diabetes, cardiovascular disease, dental caries, and osteoporosis. Strong scientific evidence on the health effects of excessive sugary drink consumption and decades of economic research on pricing incentives to change behavior have inspired many public health experts to focus specifically on sugary drinks as an appropriate target for taxation.

Another approach is to tax broad categories of foods or nutrients linked to obesity. Known as "taxes based on nutrient profiling," they target foods deemed unhealthy. One example is fast food, which often implies calorie-dense, highly processed, nutrient-poor foods that contribute saturated fat, added sugar and sodium, to the American diet. Prior economic evidence, including multiple longitudinal studies, shows that the low prices of fast food are associated with increasing body weight. Tax-induced increases in fast-food prices could potentially reverse this relationship. Other targets of obesity-related taxation proposals include snack foods, candy, and individual nutrients (saturated fat, sugar, and sodium). For example, Denmark implemented a tax on foods high in saturated fats that was later repealed.

Despite the empirical evidence on the link to obesity, taxation of unhealthy foods presents challenges with design and implementation that require additional research. First, such taxes could pose a problem based on food insecurity concerns, as inexpensive calorie-dense foods are often the primary source of calories and nutrients for low-income populations. Using the new tax revenues to subsidize healthier foods for low-income populations could help ameliorate this problem. Another challenge would be complex rules on how to define the scope of taxable unhealthy foods. A broad definition would mean considerable challenges in identifying eligible foods in the constantly evolving food market, potentially increasing administrative costs. A more limited base of unhealthy foods to be taxed could negate the effect of the tax if consumers switch to other unhealthy options that are not taxable. Finally, in contrast to sugary drinks, many unhealthy foods offer at least some good nutrients.

The Current State and Evidence

Most states already levy small (under 10%) general sales taxes on some items, including sugary drinks, snack foods, and restaurant food. State sales taxes were introduced for general revenue purposes and do not distinguish sugary drinks from healthier alternatives. Many states apply these taxes only to carbonated beverages, including diet versions, while excluding an important and fast-growing market of noncarbonated beverages (e.g., sports drinks, teas). Only a handful of states have volume-specific excise taxes on sugary drinks. Although specific excise taxes are likely to be most effective in modifying food choices (as was the case with tobacco), the existing excise taxes on beverages are very low and do not affect affordability of cheap sugary drinks. One recent exception is the city of Berkeley, California, which became the first U.S. city to implement an excise tax on sugary drinks in the amount that can matter for affordability, namely, a $0.01/ounce excise tax, which represents an approximate increase in price of 20% if businesses pass along the increase fully to consumers. A similar initiative was introduced in Mexico in January 2014, with a 1 peso/liter excise tax on sugary drinks. In November 2016, voters in San Francisco, Oakland, and Albany, which are all in California, as well as voters in Boulder, Colorado, voted in favor of a new excise tax on sugary drinks.

Evidence of the impact of the current low general sales tax on beverage consumption on obesity rates is generally weak, with most studies failing to demonstrate a measurable dent in beverage consumption and dietary and weight outcomes. Some studies find a small effect for certain population groups, such as adolescents at risk for overweight. This limited result would be expected given the low tax rate, the high affordability of sugary drinks, and the relatively low budget share of food expenditure in U.S. household income in general. Diet soft drinks and, in some states, even plain bottled water are not excluded from a sales tax, which reduces the incentive to switch to healthier options. Some consumers do not pay a sales tax on sugary drinks at all: These are purchases made using benefits of the Supplemental Food Assistance Program (SNAP). High consumption of sugary drinks is particularly prevalent in low-income populations, so the tax exclusion of the majority of sugary drink purchases among SNAP participants further undermines the potential effect of a tax to reduce unhealthy beverage purchases. The studies that have looked at prices rather than the small, nonspecific, and not comprehensive sales taxes are more likely to find more significant effects on consumption and weight outcomes.

Lack of evidence of the effects of the low sales taxes in many states has been misconstrued by some to suggest that *any* taxes on sugary drinks do not work. This proposition is unsubstantiated by the fact that the proposed tax strategies of raising prices through a specific excise tax of at least 20% offer a very different approach compared to the existing taxes. The current sales tax is on average about 5%, with some consumers not realizing that soda purchases are subject to a sales tax (because the shelf price does not reflect it) and others not paying it at all (SNAP purchases). Many economists argue that an increase in the shelf price of at least 20% for all consumers is likely to work differently from the scenarios seen in the past with the sales tax, leading to a measurable reduction in consumption (e.g., 20–25%). Preliminary data from the ongoing evaluation of excise taxes on sugary drinks in Mexico offer promising results.

Expected Effects from Modeling and Experimental Studies

Modeling studies of the tax effect on obesity and health outcomes rely on a framework that predicts (based on price elasticity) how unhealthy food/beverage consumption shifts with tax-induced changes in prices. Taking into account all dietary and physical activity changes, inclusive of substitution into untaxable products, changes in overall caloric intake are then estimated and further translated into changes in body weight. Based on shifts in the prevalence of overweight and obesity and known disease risk for obesity, one can further predict downstream changes in the incidence of major diseases linked to obesity (e.g., cardiovascular disease, diabetes mellitus, some cancers), as well as the resulting savings in health care costs and improvement in overall and disability-adjusted life expectancy. For example, a $0.01/ounce tax on sugary drinks in the United States is projected to reduce consumption by 15%, avoid many cases of chronic disease, and save over $17 billion in health care costs. Another study estimated that the same excise tax would reduce sugary drink consumption by 20%, save 32,300 life-years, and save $23.6 billion in health care costs over the 2015–2025 period. The tax intervention was predicted to become cost saving in Year 2 of the tax implementation.

A number of other modeling and experimental studies have contributed to the debate about the effect of tax policies on dietary changes, obesity, and health outcomes. Systematic literature reviews are particularly helpful in consolidating this evidence, interpreting differences in data and methodologies used, and developing a sound basis for policy evaluation. The two most recent systematic reviews concluded that tax policies (as well as subsidies) would be effective at promoting dietary and health improvements. The strength of evidence was moderately strong, with the majority of reviewed studies point-ing to the effectiveness of fiscal policy at increasing consumption of healthier foods and lowering purchases of unhealthy food across populations and settings. The most robust studies showed larger effects for taxes on noncore products that had close nontaxable substitutes, such as sugary drinks. Some uncertainty in the strength of current evidence remains, suggesting a need for longer-term studies at the population level to establish a high-quality evidence base for future policies.

Suggested Reading

Brownell, K. D., Farley, T., Willett, W. C., Popkin, B. M., Chaloupka, F. J., Thompson, J. W., et al. (2009). The public health and economic benefits of taxing sugar-sweetened beverages. *New England Journal of Medicine, 361*(16), 1599–1605.—This health policy report pres-ents evidence on the consumption of sugar-sweetened beverages and related adverse health outcomes. The authors discuss approaches to designing a tax system to promote healthy eat-ing and recover health care costs associated with the high consumption of sugar-sweetened beverages.

Faulkner, G. E., Grootendorst, P., Nguyen, V. H., Andreyeva, T., Arbour-Nicitopoulos, K., Auld, M. C., et al. (2011). Economic instruments for obesity prevention: Results of a scoping review and modified Delphi survey. *International Journal of Behavioral Nutrition and Physical Activity, 8*, 109.—This is a scoping literature review that synthesizes evidence on the impact of economic policies targeting obesity and its causal behaviors, including poor diet and lack of physical activity. The scoping review was based on a structured literature review and con-sultation with experts in the research field through a Delphi survey and an in-person expert panel meeting.

Long, M. W., Gortmaker, S. L., Ward, Z. J., Resch, S. C., Moodie, M. L., Sacks, G., et al. (2015). Cost effectiveness of a sugar-sweetened beverage excise tax in the U.S. *American Journal of Preventive Medicine, 49*(1), 112–123.—This study quantifies the expected health and economic benefits of a national sugar-sweetened beverage excise tax of $0.01/ounce over 10 years. The study provides estimates to suggest that the proposed tax could substantially reduce obesity and health care expenditures and increase healthy life expectancy.

Niebylski, M. L., Redburn, K. A., Duhaney, T., & Campbell, N. R. (2015). Healthy food sub-sidies and unhealthy food taxation: A systematic review of the evidence. *Nutrition, 31*(6), 787–795.—This systematic literature review evaluates the evidence base to assess the effect of healthy food and beverage subsidies and unhealthy food and beverage taxation. The review concludes that food taxes and subsidies should be a minimum of 10–15% and preferably used in tandem with ongoing evaluation of intended and unintended effects.

Powell, L. M., Chriqui, J. F., Khan, T., Wada, R., & Chaloupka, F. J. (2013). Assessing the poten-tial effectiveness of food and beverage taxes and subsidies for improving public health: A systematic review of prices, demand and body weight outcomes. *Obesity Reviews, 14*(2), 110–128.—This is a systematic review of recent U.S. studies on the price elasticity of demand for sugar-sweetened beverages, fast food, fruits and vegetables, as well as the associations of prices/taxes with body weight outcomes.

Thow, A. M., Downs, S., & Jan, S. (2014). A systematic review of the effectiveness of food taxes and subsidies to improve diets: Understanding the recent evidence. *Nutrition Reviews, 72*(9), 551–565.—This systematic review evaluates recent evidence for the effect of food taxes and subsidies on consumption, including an assessment of research quality. The review concludes that taxes and subsidies are likely to be an effective intervention to improve consumption pat-terns associated with obesity and chronic disease, with evidence showing a consistent effect on consumption across a range of tax rates.

Schools, Child Care, and Obesity Policy

MARLENE B. SCHWARTZ
MEGHAN L. O'CONNELL

Among the Institute of Medicine's recommended priority actions for obesity prevention, "improving the school and child care environment" is one of the most important settings for change. There are a number of reasons to focus on schools and child care settings. First, there is a precedent for adopting new health regulations in these settings before doing so in other public spaces (e.g., state laws banning smoking in public high schools preceded smoking bans in restaurants or airports). Second, there are several layers of policy change opportunities because these settings are regulated by a combination of federal, state, and local regulations. Third, schools and child care settings have a powerful set of advocates, most importantly, parents, who have been able to mobilize and promote improvements to the environments where children spend so much of their time.

Reach Children Where They Eat, Learn, and Play

Outside of home, children spend more time in school and child care than anywhere else. This creates an opportunity for schools and child care centers to influence children's diets and levels of physical activity significantly. When these settings provide healthy meals and snacks, teach children about food and nutrition, and provide positive caregiver role modeling, children have opportunities to practice healthful eating and to develop preferences for healthy foods. On the physical activity side, both child care settings and schools can provide a combination of physical education, teacher role modeling, and opportunities for structured and unstructured physical activity. Research supports the assertion that the nutrition and physical activity environments in child care and schools make a meaningful difference in children's diets and health.

The Influence of Federal Food Program Policies through Schools and Child Care

Federal laws regulate much of the food environment in schools and child care centers due to the prominence of federal food programs. The most important programs in these settings are the National School Lunch Program (NSLP), the National School Breakfast Program (NSBP), and the Child and Adult Care Food Program (CACFP). These programs are regulated at the federal level but administered at the state level, usually through the a state's Department of Education. Federal funding is provided to states to support the programs, and some states add additional financial support. Because these meals and snacks are subsidized, they are available to low-income children at either low or no cost.

The NSLP is the largest of these programs and currently reaches 30 million children each day. This program was established in 1946 to remedy the malnutrition suffered by young Americans due to a lack of access to adequate nutrients. Nutrition regulations at that time focused on providing a variety of foods in adequate portions, with calorie minimums (but not maximums). Six decades later, American children are facing a different type of malnutrition; specifically, overconsumption of calories, fat, sugar, and sodium, and underconsumption of fruits and vegetables, whole grains, low-fat dairy, and lean proteins.

Research conducted during the 1990s and early 2000s suggested that the availability of unhealthy meals and snacks in schools was contributing to poor diet and obesity risk. The regulations that had been appropriate for previous generations were now entirely out of date. Most problematically, cafeterias and school hallways had become sources of a wide range of sugary beverages and empty-calorie snacks. Only the reimbursable school lunch was regulated; the chips, candy, and baked goods from vending machines, à la carte lines, school stores, and fund-raisers were not regulated. These items are referred to as "competitive foods" because they compete with school meals. The beverage industry, in particular, took advantage of this loophole in the regulation and by the end of the 1990s had branded vending machines in the majority of American high schools. Similarly, fast food and branded snacks inundated school cafeterias, competing with the school lunch and exposing children to marketing for unhealthy foods every day.

In response, the 2010 Healthy, Hunger-Free Kids Act required the U.S. Department of Agriculture (USDA) to update the nutrition standards of the school meals programs to address the dietary shortfalls of children's diets. Significant changes were made: Meals had both minimum and maximum calorie limits; a greater variety and larger servings of fruits and vegetables were required; whole grain requirements increased; sodium limits were set; and in order for a meal to count as a reimbursable lunch, a fruit or vegetable had to be included. Early research on the influence of these changes is promising; students appear to be accepting the new meals, especially in districts that serve lower-income communities.

In 2014, another major improvement was made: the USDA Smart Snacks rule required that all competitive foods must also meet nutrition standards for calories, fat, sodium, and sugar. This change has the potential to reduce significantly the empty calories sold in schools. One challenge, however, is ensuring that the new regulation is understood and implemented. Food service providers are accustomed to assessing nutrition and following policies; however, multiple people sell snacks: administrators, teachers, parents, and other students. Education and training are needed to ensure fidelity to the new regulations.

For very young children, CACFP provides federal funding to licensed, nonprofit child care centers and for-profit centers enrolling at least 25% of children from low-income families. Like the school meal programs, CACFP sets minimum nutrition requirements that must be met for reimbursement. Currently these address the number and size of servings of meal components (meat/meat alternative, milk, fruit and vegetables, grains). While studies show that centers participating in CACFP provide healthier meals and snacks than those that do not, several studies have also documented that CACFP participating centers can meet the requirements while still serving foods that are high in saturated fat, sugar, and sodium. Improvements that have been proposed by the Institute of Medicine and the USDA are very similar to those for school meals; they require whole grains, increase servings of fruits and vegetables, and decrease servings of foods high in saturated and trans fats, sugar, and sodium.

The Role of State and Municipal Government

State and municipal regulations also have potential to impact the food quality and opportunities for physical activity in schools and child care. Some states have passed laws regulating the school environment beyond the federal laws. These can include laws about nutrition standards for competitive foods, adequate time for meals, requirements for physical education, or a minimum length of time for recess. Often policies are enacted at the state level, before the federal government addresses the issue. This allows the policy to be "tested" in one state or city, which can inform the eventual federal policy. For example, the city of Philadelphia removed soda from schools about 10 years before the federal law changed, and the state of Connecticut removed all beverages other than water, 100% juice, and milk from K–12 schools 8 years before the federal Smart Snacks regulations changed the beverage landscape in schools. The fact that these changes had been successfully implemented in some cities and states reassured policymakers that the changes were feasible and did not lead to unintended consequences.

For child care settings, state and municipality licensing regulations provide another opportunity to influence the child care nutrition and activity environment. The Public Health Law Center has developed a 50-state analysis of child care licensing laws, including state statutes and licensing regulations. This analysis suggests that nutrition, physical activity, and screen time regulations vary significantly by state, and that, overall, state regulations are often vague or lacking. There is a great opportunity for public health advocates to work with state legislatures to enact nutrition and physical activity regulations through the licensing mechanism.

Wellness Policies in Schools

At the most local level, there are opportunities to influence policy in schools through wellness policies. The concept of a "local school wellness policy" gained prominence when school districts participating in federal food programs were required by the USDA to create written policies for the 2006–2007 school year, as defined by the 2004 Child Nutrition and Special Supplemental Nutrition Program for Women, Infants, and Children (WIC) Reauthorization Act. Many school districts welcomed this new requirement as an opportunity to organize local committees of stakeholders (i.e., school administrators, teachers, school health professionals, food service personnel, community members, parents and students) to create official policy statements on nutrition education, nutrition standards for foods sold in schools, and physical activity.

Today, a decade after the original legislation was implemented, the school nutrition landscape has improved in meaningful ways. Researchers have been able to study district wellness policies as a unique natural experiment to shed light on how districts with varying characteristics prioritized different components of the policies, and how such policies could influence the school environment and, in turn, student health.

The current body of research describes the strengths and weaknesses of the national patchwork of local policies, how they can create synergy with state laws, and the realized and unrealized potential of the original legislation. The strategy of requiring districts to create their own policies was a success; national surveys suggest that nearly all (99%) districts complied and created a written policy. Some research has shown that written policies tend to be strongest in districts where children are at greatest risk of obesity; therefore, efforts to promote full implementation of strong written wellness policies may especially benefit districts that serve at-risk children, thus improving health equity.

Studies examining the relationship between written policy strength and actual policy implementation have drawn inconsistent conclusions. Some researchers have found that stronger policies lead to improved practices and environments, while others have not observed a significant relationship between policy and practice. A 2014 review by Chriqui, Pickel, and Story documents that some research has identified links between policies and student diets and weight, while other studies have not detected this association. These conflicting findings may be due in some cases to the existence of written policies that are not fully implemented or enforced, or conversely, beneficial practices that are not codified in policy.

Local Policies in Child Care

Child care centers participating in the federal food programs do not have the same wellness policy regulation as school districts; however, there are organizations that strive to influence child care providers in this domain. Specifically, the National Association for the Education of Young Children provides accreditation for early childhood programs that meet specific standards, including compliance with CACFP requirements. Examples of recommended practices with empirical support include supporting mothers' ability to breast-feed (e.g., create comfortable private areas, know how to handle breast milk), not using food as a reward, not taking away physical activity as punishment, maximizing time outdoors for play, limiting screen time, limiting juice, and communicating with families about all of these topics. Specific feeding strategies include increasing portion size and variety of fruits and vegetables, decreasing portions of nutrient-dense foods, seating small numbers of children together, staff modeling of positive eating behaviors, encouraging children to try new foods, and allowing children to serve themselves.

Future Directions

This is an exciting time for researchers and advocates interested in how schools and child care settings can be part of the national effort to address childhood obesity. In just the past few years, tremendous strides have been made by the federal government in strengthening the school and child care food programs. States, cities, school districts, and child care organizations should now focus on maximizing implementation of written policies by providing technical assistance and support to the administrators and food service professionals responsible for making changes on the ground.

The primary challenges facing those fighting for healthier school and child care environments are financial: the potentially higher cost of providing healthier foods, the cost of supporting more time and staff expertise for physical activity, and the resistance of the food industry to abandon schools and fund-raising as marketing opportunities. Encouragingly, surveys of parents over the past 6 years indicate that their support of policies to improve food in schools and reduce unhealthy food marketing has grown stronger over time. The public may believe these changes are the right thing to do, but policymakers and administrators may still need convincing. Research is needed to demonstrate that making schools and child care centers the healthiest environments possible is an investment in our children's health and wellness that will pay dividends for the rest of their lives.

Suggested Reading

American Academy of Pediatrics, American Public Health Association, National Resource Center for Health and Safety in Child Care and Early Education. (2011). *Caring for our children: National health and safety performance standards guidelines for out-of-home child care programs.* Elk Grove Village, IL: American Academy of Pediatrics; Washington, DC: American Public Health Association.—A book produced by the National Resource Center for Health and Safety in Child Care (NRC) through the collaborative efforts of the American Public Health Association, the American Academy of Pediatrics, and the Maternal and Child Health Bureau.

Chriqui, J. F., Pickel, M., & Story, M. (2014). Influence of school competitive food and beverage policies on obesity, consumption, and availability: A systematic review. *JAMA Pediatrics, 168*(3), 279–286.—This review examines the strength of the empirical evidence that competitive food policies influence the environment, consumption, and weight.

Chriqui, J., Resnick, E., Schneider, L., Schermbeck, R., Adcock, T., Carrion, V., et al. (2013). *School district wellness policies: Evaluating progress and potential for improving children's health five years after the federal mandate* (Brief Report, Vol. 3). Princeton, NJ: Robert Wood Johnson Foundation.—These reports are the most comprehensive examination of school wellness policies in the United States.

Institute of Medicine, Food and Nutrition Board. (2016). Reports, consensus statements, and workshops. Available at *www.iomnationalacademies.org.*—The IOM Food and Nutrition Board has over a dozen relevant publications that have been written by committees of experts on topics that include school meals, competitive foods, child care, nutrition education, physical activity, and how to evaluate progress in the school and child care environment.

Story, M., Nanney, M. S., & Schwartz, M. B. (2009). Schools and obesity prevention: Creating school environments and policies to promote healthy eating and physical activity. *Milbank Quarterly, 87*(1), 71–100.—This review provides an overview of the range of food and physical activity policies that are available to schools.

Trust for America's Health. (2016). The state of obesity: Better policies for a healthier America. State school based nutrition and food laws. Retrieved August 24, 2016, from *http://stateofobesity.org.*—This website includes state-by-state analysis of nutrition and food laws, as well as a wide range of obesity-related data for each state.

Addressing the Influence of Food Marketing to Children

JENNIFER L. HARRIS

In 2006, the Institute of Medicine published a comprehensive review of the literature and concluded that "food and beverage marketing practices geared to children and youth are out of balance with healthful diets and contribute to an environment that puts their health at risk" (p. 374). One year earlier, the World Health Organization similarly concluded that food advertising negatively affects children's diets and exploits their unique vulnerabilities. Research clearly showed that young people's overconsumption of the food categories most extensively marketed to youth worldwide, including soda and other sugary drinks, fast food, high-sugar cereals, candy, and snacks, significantly contributed to childhood obesity. Food companies could no longer plausibly deny that their common strategies to market these calorie-dense, nutrient-poor foods directly to children and youth was fueling the worldwide obesity crisis. Solutions directly addressing the unhealthy food environment surrounding children, including unhealthy food marketing, were required.

Since then, the debate has shifted from whether food marketing contributes to childhood obesity to a discussion of solutions that can reduce the proven negative impact of unhealthy food marketing on children's diets and health. The Institute of Medicine's report called on the food industry to demonstrate that it wants to be part of the solution by using its "creativity, resources, and full range of marketing practices" to promote more healthful diets for children and youth. More recently, First Lady Michelle Obama's Let's Move! initiative, designed to address childhood obesity, has announced partnerships with business to market healthier foods to children. Additional commonly proposed solutions include nutrition education (for children and parents), media literacy programs to teach children how to resist the influence of unhealthy food marketing, and social marketing campaigns to encourage children and parents to make healthy choices. At the same time, the food industry has responded by establishing self-regulatory programs worldwide, such as the Children's Food and Beverage Advertising Initiative (CFBAI) in the United

States, with many companies pledging to promote only healthier dietary choices and/or healthier lifestyles to children under age 12.

On the surface, then, it would appear that progress is being made. However, solutions that rely on making healthy choices more attractive and teaching children about the importance of good nutrition and/or how to defend against effects of unhealthy food marketing are based on a fundamental misperception of how food marketing works and how it affects children's health. As a result, these solutions are unlikely to substantially reduce children's preferences for and overconsumption of nutritionally poor foods, especially when supported by extensive marketing.

How Food Marketing Works

Consumers would like to believe that they are in complete control of their purchase decisions—that they consciously consider the information presented in marketing, then make the best choices to meet their needs. However, much of marketing is specifically designed to circumvent this rational consumer decision-making process and to influence consumers indirectly, using tactics borrowed from the current social-cognitive psychological literature. In fact, research shows that the most effective advertisements are those that create emotional connections to brands and convey little or no rational content. Highly persuasive marketing messages evade conscious, rational decision making about product alternatives by providing virtually no concrete information about product attributes or utility.

The primary purpose of today's marketing campaigns is to create a positive brand image that will attract the desired consumer segment. These brand images consist of associations in consumers' minds that link the brand with desirable users, core motivations, and/or positive emotions. For example, Red Bull's "Gives You Wings" campaign associates the product with extreme sports to attract a young, male consumer who wants to be daring and cool. Ads and online games for child-targeted cereals, such as Lucky Charms or Froot Loops, feature magical adventures, and the products' shapes and colors associate sugary cereals with fun in children's minds. Coca-Cola's "Open Happiness" campaign uses highly appealing images, such as cute polar bears and penguins or friendly people sharing a Coke with others, to make just about anyone feel good when they think about this sugary drink.

In addition to conveying positive emotions rather than direct product benefits, common marketing tactics are also designed to disguise the persuasive intent of the message. For example, product placements insert branded messages into the content of TV programming, movies, music, and video games; advergames incorporate branded products into child-friendly games available through websites and mobile apps; sponsorships and philanthropic tie-ins support good causes and promote positive feelings about the brands at the same time. Furthermore, the rise of marketing through social media and celebrity bloggers now enables companies to enlist peers and other influencers to deliver their marketing messages for them. These disguised forms of marketing are specifically designed to counteract increasing skepticism about traditional marketing among young people.

Companies increasingly direct these newer, disguised forms of marketing to children and adolescents. According to a Federal Trade Commission (FTC) report, food company expenditures on these forms of marketing directed at youth have increased, while traditional forms of marketing (e.g., TV, print, and radio) have declined. Legal and consumer behavior experts raise concerns that these common marketing practices may be unfair and deceptive even when aimed at adults. However, they are clearly misleading when directed toward children. The consumer development literature consistently shows that children under the age of 11 or 12 do not have the cognitive capacity to recognize, understand, and consistently resist the persuasive messages in traditional advertising, much less more covert forms of marketing. In addition, marketing often takes advantage of young people's unique developmental vulnerabilities, including their susceptibility to peer influence and reduced ability to forgo short-term rewards (e.g., unhealthy foods) in return for long-term benefits (e.g., good health).

How Food Marketing Affects Children's Health

Although research clearly demonstrates that food marketing increases children's preferences and requests to parents for unhealthy products, and that current marketing practices unfairly exploit young people's credulity, research is just beginning to demonstrate the long-term effects of food marketing on children's diets and health. Early studies indicate significant cause for concern. Experiments show that unhealthy food marketing (including TV advertising and online advergames) increases immediate consumption of any available food among children and adults. Neuroimaging studies exhibit activation of the reward regions in the brain during food ad exposure, with greater susceptibility predicting weight gain in the following year in adolescents. These studies indicate a likely causal relationship between ad exposure and body mass index (BMI; demonstrated consistently in numerous correlational studies). Additional research shows that exposure to marketing messages, including enjoyable advertising, licensed characters, and fast-food packaging, increases children's liking of the taste of promoted foods. Therefore, exposure to advertising for unhealthy foods may lead children to like these foods more than if they had never seen the advertising.

Research also demonstrates that marketing affects how parents feed their children. For example, exposure to fast-food promotion predicted parents' normative beliefs that others often eat and approve of eating fast food, mediating the positive relationship between marketing exposure and greater fast-food consumption by their children. Packaging for nutritionally poor children's foods (including cereal and fruit drinks) is more likely to feature nutrition-related claims, such as "good source of vitamin C" or "all natural ingredients" than comparable adult foods, and these claims lead parents to believe the products are healthier choices for their children. Content analyses of ads for nutritionally poor foods aimed at parents also demonstrate frequent messages about family bonding and/or grateful kids, implying that kids will love these foods and their parents for serving them.

Another growing concern about food marketing is that it exacerbates health disparities among black and Hispanic youth. These young people face greater risks of obesity and other diet-related diseases compared with white non-Hispanic youth, and they are also exposed to a "double dose" of unhealthy food marketing through higher exposure to advertising in the media and more marketing in their local communities. Furthermore, brands in some of the least nutritious product categories, including candy, sugary drinks, and fast food, are more likely to target their advertising to black and Hispanic consumers. Early research also suggests that minority youth may be more susceptible to marketing that targets them directly, as most other advertising does not show actors that look like them, and they may be more responsive to brands or use advertising to assist in assimilating to the majority culture.

Therefore, unhealthy food marketing directed to children and adolescents likely has a profound and lasting impact on children's diets and health, but additional research could strengthen the evidence base for direct causal effects. In particular, longitudinal studies that monitor children's exposure to the full extent of food marketing, as well as their diets and weight status over time, would further establish the effects of marketing beyond TV advertising.

How to Solve the Problem

The solution is clear. The overwhelming amount of marketing for highly palatable but nutritionally poor foods and beverages aimed at youth must stop. Given the subtle but powerful psychological marketing techniques utilized to make these products so appealing, teaching children to resist its influence is futile. Children eat what they think tastes good, and nutrition education cannot teach children to like the taste of healthier foods more than junk food, especially food designed by food scientists to be impossible to resist. Similarly, media literacy programs can teach children to be skeptical of advertising, but there is no evidence that skepticism provides children (or even adults) the ability to resist the strong emotional implicit appeals of advertising for highly desirable products, especially when designed to take advantage of developmental vulnerabilities or disguise the message inside another form of entertainment. Actions to shield children from exposure to this harmful influence are required.

Encouraging the food industry to reduce unhealthy food marketing to children is also unlikely to succeed. Eight years after the food industry established the CFBAI in the United States, companies continue to spend $1.8 billion annually to market almost exclusively unhealthy food directly to children and adolescents. As companies have increased the number of healthier products in their overall portfolios, virtually all products advertised to children remain high in sugar, saturated fat, or sodium. Furthermore, children's total exposure to food advertising has not declined, while adolescents' exposure has increased significantly. It appears that competition and the need to continually grow shareholder profits present an enormous barrier to change by individual companies. In addition, public health campaigns to encourage healthy eating could never receive enough funding to compete with this onslaught of unhealthy food marketing.

Therefore, action by key change agents—including researchers, consumers, and policymakers—will likely be required for companies to make the dramatic improvements required to protect children from exposure to unhealthy food marketing. Recently this approach has had some success. For example, researchers have thoroughly documented the limitations of the CFBAI in the United States, and the program responded with several improvements. Advocacy groups have implemented successful advocacy campaigns to encourage companies to improve specific child-directed food marketing practices and educate parents about the extent and poor nutritional quality of food marketing to children. Parents have responded by purchasing fewer sugary cereals, soda, and other sugary drinks for their children. The USDA's Healthy Hunger-Free Children's Act now prohibits companies from marketing products in schools that do not meet nutrition standards. Furthermore, local governments increasingly propose legislation to reduce the impact of child-directed marketing in local communities, such as setting nutrition standards for kids' meals at fast-food restaurants, placing warning labels on sugary drinks, and limiting the sale of energy drinks to minors.

With increased understanding and public recognition of the harm that unhealthy food marketing has on children's health, momentum is building to pressure companies to reduce children's exposure to these messages. Will eliminating unhealthy food marketing solve the problem of poor diet and obesity in children? Of course not. The problem is too complex and multidimensional to rely on just one solution. However, it will be impossible to substantially improve children's diets without also protecting them from marketing messages for junk food that drown out and outmaneuver the messages from parents, schools, and others who care about children's health.

Suggested Reading

Federal Trade Commission. (2012). *A review of food marketing to children and adolescents: Follow-up report*. Washington DC: Author. Available at *www.ftc.gov/os/2012/12/12122 1foodmarketingreport.pdf.*—The FTC subpoenaed major food and beverage companies to obtain detailed expenditure data on marketing to children and adolescents by type in 2006 and 2009.

Harris, J. L., Brownell, K. D., & Bargh, J. A. (2009). The food marketing defense model: Integrating psychological research to protect youth and inform public policy. *Social Issues and Policy Review, 3*(1), 211–271.—Reviews the literature to examine the psychological mechanisms through which marketing affects young people and how to defend against unwanted influence, and proposes a research agenda to inform public policy to effectively protect youth from harmful effects of food marketing.

Harris, J. L., & Graff, S. K. (2012). Protecting young people from junk food advertising: Implications of psychological research for First Amendment law. *American Journal of Public Health, 102*, 214–222.—Discusses potential options to regulate unhealthy food marketing to young people within Constitutional constraints in the United States.

Institute of Medicine, National Academy of Sciences, Committee on Food Marketing and the Diets of Children and Youth. (2006). *Food marketing to children and youth: Threat or opportunity?* (J. M. McGinnis, J. Gootman, & V. I. Kraak, Eds.). Washington, DC: National Academies Press.—Provides a comprehensive review of the literature on children's diets, food marketing to children, and its effects.

Powell, L. M., Harris, J. L., & Fox, T. (2013). Food marketing expenditures aimed at youth: Putting the numbers in context. *American Journal of Preventive Medicine, 45*(4), 453–461.—Summarizes the research on the extent and amount of food marketing to children and adolescents and the nutritional quality of advertised products to evaluate the impact of the CFBAI and explain changes in expenditures detailed in the FTC report.

Changing Physical Activity Environments

JAMES F. SALLIS

Defining Physical Activity Environments

Physical activity is usually done in specific settings that can be thought of as physical activity environments. Parks and private recreation facilities such as health clubs and dance studios are common places for leisure-time physical activity. Walking and bicycling for transportation is done on sidewalks and bicycle infrastructure such as trails, bike lanes, and separate cycleways. These transportation facilities also are used for leisure and exercise purposes. Children are active at schools, preschools, and child care programs. Workplaces and buildings in general can be designed to promote physical activity, for example, by making stairs highly visible, convenient, and attractive. Homes can become physical activity environments with the addition of exercise equipment or weight-lifting supplies.

The problem is that many of these settings are not designed to promote physical activity, especially in the United States. Many neighborhoods lack parks and sidewalks. Roads are designed to optimize travel by car, with a side effect of making walking and bicycling dangerous. Many education and child care settings have limited space for physical activity. Stairs are hidden and unappealing in many buildings. Absent or poorly designed physical activity environments present a wide range of barriers to physical activity, so there are many opportunities to intervene.

It is worthwhile to consider three levels of environmental interventions. Presence or proximity is the first goal, such as having a park and shops within walking distance and having good coverage of sidewalks and bicycle facilities. A second goal is to design the setting to support or facilitate physical activity. This can be done by putting a playground and walking track in the park, making sidewalks wide and shaded by trees or awnings, and building shops to open onto the sidewalk instead of a parking lot, so that they encourage walking. A third goal is to promote use of physical activity environments through events and physical activity classes in parks, family bicycling days on trails, and opening school grounds for community use.

The nature of physical activity environments requires both researchers and practitioners to collaborate with professionals in multiple sectors. Partnerships with city planners, urban designers, transportation engineers, park and recreation professionals, landscape architects, architects, and education professionals have become common. Professionals trained in public health, medicine, behavioral science, and exercise science rarely have expertise in physical activity environments and are not involved in decisions about the design of those environments, so health professionals must work with leaders in other disciplines and sectors to achieve health goals.

The Role of Environments in Shaping Physical Activity

Because it is difficult to randomly assign people to live in specific neighborhoods or to randomize neighborhoods for environmental renovation, the vast majority of the literature on physical activity environments is observational and cross-sectional. Though there are important limitations of such studies, much has been learned. The most studied variables have been at the "macro" level, dealing with the layout of communities and land use. Adrian Bauman and colleagues (2012) conducted a review of reviews and identified several environmental variables with the best evidence of correlations with physical activity of adults. These included walkability of neighborhoods, such that residents of higher-density mixed land use areas, with destinations such as shops and schools within walking distance of homes, were substantially more active than people who lived in suburban-style areas with homes far from shopping areas. One study indicated that adults in high-walkability neighborhoods did 35–49 more minutes of physical activity per week than people in low-walkability areas. Thus, improving walkability of a neighborhood could help residents obtain up to one-third of the 150 minutes/week physical activity recommendation. The review by Bauman and colleagues also found that facilities for walking and bicycling, proximity to recreation facilities, and neighborhood aesthetics were related to physical activity of adults, children, and adolescents.

Newer evidence points to the importance of micro-scale environmental variables in shaping physical activity. "Micro-scale" refers to the design of streetscapes that might affect the experience of people being active there. Example attributes include sidewalk width and maintenance; trees and shade; design of street crossings; and indicators of social disorder, such as graffiti. These environmental details can be assessed by trained observers. Sallis and colleagues (2012) found that total streetscape quality scores were related to walking for transportation among children, adolescents, adults, and older adults. Aesthetic attributes were related to leisure-time physical activity. Micro-scale attributes can be feasibly changed with realistic budgets and time lines.

A disturbing finding is that the quality of physical activity environments is often lower in communities with highest risk for obesity and chronic diseases. Lack of parks is twice as common in mostly African American and Latino neighborhoods than in mostly non-Hispanic white neighborhoods. Sidewalks and safe street crossings have been found to be less common in low-income neighborhoods. These environmental disparities provide an evidence-based rationale for interventions to improve the activity-supportiveness of environments in low-income and mostly minority neighborhoods.

Evaluating Environmental Changes

To improve the rigor of evidence, a priority is being placed on studies that evaluate the impact of environmental changes on physical activity. Almost all such studies are considered "natural experiments" or evaluations of changes that the investigators do not control. Some studies include comparison conditions; others do not.

The first painted bike lane in the city of New Orleans, Louisiana, was evaluated by counting bicyclists and pedestrians before and after the installation. Some nearby streets were also evaluated to determine whether the new lane actually attracted new riders or bicyclists merely changed their routes. Results indicated the net increase in bicycling on the street with bike lane was about 250%.

The Trust for Public Land installed Family Fitness Zones in 10 parks in low-income Los Angeles neighborhoods. The zones are outfitted with outdoor equipment that can be used for aerobic and strengthening exercise by anyone age 13 years and older. The evaluation was conducted by Deborah Cohen and colleagues (2012), who compared the intervention parks with 10 control parks before and after the installations. Observations revealed that the new equipment was used, though use declined somewhat over time. Overall park use increased in the intervention parks located in densely populated areas. More physical activity was observed in intervention parks.

Safe Routes to School is a federal initiative to provide funding to schools to encourage walking and biking to school through several strategies, including encouragement and environmental changes such as adding or improving sidewalks, crosswalks, and signage around schools. Recent uncontrolled evaluations across several states showed active transport to school increased about 40%, and the impact increased over time.

An ambitious study was undertaken in Perth, Western Australia, by Billie Giles-Corti and colleagues (2014) to evaluate the impact of moving to new neighborhoods that varied on walkability. This is one of very few studies that answered the question of whether the same person's behavior is different when he or she moves to a different type of neighborhood. The authors found that the extent of walkable community design and pedestrian-oriented transportation facilities were strongly related to walking for transportation.

Studies on bicycling interventions have important lessons. Controlled studies of single interventions, such as provision of bike lanes, separated paths, bicycle traffic signals, bike sharing programs, bike parking, and education, usually indicate that the interventions have little impact. By contrast, John Pucher and colleagues (2010) reported rates of bicycling for transportation before and after more than 20 cities around the world made many significant changes over several years to increase bicycling. Rates of bicycling increased substantially in all cities except one, Groningen, The Netherlands, which had 40% of all trips by bicycle at the beginning. Thus, it appears that major and multiple environmental changes may be needed to change physical activity.

In summary, the extensive correlational evidence linking built environments and physical activity is extended by evaluations of environmental changes. Environmental changes in parks, roadways, and communities have been related to physical activity for both recreation and transportation purposes.

The Practice of Changing Physical Activity Environments

Communities around the United States and abroad are making changes designed to increase physical activity. Whereas some are motivated by improving health, others are more motivated by the economic development benefits. Some efforts have been supported by foundations, such as Active Living by Design, funded by the Robert Wood Johnson Foundation. This demonstration program involved 49 mostly disadvantaged communities. Multisector groups were assisted in creating environmental and policy changes supported by promotional activities, and informed by community engagement.

The U.S. Centers for Disease Control and Prevention has funded states, communities, and tribes to make policy, systems, and environment changes designed to improve physical activity, improve eating habits, and prevent obesity. Communities Putting Prevention to Work and Community Transformation Grants provided hundreds of millions of dollars to support communitywide changes. These grants built capacity for creating communitywide change and provided models about how to make permanent environmental changes that promote health.

Conclusions

The public health importance of physical activity environments is that optimizing the design of these environments is expected to have effects on virtually all residents for as long as they are in those settings. Many consider the massive investments in automobile-centric transportation and sprawling development with large distances between homes and destinations to be critical root causes of the inactivity and obesity epidemics. Within the public health field, changing physical activity environments has become a central focus of initiatives to increase physical activity and to prevent and manage obesity. There have been increasing efforts over the past 15 years to understand through research how the environment shapes physical activity and identify which attributes of environments are most important. Multisector partnerships and collaborations are now common at the local, state, and national levels. Public health departments are developing expertise in working with partners in other sectors to pursue strategies that improve environments for physical activity, while achieving other goals, such as reducing traffic, pollution, and carbon emissions, and enhancing economic vitality. There are many examples of communities making major changes to physical activity environments such as parks, schools, roads, and community design, and evidence is accumulating that these environmental changes can increase physical activity. Environmental change is a central part of all national physical activity plans and the World Health Organization's efforts to increase physical activity internationally.

Acknowledgment

This work was supported by National Institutes of Health Grant No, HL111378 and by the Robert Wood Johnson Foundation.

Suggested Reading

Bauman, A. E., Reis, R. S., Sallis, J. F., Wells, J. C., Loos, R. J., Martin, B. W., et al. (2012). Correlates of physical activity: Why are some people physically active and others not? *Lancet, 380,* 258–271.—This article includes a review of reviews indicating that there is good evidence that several built environment variables are related to physical activity of both youth and adults.

Cohen, D. A., Marsh, T., Williamson, S., Golinelli, D., & McKenzie, T. L. (2012). Impact and cost-effectiveness of Family Fitness Zones: A natural experiment in urban parks. *Health and Place, 18,* 39–45.—This study found that adding outdoor fitness equipment in parks increased physical activity in those parks, especially those in densely populated neighborhoods.

Hooper, P., Giles-Corti, B., & Knuiman, M. (2014). Evaluating the implementation and active living impacts of a state government planning policy designed to create walkable neighborhoods in Perth, Western Australia. *American Journal of Health Promotion, 28*(Suppl. 3), S5–S18.—A natural experiment demonstrated that people who moved to more physical activity–supportive environments did more walking as a means of transportation.

McDonald, N. (2015). *Impact of Safe Routes to School programs on walking and biking* (Research brief). San Diego, CA: Active Living Research. Retrieved from *http://activelivingresearch.org/impact-safe-routes-school-programs-walking-and-biking.*—This brief summarizes recent evaluations showing that Safe Routes to School interventions increased active transport to school.

Parker, K. M., Rice, J., Gustat, J., Ruley, J., Spriggs, A., & Johnson, C. (2013). Effect of bike lane infrastructure improvements on ridership in one New Orleans neighborhood. *Annals of Behavioral Medicine, 45*(1), 101–107.—This natural experiment indicates that the first bike lane in New Orleans substantially increased bicycling in the area.

Pucher, J., Dill, J., & Handy, S. (2010). Infrastructure, programs, and policies to increase bicycling: An international review. *Preventive Medicine, 50,* S106–S125.—Though controlled studies of single bicycle intervention strategies did not have good evidence of effects, case studies of cities implementing multiple interventions showed substantial increases in bicycling.

Sallis, J. F., Cain, K. L., Conway, T. L., Gavand, K. A., Millstein, R. A., Geremia, C. M., et al. (2015). Is your neighborhood designed to support physical activity?: A brief streetscape audit tool. *Preventing Chronic Disease, 12,* e41.—Scores on a direct observation instrument of streetscape characteristics were related to walking for transportation in children, adolescents, adults, and older adults.

Sallis, J. F., Floyd, M. F., Rodríguez, D. A., & Saelens, B. E. (2012). Role of built environments in physical activity, obesity, and cardiovascular disease. *Circulation, 125*(5), 729–737.—This article provides an overview of the rationale for studying built environments and summarizes the literature.

Sallis, J. F., Saelens, B. E., Frank, L. D., Conway, T. L., Slymen, D. J., Cain, K. L., et al. (2009). Neighborhood built environment and income: Examining multiple health outcomes. *Social Science and Medicine, 68*(7), 1285–1293.—Adult residents of high-walkable neighborhoods had more total physical activity those living in low-walkable neighborhoods, and results were similar across income groups.

Strunk, S. L. (2009). Active Living by Design: Building and sustaining a national program. *American Journal of Preventive Medicine, 37*(6), S457–S460.—This article provides an overview of Active Living by Design community-based interventions and is part of a journal supplement devoted to the program.

Taylor, W., & Lou, D. (2011). *Do all children have places to be active?: Disparities in access to physical activity environments in racial and ethnic minority and lower-income communities* (Research synthesis). San Diego, CA: Active Living Research.—This document summarizes evidence indicating disparities in access to, and quality of, physical activity environments.

Food Labeling and Obesity

CHRISTINA A. ROBERTO
NEHA KHANDPUR
ERIC M. VANEPPS

Obesity is a complex problem with many different causes. One contributing factor may be that people do not have accurate knowledge about the nutritional content of the foods and beverages they consume. For example, Block and colleagues (2013) asked 1,877 adults, 1,178 adolescents, and 330 school-age children exiting 89 restaurants across six major fast-food chains to estimate the kilocalorie (calorie) content of their purchases. They found that adults and adolescents underestimated by 175 calories on average, while school-age children underestimated by 259 calories on average.

One way to educate consumers about the nutrition content of food is through labeling. From a public health perspective, nutrition labels can help improve people's diets in two ways. First, labels are designed to inform consumers of the nutritional value of food, which may encourage healthier dietary decisions. Second, labels can encourage food companies to reformulate products to be healthier. Currently, nutrition labeling takes a variety of forms, some mandated by government and others voluntarily implemented by food companies. In this chapter, we discuss how three of the most common types of nutrition labels—(1) nutrition facts panels on the side or back of food packaging, (2) front-of-package nutrition labels, and (3) restaurant menu labels—influence consumer understanding and behavior, as well as product reformulation.

Nutrition Facts Panels

In the United States, the Nutrition Labeling and Education Act (NLEA) of 1990 required that packaged food products display a nutrition facts panel that provides standardized information on serving size, calories, and calories from fat; total, saturated, and trans fat; and cholesterol, sodium, total carbohydrates, dietary fiber, sugars, and protein. The panel also displays information for certain vitamins and minerals. Nutrient amounts for a single serving are presented in grams and milligrams, and are accompanied by percent daily values (% DV), derived from recommended daily allowances based on a 2,000 calorie diet. Many countries around the world, such as Australia, Chile, China, Guatemala, and Mexico, mandate a similar nutrition label on packaged foods.

Depending on the survey, it is estimated that between 40 and 85% of American consumers report using food labels to inform dietary choices, although research using eye-tracking technology to objectively measure consumer use of nutrition facts panels suggests these self-reports likely overestimate actual label use. Graham and Jeffery (2011) found that 33% of 203 adults reported "almost always" looking at calorie information on nutrition panels when shopping for groceries. However, eye-tracking data from those same participants showed that only 9% of study participants looked at the calorie information during a simulated grocery shopping task.

Even so, these self-reports of label use may predict actual label use and attention to nutrition in one's diet. According to the 2005–2006 National Health and Nutrition Examination Survey, 62% of 5,502 Americans reported using the nutrition facts panel at least sometimes when deciding to buy a food product. In the same study, two dietary recall interviews with 4,454 individuals revealed that participants who reported nutrition label use had significantly lower intake of total energy, total fat, saturated fat, and sugars, as well as higher fiber intake relative to label nonusers. An analysis by Variyam (2008) of in-person and telephone interviews with over 5,400 participants from two nationally representative samples (the 1994–1996 Continuing Survey of Food Intakes by Individuals and the companion Diet and Health Knowledge Survey) found that the introduction of nutrition labels helped label users consume more iron and dietary fiber relative to nonusers. This analysis also revealed that label users generally consumed less fat, saturated fat, and cholesterol than nonusers. However, these latter patterns existed both for labeled foods and for nonlabeled foods consumed outside the home, suggesting that label use is likely correlated with individual characteristics, such as health consciousness or nutrition knowledge, and those characteristics lead to healthy eating behaviors.

Although nutrition facts labels might only influence purchasing decisions among the minority of consumers who regularly use them, they are also credited with prompting product reformulation. Unfortunately, research by Moorman, Ferraro, and Huber (2012) suggests that the NLEA actually led to an unintended *decrease* in the nutrition quality (a combination of fat, cholesterol, sodium, and fiber per serving) of most labeled products. However, there is some evidence that labeling can promote healthier reformulation of those item categories that are particularly unhealthy. Moorman and colleagues showed that firms selling products in low-health categories (e.g., french fries, hot dogs, and pancake syrup) increased their nutrition quality in response to the NLEA. In addition, when the U.S. government mandated that trans-fat content be disclosed on the nutrition panel in January 2006, food manufacturers and restaurants began reformulating certain items. One U.S. study found that 178 of 270 (66%) products containing .5 g or more of trans fatty acids had reduced the levels of trans fat between 2007 and 2011.

Front-of-Package Nutrition Labels

Labels designed to appear on the front of food packaging generally provide less detailed information than nutrition facts panels to help consumers make quick judgments about food products. These labeling schemes vary in the degree to which the label helps consumers. One approach adopted by some food manufacturers in the United States is called Facts Up Front. This label displays information about calories, saturated fat, sodium, and sugars per serving, as well as up to two nutrients to encourage (e.g., fiber, vitamin A), in both absolute quantities (grams or milligrams) and in %DV. Public health researchers and scientists have raised concerns about systems like Facts Up Front based on research indicating that consumers find percentages on front-of-package labels confusing and prefer simpler labeling schemes. In addition, the highlighting of beneficial nutrients, such as fiber, might make unhealthy products appear healthier than is actually the case.

Other interpretive labeling systems strive to make nutrition information more accessible. For example, in the United Kingdom, some food manufacturers use a traffic light labeling system that uses red (high), yellow (medium), or green (low) colored circles to signify amounts of unhealthy nutrients such as sugar, salt, and saturated fat in a product. Thorndike and colleagues (2014) conducted an intervention study in a hospital cafeteria using a traffic light system to indicate the overall healthfulness of items coupled with a choice architecture intervention that placed bottled water and other healthy items in highly visible places. Two years later, they found that the proportion of sales of red items decreased by 4% and sales of green items increased by 6%; results were more marked for beverages. Although this study was done in conjunction with structural changes to item placement in the cafeteria, it provides some of the most compelling data that traffic lights might help to encourage healthier purchases.

Another common interpretive labeling format is the use of a rank-ordered symbol, such as the three-star Guiding Stars system used by the U.S-based Hannaford supermarket chain or the five-star voluntary system announced in Australia. These systems use fewer stars to indicate less healthy products and more stars to indicate healthier products. An even simpler approach is to place a symbol on the front of a product to signify that a product meets a specific nutritional threshold or has been approved by a health-related organization, such as the American Heart Association. One such example is the Choices checkmark symbol used in the Netherlands, Poland, and the Czech Republic, which identifies items with relatively less sodium, fat, and sugar than other items in the same product category.

Front-of-package labels, whether by virtue of their location, simplicity, or presentation format, may be better able to capture consumers' attention than nutrition facts panels on the side and back of food packaging. Related evidence from studies that have evaluated supermarket shelf-tag labeling systems, which are labels placed on supermarket shelves rather than on actual products, suggests that these simple labeling strategies can promote the sale of healthier foods.

Studies have also found that disclosing nutrition information via a front-of-package label has been associated with product reformulation. For example, the Pick the Tick program in New Zealand was credited with the reduction of nearly 33 tons of salt in the food supply over a 1-year period. In the Netherlands, Vyth and colleagues (2010) collected data from 40% of the 119 food manufacturers participating in the Choices program. They found that 168 products were reformulated after the Choices front-of-package logo was introduced and 236 newly developed products meeting the Choices criteria were introduced into the market. The study reported significant decreases in sodium, saturated fatty acids, and added sugars across various product categories. Sodium was the most frequently reformulated nutrient, particularly in processed meats and soups, suggesting that sodium content can change, and that front-of-package labels may motivate healthier product reformulation.

Menu Labeling

Menu labeling refers to displaying nutrition information on restaurant menus and menu boards, so that it is visible at the point of purchase. In the United States, the Patient Protection and Affordable Care Act of 2010 mandates that chain restaurants with 20 or more locations post calorie information on menus, although nationwide implementation has been delayed. However, several cities and states have already required menu labeling, and it has been mandated and implemented in other countries, such as Australia and South Korea, and adopted on a voluntary basis across the United Kingdom. Research has shown that consumers often struggle to estimate the calorie content of restaurant items, suggesting that clearer provision of this information is needed to facilitate lower-calorie choices. Although nutrition information in some chain restaurants has been available for some time, through posters, brochures, or computer kiosks, one study found that only six out of 4,311 (0.1%) people sought out this information while in the restaurant, suggesting a need for more salient displays of nutrition information.

Several national polls in the United States have shown strong public support for menu labeling policies, revealing that over 70% of the respondents favor restaurant calorie labeling. However, research on the impact of labeling on consumer choice is mixed. Two observational studies conducted in New York City ($N = 1,156$) and Philadelphia ($N = 2,083$) compared individuals at fast-food restaurants before and after the implementation of menu labeling, and did not show differences in calories ordered. These studies controlled for gender, age, ethnicity, and education and had comparison cities (Newark and Baltimore, respectively) as controls. Another observational study in Seattle of chain taco restaurants with and without labeling also did not detect an effect of labeling. In contrast, a study of 316 Starbucks outlets, with data on over 100 million transactions that included control stores, observed a 6% average decrease in calories purchased per transaction in the presence of calorie labeling. The decrease in calories was driven largely by a decrease in food calories purchased, while calories from beverages stayed the same. Although revenue per transaction was slightly reduced in the presence of calorie labels, the total number of transactions per day slightly increased, causing no net change in average revenue generated. In addition, a cross-sectional study of 648 consumers at a large, casual dining restaurant chain showed that diners in Philadelphia (where menu labeling requirements include calories, sodium, fat, saturated fat, and carbohydrates) purchased 151 fewer calories and significantly less saturated fat and carbohydrates than diners outside of Philadelphia (where menus were unlabeled). Finally, an experimental study had corporate employees place lunch orders from their company's onsite cafeteria through a newly launched website. They found that orders placed using calorie labeling reduced calories by 10% compared to orders placed in the absence of calorie labels, suggesting a benefit of calorie labeling in non-fast-food settings.

The effect of menu labeling on calories purchased will become clearer as more data are gathered over time across diverse settings. The current evidence suggests that certain consumers (e.g., women, higher-income patrons) are more likely to use calorie labels when making purchasing decisions, but more research is needed to better understand where and for whom calorie labels encourage healthier choices. However, even if only a small segment of the population uses calorie labeling to inform their food choices, many more people will benefit if labeling encourages healthier menu offerings.

Early analyses suggest that menu labeling may be prompting reformulation. Bruemmer and colleagues (2012) audited the calorie, saturated fat, and sodium content of entrees in 37 sit-down and quick-service chains 6 months and 18 months after the implementation of menu labeling legislation. With the exception of pizza chains, entrees that were included at both time periods had significantly fewer calories at 18 months than at 6 months, demonstrating reformulation among these items. In addition, the total proportion of entrees that exceeded recommended calorie levels decreased from 60 to 56%, saturated fat from 79 to 77%, and sodium from 91 to 89%. Similarly, the introduction of menu calorie labeling laws in certain cities, counties, and states between 2005 and 2011 may have prompted fast-food chains operating in those jurisdictions to increase the proportion of healthy food options on menus from 13 to 20%, whereas the proportion of healthy items at fast-food chains operating outside those jurisdictions has remained constant at 8%. There is always a worry that food reformulation will fail to lead to healthier overall offerings. For instance, although a restaurant might reduce the calorie and fat content of an item, it may compensate by simultaneously increasing sodium content. Thus, it will be important to evaluate the overall nutritional profile of foods offered following the nationwide implementation of menu labeling in the United States and in other countries.

Moving Toward Better Labeling Systems

Despite the substantial effort and resources invested in nutrition labels, people still may fail to use them as often as public health advocates would like, in part because nutrition information remains complex. Consumers with limited literacy and numeracy often have difficulty understanding numerical information on labels, especially for products with multiple servings. Research indicates that specific groups are less likely to understand and use labels, including older adults, black non-Hispanics and other ethnic minorities, those with a low annual household income, and those without a college education. Such trends are concerning because these groups are at higher risk for poor diet and obesity.

Nutrition labels have an essential role to play in improving public health, and attention needs to be paid to the best means of delivering nutrition information to facilitate healthier consumer choice and to encourage healthier product offerings. Nutrition labeling may not be the "silver bullet" to defeat obesity, but it should be part of any comprehensive plan to improve population diet.

Suggested Reading

Bruemmer, B., Krieger, J., Saelens, B. E., & Chan, N. (2012). Energy, saturated fat, and sodium were lower in entrées at chain restaurants at 18 months compared with 6 months following the implementation of mandatory menu labeling regulation in King County, Washington. *Journal of the Academy of Nutrition and Dietetics, 112*(8), 1169–1176.—This article evaluates the nutrient content of entrées at eligible restaurants 6 and 18 months after mandatory menu labeling in King County, Washington.

Campos, S., Doxey, J., & Hammond, D. (2011). Nutrition labels on pre-packaged foods: A systematic review. *Public Health Nutrition, 14*(8), 1496–1506.—This study reviews use and impact of nutrition facts labels on packaged foods.

Graham, D. J., & Jeffery, R. W. (2011). Location, location, location: Eye-tracking evidence that consumers preferentially view prominently positioned nutrition information. *Journal of the American Dietetic Association, 111*(11), 1704–1711.—This study uses eye-tracking to detect where people focus their visual attention in a simulated grocery shopping task.

Hawley, K. L., Roberto, C. A., Bragg, M. A., Liu, P. J., Schwartz, M. B., & Brownell, K. D. (2013). The science on front-of-package food labels. *Public Health Nutrition, 16*(3), 430–439.—This article reviews the evidence on front-of-package labeling systems and discusses components of an optimal labeling system.

Kiesel, K., McCluskey, J. J., & Villas-Boas, S. B. (2011). Nutritional labeling and consumer choices. *Annual Review of Resource Economics, 3,* 141–158.—This article reviews the evidence on how consumers value and respond to nutrition facts labels on packaged foods.

Malam, S., Clegg, S., Kirwan, S., McGinigal, S., Raats, M., Shepherd, R., et al. (2009). *Comprehension and use of UK nutrition signpost labelling schemes.* London: Food Standards Agency.—This report details a number of studies evaluating comprehension and use of the UK's traffic light labeling system.

Moorman, C., Ferraro, R., & Huber, J. (2012). Unintended nutrition consequences: Firm responses to the nutrition labeling and education act. *Marketing Science, 31,* 717–737.—This study reports on category, brand, and firm conditions associated with improvement and declines in the nutritional profile of foods following the U.S. NLEA.

Thorndike, A. N., Riis, J., Sonnenberg, L. M., & Levy, D. E. (2014). Traffic-light labels and choice architecture promoting healthy food choices. *American Journal of Preventive Medicine, 46*(2), 143–149.—This longitudinal study showed that traffic-light labeling of items in a hospital cafeteria decreased sales of red-labeled items and increased sales of green-labeled items over a 2-year period.

VanEpps E. M., Roberto, C. A., Park, S., Economos, C. D., & Bleich S. N. (2016). Restaurant menu labeling policy: Review of evidence and controversies. *Current Obesity Reports, 5,* 72–80.—This review summarizes literature evaluating the influence of restaurant menu labeling on consumer behavior.

Variyam, J. N. (2008). Do nutrition labels improve dietary outcomes? *Health Economics, 17*(6), 695–708.—This study tests whether nutrition facts labels mandated by the NLEA affected nutrient intake among label users and label nonusers.

Volkova, E., & Mhurchu, C. N. (2015). The influence of nutrition labeling and point-of-purchase information on food behaviours. *Current Obesity Reports, 4,* 19–29.—This provides a summary of real-world effectiveness of point-of-purchase labeling strategies on consumer behavior.

Vyth, E. L., Steenhuis, I. H. M., Roodenburg, A. J. C., Brug, J., & Seidell, J. C. (2010). Front-of-pack nutrition label stimulates healthier product development: A quantitative analysis. *International Journal of Behavioral Nutrition and Physical Activity, 7*(1), 65.—This article identifies the extent and types of product reformulation and new product development by Dutch food manufacturers who used the Choices nutrition labels.

The Centers for Disease Control and Prevention's Role as a Federal Agency in Reversing U.S. Trends in Obesity

HEIDI M. BLANCK

Many federal agencies are involved in supporting priority behaviors related to obesity, which include healthy eating, breastfeeding, and active living strategies for Americans. Key roles in the obesity epidemic for the Centers for Disease Control and Prevention (CDC) as the leading federal government public health agency include monitoring and disseminating data, applied research, guidelines development, public health agency support, public health to health care linkages, and partnerships. For example, the CDC plays a role in reviewing the evidence, including through the Guide to Community Preventive Services process to better identify targets for interventions, as well as providing evidence-based guidance to stakeholders. The CDC also provides funding and technical support to state, territorial, tribal, and local public health agencies for the implementation of setting-specific interventions designed for early care and education, schools, hospitals, worksites, and the community. Collaborative federal government efforts for reducing obesity have emerged over the past decade to speed progress and ensure efficiency across agencies, including the National Prevention Council and the National Collaborative on Childhood Obesity Research.

Monitoring and Disseminating Data

Many federal agencies have played a role in building awareness about the burden of obesity, its consequences, and strategies to reverse the rising trends. The CDC's role as a federal government agency in the obesity epidemic included early work focused on nutrition and physical activity behaviors, but the agency moved to the forefront with its efforts to increase awareness of rising rates through national and state monitoring data, including the National Health and Nutrition Examination Survey, the National Health

Interview Survey, the Behavioral Risk Factor Surveillance System, and the Youth Risk Behavior Surveillance System. These surveillance data, beyond raising awareness, also help to set goals and objectives, including through the *Healthy People* initiative, and are used for evaluation of progress on implementing strategies. Dissemination efforts of the monitoring data include dashboards with metrics and state indicator reports, as well as periodic manuscripts on national trends, and state obesity maps from the National Center for Health Statistics (*www.cdc.gov/nchs/data/factsheets/factsheet_obesity.htm*) and the National Center for Chronic Disease Prevention and Health Promotion (*www. cdc.gov/obesity/data/prevalence-maps.html*), respectively. The first obesity map showing state-by-state prevalence was released in 1999, with annual releases in subsequent years. The CDC maintains an interactive database on select national, state, and territorial data on weight status and key behavioral and environmental indicators for breast-feeding, nutrition, and physical activity (*www.cdc.gov/obesity/data/databases.html*). An example, of specific, ongoing monitoring is the CDC's national survey of Maternity Practices in Infant Nutrition and Care (mPINC), which is administered every 2 years to monitor and examine changes in supportive breastfeeding practices over time at all hospitals and birth centers with registered maternity beds in the United States and its territories (*www.cdc.gov/breastfeeding/data/mpinc/index.htm*). The CDC also supports the School Health Policies and Practices Study (SHPPS), a national survey that is periodically conducted to assess school health policies and practices at the state, district, school, and classroom levels. The survey was first conducted in 1994. SHPPS assesses the characteristics of eight components of school health: health education, physical education and activity, health services, mental health and social services, nutrition services, healthy and safe school environment, faculty and staff health promotion, and family and community involvement. In addition to SHPPS, the CDC also supports the School Health Profiles (Profiles) surveys. Profiles is a system of surveys assessing school health policies and practices in states, large urban school districts, territories, and tribal governments. Profiles surveys are conducted with middle and high school principals and leading health education teachers every 2 years by education and health agencies. Areas assessed include physical education and physical activity, and nutrition.

In addition to monitoring behavior and setting specific surveys, the Chronic Disease State Tracking System is a searchable database that provides state-level legislative information pertaining to nutrition, physical activity, and obesity (*www.cdc.gov/obesity/data/databases.html*). It provides bill numbers, year, Congressional sponsor, a short summary of the legislation, and its current status.

State and Community Program Support

From the early documentation of the health burden experienced by persons with obesity came a federal response about key behaviors and community strategies. Operating within the Department of Health and Human Services (DHHS), the CDC and other federal agencies provided technical expertise for recommendations to address obesity within The Surgeon General's 2001 Call to Action to Prevent and Decrease Overweight and Obesity (*www.ncbi.nlm.nih.gov/books/nbk44206*). This document put forth a variety of strategies across key sectors and settings. It also called on a diverse array of stakeholders to take part in reversing trends. For example, the Call to Action (CTA) called for environmental changes and public–private partnerships. The CTA also focused on specific behavior targets that could be addressed in the population, including increasing fruit and vegetable intake and breastfeeding initiation and duration, reducing television viewing and sedentary behaviors, and increasing physical activity. This document served as an early framework for state and local programs and stakeholders.

The CDC's Division of Adolescent and School Health (DASH) and Division of Population Health, School Health Branch, also has a long tenure in supporting coordinated school health efforts in states through local school districts to include nutrition and physical activity through its programs, partnerships, surveillance, and guidance tools. The CDC also synthesizes research and best practices related to promoting healthy eating and physical activity in schools, which has culminated first in 1996 with the *School Health Guidelines to Promote Lifelong Healthy Eating and Physical Activity* and recently in nine guidelines released in 2011 (*www.cdc.gov/healthyyouth/npao/strategies.htm*). The guidelines serve as the foundation for developing, implementing, and evaluating school-based healthy eating and physical activity policies and practices for students. Similar to the work in schools, the CDC supports early care and education (ECE) programs for obesity prevention. Among the state and local programs in ECE is a Learning Collaboratives Project. This 5-year project funds a national partner to implement learning collaboratives in 10 states to support obesity prevention in ECE programs that leverage state-level policy and systems improvements such as licensing regulations and quality rating systems.

In 2000, the CDC's Division of Nutrition, Physical Activity, and Obesity (DNPAO) funded six state health departments to support programs to improve diet and physical activity. This effort expanded to 20 state programs in 2003, and in the following year the program covered 28 states. The CDC supported the state programs through cooperative agreement funding and provided resources to help states develop skills to implement strategies to improve the target behaviors. In 2008, a new round of program funds led to a reduction in the number of states ($n = 23$) with the intent to bolster more intense work in changing environments to support healthier food and physical activity offerings. In 2013, support for state health department work on obesity prevention and control became housed within a new 5-year program that integrates work across obesity, diabetes, heart disease, and school health. The latest program, called "State Public Health Actions to Prevent and Control Diabetes, Heart Disease, Obesity, and Associated Risk Factors and Promote School Health," provides funding to all states (Centers for Disease Control and Prevention, Chronic Disease Prevention and Health Promotion, State Profiles; available at *www.cdc.gov/chronicdisease/states/index.htm*).

This was the first time that all 50 states and Washington, D.C., had a 5-year program that included coordinated school health and nutrition, physical activity, and obesity strategies to support prevention. The current program funds all entities at a small base level (e.g., $150,000) for specific nutrition and physical activity strategies (*www.cdc.gov/nccdphp/dnpao/state-local-programs/funding.html*), with some states receiving additional enhancement funds (e.g., an additional $250,000). The enhanced funding supports healthy eating options and active living opportunities in early care and education (ECE), schools, hospitals, worksites, and community venues (*www.cdc.gov/obesity/resources/strategies-guidelines.html*). Improving health equity through reduction of health disparities is included in these program efforts as a goal, and resources have been created to aid state health departments (*www.cdc.gov/obesity/health_equity/index.html*).

In addition to state programs, the CDC supports community-level programs to reduce chronic disease, with many including healthy eating and active living strategies. These include the 2003–2009 STEPS program (*www.cdc.gov/nccdphp/dch/programs/*

healthycommunitiesprogram/communities/steps/index.htm); Communities Putting Prevention to Work (2010–2013); the Racial and Ethnic Approaches to Community Health (REACH) programs (1999–present) (*www.cdc.gov/nccdphp/dch/programs/reach/pdf/2-reach_factsheet-for-web.pdf*), including the REACH Obesity and Hypertension Demonstration Projects (2012–2014); and the Community Transformation Grants (CTG; Centers for Disease Control and Prevention, Division of Community Health; available at *www.cdc.gov/nccdphp/dch/programs/index.htm*). CTG awardees worked on tobacco-free living, healthy eating and active living, and clinical and community services to prevent and control high cholesterol and high blood pressure. In 2011, CTG awarded $103 million to 61 state and local government agencies, tribes and territories, and nonprofit organizations. In 2012, CTG, Small Communities Grants, awarded approximately $70 million to communities with a population size of less than 500,000 residents. The CTG grants ended in 2014 but REACH grants (2014–2017) have continued to support local community efforts. Also, Partnerships to Improve Community Health (PICH), launched in 2014, is an initiative that supports implementation of evidence-based strategies to improve the health of communities and reduce the prevalence of chronic disease. PICH builds on a body of knowledge developed through previously funded CDC programs and encourages collaborations with a multisectoral coalition to implement sustainable changes in communities where people live, learn, work, and play. To improve health and wellness in their communities, PICH awardees focus on four risk factors: poor nutrition; physical inactivity; tobacco use and exposure; and lack of access to opportunities for chronic disease prevention, risk reduction, and disease management. Finally, a new initiative called Programs to Reduce Obesity in High-Obesity Areas funds land grant universities in states with counties that have more than 40% prevalence of adult obesity. Physical activity and nutrition intervention strategies are being implemented through existing cooperative extension and outreach services at the county level (*www.cdc.gov/nccdphp/dnpao/state-local-programs/funding.html*).

As another supportive lever, the CDC, under leadership of its Director, Dr. Thomas Frieden, identified six domestic, winnable battles in 2010 based on public health burden and the ability to hasten progress by expanding evidence-based interventions. Nutrition, physical activity, and obesity, along with food safety, was identified as one of the battles. The CDC has established short- and long-term goals, performance measures, and strategic actions. For each battle, key strategies and a process to leverage resources and partnerships have been identified. The CDC's plan for nutrition, physical activity, and obesity includes working with partners to (1) increase breastfeeding support in early care settings, hospitals, worksites, and communities; (2) reduce artificial trans fat in the food supply; (3) reduce sodium in the food supply; (4) reduce consumption of calories from added sugars; (5) promote food service guidelines in cafeterias, concessions, vending machines; and (6) promote healthy eating and physical activity in child care centers, schools, hospitals, workplaces, and communities (*www.cdc.gov/winnablebattles/targets/pdf/nutrition-physicalactivity-obesity-winnablebattles-progressreport.pdf*). Leadership support includes reviewing progress and eliminating barriers through the involvement of senior policy, communications, and science offices. Collaborative federal government efforts to aid these top strategies also occurs through engagement of the National Prevention Council and its oversight of the National Prevention Strategy. In addition to specific work by programs and the Winnable Battle projects, the Guide to Community Preventive Services processes aid work across the agency to provide evidence-based guidance to stakeholders on obesity-related behaviors and obesity.

Health Care and Public Health Linkage

To better inform clinical–community efforts, the CDC has created a Health Level Seven International (HL7) electronic health record (EHR) standard for healthy weight and an Integrating the Healthcare Enterprise (IHE) Healthy Weight Profile (*http://wiki.ihe.net/ index.php/Healthy_Weight*). The standard can be utilized by various health information technology platforms and has the ability to capture high-quality, standardized height and weight data that can be used to improve health care site and system quality measurement and service delivery. In addition, the electronic clinical decision support (CDS) tools used at pediatric offices can include automatic alerts for a child with a high BMI, links to growth charts, screening guidelines, and referrals for weight management programs. Fast Healthcare Interoperability Resources (FHIR; pronounced "fire") allow for a set of information technology (IT) tools to aid steps in clinical engagement with patients including CDS. Information from the clinic can also be exchanged between secure systems linking health care and public health for better patient care coordination, local-level surveillance, and population health improvement activities (Healthy Weight IT standards for all stakeholders; available online at *www.ihe.net/uploadedfiles/documents/ qrph/ihe_qrph_suppl_hw.pdf* and *www.hl7.org/implement/standards/product_brief. cfm?product_id=315*).

Research

The CDC supports extramural applied research to determine effective models of health care delivery, including a project called the Childhood Obesity Research Demonstration (CORD 2011–2015) project. This community-based study assesses multiple-level, multiple-setting integration of primary care and community-based interventions to prevent and manage childhood obesity among underserved children ages 2–12 years in three U.S. communities. In 2011, with funds from the Affordable Care Act, the CDC provided funding to four grantees to conduct the 4-year Childhood Obesity Research Demonstration project (CORD), which aims to improve children's nutrition and physical activity behaviors in the places where they live, learn, and play (*www.cdc.gov/nccdphp/dnpao/ division-information/programs/researchproject.html*). The grantees are engaged with community coalitions and community health workers, and are working with partners to carry out interventions in health care centers, schools, early care and education centers, and communities. A new study effort called CORD 2.0 began in the summer of 2016, with a focus on pediatric weight management programs for low-income children, in two states, that meet the United States Preventive Services Task Force (USPSTF) recommendations of screening children age 6 years and older for obesity and offering or referring them to intensive behavioral interventions. The new efforts will focus on low-income children with obesity through family-based behavioral management programs, with the aim of improving behaviors and weight status through an affordable, effective program that meets guidelines and that could be replicated by other sites and payer modes.

   The CDC supports two policy research networks, the Physical Activity Policy Research Network and the Nutrition and Obesity Policy Research and Evaluation Network, both of which are thematic networks and part of the Prevention Research Center program. The research networks aim to conduct relevant evaluation of policy approaches happening across various policy strategies (e.g., executive order, regulation, legislation), as well as jurisdiction. The CDC also partners with other major funders through the National Collaborative on Childhood Obesity Research (NCCOR), which comprises the CDC, the National Institutes of Health, the U.S. Department of Agriculture (USDA), and the Robert Wood Johnson Foundation. These leading national organizations share insights and expertise to strengthen surveillance, evaluation, research, and guidance. NCCOR focuses on efforts that have the potential to benefit children, teens, and their families, and the communities in which they live. A special emphasis is placed on the populations and communities in which obesity rates are highest and rising the fastest.

Obesity remains high across most subgroups of Americans, with prevalence even higher among some low-income and minority populations. Although recent reports of small obesity declines in U.S. youth are encouraging (*www.cdc.gov/vitalsigns/childhoodobesity/index.html*), much remains to be done across the United States to ensure that all Americans have access to affordable, healthy eating and active living opportunities as two broad factors related to weight management. As part of its mission, the CDC will continue to conduct needed surveillance and applied research, and support state and local public health agencies to deliver effective interventions in order to foster healthy nutrition and physical activity behaviors.

Acknowledgment

The views expressed in this chapter are solely those of the author and do not represent the official views of the Centers for Disease Control and Prevention.

Suggested Reading

Centers for Disease Control and Prevention. (2015). National Center for Chronic Disease Prevention and Health Promotion. Retrieved from *www.cdc.gov/chronicdisease/index.htm.*—Overview site for the CDC National Center for Chronic Disease Prevention and Health Promotion, including Chronic Program Sites.

Centers for Disease Control and Prevention. (2015). Winnable Battles. Retrieved from *www.cdc.gov/winnablebattles/targets/index.html.*—Overview materials for the CDC's Winnable Battles, including strategies, actionable targets, and progress reports.

Dietz, W. H. (2015). The response of the U.S. Centers for Disease Control and Prevention to the obesity epidemic. *Annual Review of Public Health, 36,* 575–596.—This article provides an extensive historical overview of the CDC's recognition and response to the nation's obesity epidemic.

Dooyema, C. A., Belay, B., Foltz, J. L., Williams, N., & Blanck, H. M. (2013). The childhood obesity research demonstration project: A comprehensive community approach to reduce childhood obesity. *Childhood Obesity, 9*(5), 454–459.—This article provides an overview of the CDC's Childhood Obesity Research Demonstration Project, which includes interventions across the socioecological model in both health care and public health settings.

Foltz, J. L., May, A. L., Belay, B., Nihiser, A. J., Dooyema, C. A., & Blanck, H. M. (2012). Population-level intervention strategies and examples for obesity prevention in children. *Annual Review of Nutrition, 32,* 391–415.—This review of research- and practice-tested interventions and innovative approaches for childhood obesity prevention is divided by setting to provide a practical set of approaches.

Modeling the Impact of Public Policies

STEVEN L. GORTMAKER

Many public policies have been developed to improve diet, increase physical activity, and reduce the population prevalence of obesity and eating disorders. Likewise, extant policies likely contribute to the current levels of obesity prevalence and eating disorders in countries throughout the world. It is therefore critical to evaluate the impact of policy changes, and decision makers are now moving beyond asking simply whether something works, and are looking to quantify further the impact on population health. This means taking into account evidence for effectiveness in not only changing outcomes such as relative weight or obesity, but also in quantifying population reach (e.g., whether the intervention reaches 1,000 or 1 million people), the economic costs of implementing the policy, longer-term cost consequences (e.g., policies may change long-term health care costs), effects on equity, and the relative cost-effectiveness of different approaches.

Simulation modeling of policy changes can produce analyses relevant to all these issues and provide useful metrics for decision makers to use in comparing the population impact of different policies. Simulation models are therefore growing in importance because they are able to integrate a wide variety of available data, and to project "what if" scenarios: How would population health change if a policy were implemented at the state or national level? What policy will produce the "biggest bang for the buck"?

Modeling the Impact of Public Policies on Obesity and Eating Disorders

Simulation models can be described as a collection of mathematical equations that relate inputs (e.g., population characteristics, dietary intake levels, baseline levels of body mass index [BMI] and obesity prevalence, evidence for intervention effectiveness and cost) and outputs (e.g., changes in cases of obesity, obesity prevalence, eating disorder prevalence, quality-adjusted life years [QALYS]). Simulation models of policy impacts have been used to project the comparative effectiveness of policies aimed at reducing smoking. These approaches are now being applied to the comparative analysis of policies that impact dietary intake, physical activity, obesity and its consequences, and are beginning to be applied to the analysis of policies designed to prevent and treat eating disorders.

A variety of simulation models have been used: Some cohort simulations follow a particular cohort over time, while other microsimulation models have been developed to simulate policy effects for an entire population. The simulation models referenced in the "Suggested Reading" section were used to evaluate a large number of different policy changes using the same simulation modeling approach, so that the comparative effectiveness of these approaches was enhanced.

The utility of simulation models of policy change depends on the input data to the model, and the model assumptions. Simulation models of policy changes generally require many assumptions, and our experience has been that it is important to carefully review the inputs, outputs, and assumptions. The following list offers key aspects of model input and design that need to be carefully considered.

Specification of the Policy Intervention

The modeled intervention should closely approximate the policy of interest, and this specification is often helped by a logic model of how the intervention works, including setting, target population, and intervention activities.

Evidence for Cause

Establishing the effects of a policy change on outcomes such as obesity prevalence or BMI change ("effect size") is generally not simple. Rarely can public policies be evaluated using the "gold standard" approach of randomized trials, where the policy is randomly assigned to representative samples of individuals or groups of individuals, but not to others who are similar in all respects. Sometimes natural experimental evaluations may be possible, in which a new policy is implemented in a large population, with before and after data gathered (and a control population available) so that impact can be assessed. Most often, more local results need to be used, and these results then need to be scaled up to be useful to policymakers: This process of scaling up requires further assumptions about implementation.

I believe it is most useful to focus on experimental and natural experimental results, with careful reviews of the evidence for effectiveness. Observational studies of change in behavior and change in outcome can also be valuable. While a policy change may have a primary focus on change in diet or change in physical activity, if the outcome variable of primary interest is BMI or obesity rates, I believe it is important to focus on change in relative weight as the outcome. I emphasize the importance of direct effects on relative weight because these analyses take into account potential compensation issues. For example, if a person consumes more calories at one meal, he or she may consume fewer at the next meal, or compensate. Models certainly can be used with change in energy intake or change in energy expenditures as an outcome, but to translate changes in energy intake or expenditure to changes in relative weight requires further assumptions about lack of compensation.

Costs of the Intervention

Policy implementation requires resources, and costing should follow standard guidelines. Many of the costs associated with policy interventions are costs of time for workers to administer the policy and check for adherence, and are therefore relatively straightforward to estimate. Longer-term cost offsets, such as reduced obesity-related health care costs, can also be calculated.

Population Reach of Interventions

Reach can vary greatly: Some policy changes affect only a small number of individuals, while others affect millions.

Short-Term or Lifetime Effects?

Some policy simulation models project results over the lifetime of a cohort, while others focus on a shorter term, such as 10 years. In my experience, shorter time frames are more useful to policymakers because they represent a more relevant time frame similar to those used, for example, by legislators and the federal Office of Management and Budget. In addition, long-term (or lifetime) projections of the impact of policies, of necessity, will be less accurate than shorter-term projections.

Outcome Metrics

A wide variety of different useful outcome metrics can be developed with policy simulation models: These include specific measures documenting impact—for example, a microsimulation model can be used to estimate the number of cases of childhood obesity prevented in a particular year. Incremental cost-effectiveness ratios (ICERs) can be calculated, including those that are specific to the topic of study. For example, my colleagues and I have found it useful in our work to estimate the cost per BMI unit change and costs saved per dollar invested. Particularly useful are ICERS that can be compared across policies in many intervention areas: two examples are QALYs) and disability-adjusted life years (DALYs). These measures allow the comparison of relative cost-effectiveness of very different interventions—for example, obesity prevention and eating disorder treatment—using the same metric. However, QALYs and DALYs are driven to a large extent by differences in morbidity and mortality rates, and few children die because of obesity-related health issues (most morbidity and mortality onset occurs at ages 35 and above). In addition, it is difficult to measure quality of life in children. Our experience has been that QALYs and DALYs are less useful in the short-run analysis of childhood obesity interventions, compared to more sensitive short-term measures reflecting obesity more directly.

Uncertainty

Uncertainty and sensitivity analyses need to be calculated for all modeled results to describe uncertainty in the outcome measures as a result of the joint uncertainties surrounding model inputs.

Comparing Multiple Policies

One useful approach is to model many policies using the same simulation model. This controls for methodological differences among studies and therefore enhances comparison of policies.

Equity

Equity and implementation considerations, including the acceptability of policies, implementation success and failure, the sustainability of the policy change, and effects on equity and disparities of outcomes can be combined with cost-effectiveness results to provide a more complete picture for decision makers.

Recommendations

Decision makers need to move beyond simple yes–no notions of policy effectiveness, and move to richer analysis of effectiveness, population impact, and cost and cost-effectiveness of proposed policy changes. Simulation models of policy changes have much to offer policymakers, and they will grow in value as more are implemented and researchers conform to common standards of evidence, costing, and modeling, and as projections about future policy changes are eventually validated against actual policy implementation and results.

Simulation models of the impact of policy changes allow the analyst simultaneously to take into account evidence regarding intervention effects, reach, and cost. These models can produce many relevant and useful outcome metrics, but, of course, the models also are dependent on their assumptions, the details of the specification of the policy, its implementation, and the evidence for effect and cost. Particularly useful are metrics that focus on the cost-effectiveness of interventions. The focus is therefore generally on "best value for money" and features incremental cost-effectiveness measures.

Acknowledgment

Preparation of this chapter was supported, in part, by grants from The JPB Foundation.

Suggested Reading

Carter, R., Vos, T., Moodie, M., Haby, M., Magnus, A., & Mihalopoulos, C. (2008). Priority setting in health: Origins, description and application of the Australian Assessing Cost-Effectiveness initiative. *Expert Review of Pharmacoeconomics and Outcomes Research, 8*(6), 593–617.—A framework for organizing cost-effectiveness modeling work, including discussion of further concerns, including equity, feasibility and sustainability.

Gortmaker, S. L., Long, M. W., Resch, S. C., Ward, Z. J., Cradock, A. L., Barrett, J. L., et al. (2015). Cost effectiveness of childhood obesity interventions: Evidence and methods for CHOICES. *American Journal of Preventive Medicine, 49*(1), 102–111.—A cohort simulation model along with evidence reviews and cost analyses are used to evaluate the relative cost-effectiveness of four different childhood obesity preventive interventions over a 10-year period, with estimates of population effectiveness, reach, cost, and cost-effectiveness.

Gortmaker, S. L., Wang, Y. C., Long, M. W., Giles, C. M., Ward, Z. J., Barrett, J. L., et al. (2015). Three interventions that reduce childhood obesity are projected to save more than they cost to implement. *Health Affairs, 34*(11), 1932–1939.—A microsimulation model combined with systematic evidence reviews and costing of interventions is used to project over 10 years the relative cost-effectiveness, reach, and population impact of six preventive and one treatment intervention for childhood obesity. The evidence strongly suggests that prevention is the treatment of choice.

Guyatt, G. H., Oxman, A. D., Kunz, R., Vist, G. E., Falck-Ytter, Y., & Schünemann, H. J. (2008). What is "quality of evidence" and why is it important to clinicians? *British Medical Journal, 336,* 995–998.—Evidence guidelines used in Cochrane studies that can be applied to evidence used in simulation modeling.

Levy, D. T., Mabry, P. L., Wang, Y. C., Gortmaker, S., Huang, T. K., Marsh, T., et al. (2011). Simulation models of obesity: A review of the literature and implications for research and policy. *Obesity Reviews, 12*(5), 378–394.—The authors provide a thorough discussion of the elements of policy simulation models, with references to both the tobacco and the obesity literature.

Siegel, J. E., Weinstein, M. C., Russell, L. B., & Gold, M. R. (1996). Recommendations for reporting cost-effectiveness analyses. *Journal of the American Medical Association, 276*(16), 1339–1341.—Guidelines for reporting cost-effectiveness data and results.

Vos, T., Carter, R., Barendregt, J., Mihalopoulos, C., Veerman, L., Magnus, A., et al. (2010). *Assessing cost-effectiveness in prevention: ACE–prevention: Final report.* Brisbane, Australia: University of Queensland.—A groundbreaking study of a cohort over members' lifetimes that examines the relative cost-effectiveness of 150 preventive and treatment interventions in Australia, including those targeting obesity.

Wright, D. R., Austin, S. B., LeAnn Noh, H., Jiang, Y., & Sonneville, K. R. (2014). The cost-effectiveness of school-based eating disorder screening. *American Journal of Public Health, 104*(9), 1774–1782.—An example of a microsimulation model applied to estimating the cost effectiveness of school-based screening of eating disorders.

Index